AIR FRYER
COOKBOOK

1000 delicious, quick and hassle-free recipes for crispy and crunchy dishes with guilt-free.

BESS NOWAK

1. Basil Tomato Frittata
ტ Prep Time 10 m | ტ Cooking Time 35 m | 6 Servings

Ingredients
- 12 eggs
- 1/2 cup cheddar cheese, grated
- 1 1/2 cups cherry tomatoes, cut in half
- 1/2 cup fresh basil, chopped
- 1 cup baby spinach, chopped
- 1/2 cup yogurt
- Pepper
- Salt

Directions
1. Spray a baking dish using cooking spray and set aside.
2. Insert wire rack in rack position 6. Select bake, set temperature 390 F, timer for 35 minutes. Press start to preheat the oven.
3. Whisk eggs and yogurt inside a large bowl.
4. Layer spinach, basil, tomatoes, and cheese in prepared baking dish. Pour egg mixture over spinach mixture. Season with pepper and salt.
5. Bake in the oven for 35 minutes.
6. Serve and enjoy.

Nutrition
Calories 188 | Fat 12.2 g | Carbohydrates 4.2 g | Sugar 3.4 g | Protein 15.2 g | Cholesterol 338 mg

2. Italian Breakfast Frittata
ტ Prep Time 10 m | ტ Cooking Time 30 m | 4 Servings

Ingredients
- 8 eggs
- 1 tbsp. fresh parsley, chopped
- 3 tbsp. parmesan cheese, grated
- 2 small zucchinis, chopped and cooked
- 1/2 cup pancetta, chopped and cooked
- Pepper
- Salt

Directions
1. Spray a baking dish using cooking spray and set aside.
2. Insert wire rack in rack position 6. Select bake, set temperature 350 F, timer for 20 minutes. Press start to preheat the oven.
3. In a mixing bowl, whisk eggs with pepper and salt. Add parsley, cheese, zucchini, and pancetta and stir well.
4. Pour egg mixture into the baking dish that was prepared.
5. Bake frittata for 20 minutes.
6. Serve and enjoy.

Nutrition
Calories 327 | Fat 23.2 g | Carbohydrates 3.5 g | Sugar 1.7 g | Protein 26 g | Cholesterol 367 mg

3. Healthy Baked Omelette
ტ Prep Time 10 m | ტ Cooking Time 45 m | 6 Servings

Ingredients
- 8 eggs
- 1 cup bell pepper, chopped
- 1/2 cup onion, chopped
- 1/2 cup cheddar cheese, shredded
- 6 oz. ham, diced and cooked
- 1 cup milk
- Pepper
- Salt

Directions
1. Spray an 8-inch baking dish using cooking spray and set aside.
2. Insert wire rack in rack position 6. Select bake, set temperature 350 F, timer for 45 minutes. Press start to preheat the oven.
3. In a large bowl, whisk milk with egg, pepper, and salt. Add remaining ingredients and stir well.
4. Pour egg mixture into the baking dish that was prepared.
5. Bake omelet for 45 minutes.
6. Slice and serve.

Nutrition
Calories 199 | Fat 12.3 g | Carbohydrates 6.1 g | Sugar 3.7 g | Protein 16.1 g | Cholesterol 248 mg

4. Easy Egg Casserole
ტ Prep Time 10 m | ტ Cooking Time 55 m | 8 Servings

Ingredients
- 8 eggs
- 1/2 tsp garlic powder
- 2 cups cheddar cheese, shredded
- 1 cup milk
- 24 oz. frozen hash browns, thawed
- 1/2 onion, diced
- 1 red pepper, diced
- 4 bacon slices, diced
- 1/2 lb. turkey breakfast sausage
- Pepper
- Salt

Directions
1. Spray a 9*13-inch baking dish using cooking spray and set aside.
2. Insert wire rack in rack position 6. Select bake, set temperature 350 F, timer for 50 minutes. Press start to preheat the oven.
3. Cook the breakfast sausage in a pan over medium heat until cooked through. Drain well and set aside.
4. Cook bacon in the same pan. Drain well and keep aside.
5. In a mixing bowl, whisk eggs with milk, garlic powder, pepper, and salt. Add 1 cup cheese, hash browns, onion, red pepper, bacon, and sausage and stir well.
6. Pour the entire egg mixture into the baking dish. Sprinkle remaining cheese on top.
7. Cover dish with foil and bake for 50 minutes. Remove foil and bake for 5 more minutes.
8. Serve and enjoy.

Nutrition
Calories 479 | Fat 29.1 g | Carbohydrates 34.1 g | Sugar 4.2 g | Protein 20.2 g | Cholesterol 207 mg

5. Flavor Packed Breakfast Casserole
⏰ Prep Time 10 m | ⏲ Cooking Time 40 m | 8 Servings

Ingredients
- 12 eggs
- 1/2 cup cheddar cheese, shredded
- 1 tsp garlic powder
- 1 cup milk
- 1/4 cup onion, diced

- 2 bell pepper, cubed
- 4 small potatoes, cubed
- 2 cups sausage, cooked and diced
- Pepper
- Salt

Directions
1. Spray a 9*13-inch baking dish using cooking spray and keep aside.
2. Insert wire rack in rack position 6. Select bake, set temperature 350 F, timer for 40 minutes. Press start to preheat the oven.
3. In a large bowl, whisk eggs with milk, garlic powder, pepper, and salt.
4. Add sausage, bell peppers, and potatoes into the baking dish. Pour egg mixture over sausage mixture. Sprinkle with cheese and onion.
5. Bake casserole for 40 minutes.
6. Slice and serve.

Nutrition
Calories 232 | Fat 11.6 g | Carbohydrates 18.3 g | Sugar 4.6 g | Protein 14.2 g | Cholesterol 261 mg

6. Vegetable Sausage Egg Bake
⏰ Prep Time 10 m | ⏲ Cooking Time 35 m | 4 Servings

Ingredients
- 10 eggs
- 1 cup spinach, diced
- 1 cup onion, diced
- 1 cup pepper, diced
- 1 lb. sausage, cut into 1/2-inch pieces

- 1 tsp garlic powder
- 1/2 cup almond milk
- Pepper
- Salt

Directions
1. Spray an 8*8-inch baking dish with cooking spray and set aside.
2. Insert wire rack in rack position 6. Select bake, set temperature 390 F, timer for 35 minutes. Press start to preheat the oven.
3. In a bowl, whisk milk with eggs and spices. Add vegetables and sausage and stir to combine.
4. Pour the mixture of egg into the prepared baking dish. Bake for 35 minutes.
5. Slice and serve.

Nutrition
Calories 653 | Fat 50.6 g | Carbohydrates 12.6 g | Sugar 3.3 g | Protein 38.3 g | Cholesterol 504 mg

7. Cheese Broccoli Bake
⏰ Prep Time 10 m | ⏲ Cooking Time 30 m | 12 Servings

Ingredients
- 12 eggs
- 1 1/2 cup cheddar cheese, shredded
- 2 cups broccoli florets, chopped
- 1 small onion, diced

- 1 cup milk
- Pepper
- Salt

Directions
1. Spray a 9*13-inch baking dish using cooking spray and set aside.
2. Insert wire rack in rack position 6. Select bake, set temperature 390 F, timer for 30 minutes. Press start to preheat the oven.
3. In a large bowl, whisk eggs with milk, pepper, and salt. Add cheese, broccoli, and onion and stir well.
4. Pour the mixture of eggs into the prepared baking dish and bake for 30 minutes.
5. Slice and serve.

Nutrition
Calories 138 | Fat 9.5 g | Carbohydrates 3.1 g | Sugar 1.8 g | Protein 10.2 g | | Cholesterol 180 mg

8. Cheese Ham Omelette
⏰ Prep Time 10 m | ⏲ Cooking Time 25 m | 6 Servings

Ingredients
- 8 eggs
- 1 cup ham, chopped
- 1 cup cheddar cheese, shredded

- 1/3 cup milk
- Pepper
- Salt

Directions
1. Spray a 9*9-inch baking dish using cooking spray and set aside.
2. Insert wire rack in rack position 6. Select bake, set temperature 390 F, timer for 25 minutes. Press start to preheat the oven.
3. In a large bowl, whisk eggs with milk, pepper, and salt. Stir in ham and cheese.
4. Pour the mixture of eggs into the prepared baking dish and bake for 25 minutes.
5. Slice and serve.

Nutrition
Calories 203 | Fat 14.3 g | Carbohydrates 2.2 g | Sugar 1.2 g | Protein 16.3 g | Cholesterol 252 mg

9. Sweet Potato Frittata
Prep Time 10 m | Cooking Time 30 m | 6 Servings

Ingredients
- 10 eggs
- 1/4 cup goat cheese, crumbled
- 1 onion, diced
- 1 sweet potato, diced
- 2 cups broccoli, chopped
- 1 tbsp. olive oil
- Pepper
- Salt

Directions
1. Spray a baking dish using cooking spray and set aside.
2. Insert wire rack in rack position 6. Select bake, set temperature 390 F, timer for 20 minutes. Press start to preheat the oven.
3. Heat oil in a pan over medium heat. Add sweet potato, broccoli, and onion and cook for 10-15 minutes or until sweet potato is tender.
4. In a large bowl, whisk eggs with pepper and salt.
5. Transfer cooked vegetables into the baking dish. Pour egg mixture over vegetables. Spray in goat cheese and bake for 15-20 minutes.
6. Slice and serve.

Nutrition
Calories 201 | Fat 13 g | Carbohydrates 8.4 g | Sugar 3.3 g | Protein 13.5 g | Cholesterol 282 mg

10. Squash Oat Muffins
Prep Time 10 m | Cooking Time 20 m | 12 Servings

Ingredients
- 2 eggs
- 1 tbsp. pumpkin pie spice
- 2 tsp baking powder
- 1 cup oats
- 1 cup all-purpose flour
- 1 tsp vanilla
- 1/3 cup olive oil
- 1/2 cup yogurt
- 1/2 cup maple syrup
- 1 cup butternut squash puree
- 1/2 tsp sea salt

Directions
1. Line 12 cups muffin pan with cupcake liners.
2. Insert wire rack in rack position 6. Select bake, set temperature 390 F, timer for 20 minutes. Press start to preheat the oven.
3. In a large bowl, whisk together eggs, vanilla, oil, yogurt, maple syrup, and squash puree.
4. In a small bowl, mix together flour, pumpkin pie spice, baking powder, oats, and salt.
5. Add flour mixture into the moist mixture and stir to combine.
6. Scoop the batter to the prepared muffin pan and bake for 20 minutes.
7. Serve and enjoy.

Nutrition
Calories 171 | Fat 7.1 g | Carbohydrates 23.8 g | Sugar 9.4 g | Protein 3.6 g | Cholesterol 28 mg

11. Hashbrown Casserole
Prep Time 10 m | Cooking Time 60 m | 10 Servings

Ingredients
- 2 cups cheddar cheese, shredded
- 15 eggs, lightly beaten
- 5 bacon slices, cooked and chopped
- 32 oz. frozen hash browns with onions and peppers
- Pepper
- Salt

Directions
1. Spray 9*13-inch casserole dish with cooking spray and set aside.
2. Insert wire rack in rack position 6. Select bake, set temperature 350 F, timer for 60 minutes. Press start to preheat the oven.
3. In a large bowl, whisk eggs with pepper and salt. Add 1 cup of cheese, bacon, and hash browns and mix well.
4. Pour egg mixture into the prepared casserole dish and sprinkle with remaining cheese.
5. Bake for 60 minutes or until the top is golden brown.
6. Slice and serve.

Nutrition
Calories 403 | Fat 27.1 g | Carbohydrates 23.6 g | Sugar 0.6 g | Protein 19 g | Cholesterol 280 mg

12. Mexican Breakfast Frittata
Prep Time 10 m | Cooking Time 25 m | 6 Servings

Ingredients
- 8 eggs, scrambled
- 1/2 cup cheddar cheese, grated
- 3 scallions, chopped
- 1/3 lb. tomatoes, sliced
- 1 green pepper, chopped
- 1/2 cup salsa
- 2 tsp taco seasoning
- 1 tbsp. olive oil
- 1/2 lb. ground beef
- Pepper
- Salt

Directions
1. Spray a baking dish using cooking spray and set aside.
2. Insert wire rack in rack position 6. Select bake, set temperature 375 F, timer for 25 minutes. Press start to preheat the oven.
3. Heat oil in a pan over low heat. Add ground beef in a pan and cook until brown.
4. Add salsa, taco seasoning, scallions, and green pepper into the pan and stir well.
5. Transfer meat into the prepared baking dish. Arrange slices of tomato on top of the meat mixture.
6. In a bowl, whisk eggs with cheese, pepper, and salt. Pour egg mixture over the meat mixture and bake for 25 minutes.
7. Serve and enjoy.

Nutrition
Calories 231 | Fat 13.9 g | Carbohydrates 4.5 g | Sugar 2.5 g | Protein 22.2 g | Cholesterol 262 mg

13. *Perfect Brunch Baked Eggs*
🕐 Prep Time 10 m | 🕐 Cooking Time 20 m | 4 Servings

Ingredients
- 4 eggs
- 1/2 cup parmesan cheese, grated
- 2 cups marinara sauce
- Pepper
- Salt

Directions
1. Spray 4 shallow baking dishes using cooking spray and set aside.
2. Insert wire rack in rack position 6. Select bake, set temperature 390 F, timer for 20 minutes. Press start to preheat the oven.
3. Divide marinara sauce into four baking dishes.
4. Break the egg into each baking dish. Sprinkle cheese, pepper, and salt on top of eggs and bake for 20 minutes.
5. Serve and enjoy.

Nutrition

Calories 208 | Fat 10.1 g | Carbohydrates 18 g | Sugar 11.4 g | Protein 11.4 g | Cholesterol 174 mg

14. *Green Chile Cheese Egg Casserole*
🕐 Prep Time 10 m | 🕐 Cooking Time 40 m | 12 Servings

Ingredients
- 12 eggs
- 8 oz. can green chilies, diced
- 6 tbsp. butter, melted
- 3 cups cheddar cheese, shredded
- 2 cups curd cottage cheese
- 1 tsp baking powder
- 1/2 cup flour
- Pepper
- Salt

Directions
1. Spray a 9*13-inch baking dish using cooking spray and set aside.
2. Insert wire rack in rack position 6. Select bake, set temperature 350 F, timer for 40 minutes. Press start to preheat the oven.
3. In a large mixing bowl, beat eggs until fluffy. Add baking powder, flour, pepper, and salt.
4. Stir in green chilies, butter, cheddar cheese, and cottage cheese.
5. Pour the mixture of eggs into the prepared baking dish and bake for 40 minutes.
6. Slice and serve.

Nutrition

Calories 284 | Fat 21.3 g | Carbohydrates 7.4 g | Sugar 1.8 g | Protein 17 g | Cholesterol 217 mg

15. *Breakfast Salmon Patties*
🕐 Prep Time 10 m | 🕐 Cooking Time 8 m | 6 Servings

Ingredients
- 14 oz. can salmon, drained and minced
- 1 tsp paprika
- 2 tbsp. green onion, minced
- 2 tbsp. fresh coriander, chopped
- 1 egg, lightly beaten
- Pepper
- Salt

Directions
1. Preheat the instant vortex air fryer to 360 F.
2. Add all ingredients into the bowl and mix until well combined.
3. Spray air fryer oven pan with cooking spray.
4. Make six even shape patties from salmon mixture and place on pan and air fry for 6-8 minutes. Turn halfway through.
5. Serve and enjoy.

Nutrition

Calories 122 | Fat 5.6 g | Carbohydrates 0.4 g | Sugar 0.2 g | Protein 16.5 g | Cholesterol 56 mg

16. *Zucchini Fries*
🕐 Prep Time 10 m | 🕐 Cooking Time 10 m | 4 Servings

Ingredients
- 2 medium zucchini, cut into fries shape
- ½ tsp garlic powder
- 1 tsp Italian seasoning
- ½ cup parmesan cheese, grated
- ½ cup breadcrumbs
- 1 egg, lightly beaten
- Pepper
- Salt

Directions
1. In a shallow bowl, mix together parmesan cheese, breadcrumbs, Italian seasoning, garlic powder, pepper, and salt.
2. Coat zucchini pieces with egg then coat with breadcrumb mixture.
3. Spray air fryer oven tray with cooking spray.
4. Arrange coated zucchini fries on a tray and air fry at 400 F for 10 minutes.
5. Serve and enjoy.

Nutrition

Calories 240 | Fat 11.3 g | Carbohydrates 13.5 g | Sugar 2.8 g | Protein 16.5 g | Cholesterol 72 mg

17. Breakfast Stuffed Peppers
🕐 Prep Time 10 m | 🕐 Cooking Time 13 m | 2 Servings

Ingredients
- 4 eggs
- 1 bell pepper, halved and seed removed
- ¼ tsp red chili flakes
- Pepper
- Salt

Directions
1. Crack 2 eggs into each bell pepper half and season with pepper and salt.
2. Sprinkle red chili flakes on top.
3. Arrange peppers on air fryer oven tray and cook at 390 F for 13 minutes.
4. Serve and enjoy.

Nutrition
Calories 165 | Fat 11.2 g | Carbohydrates 5.2 g | Sugar 3.7 g | Protein 11.7 g | Cholesterol 327 mg

18. Crispy Breakfast Potatoes
🕐 Prep Time 10 m | 🕐 Cooking Time 20 m | 6 Servings

Ingredients
- 1 ½ lbs. potatoes, diced into ½-inch cubes
- 1 tsp paprika
- 1 tsp garlic powder
- 1 tbsp. olive oil
- ½ tbsp. dried parsley
- ¼ tsp chili powder
- ¼ tsp pepper
- 2 tsp salt

Directions
1. Add potatoes into the mixing bowl. Add remaining ingredients over the potatoes and toss until evenly coated.
2. Arrange potatoes on air fryer oven tray and air fry at 400 F for 20 minutes. Turn potatoes to the other side halfway through.
3. Serve and enjoy.

Nutrition
Calories 102 | Fat 2.5 g | Carbohydrates 18.5 g | Sugar 1.5 g | Protein 2.1 g | Cholesterol 0 mg

19. Quick Cheese Omelet
🕐 Prep Time 5 m | 🕐 Cooking Time 9 m | 1 Servings

Ingredients
- 2 eggs, lightly beaten
- ¼ cup cheddar cheese, shredded
- ¼ cup milk
- Pepper
- Salt

Directions
1. In a bowl, whisk milk, eggs with pepper, and salt.
2. Spray small air fryer pan with cooking spray.
3. Pour egg mixture into the prepared pan and cook at 350 F for 6 minutes.
4. Sprinkle cheese on top and cook for 3 minutes more.
5. Serve and enjoy.

Nutrition
Calories 270 | Fat 19.4 g | Carbohydrates 4.1 g | Sugar 3.6 g | Protein 20.1 g | Cholesterol 362 mg

20. Tomato Spinach Frittata
🕐 Prep Time 10 m | 🕐 Cooking Time 7 m | 1 Servings

Ingredients
- 2 eggs, lightly beaten
- ¼ cup spinach, chopped
- ¼ cup tomatoes, chopped
- 2 tbsp. milk
- 1 tbsp. parmesan cheese, grated
- Pepper
- Salt

Directions
1. In a medium bowl, whisk eggs. Add other ingredients and mix until well combined.
2. Spray small air fryer pan with cooking spray.
3. Pour egg mixture into the prepared pan and cook at 330 F for 7 minutes.
4. Serve and enjoy.

Nutrition
Calories 189 | Fat 11.7 g | Carbohydrates 4.3 g | Sugar 3.3 g | Protein 15.7 g | Cholesterol 337 mg

21. Ham Egg Brunch Bake

⏱ Prep Time 10 m | ⏱ Cooking Time 60 m | 6 Servings

Ingredients

- 4 eggs
- 20 oz. hash browns
- 1 onion, chopped
- 2 cups ham, chopped
- 3 cups cheddar cheese, shredded
- 1 cup sour cream
- 1 cup milk
- Pepper
- Salt

Directions

1. Spray a 9*13-inch baking dish using cooking spray and set aside.
2. Insert wire rack in rack position 6. Select bake, set temperature 375 F, timer for 35 minutes. Press start to preheat the oven.
3. In a large bowl, whisk eggs with sour cream, milk, pepper, and salt. Add 2 cups cheese and stir well.
4. Cook onion and ham in a medium pan until onion is softened.
5. Add hash brown to the pan and cook for 5 minutes.
6. Add onion ham mixture into the egg mixture and mix well.
7. Pour the mixture of eggs into the prepared baking dish. Cover dish with foil and bake for 35 minutes.
8. Remove foil and bake for 25 minutes more.
9. Slice and serve.

Nutrition

Calories 703 | Fat 46.2 g | Carbohydrates 41.2 g | Sugar 4.6 g | Protein 30.8 g | Cholesterol 214 mg

22. Roasted Brussels Sprouts & Sweet Potatoes

⏱ Prep Time 10 m | ⏱ Cooking Time 20 m | 4 Servings

Ingredients

- 1 lb. Brussels sprouts, cut in half
- 2 sweet potatoes, wash and cut into 1-inch pieces
- 2 tbsp. olive oil
- ¼ tsp garlic powder
- ½ tsp pepper
- 1 tsp salt

Directions

1. Add sweet potatoes and Brussels sprouts in the mixing bowl.
2. Add remaining ingredients over sweet potatoes and Brussels sprouts and toss until well coated.
3. Transfer sweet potatoes and Brussels sprouts on air fryer oven tray and roast at 400 F for 10 minutes.
4. Turn sweet potatoes and Brussels sprouts to the other side and roast for 10 minutes more.
5. Serve and enjoy.

Nutrition:

Calories 138 | Fat 7.4 g | Carbohydrates 17.2 g | Sugar 3.9 g | Protein 4.4 g | Cholesterol 0 mg

23. Roasted Potato Wedges

⏱ Prep Time 10 m | ⏱ Cooking Time 10 m | 6 Servings

Ingredients

- 2 lbs. potatoes, cut into wedges
- 2 tbsp. McCormick's chipotle seasoning
- ¼ cup olive oil

Directions

1. Add potato wedges into the mixing bowl.
2. Add remaining ingredients over potato wedges and toss until well coated.
3. Transfer potato wedges onto the air fryer oven tray roast at 400 F for 5 minutes.
4. Turn potato wedges to the other side and roast for 5 minutes more.
5. Serve and enjoy.

Nutrition

Calories 176 | Fat 8.6 g | Carbohydrates 23.8 g | Sugar 1.7 g | Protein 2.5 g | Cholesterol 0 mg

24. Breakfast Egg Bites

⏱ Prep Time 10 m | ⏱ Cooking Time 13 m | 4 Servings

Ingredients

- 4 eggs, lightly beaten
- ¼ cup ham, diced
- ¼ cup cheddar cheese, shredded
- ¼ cup bell pepper, diced
- ½ cup milk
- Pepper
- Salt

Directions

1. Add all necessary ingredients into the mixing bowl and whisk until well combined.
2. Spray muffin silicone mold with cooking spray.
3. Pour egg mixture into the silicone muffin mold and place it in the air fryer oven and bake at 350 F for 10 minutes.
4. After 10 minutes flip egg bites and cook for 3 minutes more.
5. Serve and enjoy.

Nutrition

Calories 123 | Fat 8.1 g | Carbohydrates 2.8 g | Sugar 2.1 g | Protein 9.8 g | Cholesterol 178 mg

25. Grilled Cheese Sandwich
🕐 Prep Time 5 m | 🕐 Cooking Time 4 m | 2 Servings

Ingredients
- 4 Texas toast slices
- 4 Colby jack cheese slices

Directions
1. Spray air fryer oven tray with cooking spray.
2. Place two toast slices on a tray then top with cheese slices.
3. Now place remaining toast slices on top of the cheese.
4. Air fry at 400 F for 4 minutes.
5. Serve and enjoy.

Nutrition
Calories 225 | Fat 4 g | Carbohydrates 38.5 g | Sugar 4 g | Protein 8.5 g | Cholesterol 5 mg

26. Eggs in Avocado Cups
🕐 Prep Time 10 m | 🕐 Cooking Time 10 m | 2 Servings

Ingredients:
- 1 avocado, halved and pitted
- 2 large eggs
- Salt and ground black pepper, as required
- 2 cooked bacon slices, crumbled

Directions:
1. Carefully, scoop out about 2 teaspoons of flesh from each avocado half.
2. Crack 1 egg in each avocado half and sprinkle with salt and black pepper.
3. Press "Power Button" of Air Fry Oven and turn the dial to select the "Air Roast" mode.
4. Press the Time button and again turn the dial to set the cooking time to 10 minutes.
5. Now push the Temp button and rotate the dial to set the temperature at 375 degrees F.
6. Press "Start/Pause" button to start.
7. When the unit beeps to show that it is preheated, open the lid and line the "Sheet Pan" with a lightly, grease piece of foil.
8. Arrange avocado halves into the "Sheet Pan" and insert in the oven.
9. Top each avocado half with bacon pieces and serve.

Nutrition:
Calories 300 | Fat 26.6 g | Cholesterol 190 mg | Sodium 229 mg | Carbs 9 g | Fiber 6.7 g | Protein 9.7g

27. Cinnamon French Toasts
🕐 Prep Time 10 m | 🕐 Cooking Time 5 m | 2 Servings

Ingredients:
- 2 eggs
- ¼ cup whole milk
- 3 tablespoons sugar
- 2 teaspoons olive oil
- 1/8 teaspoon vanilla extract
- 1/8 teaspoon ground cinnamon
- 4 bread slices

Directions:
1. In a large bowl, mix together all the ingredients except bread slices.
2. Coat the bread slices with egg mixture evenly.
3. Press "Power Button" of Air Fry Oven and turn the dial to select the "Air Fry" mode.
4. Press the Time button and again turn the dial to set the cooking time to 6 minutes.
5. Now push the Temp button and rotate the dial to set the temperature at 390 degrees F.
6. Press "Start/Pause" button to start.
7. When the unit beeps to show that it is preheated, open the lid and lightly, grease the sheet pan.
8. Arrange the bread slices into "Air Fry Basket" and insert in the oven.
9. Flip the bread slices once halfway through.
10. Serve warm.

Nutrition
Calories 238 | Fat 10.6 g | Cholesterol 167 mg | Sodium 122 mg | Carbs 0.8 g | Fiber 0.5 | Protein 7.9g

28. Sweet Spiced Toasts
🕐 Prep Time 10 m | 🕐 Cooking Time 5 m | 3 Servings

Ingredients:
- ¼ cup sugar
- ½ teaspoon ground cinnamon
- 1/8 teaspoon ground cloves
- 1/8 teaspoon ground ginger
- ½ teaspoons vanilla extract
- ¼ cup salted butter, softened
- 6 bread slices

Directions:
1. In a bowl, add the sugar, vanilla, cinnamon, pepper, and butter. Mix until smooth.
2. Spread the butter mixture evenly over each bread slice.
3. Press "Power Button" of Air Fry Oven and turn the dial to select the "Air Fry" mode.
4. Press the Time button and again turn the dial to set the cooking time to 4 minutes.
5. Now push the Temp button and rotate the dial to set the temperature at 400 degrees F.
6. Press "Start/Pause" button to start.
7. When the unit beeps to show that it is preheated, open the lid and lightly, grease the sheet pan.
8. Arrange the bread slices into "Air Fry Basket" buttered-side up and insert in the oven.

Nutrition
Calories 250 | Fat 16 g | Cholesterol 41 mg | Sodium 232 mg | Carbs 26.3 g | Fiber 0.7 g | Protein 1.6 g

29. Savory French Toast

☺ Prep Time 10 m | ☺ Cooking Time 5 m | 2 Servings

Ingredients:

- ¼ cup chickpea flour
- 3 tablespoons onion, finely chopped
- 2 teaspoons green chili, seeded and finely chopped
- ½ teaspoon red chili powder
- ¼ teaspoon ground turmeric
- ¼ teaspoon ground cumin
- Salt, to taste
- Water, as needed
- 4 bread slices

Directions:

1. Add all the ingredients except bread slices in a large bowl and mix until a thick mixture form.
2. With a spoon, spread the mixture over both sides of each bread slice.
3. Arrange the bread slices into the lightly greased the sheet pan.
4. Press "Power Button" of Air Fry Oven and turn the dial to select the "Air Fry" mode.
5. Press the Time button and again turn the dial to set the cooking time to 5 minutes.
6. Now push the Temp button and rotate the dial to set the temperature at 390 degrees F.
7. Press "Start/Pause" button to start.
8. When the unit beeps to show that it is preheated, open the lid and lightly, grease sheet pan.
9. Arrange the bread slices into "Air Fry Basket" and insert in the oven.
10. Flip the bread slices once halfway through.
11. Serve warm.

Nutrition:

Calories 151| Fat 2.3 g |Cholesterol 0 mg |Sodium 234 mg |Carbs 26.7 g| Fiber 5.4 g|Protein 6.5g

30. Cheddar Mustard Toasts

☺ Prep Time 10 m | ☺ Cooking Time 10 m | 2 Servings

Ingredients:

- 4 bread slices
- 2 tablespoons cheddar cheese, shredded
- 2 eggs, whites and yolks, separated
- 1 tablespoon mustard
- 1 tablespoon paprika

Directions:

1. In a clean glass bowl, add the egg whites in and beat until they form soft peaks.
2. In another bowl, mix together the cheese, egg yolks, mustard, and paprika.
3. Gently, fold in the egg whites.
4. Spread the mustard mixture over the toasted bread slices.
5. Press "Power Button" of Air Fry Oven and turn the dial to select the "Air Fry" mode.
6. Press the Time button and again turn the dial to set the cooking time to 10 minutes.
7. Now push the Temp button and rotate the dial to set the temperature at 355 degrees F.
8. Press "Start/Pause" button to start.
9. When the unit beeps to show that it is preheated, open the lid and lightly, grease the sheet pan.
10. Arrange the bread slices into "Air Fry Basket" and insert in the oven.
11. Serve warm.

Nutrition:

Calories 175|Fat 9.4 g|Cholesterol 171 mg|Sodium 229 mg|Carbs 13.4 g|Fiber 2.5 g|Protein10.6 g

31. Pickled Toasts

☺ Prep Time 10 m | ☺ Cooking Time 5 m | 2 Servings

Ingredients:

- 4 bread slices, toasted
- 2 tablespoons unsalted butter, softened
- 2 tablespoons Branston pickle
- ¼ cup Parmesan cheese, grated

Directions:

1. Spread butter over bread slices evenly, followed by Branston pickle.
2. Top with cheese evenly.
3. Press "Power Button" of Air Fry Oven and turn the dial to select the "Air Fry" mode.
4. Press the Time button and again turn the dial to set the cooking time to 5 minutes.
5. Now push the Temp button and rotate the dial to set the temperature at 390 degrees F.
6. Press "Start/Pause" button to start.
7. When the unit beeps to show that it is preheated, open the lid and lightly, grease the sheet pan.
8. Arrange the bread slices into "Air Fry Basket" and insert in the oven.
9. Serve warm.

Nutrition:

Calories 211|Fat 14.5 g|Cholesterol 39 mg|Sodium 450 mg|Carbs 16.1 g|Fiber 0.4 g|Protein 5.5 g

32. Ricotta Toasts with Salmon

⏱ Prep Time 10 m | ⏱ Cooking Time 4 m | 2 Servings

Ingredients:

- 4 bread slices
- 1 garlic clove, minced
- 8 oz. ricotta cheese
- 1 teaspoon lemon zest
- Freshly ground black pepper, to taste
- 4 oz. smoked salmon

Directions:

1. In a food processor, add the garlic, ricotta, lemon zest and black pepper and pulse until smooth.
2. Spread ricotta mixture over each bread slices evenly.
3. Press "Power Button" of Air Fry Oven and turn the dial to select the "Air Fry" mode.
4. Press the Time button and again turn the dial to set the cooking time to 4 minutes.
5. Now push the Temp button and rotate the dial to set the temperature at 355 degrees F.
6. Press "Start/Pause" button to start.
7. When the unit beeps to show that it is preheated, open the lid and lightly, grease the sheet pan.
8. Arrange the bread slices into "Air Fry Basket" and insert in the oven.
9. Top with salmon and serve.

Nutrition:

Calories 274 | Fat 12 g | Cholesterol 48 mg | Sodium 1300 mg | Carbs 15.7 g | Fiber 0.5 g | Protein 4.8 g

33. Pumpkin Pancakes

⏱ Prep Time 15 m | ⏱ Cooking Time 12 m | 4 Servings

Ingredients:

- 1 square puff pastry
- 3 tablespoons pumpkin filling
- 1 small egg, beaten

Directions:

1. Roll out a square of puff pastry and layer it with pumpkin pie filling, leaving about ¼-inch space around the edges.
2. Cut it up into 8 equal sized square pieces and coat the edges with beaten egg.
3. Press "Power Button" of Air Fry Oven and turn the dial to select the "Air Fry" mode.
4. Press the Time button and again turn the dial to set the cooking time to 12 minutes.
5. Now push the Temp button and rotate the dial to set the temperature at 355 degrees F.
6. Press "Start/Pause" button to start.
7. When the unit beeps to show that it is preheated, open the lid.
8. Arrange the squares into a greased "Sheet Pan" and insert in the oven.
9. Serve warm.

Nutrition:

Calories 109 | Fat 6.7 g | Cholesterol 34 mg | Sodium 87 mg | Carbs 9.8 g | Fiber 0.5 g | Protein 2.4 g

34. Zucchini Fritters

⏱ Prep Time 15 m | ⏱ Cooking Time 7 m | 4 Servings

Ingredients:

- 10½ oz. zucchini, grated and squeezed
- 7 oz. Halloumi cheese
- ¼ cup all-purpose flour
- 2 eggs
- 1 teaspoon fresh dill, minced
- Salt and ground black pepper, as required

Directions:

1. In a large bowl and mix together all the ingredients.
2. Make a small-sized fritter from the mixture.
3. Press "Power Button" of Air Fry Oven and turn the dial to select the "Air Fry" mode.
4. Press the Time button and again turn the dial to set the cooking time to 7 minutes.
5. Now push the Temp button and rotate the dial to set the temperature at 355 degrees F.
6. Press "Start/Pause" button to start.
7. When the unit beeps to show that it is preheated, open the lid.
8. Arrange fritters into grease "Sheet Pan" and insert in the oven.
9. Serve warm.

Nutrition:

Calories 253 | Fat 17.2 g | Cholesterol 121 mg | Sodium 333 mg | Carbs 10 g | Fiber 1.1 g | Protein 15.2g

35. Sweet Potato Rosti

⏱ Prep Time 15 m | ⏱ Cooking Time 15 m | 2 Servings

Ingredients:

- ½ lb. sweet potatoes, peeled, grated and squeezed
- 1 tablespoon fresh parsley, chopped finely
- Salt and ground black pepper, as required
- 2 tablespoons sour cream

Directions:

1. In a large bowl, mix together the grated sweet potato, parsley, salt, and black pepper.
2. Press "Power Button" of Air Fry Oven and turn the dial to select the "Air Fry" mode.
3. Press the Time button and again turn the dial to set the cooking time to 15 minutes.
4. Now push the Temp button and rotate the dial to set the temperature at 355 degrees F.
5. Press "Start/Pause" button to start.
6. When the unit beeps to show that it is preheated, open the lid and lightly, grease the sheet pan.
7. Arrange the sweet potato mixture into the "Sheet Pan" and shape it into an even circle.
8. Insert the "Sheet Pan" in the oven.
9. Cut the potato rosti into wedges.
10. Top with the sour cream and serve immediately.

Nutrition:

Calories 160 | Fat 2.7 g | Cholesterol 5 mg | Sodium 95mg | Carbs 32.3 g | Fiber 4.7 g | Protein 2.2 g

36. Cheddar & Cream Omelet
⏲ Prep Time 10 m | ⏲ Cooking Time 8 m | 2 Servings

Ingredients:
- 4 eggs
- ¼ cup cream
- Salt and ground black pepper, as required
- ¼ cup Cheddar cheese, grated

Directions:
1. In a bowl, add the eggs, cream, salt, and black pepper and beat well.
2. Place the egg mixture into a small baking pan.
3. Press "Power Button" of Air Fry Oven and turn the dial to select the "Air Fry" mode.
4. Press the Time button and again turn the dial to set the cooking time to 8 minutes.
5. Now push the Temp button and rotate the dial to set the temperature at 350 degrees F.
6. Press "Start/Pause" button to start.
7. When the unit beeps to show that it is preheated, open the lid.
8. Arrange pan over the "Wire Rack" and insert in the oven.
9. After 4 minutes, sprinkle the omelet with cheese evenly.
10. Cut the omelet into 2 portions and serve hot.
11. Cut into equal-sized wedges and serve hot.

Nutrition:
Calories 202| Fat 15.1 g|Cholesterol 348 mg|Sodium 298 mg|Carbs 1.8 g|Fiber 0 g|Protein 14.8 g

37. Onion Omelet
⏲ Prep Time 10 m | ⏲ Cooking Time 15 m | 2 Servings

Ingredients:
- 4 eggs
- ¼ teaspoon low-sodium soy sauce
- Ground black pepper, as required
- 1 teaspoon butter
- 1 medium yellow onion, sliced
- ¼ cup Cheddar cheese, grated

Directions:
1. In a skillet, melt the butter over medium heat and cook the onion and cook for about 8-10 minutes.
2. Remove from the heat and set aside to cool slightly.
3. Meanwhile, in a bowl, add the eggs, soy sauce and black pepper and beat well.
4. Add the cooked onion and gently, stir to combine.
5. Place the zucchini mixture into a small baking pan.
6. Press "Power Button" of Air Fry Oven and turn the dial to select the "Air Fry" mode.
7. Press the Time button and again turn the dial to set the cooking time to 5 minutes.
8. Now push the Temp button and rotate the dial to set the temperature at 355 degrees F.
9. Press "Start/Pause" button to start.
10. When the unit beeps to show that it is preheated, open the lid.
11. Arrange pan over the "Wire Rack" and insert in the oven.
12. Cut the omelet into 2 portions and serve hot.

Nutrition:
Calories 222|Fat 15.4 g|Cholesterol 347 mg|Sodium 264 mg|Carbs 6.1 g|Fiber 1.2 g|Protein 15 g

38. Zucchini Omelet
⏲ Prep Time 15 m | ⏲ Cooking Time 14 m | 2 Servings

Ingredients:
- 1 teaspoon butter
- 1 zucchini, julienned
- 4 eggs
- ¼ teaspoon fresh basil, chopped
- ¼ teaspoon red pepper flakes, crushed
- Salt and ground black pepper, as required

Directions:
1. In a skillet, melt the butter over medium heat and cook the zucchini for about 3-4 minutes.
2. Remove from the heat and set aside to cool slightly.
3. Meanwhile, in a bowl, mix together the eggs, basil, red pepper flakes, salt, and black pepper.
4. Add the cooked zucchini and gently, stir to combine.
5. Place the zucchini mixture into a small baking pan.
6. Press "Power Button" of Air Fry Oven and turn the dial to select the "Air Fry" mode.
7. Press the Time button and again turn the dial to set the cooking time to 10 minutes.
8. Now push the Temp button and rotate the dial to set the temperature at 355 degrees F.
9. Press "Start/Pause" button to start.
10. When the unit beeps to show that it is preheated, open the lid.
11. Arrange pan over the "Wire Rack" and insert in the oven.
12. Cut the omelet into 2 portions and serve hot.

Nutrition:
Calories 159|Fat 10.9 g|Cholesterol 332 mg|Sodium 224 mg|Carbs 4.1 g|Fiber 1.1 g|Protein 12 g

39. Mushroom & Pepperoncini Omelet
⏰ Prep Time 15 m | ⏰ Cooking Time 20 m | 2 Servings

Ingredients:

- 3 large eggs
- ¼ c milk
- Salt and ground black pepper, as required
- ½ cup cheddar cheese, shredded
- ¼ cup cooked mushrooms
- 3 pepperoncini peppers, sliced thinly
- ½ tablespoon scallion, sliced thinly

Directions:

1. In a bowl, add the eggs, milk, salt and black pepper and beat well.
2. Place the mixture into a greased baking pan.
3. Press "Power Button" of Air Fry Oven and turn the dial to select the "Air Bake" mode.
4. Press the Time button and again turn the dial to set the cooking time to 20 minutes.
5. Now push the Temp button and rotate the dial to set the temperature at 350 degrees F.
6. Press "Start/Pause" button to start.
7. When the unit beeps to show that it is preheated, open the lid.
8. Arrange pan over the "Wire Rack" and insert in the oven.
9. Cut into equal-sized wedges and serve hot.

Nutrition:

Calories 254 | Fat 17.5 g | Cholesterol 311 mg | Sodium 793 mg | Carbs 7.3 g | Fiber 0.1 g | Protein 8.2 g

40. Chicken Omelet
⏰ Prep Time 10 m | ⏰ Cooking Time 16 m | 2 Servings

Ingredients:

- 1 teaspoon butter
- 1 small yellow onion, chopped
- ½ jalapeño pepper, seeded and chopped
- 3 eggs
- Salt and ground black pepper, as required
- ¼ cup cooked chicken, shredded

Directions:

1. In a frying pan, melt the butter over medium heat and cook the onion for about 4-5 minutes.
2. Add the jalapeño pepper and cook for about 1 minute.
3. Remove from the heat and set aside to cool slightly.
4. Meanwhile, in a bowl, add the eggs, salt, and black pepper and beat well.
5. Add the onion mixture and chicken and stir to combine.
6. Place the chicken mixture into a small baking pan.
7. Press "Power Button" of Air Fry Oven and turn the dial to select the "Air Fry" mode.
8. Press the Time button and again turn the dial to set the cooking time to 6 minutes.
9. Now push the Temp button and rotate the dial to set the temperature at 355 degrees F.
10. Press "Start/Pause" button to start.
11. When the unit beeps to show that it is preheated, open the lid.
12. Arrange pan over the "Wire Rack" and insert in the oven.
13. Cut the omelet into 2 portions and serve hot.

Nutrition:

Calories 153 | Fat 9.1 g | Cholesterol 264 mg | Sodium 196 mg | Carbs 4 g | Fiber 0.9 g | Protein 13.8 g

41. Chicken & Zucchini Omelet
⏰ Prep Time 15 m | ⏰ Cooking Time 35 m | 6 Servings

Ingredients:

- 8 eggs
- ½ cup milk
- Salt and ground black pepper, as required
- 1 cup cooked chicken, chopped
- 1 cup Cheddar cheese, shredded
- ½ cup fresh chives, chopped
- ¾ cup zucchini, chopped

Directions:

1. In a bowl, add the eggs, milk, salt and black pepper and beat well.
2. Add the remaining ingredients and stir to combine.
3. Place the mixture into a greased baking pan.
4. Press "Power Button" of Air Fry Oven and turn the dial to select the "Air Bake" mode.
5. Press the Time button and again turn the dial to set the cooking time to 35 minutes.
6. Now push the Temp button and rotate the dial to set the temperature at 315 degrees F.
7. Press "Start/Pause" button to start.
8. When the unit beeps to show that it is preheated, open the lid.
9. Arrange pan over the "Wire Rack" and insert in the oven.
10. Cut into equal-sized wedges and serve hot.

Nutrition:

Calories 209 | Fat 13.3 g | Cholesterol 258 mg | Sodium 252 mg | Carbs 2.3 g | Fiber 0.3 g | Protein 9.8 g

42. Pepperoni Omelet

Prep Time 15 m | Cooking Time 12 m | 2 Servings

Ingredients:

- 4 eggs
- 2 tablespoons milk
- Pinch of salt
- Ground black pepper, as required
- 8-10 turkey pepperoni slices

Directions:

1. In a bowl, crack the eggs and beat well.
2. Add the remaining ingredients and gently, stir to combine.
3. Place the mixture into a baking pan.
4. Press "Power Button" of Air Fry Oven and turn the dial to select the "Air Fry" mode.
5. Press the Time button and again turn the dial to set the cooking time to 12 minutes.
6. Now push the Temp button and rotate the dial to set the temperature at 355 degrees F.
7. Press "Start/Pause" button to start.
8. When the unit beeps to show that it is preheated, open the lid.
9. Arrange pan over the "Wire Rack" and insert in the oven.
10. Cut into equal-sized wedges and serve hot.

Nutrition:

Calories 149 | Fat 10 g | Cholesterol 337 mg | Sodium 350 mg | Carbs 1.5 g | Fiber 0 g | Protein 13.6 g

43. Sausage Omelet

Prep Time 10 m | Cooking Time 13 m | 2 Servings

Ingredients:

- 4 eggs
- 1 bacon slice, chopped
- 2 sausages, chopped
- 1 yellow onion, chopped

Directions:

1. In a bowl, crack the eggs and beat well.
2. Add the remaining ingredients and gently, stir to combine.
3. Place the mixture into a baking pan.
4. Press "Power Button" of Air Fry Oven and turn the dial to select the "Air Fry" mode.
5. Press the Time button and again turn the dial to set the cooking time to 13 minutes.
6. Now push the Temp button and rotate the dial to set the temperature at 320 degrees F.
7. Press "Start/Pause" button to start.
8. When the unit beeps to show that it is preheated, open the lid.
9. Arrange pan over the "Wire Rack" and insert in the oven.
10. Cut into equal-sized wedges and serve hot.

Nutrition:

Calories 325 | Fat 23.1 g | Cholesterol 368 mg | Sodium 678 mg | Carbs 6 g | Fiber 1.2 g | Protein 22.7 g

44. Pancetta & Hot Dogs Omelet

Prep Time 10 m | Cooking Time 10 m | 2 Servings

Ingredients:

- 4 eggs
- ¼ teaspoon dried parsley
- ¼ teaspoon dried rosemary
- 1 pancetta slice, chopped
- 2 hot dogs, chopped
- 2 small onions, chopped

Directions:

1. In a bowl, crack the eggs and beat well.
2. Add the remaining ingredients and gently, stir to combine.
3. Place the mixture into a baking pan.
4. Press "Power Button" of Air Fry Oven and turn the dial to select the "Air Fry" mode.
5. Press the Time button and again turn the dial to set the cooking time to 10 minutes.
6. Now push the Temp button and rotate the dial to set the temperature at 320 degrees F.
7. Press "Start/Pause" button to start.
8. When the unit beeps to show that it is preheated, open the lid.
9. Arrange pan over the "Wire Rack" and insert in the oven.
10. Cut into equal-sized wedges and serve hot.

Nutrition: Calories 282 | Fat 19.3 g | Cholesterol 351mg | Sodium 632 mg | Carbs 8.2 g | Fiber 1.6 g | Protein 18.9 g

45. Egg & Tofu Omelet

Prep Time 15 m | Cooking Time 10 m | 2 Servings

Ingredients:

- 1 teaspoon arrowroot starch
- 2 teaspoons water
- 3 eggs
- 2 teaspoons fish sauce
- 1 teaspoon olive oil
- Ground black pepper, as required
- 8 oz. silken tofu, pressed and sliced

Directions:

1. In a large bowl, dissolve arrowroot starch in water.
2. Add the eggs, fish sauce, oil and black pepper and beat well.
3. Place tofu in the bottom of a greased baking pan and top with the egg mixture.
4. Press "Power Button" of Air Fry Oven and turn the dial to select the "Air Fry" mode.
5. Press the Time button and again turn the dial to set the cooking time to 10 minutes.
6. Now push the Temp button and rotate the dial to set the temperature at 390 degrees F.
7. Press "Start/Pause" button to start.
8. When the unit beeps to show that it is preheated, open the lid.
9. Arrange pan over the "Wire Rack" and insert in the oven.
10. Cut into equal-sized wedges and serve hot.

Nutrition: Calories 192 | Fat 12 g | Cholesterol 246mg | Sodium 597 mg | Carbs 4.6 g | Fiber 0.2 g | Protein 16.4 g

46. Eggs, Tofu & Mushroom Omelet

⏱ Prep Time 15 m | ⏱ Cooking Time 35 m | 2 Servings

Ingredients:

- 2 teaspoons canola oil
- ¼ of onion, chopped
- 1 garlic clove, minced
- 8 oz. silken tofu, pressed and sliced
- 3½ oz. fresh mushrooms, sliced
- Salt and ground black pepper, as needed
- 3 eggs, beaten

Directions:

1. In a skillet, heat the oil over medium heat and sauté the onion, and garlic for about 4-5 minutes.
2. Add the mushrooms and cook for about 4-5 minutes.
3. Remove from the heat and stir in the tofu, salt and black pepper.
4. Place the tofu mixture into a pan and top with the beaten eggs.
5. Press "Power Button" of Air Fry Oven and turn the dial to select the "Air Fry" mode.
6. Press the Time button and again turn the dial to set the cooking time to 25 minutes.
7. Now push the Temp button and rotate the dial to set the temperature at 355 degrees F.
8. Press "Start/Pause" button to start.
9. When the unit beeps to show that it is preheated, open the lid.
10. Arrange pan over the "Wire Rack" and insert in the oven.
11. Cut into equal-sized wedges and serve hot.

Nutrition:

Calories 224 | Fat 14.5 g | Cholesterol 246 mg | Sodium 214 mg | Carbs 6.6 g | Fiber 0.9 g | Protein 18g

47. Mini Mushroom Frittatas

⏱ Prep Time 15 m | ⏱ Cooking Time 17 m | 2 Servings

Ingredients:

- 1 tablespoon olive oil
- ½ of onion, sliced thinly
- 2 cups button mushrooms, sliced thinly
- 3 eggs
- Salt and ground black pepper, as required
- 3 tablespoons feta cheese, crumbled

Directions:

1. In a frying pan, heat the oil over medium heat and cook the onion and mushroom for about 5 minutes.
2. Remove from the heat and set aside to cool slightly.
3. Meanwhile, in a small bowl, add the eggs, salt and black pepper and beat well.
4. Divide the beaten eggs in 2 greased ramekins evenly and top with the mushroom mixture.
5. Press "Power Button" of Air Fry Oven and turn the dial to select the "Air Fry" mode.
6. Press the Time button and again turn the dial to set the cooking time to 12 minutes.
7. Now push the Temp button and rotate the dial to set the temperature at 330 degrees F.
8. Press "Start/Pause" button to start.
9. When the unit beeps to show that it is preheated, open the lid.
10. Arrange the ramekins over the "Wire Rack" and insert in the oven.
11. Serve hot.

Nutrition:

Calories 218 | Fat 16.8 g | Cholesterol 258 mg | Sodium 332 mg | Carbs 6 g | Fiber 1.3 g | Protein 12.8 g

48. Tomato Frittata

⏱ Prep Time 10 m | ⏱ Cooking Time 30 m | 2 Servings

Ingredients:

- 4 eggs
- ¼ cup onion, chopped
- ½ cup tomatoes, chopped
- ½ cup milk
- 1 cup Gouda cheese, shredded
- Salt, as required

Directions:

1. In a small baking pan, add all the ingredients and mix well.
2. Press "Power Button" of Air Fry Oven and turn the dial to select the "Air Fry" mode.
3. Press the Time button and again turn the dial to set the cooking time to 30 minutes.
4. Now push the Temp button and rotate the dial to set the temperature at 340 degrees F.
5. Press "Start/Pause" button to start.
6. When the unit beeps to show that it is preheated, open the lid.
7. Arrange the baking pan over the "Wire Rack" and insert in the oven.
8. Cut into 2 wedges and serve.

Nutrition:

Calories 247 | Fat 16.1 g | Cholesterol 332 mg | Sodium 417 mg | Carbs 7.3 g | Fiber 1 g | Protein 18.6 g

49. Mushroom Frittata

🕐 Prep Time 15 m | 🕐 Cooking Time 36 m | 4 Servings

Ingredients:

- 2 tablespoons olive oil
- 1 shallot, sliced thinly
- 2 garlic cloves, minced
- 4 cups white mushrooms, chopped
- 6 large eggs
- ¼ teaspoon red pepper flakes, crushed
- Salt and ground black pepper, as required
- ½ teaspoon fresh dill, minced
- ½ cup cream cheese, softened

Directions:

1. In a skillet, heat the oil over medium heat and cook the shallot, mushrooms and garlic for about 5-6 minutes, stirring frequently.
2. Remove from the heat and transfer the mushroom mixture into a bowl.
3. In another bowl, add the eggs, red pepper flakes, salt and black peppers and beat well.
4. Add the mushroom mixture and stir to combine.
5. Place the egg mixture into a greased baking pan and sprinkle with the dill.
6. Spread cream cheese over egg mixture evenly.
7. Press "Power Button" of Air Fry Oven and turn the dial to select the "Air Fry" mode.
8. Press the Time button and again turn the dial to set the cooking time to 30 minutes.
9. Now push the Temp button and rotate the dial to set the temperature at 330 degrees F.
10. Press "Start/Pause" button to start.
11. When the unit beeps to show that it is preheated, open the lid.
12. Arrange pan over the "Wire Rack" and insert in the oven.
13. Cut into equal-sized wedges and serve

Nutrition:

Calories 290 | Fat 24.8g | Cholesterol 311 mg | Sodium 236 mg | Carbs 5 g | Fiber 0.8 g | Protein 14.1 g

50. Mixed Veggies Frittata

🕐 Prep Time 15 m | 🕐 Cooking Time 21 m | 4 Servings

Ingredients:

- ½ teaspoon olive oil
- 4 fresh mushrooms, sliced
- 4 eggs
- 3 tablespoons heavy cream
- Salt, as required
- 4 tablespoons Cheddar cheese, grated
- 4 tablespoons fresh spinach, chopped
- 3 grape tomatoes, halved
- 2 tablespoons fresh mixed herbs, chopped
- 1 scallion, sliced

Directions:

1. In a skillet, heat the oil over medium heat and cook the mushrooms for about 5-6 minutes, stirring frequently.
2. Remove from the heat and transfer the mushroom into a bowl.
3. In a bowl, add the eggs, cream and salt and beat well.
4. Add the mushroom and remaining ingredients and stir to combine.
5. Place the mixture into a greased baking pan evenly.
6. Press "Power Button" of Air Fry Oven and turn the dial to select the "Air Fry" mode.
7. Press the Time button and again turn the dial to set the cooking time to 15 minutes.
8. Now push the Temp button and rotate the dial to set the temperature at 350 degrees F.
9. Press "Start/Pause" button to start.
10. When the unit beeps to show that it is preheated, open the lid.
11. Arrange pan over the "Wire Rack" and insert in the oven.
12. Cut into equal-sized wedges and serve.

Nutrition:

Calories 159 | Fat 11.7 g | Cholesterol 187 mg | Sodium 156 mg | Carbs 5.6 g | Fiber 1.7 g | Protein 9.1 g

51. Pancetta & Spinach Frittata

🕐 Prep Time 15 m | 🕐 Cooking Time 16 m | 2 Servings

Ingredients:

- ¼ cup pancetta
- ½ of tomato, cubed
- ¼ cup fresh baby spinach
- 3 eggs
- Salt and ground black pepper, as required
- ¼ cup Parmesan cheese, grated

Directions:

1. Heat a nonstick skillet over medium heat and cook the pancetta for about 5 minutes.
2. Add the tomato and spinach cook for about 2-3 minutes.
3. Remove from the heat and drain the grease from skillet.
4. Set aside to cool slightly.
5. Meanwhile, in a small bowl, add the eggs, salt and black pepper and beat well.
6. In the bottom of a greased baking pan, place the pancetta mixture and top with the eggs, followed by the cheese.
7. Press "Power Button" of Air Fry Oven and turn the dial to select the "Air Fry" mode.
8. Press the Time button and again turn the dial to set the cooking time to 8 minutes.
9. Now push the Temp button and rotate the dial to set the temperature at 355 degrees F.
10. Press "Start/Pause" button to start.
11. When the unit beeps to show that it is preheated, open the lid.
12. Arrange pan over the "Wire Rack" and insert in the oven.
13. Cut into equal-sized wedges and serve.

Nutrition:

Calories 287 | Fat 20.8g | Cholesterol 285 mg | Sodium 915 mg | Carbs 1.7 g | Fiber 0.3 g | Protein 23.1 g

52. Trout Frittata
Prep Time 15 m | Cooking Time 25 m | 4 Servings

Ingredients:

- 1 tablespoon olive oil
- 1 onion, sliced
- 6 eggs
- ½ tablespoon horseradish sauce

- 2 tablespoons crème fraiche
- 2 hot-smoked trout fillets, chopped
- ¼ cup fresh dill, chopped

Directions:

1. In a skillet, heat the oil over medium heat and cook the onion for about 4-5 minutes.
2. Remove from the heat and set aside.
3. Meanwhile, in a bowl, add the eggs, horseradish sauce, and crème fraiche and mix well.
4. In the bottom of a baking pan, place the cooked onion and top with the egg mixture, followed by trout.
5. Press "Power Button" of Air Fry Oven and turn the dial to select the "Air Fry" mode.
6. Press the Time button and again turn the dial to set the cooking time to 20 minutes.
7. Now push the Temp button and rotate the dial to set the temperature at 320 degrees F.
8. Press "Start/Pause" button to start.
9. When the unit beeps to show that it is preheated, open the lid.
10. Arrange pan over the "Wire Rack" and insert in the oven.
11. Cut into equal-sized wedges and serve with the garnishing of dill.

Nutrition:

Calories 258 | Fat 15.7 g | Cholesterol 288 mg | Sodium 141 mg | Carbs 5.1 g | Fiber 1 g | Protein 24.4 g

53. Bacon, Mushroom & Tomato Frittata
Prep Time 15 m | Cooking Time 16 m | 2 Servings

Ingredients:

- 1 cooked bacon slice, chopped
- 6 cherry tomatoes, halved
- 6 fresh mushrooms, sliced
- Salt and ground black pepper, as required

- 3 eggs
- 1 tablespoon fresh parsley, chopped
- ¼ cup Parmesan cheese, grated

Directions:

1. In a baking pan, add the bacon, tomatoes, mushrooms, salt, and black pepper and mix well.
2. Press "Power Button" of Air Fry Oven and turn the dial to select the "Air Fry" mode.
3. Press the Time button and again turn the dial to set the cooking time to 16 minutes.
4. Now push the Temp button and rotate the dial to set the temperature at 320 degrees F.
5. Press "Start/Pause" button to start.
6. When the unit beeps to show that it is preheated, open the lid.
7. Arrange pan over the "Wire Rack" and insert in the oven.
8. Meanwhile, in a bowl, add the eggs and beat well.
9. Add the parsley and cheese and mix well.
10. After 6 minutes of cooking, top the bacon mixture with egg mixture evenly.
11. Cut into equal-sized wedges and serve.

Nutrition:

Calories 228 | Fat 15.5 g | Cholesterol 270 mg | Sodium 608 mg | Carbs 3.5 g | Fiber 1 g | Protein 19.8 g

54. Sausage, Spinach & Broccoli Frittata
Prep Time 15 m | Cooking Time 30 m | 4 Servings

Ingredients:

- 1 teaspoon butter
- 6 turkey sausage links, cut into small pieces
- 1 cup broccoli florets, cut into small pieces
- ½ cup fresh spinach, chopped up
- 6 eggs

- 1/8 teaspoon hot sauce
- 2 tablespoons half-and-half
- 1/8 teaspoon garlic salt
- Salt and ground black pepper, as required
- ¾ cup Cheddar cheese, shredded

Directions:

1. In a skillet, melt the butter over medium heat and cook the sausage for about 7-8 minutes or until browned.
2. Add the broccoli and cook for about 3-4 minutes.
3. Add the spinach and cook for about 2-3 minutes.
4. Remove from the heat and set aside to cool slightly.
5. Meanwhile, in a bowl, add the eggs, half-and-half, hot sauce, garlic salt, salt and black pepper and beat until well combined.
6. Add the cheese and stir to combine.
7. In the bottom of a lightly greased pan, place the broccoli mixture and to with the egg mixture.
8. Press "Power Button" of Air Fry Oven and turn the dial to select the "Air Bake" mode.
9. Press the Time button and again turn the dial to set the cooking time to 15 minutes.
10. Now push the Temp button and rotate the dial to set the temperature at 400 degrees F.
11. Press "Start/Pause" button to start.
12. When the unit beeps to show that it is preheated, open the lid.
13. Arrange pan over the "Wire Rack" and insert in the oven.
14. Cut into equal-sized wedges and serve hot.

Nutrition:

Calories 339 | Fat 27.4g | Cholesterol 229 mg | Sodium 596 mg | Carbs 3.7 g | Fiber 0.7 g | Protein 19.6 g

55. Sausage & Scallion Frittata
⏰ Prep Time 15 m | ⏰ Cooking Time 20 m | 2 Servings

Ingredients:

- ¼ lb. cooked breakfast sausage, crumbled
- ½ cup Cheddar cheese, shredded
- 4 eggs, beaten lightly
- 2 scallions, chopped
- Pinch of cayenne pepper

Directions:

1. In a bowl, add the sausage, cheese, eggs, scallion and cayenne and mix until well combined.
2. Place the mixture into a greased baking pan.
3. Press "Power Button" of Air Fry Oven and turn the dial to select the "Air Fry" mode.
4. Press the Time button and again turn the dial to set the cooking time to 20 minutes.
5. Now push the Temp button and rotate the dial to set the temperature at 360 degrees F.
6. Press "Start/Pause" button to start.
7. When the unit beeps to show that it is preheated, open the lid.
8. Arrange pan over the "Wire Rack" and insert in the oven.
9. Cut into equal-sized wedges and serve hot.

Nutrition:

Calories 437 | Fat 32 g | Cholesterol 405 mg | Sodium 726 mg | Carbs 2.2 g | Fiber 0.4 g | Protein 29.4 g

56. Tomato Quiche
⏰ Prep Time 15 m | ⏰ Cooking Time 30 m | 2 Servings

Ingredients:

- 4 eggs
- ¼ cup onion, chopped
- ½ cup tomatoes, chopped
- ½ cup milk
- 1 cup Gouda cheese, shredded
- Salt, as required

Directions:

1. In a small baking pan, add all the ingredients and mix well.
2. Press "Power Button" of Air Fry Oven and turn the dial to select the "Air Fry" mode.
3. Press the Time button and again turn the dial to set the cooking time to 30 minutes.
4. Now push the Temp button and rotate the dial to set the temperature at 340 degrees F.
5. Press "Start/Pause" button to start.
6. When the unit beeps to show that it is preheated, open the lid.
7. Arrange pan over the "Wire Rack" and insert in the oven.
8. Cut into equal-sized wedges and serve.

Nutrition:

Calories 247 | Fat 16.1 g | Cholesterol 332 mg | Sodium 417 mg | Carbs 7.3 g | Fiber 0.9 g | Protein 18.6 g

57. Mini Macaroni Quiches
⏰ Prep Time 15 m | ⏰ Cooking Time 20 m | 4 Servings

Ingredients:

- 1 short crust pastry
- ½ cup leftover macaroni n' cheese
- 2 tablespoons plain Greek yogurt
- 1 teaspoon garlic puree
- 11 oz. milk
- 2 large eggs
- 2 tablespoons Parmesan cheese, grated

Directions:

1. Dust 4 ramekins with a little flour.
2. Line the bottom of prepared ramekins with short crust pastry.
3. In a bowl, mix together macaroni, yogurt and garlic.
4. Transfer the macaroni mixture between ramekins about ¾ full.
5. In a small bowl, add the milk and eggs and beat well.
6. Place the egg mixture over the macaroni mixture and top with the cheese evenly.
7. Press "Power Button" of Air Fry Oven and turn the dial to select the "Air Fry" mode.
8. Press the Time button and again turn the dial to set the cooking time to 20 minutes.
9. Now push the Temp button and rotate the dial to set the temperature at 355 degrees F.
10. Press "Start/Pause" button to start.
11. When the unit beeps to show that it is preheated, open the lid.
12. Arrange the ramekins over the "Wire Rack" and insert in the oven.

Nutrition:

Calories 209 | Fat 10.4 g | Cholesterol 102 mg | Sodium 135 mg | Carbs 19 g | Fiber 0.6 g | Protein 9.6 g

58. Chicken & Broccoli Quiche

🕐 Prep Time 15 m | 🕐 Cooking Time 12 m | 2 Servings

Ingredients:

- ½ of frozen ready-made pie crust
- ¼ tablespoon olive oil
- 1 small egg
- 3 tablespoons cheddar cheese, grated
- 1½ tablespoons whipping cream
- Salt and freshly ground black pepper, as needed
- 3 tablespoons boiled broccoli, chopped
- 2 tablespoons cooked chicken, chopped

Directions:

1. Cut 1 (5-inch) round from the pie crust.
2. Arrange the pie crust round in a small pie pan and gently, press in the bottom and sides.
3. In a bowl, mix together the egg, cheese, cream, salt, and black pepper.
4. Pour the egg mixture over dough base and top with the broccoli and chicken.
5. Press "Power Button" of Air Fry Oven and turn the dial to select the "Air Fry" mode.
6. Press the Time button and again turn the dial to set the cooking time to 12 minutes.
7. Now push the Temp button and rotate the dial to set the temperature at 390 degrees F.
8. Press "Start/Pause" button to start.
9. When the unit beeps to show that it is preheated, open the lid.
10. Arrange pan over the "Wire Rack" and insert in the oven.
11. Cut into equal-sized wedges and serve.

Nutrition:

Calories 197 | Fat 15 g | Cholesterol 99 mg | Sodium 184 mg | Carbs 7.4 g | Fiber 0.4 g | Protein 8.6 g

59. Bacon & Spinach Quiche

🕐 Prep Time 15 m | 🕐 Cooking Time 10 m | 4 Servings

Ingredients:

- 2 cooked bacon slices, chopped
- ½ cup fresh spinach, chopped
- ¼ cup mozzarella cheese, shredded
- ½ cup Parmesan cheese, shredded
- 2 tablespoons milk
- 2 dashes Tabasco sauce
- Salt and ground black pepper, as required

Directions:

1. In a bowl, add all ingredients and mix well.
2. Transfer the mixture into a baking pan.
3. Press "Power Button" of Air Fry Oven and turn the dial to select the "Air Fry" mode.
4. Press the Time button and again turn the dial to set the cooking time to 10 minutes.
5. Now push the Temp button and rotate the dial to set the temperature at 320 degrees F.
6. Press "Start/Pause" button to start.
7. When the unit beeps to show that it is preheated, open the lid.
8. Arrange pan over the "Wire Rack" and insert in the oven.

Nutrition:

Calories 130 | Fat 9.3 g | Cholesterol 25 mg | Sodium 561 mg | Carbs 1.1 g | Fiber 0.1 g | Protein 10 g

60. Salmon Quiche

🕐 Prep Time 15 m | 🕐 Cooking Time 20 m | 2 Servings

Ingredients:

- 5½ oz. salmon fillet, chopped
- Salt and ground black pepper, as required
- ½ tablespoon fresh lemon juice
- 1 egg yolk
- 3½ tablespoons chilled butter
- 2/3 cup flour
- 1 tablespoon cold water
- 2 eggs
- 3 tablespoons whipping cream
- 1 scallion, chopped

Directions:

1. In a bowl, mix together the salmon, salt, black pepper and lemon juice.
2. In another bowl, add the egg yolk, butter, flour and water and mix until a dough forms.
3. Place the dough onto a floured smooth surface and roll into about 7-inch round.
4. Place the dough in a quiche pan and press firmly in the bottom and along the edges.
5. Trim the excess edges.
6. In a small bowl, add the eggs, cream, salt and black pepper and beat until well combined.
7. Place the cream mixture over crust evenly and top with the salmon mixture, followed by the scallion.
8. Press "Power Button" of Air Fry Oven and turn the dial to select the "Air Fry" mode.
9. Press the Time button and again turn the dial to set the cooking time to 20 minutes.
10. Now push the Temp button and rotate the dial to set the temperature at 355 degrees F.
11. Press "Start/Pause" button to start.
12. When the unit beeps to show that it is preheated, open the lid.
13. Arrange pan over the "Wire Rack" and insert in the oven.
14. Cut into equal-sized wedges and serve.

Nutrition:

Calories 592 | Fat 39 g | Cholesterol 381 mg | Sodium 331 mg | Carbs 33.8 g | Fiber 1.4 g | Protein 27.2g

61. Sausage & Mushroom Casserole
☉ Prep Time 15 m | ☉ Cooking Time 19 m | 6 Servings

Ingredients:

- 1 tablespoon olive oil
- ½ lb. spicy ground sausage
- ¾ cup yellow onion, chopped
- 5 fresh mushrooms, sliced

- 8 eggs, beaten
- ½ teaspoon garlic salt
- ¾ cup Cheddar cheese, shredded and divided
- ¼ cup Alfredo sauce

Directions:

1. In a skillet, heat the oil over medium heat and cook the sausage and onions for about 4-5 minutes.
2. Add the mushrooms and cook for about 6-7 minutes.
3. Remove from the oven and drain the grease from skillet.
4. In a bowl, add the sausage mixture, beaten eggs, garlic salt, ½ cup of cheese and Alfredo sauce and stir to combine.
5. Place the sausage mixture into a baking pan.
6. Press "Power Button" of Air Fry Oven and turn the dial to select the "Air Fry" mode.
7. Press the Time button and again turn the dial to set the cooking time to 12 minutes.
8. Now push the Temp button and rotate the dial to set the temperature at 390 degrees F.
9. Press "Start/Pause" button to start.
10. When the unit beeps to show that it is preheated, open the lid.
11. Arrange pan over the "Wire Rack" and insert in the oven.
12. After 6 minutes of cooking, stir the sausage mixture well.
13. Cut into equal-sized wedges and serve with the topping of remaining cheese.

Nutrition:

Calories 319 | Fat 24.5 g | Cholesterol 267 mg | Sodium 698 mg | Carbs 5 g | Fiber 0.5 g | Protein 19.7 g

62. Sausage & Bell Pepper Casserole
☉ Prep Time 15 m | ☉ Cooking Time 25 m | 6 Servings

Ingredients:

- 1 teaspoon olive oil
- 1 lb. ground sausage
- 1 green bell pepper, seeded and chopped
- ¼ cup onion, chopped

- 8 eggs, beaten
- ½ cup Colby Jack cheese, shredded
- 1 teaspoon fennel seed
- ½ teaspoon garlic salt

Directions:

1. In a skillet, heat the oil over medium heat and cook the sausage for about 4-5 minutes.
2. Add the bell pepper and onion and cook for about 4-5 minutes.
3. Remove from the heat and transfer the sausage mixture into a bowl to cool slightly.
4. In a baking pan, place the sausage mixture and top with the cheese, followed by the beaten eggs, fennel seed and garlic salt.
5. Press "Power Button" of Air Fry Oven and turn the dial to select the "Air Fry" mode.
6. Press the Time button and again turn the dial to set the cooking time to 15 minutes.
7. Now push the Temp button and rotate the dial to set the temperature at 390 degrees F.
8. Press "Start/Pause" button to start.
9. When the unit beeps to show that it is preheated, open the lid.
10. Arrange pan over the "Wire Rack" and insert in the oven.
11. Cut into equal-sized wedges and serve hot.

Nutrition:

Calories 394 | Fat 1.1 g | Cholesterol 290 mg | Sodium 709 mg | Carbs 3.1 g | Fiber 0.5 g | Protein 24.4 g

63. Turkey & Yogurt Casserole
☉ Prep Time 10 m | ☉ Cooking Time 25 m | 4 Servings

Ingredients:

- 6 eggs
- ½ cup plain Greek yogurt
- ½ cup cooked turkey meat, chopped

- Salt and ground black pepper, as required
- ½ cup sharp Cheddar cheese, shredded

Directions:

1. In a bowl, add the egg and yogurt and beat well.
2. Add the remaining ingredients and stir to combine.
3. In a greased baking pan, place the egg mixture.
4. Press "Power Button" of Air Fry Oven and turn the dial to select the "Air Bake" mode.
5. Press the Time button and again turn the dial to set the cooking time to 25 minutes.
6. Now push the Temp button and rotate the dial to set the temperature at 375 degrees F.
7. Press "Start/Pause" button to start.
8. When the unit beeps to show that it is preheated, open the lid.
9. Arrange pan over the "Wire Rack" and insert in the oven.
10. Cut into equal-sized wedges and serve.

Nutrition:

Calories 203 | Fat 12.5 g | Cholesterol 275 mg | Sodium 253 mg | Carbs 2.9 g | Fiber 0 g | Protein 18.7 g

64. Eggs with Ham

⏱ Prep Time 15 m | ⏱ Cooking Time 13 m | 2 Servings

Ingredients:

- 2 teaspoons unsalted butter, softened
- 2 oz. ham, sliced thinly
- 4 large eggs, divided
- Salt and ground black pepper, as required
- 2 tablespoons heavy cream
- 1/8 teaspoon smoked paprika
- 3 tablespoons Parmesan cheese, grated finely
- 2 teaspoons fresh chives, minced

Directions:

1. In the bottom of a baking pan, spread butter.
2. Arrange the ham slices over the butter.
3. In a bowl, add 1egg, salt, black pepper and cream and beat until smooth.
4. Place the egg mixture over the ham slices evenly.
5. Carefully, crack the remaining eggs on top and sprinkle with paprika, salt, black pepper, cheese and chives evenly.
6. Press "Power Button" of Air Fry Oven and turn the dial to select the "Air Fry" mode.
7. Press the Time button and again turn the dial to set the cooking time to 13 minutes.
8. Now push the Temp button and rotate the dial to set the temperature at 320 degrees F.
9. Press "Start/Pause" button to start.
10. When the unit beeps to show that it is preheated, open the lid.
11. Arrange pan over the "Wire Rack" and insert in the oven.
12. Cut into equal-sized wedges and serve.

Nutrition:

Calories 302 | Fat 23.62 g | Cholesterol 425 mg | Sodium 685 mg | Carbs 2.4g | Fiber 0.5g | Protein 20.7g

65. Ham & Hashbrown Casserole

⏱ Prep Time 15 m | ⏱ Cooking Time 35 m | 2 Servings

Ingredients:

- 1½ tablespoons olive oil
- ½ of large onion, chopped
- 24 oz. frozen hashbrowns
- 3 eggs
- 2 tablespoons milk
- Salt and ground black pepper, as required
- ½ lb. ham, chopped
- ¼ cup Cheddar cheese, shredded

Directions:

1. In a skillet, heat the oil over medium heat and sauté the onion for about 4-5 minutes.
2. Remove from the heat and transfer the onion into a bowl.
3. Add the hashbrowns and mix well.
4. Place the mixture into a baking pan.
5. Press "Power Button" of Air Fry Oven and turn the dial to select the "Air Bake" mode.
6. Press the Time button and again turn the dial to set the cooking time to 32 minutes.
7. Now push the Temp button and rotate the dial to set the temperature at 350 degrees F.
8. Press "Start/Pause" button to start.
9. When the unit beeps to show that it is preheated, open the lid.
10. Arrange pan over the "Wire Rack" and insert in the oven.
11. Stir the mixture once after 8 minutes.
12. Meanwhile, in a bowl, add the eggs, milk, salt and black pepper and beat well.
13. After 15 minutes of cooking, place the egg mixture over hashbrown mixture evenly and top with the ham.
14. After 30 minutes of cooking, sprinkle the casserole with the cheese.
15. Cut into equal-sized wedges and serve.

Nutrition:

Calories 540 | Fat 29.8 g | Cholesterol 131 mg | Sodium 1110mg | Carbs 51.5g | Fiber 5.3g | Protein16.7g

66. Eggs with Turkey & Spinach

⏱ Prep Time 15 m | ⏱ Cooking Time 23 m | 4 Servings

Ingredients:

- 1 tablespoon unsalted butter
- 1 lb. fresh baby spinach
- 4 eggs
- 7 oz. cooked turkey, chopped
- 4 teaspoons milk
- Salt and ground black pepper, as required

Directions:

1. In a skillet, melt the butter over medium heat and cook the spinach for about 2-3 minutes or until just wilted.
2. Remove from the heat and transfer the spinach into a bowl.
3. Set aside to cool slightly.
4. Divide the spinach into 4 greased ramekins, followed by the turkey.
5. Crack 1 egg into each ramekin and drizzle with milk.
6. Sprinkle with salt and black pepper.
7. Press "Power Button" of Air Fry Oven and turn the dial to select the "Air Fry" mode.
8. Press the Time button and again turn the dial to set the cooking time to 20 minutes.
9. Now push the Temp button and rotate the dial to set the temperature at 355 degrees F.
10. Press "Start/Pause" button to start.
11. When the unit beeps to show that it is preheated, open the lid.
12. Arrange ramekins over the "Wire Rack" and insert in the oven.
13. Serve hot.

Nutrition:

Calories 201 | Fat 10.3 g | Cholesterol 209 mg | Sodium 248 mg | Carbs 4.7 g | Fiber 2.5g | Protein 23.5 g

67. Eggs with Ham & Veggies
Prep Time 15 m | Cooking Time 15 m | 2 Servings

Ingredients:

- 1 teaspoon olive oil
- 6 small button mushroom, quartered
- 6 cherry tomatoes, halved
- 4 slices shaved ham
- 2 tablespoons spinach, chopped
- 1 cup cheddar cheese, shredded
- 2 eggs
- 1 tablespoon fresh rosemary, chopped
- Salt and ground black pepper, as required

Directions:

1. In a skillet, heat the oil over medium heat and cook the mushrooms for about 6-7 minutes.
2. Remove from the heat and set aside to cool slightly.
3. In a bowl, mix together the mushrooms, tomatoes, ham and greens.
4. Place half of the vegetable mixture in a greased baking pan and top with half of the cheese.
5. Repeat the layers once.
6. Make 2 wells in the mixture.
7. Carefully, crack 1 eggs in each well and sprinkle with rosemary, salt and black pepper.
8. Press "Power Button" of Air Fry Oven and turn the dial to select the "Air Fry" mode.
9. Press the Time button and again turn the dial to set the cooking time to 8 minutes.
10. Now push the Temp button and rotate the dial to set the temperature at 390 degrees F.
11. Press "Start/Pause" button to start.
12. When the unit beeps to show that it is preheated, open the lid.
13. Arrange ramekins over the "Wire Rack" and insert in the oven.
14. Serve hot.

Nutrition:

Calories 424 | Fat 30.7 g | Cholesterol 255 mg | Sodium 1140 mg | Carbs 7 g | Fiber 2.3 g | Protein 31 g

68. Eggs in Bread & Tomato Cups
Prep Time 15 m | Cooking Time 12 m | 2 Servings

Ingredients:

- ½ teaspoon butter
- 2 bread slices
- 1 pancetta slice, chopped
- 4 tomato slices
- 1 tablespoon Mozzarella cheese, shredded
- 2 eggs
- 1/8 teaspoon maple syrup
- 1/8 teaspoon balsamic vinegar
- ¼ teaspoon fresh parsley, chopped
- Salt and freshly ground pepper, to taste

Directions:

1. Line each prepared ramekin with 1 bread slice.
2. Divide bacon and tomato slices over bread slice evenly in each ramekin.
3. Top with the cheese evenly.
4. Crack 1 egg in each ramekin over cheese.
5. Drizzle with maple syrup and balsamic vinegar and then sprinkle with parsley, salt and black pepper.
6. Press "Power Button" of Air Fry Oven and turn the dial to select the "Air Fry" mode.
7. Press the Time button and again turn the dial to set the cooking time to 12 minutes.
8. Now push the Temp button and rotate the dial to set the temperature at 320 degrees F.
9. Press "Start/Pause" button to start.
10. When the unit beeps to show that it is preheated, open the lid.
11. Arrange the ramekins over the "Wire Rack" and insert in the oven.
12. Serve warm.

Nutrition:

Calories 219 | Fat 14.2 g | Cholesterol 190 mg | Sodium 628 mg | Carbs 6.8 g | Fiber 0.5g | Protein 15.8 g

69. Eggs in Bread & Sausage Cups
Prep Time 10 m | Cooking Time 22 m | 2 Servings

Ingredients:

- ¼ cup cream
- 3 eggs
- 2 cooked sausages, sliced
- 1 bread slice, cut into sticks
- ¼ cup mozzarella cheese, grated

Directions:

1. In a bowl, add the cream and eggs and beat well.
2. Transfer the egg mixture into ramekins.
3. Place the sausage slices and bread sticks around the edges and gently push them in the egg mixture.
4. Sprinkle with the cheese evenly.
5. Press "Power Button" of Air Fry Oven and turn the dial to select the "Air Fry" mode.
6. Press the Time button and again turn the dial to set the cooking time to 22 minutes.
7. Now push the Temp button and rotate the dial to set the temperature at 355 degrees F.
8. Press "Start/Pause" button to start.
9. When the unit beeps to show that it is preheated, open the lid.
10. Arrange the ramekins over the "Wire Rack" and insert in the oven.
11. Serve warm.

Nutrition:

Calories 229 | Fat 18.6 g | Cholesterol 278 mg | Sodium 360 mg | Carbs 3.9 g | Fiber 0.1g | Protein 15.2 g

70. Eggs in Bread & Bacon Cups

🕐 Prep Time 10 m | 🕐 Cooking Time 15 m | 4 Servings

Ingredients:
- 4 bacon slices
- 4 bread slices
- 1 scallion, chopped
- 2 tablespoons bell pepper, seeded and chopped
- 1½ tablespoons mayonnaise
- 4 eggs

Directions:
1. Grease 6 cups muffin tin with cooking spray.
2. Line the sides of each prepared muffin cup with 1 bacon slice.
3. Cut bread slices with round cookie cutter.
4. Arrange the bread slice in the bottom of each muffin cup.
5. Top with, scallion, bell pepper and mayonnaise evenly.
6. Carefully, crack one egg in each muffin cup.
7. Press "Power Button" of Air Fry Oven and turn the dial to select the "Air Fry" mode.
8. Press the Time button and again turn the dial to set the cooking time to 15 minutes.
9. Now push the Temp button and rotate the dial to set the temperature at 375 degrees F.
10. Press "Start/Pause" button to start.
11. When the unit beeps to show that it is preheated, open the lid.
12. Arrange the ramekins over the "Wire Rack" and insert in the oven.
13. Serve warm.

Nutrition:
Calories 298 | Fat 20.7 g | Cholesterol 197 mg | Sodium 829mg | Carbs 10.1g | Fiber 1.1g | Protein 17.6 g

71. Spinach & Mozzarella Muffins

🕐 Prep Time 10 m | 🕐 Cooking Time 10 m | 2 Servings

Ingredients:
- 2 large eggs
- 2 tablespoons half-and-half
- 2 tablespoons frozen spinach, thawed
- 4 teaspoons mozzarella cheese, grated
- Salt and ground black pepper, as required

Directions:
1. Grease 2 ramekins.
2. In each prepared ramekin, crack 1 egg.
3. Divide the half-and-half, spinach, cheese, salt and black pepper and each ramekin and gently stir to combine, without breaking the yolks.
4. Press "Power Button" of Air Fry Oven and turn the dial to select the "Air Fry" mode.
5. Press the Time button and again turn the dial to set the cooking time to 10 minutes.
6. Now push the Temp button and rotate the dial to set the temperature at 330 degrees F.
7. Press "Start/Pause" button to start.
8. When the unit beeps to show that it is preheated, open the lid.
9. Arrange the ramekins over the "Wire Rack" and insert in the oven.
10. Serve warm.

Nutrition:
Calories 251 | Fat 16.7 g | Cholesterol 222 mg | Sodium 495 mg | Carbs 3.1 g | Fiber 0 g | Protein 22.8 g

72. Bacon & Spinach Muffins

🕐 Prep Time 10 m | 🕐 Cooking Time 17 m | 6 Servings

Ingredients:
- 6 eggs
- ½ cup milk
- Salt and ground black pepper, as required
- 1 cup fresh spinach, chopped
- 4 cooked bacon slices, crumbled

Directions:
1. In a bowl, add the eggs, milk, salt and black pepper and beat until well combined.
2. Add the spinach and stir to combine.
3. Divide the spinach mixture into 6 greased cups of an egg bite mold evenly.
4. Press "Power Button" of Air Fry Oven and turn the dial to select the "Air Fry" mode.
5. Press the Time button and again turn the dial to set the cooking time to 17 minutes.
6. Now push the Temp button and rotate the dial to set the temperature at 325 degrees F.
7. Press "Start/Pause" button to start.
8. When the unit beeps to show that it is preheated, open the lid.
9. Arrange the mold over the "Wire Rack" and insert in the oven.
10. Place the mold onto a wire rack to cool for about 5 minutes.
11. Top with bacon pieces and serve warm.

Nutrition:
Calories 179 | Fat 12.9 g | Cholesterol 187 mg | Sodium 549 mg | Carbs 1.8 g | Fiber 0.1g | Protein 13.5 g

73. Ham Muffins

⏱ Prep Time 10 m | ⏱ Cooking Time 18 m | 6 Servings

Ingredients:

- 6 ham slices
- 6 eggs
- 6 tablespoons cream
- 3 tablespoon mozzarella cheese, shredded
- ¼ teaspoon dried basil, crushed

Directions:

1. Lightly, grease 6 cups of a silicone muffin tin.
2. Line each prepared muffin cup with 1 ham slice.
3. Crack 1 egg into each muffin cup and top with cream.
4. Sprinkle with cheese and basil.
5. Press "Power Button" of Air Fry Oven and turn the dial to select the "Air Fry" mode.
6. Press the Time button and again turn the dial to set the cooking time to 18 minutes.
7. Now push the Temp button and rotate the dial to set the temperature at 350 degrees F.
8. Press "Start/Pause" button to start.
9. When the unit beeps to show that it is preheated, open the lid.
10. Arrange the muffin tin over the "Wire Rack" and insert in the oven.
11. Place the muffin tin onto a wire rack to cool for about 5 minutes.
12. Carefully, invert the muffins onto the platter and serve warm.

Nutrition:

Calories 156 | Fat 10 g | Cholesterol 189 mg | Sodium 516 mg | Carbs 2.3 g | Fiber 0.4g | Protein 14.3 g

74. Savory Carrot Muffins

⏱ Prep Time 15 m | ⏱ Cooking Time 7 m | 6 Servings

Ingredients:

- For Muffins:
- ¼ cup whole-wheat flour
- ¼ cup all-purpose flour
- ½ teaspoon baking powder
- 1/8 teaspoon baking soda
- ½ teaspoon dried parsley, crushed
- ½ teaspoon salt
- ½ cup plain yogurt
- 1 teaspoon vinegar
- 1 tablespoon vegetable oil
- 3 tablespoons cottage cheese, grated
- 1 carrot, peeled and grated
- 2-4 tablespoons water (if needed)
- For Topping:
- 7 oz. Parmesan cheese, grated
- ¼ cup walnuts, chopped

Directions:

1. For muffin: in a large bowl, mix together the flours, baking powder, baking soda, parsley, and salt.
2. In another large bowl, mix well the yogurt, and vinegar.
3. Add the remaining ingredients except water and beat them well. (add some water if needed)
4. Make a well in the center of the yogurt mixture.
5. Slowly, add the flour mixture in the well and mix until well combined.
6. Place the mixture into lightly greased muffin molds evenly and top with the Parmesan cheese and walnuts.
7. Press "Power Button" of Air Fry Oven and turn the dial to select the "Air Fry" mode.
8. Press the Time button and again turn the dial to set the cooking time to 7 minutes.
9. Now push the Temp button and rotate the dial to set the temperature at 355 degrees F.
10. Press "Start/Pause" button to start.
11. When the unit beeps to show that it is preheated, open the lid.
12. Arrange the ramekins over "Wire Rack" and insert in the oven.
13. Place the muffin molds onto a wire rack to cool for about 5 minutes.
14. Carefully, invert the muffins onto the platter and serve warm.

Nutrition:

Calories 292 | Fat 13.1 g | Cholesterol 25 mg | Sodium 579 mg | Carbs 27.2 g | Fiber 1.5g | Protein 17.7 g

75. Savory Barley

⏱ Prep Time 10 m | ⏱ Cooking Time 18 m | 4 Servings

Ingredients:

- 1 cup pearl barley
- 4 oz. baby kale
- 4 cups vegetable broth
- 1/4 cup onion, chopped
- 1 tbsp. olive oil
- 1/2 tsp sea salt

Directions:

1. Add oil into the instant pot and set the pot on sauté mode.
2. Add onion and barley and sauté for 3 minutes.
3. Add broth and salt and stir everything well.
4. Seal pot with lid and cook on manual high pressure for 15 minutes.
5. Once done then allow to release pressure naturally then open the lid.
6. Add kale and stir until kale is wilted.
7. Serve and enjoy.

Nutrition:

Calories 262 Fat 5.6 g Carbohydrates 43.4 g Sugar 1.4 g Protein 10.9 g Cholesterol 0 mg

76. Potato & Bell Pepper Hash
⏰ Prep Time 15 m | ⏰ Cooking Time 25 m | 4 Servings

Ingredients:

- 2 cups water
- 5 russet potatoes, peeled and cubed
- ½ tablespoon extra-virgin olive oil
- ½ of onion, chopped
- ½ of jalapeño, chopped
- 1 green bell pepper, seeded and chopped
- ¼ teaspoon dried oregano, crushed
- ¼ teaspoon garlic powder
- ¼ teaspoon ground cumin
- ¼ teaspoon red chili powder
- Salt and freshly ground black pepper, as needed

Directions:

1. In a large bowl, add the water and potatoes and set aside for about 30 minutes.
2. Drain well and pat dry with the paper towels.
3. In a bowl, add the potatoes and oil and toss to coat well.
4. Press "Power Button" of Air Fry Oven and turn the dial to select the "Air Fry" mode.
5. Press the Time button and again turn the dial to set the cooking time to 5 minutes.
6. Now push the Temp button and rotate the dial to set the temperature at 330 degrees F.
7. Press "Start/Pause" button to start.
8. When the unit beeps to show that it is preheated, open the lid.
9. Arrange the potato cubes in "Air Fry Basket" and insert in the oven.
10. Transfer the potatoes onto a plate.
11. In a bowl, add the potatoes and remaining ingredients and toss to coat well.
12. Press "Power Button" of Air Fry Oven and turn the dial to select the "Air Fry" mode.
13. Press the Time button and again turn the dial to set the cooking time to 20 minutes.
14. Now push the Temp button and rotate the dial to set the temperature at 390 degrees F.
15. Press "Start/Pause" button to start.
16. When the unit beeps to show that it is preheated, open the lid.
17. Arrange the veggie mixture in "Air Fry Basket" and insert in the oven.
18. Serve hot.

Nutrition: Calories 216 | Fat 2.2 g | Cholesterol 0 mg | Sodium 58 mg | Carbs 45.7 g | Fiber 7.2 g | Protein 5 g

77. Fajita Casserole
⏰ Prep Time 10 m | ⏰ Cooking Time 7 m | 2 Servings

Ingredients:

- 4 eggs
- 1 tbsp. olive oil
- 1 1/2 cups bell peppers, sliced
- 1/2 medium onion, sliced
- Pepper
- Salt

Directions:

1. Add oil into the instant pot and set the pot on sauté mode.
2. Add bell peppers and onions and sauté for 5 minutes. Transfer bell peppers and onion mixture into the baking dish.
3. Crack eggs and place them on top of onion and bell pepper mixture. Season with pepper and salt.
4. Pour 1 cup of water into the instant pot then place the trivet in the pot.
5. Place baking dish on top of the trivet.
6. Seal pot with lid and cook on high pressure for 2 minutes.
7. Once done then release pressure using the quick-release method than open the lid.
8. Serve and enjoy.

Nutrition: Calories 225 Fat 16 g Carbohydrates 10 g Sugar 6.4 g Protein 12.3 g Cholesterol 327 mg

78. Latte Oatmeal
⏰ Prep Time 10 m | ⏰ Cooking Time 10 m | 4 Servings

Ingredients:

- 1 cup steel-cut oats
- 1 1/2 tsp vanilla
- 1 tsp espresso powder
- 2 tbsp. sugar
- 1 cup milk
- 2 1/2 cups water
- 1/4 tsp salt

Directions:

1. Add oats, espresso powder, sugar, milk, water, and salt into the instant pot and stir well.
2. Seal pot with lid and cook on high pressure for 10 minutes.
3. Once done then allow to release pressure naturally for 10 minutes then release using the quick-release method. Open the lid.
4. Stir in vanilla and serve.

Nutrition: Calories 135 Fat 2.6 g Carbohydrates 23 g Sugar 9.2 g Protein 4.7 g Cholesterol 5 mg

79. Coconut Blueberry Oatmeal
⏰ Prep Time 10 m | ⏰ Cooking Time 30 m | 6 Servings

Ingredients:

- 2 1/4 cups oats
- 1 cup blueberries
- 1/4 cup gluten-free flour
- 1/2 tsp vanilla
- 3 cups of water
- 14 oz. coconut milk
- 6 tbsp. brown sugar
- 1/8 tsp salt

Directions:

1. Add all ingredients into the instant pot and stir well.
2. Seal pot with lid and cook on manual mode for 30 minutes.
3. Once done then release pressure using the quick-release method than open the lid.
4. Stir well and serve.

Nutrition: Calories 337 Fat 18.1 g Carbohydrates 40.3 g Sugar 13.7 g Protein 6.4 g Cholesterol 0 mg

80. Pumpkin Cranberry Oatmeal
⏱ Prep Time 10 m | ⏱ Cooking Time 3 m | 4 Servings

Ingredients:

- 1 cup steel-cut oats
- 2 tbsp. honey
- 1/2 cup dried cranberries
- 3/4 cup pumpkin puree
- 1 cup milk
- 2 cups of water
- 1 1/2 tsp pumpkin pie spice
- Pinch of salt

Directions:

1. Add oats, cranberries, pumpkin puree, milk, water, pumpkin pie spice, and salt and stir well.
2. Seal pot with lid and cook on manual high pressure for 3 minutes.
3. Once done then release pressure using the quick-release method than open the lid.
4. Add honey and stir well.
5. Serve and enjoy.

Nutrition:
Calories 165 Fat 2.8 g Carbohydrates 30.9 g Sugar 13.6 g Protein 5.3 g Cholesterol 5 mg

81. Cranberry Farro
⏱ Prep Time 10 m | ⏱ Cooking Time 20 m | 8 Servings

Ingredients:

- 15 oz. farro
- 1/2 cup dried cranberries
- 1 tsp lemon extract
- 1/2 cup brown sugar
- 4 1/2 cups water
- 1/4 tsp salt

Directions:

1. Add farro, lemon extract, brown sugar, water, and salt into the instant pot and stir well.
2. Seal pot with lid and cook on high pressure for 20 minutes.
3. Once done then allow to release pressure naturally for 10 minutes then release using the quick-release method. Open the lid.
4. Add cranberries and stir well.
5. Serve and enjoy.

Nutrition:
Calories 130 Fat 3.9 g Carbohydrates 21.2 g Sugar 10.4 g Protein 3.9 g Cholesterol 6 mg

82. Tropical Oatmeal
⏱ Prep Time 10 m | ⏱ Cooking Time 4 m | 4 Servings

Ingredients:

- 1 cup steel-cut oats
- 3 tbsp. hemp seeds
- 1/2 papaya, chopped
- 1/2 cup coconut cream
- 2 cups of water

Directions:

1. Add oats, coconut cream, and water into the instant pot and stir well.
2. Seal pot with lid and cook on manual high pressure for 4 minutes.
3. Once done then allow to release pressure naturally for 10 minutes then release using the quick-release method. Open the lid.
4. Stir in hemp seeds and papaya.
5. Serve and enjoy.

Nutrition:
Calories 195 Fat 11.2 g Carbohydrates 20.1 g Sugar 4.3 g Protein 5.5 g Cholesterol 0 mg

83. Simple & Easy Breakfast Casserole
⏱ Prep Time 10 m | ⏱ Cooking Time 20 m | 4 Servings

Ingredients:

- 2 1/2 cups egg whites
- 1/2 cup Mexican blend cheese
- 1/4 cup cream cheese
- 1/2 cup onion, chopped
- 1 cup bell pepper, chopped
- 1/2 tsp onion powder
- 1/4 tsp garlic powder
- 1/4 tsp pepper
- 1/4 tsp salt

Directions:

1. Spray instant pot from inside with cooking spray.
2. Add onion and bell pepper to the pot and cook until softened, about 5 minutes.
3. Transfer onion and bell pepper to the baking dish.
4. Add egg whites, seasonings, and cream cheese and stir well. Top with Mexican blend cheese.
5. Pour 1 cup of water into the instant pot then place the trivet in the pot.
6. Place baking dish on top of the trivet.
7. Seal pot with lid and cook on manual mode for 15 minutes.
8. Once done then release pressure using the quick-release method than open the lid.
9. Slice and serve.

Nutrition:
Calories 208 Fat 10.4 g Carbohydrates 6.3 g Sugar 4.1 g Protein 21.7 g Cholesterol 33 mg

84. Creamy Mac n Cheese
⏱ Prep Time 10 m | ⏱ Cooking Time 5 m | 8 Servings

Ingredients:

- 15 oz. elbow macaroni
- 1 cup milk
- 1/2 cup parmesan cheese, shredded
- 1 cup mozzarella cheese, shredded
- 2 cups cheddar cheese, shredded
- 1 tsp garlic powder

- 1 tsp hot pepper sauce
- 2 tbsp. butter
- 4 cups vegetable broth
- 1/4 tsp pepper
- 1/2 tsp salt

Directions:

1. Add macaroni, garlic powder, hot sauce, butter, broth, pepper, and salt into the instant pot and stir well.
2. Seal pot with lid and cook on manual high pressure for 5 minutes.
3. Once done then release pressure using the quick-release method than open the lid.
4. Add cheese and milk and stir until cheese is melted.
5. Serve and enjoy.

Nutrition:

Calories 388 Fat 15.3 g Carbohydrates 42.5 g Sugar 3.4 g Protein 19 g Cholesterol 43 mg

85. Cherry Risotto
⏱ Prep Time 10 m | ⏱ Cooking Time 10 m | 4 Servings

Ingredients:

- 1 1/2 cups Arborio rice
- 1/2 cup dried cherries
- 3 cups of milk
- 1 cup apple juice
- 1/3 cup brown sugar

- 1 1/2 tsp cinnamon
- 2 apples, cored and diced
- 2 tbsp. butter
- 1/4 tsp salt

Directions:

1. Add butter into the instant pot and set the pot on sauté mode.
2. Add rice and cook for 3-4 minutes.
3. Add brown sugar, spices, apples, milk, and apple juice and stir well.
4. Seal pot with lid and cook on manual high pressure for 6 minutes.
5. Once done then release pressure using the quick-release method than open the lid.
6. Stir in dried cherries and serve.

Nutrition:

Calories 544 Fat 10.2 g Carbohydrates 103.2 g Sugar 37.6 g Protein 11.2 g Cholesterol 30 mg

86. Almond Coconut Risotto
⏱ Prep Time 10 m | ⏱ Cooking Time 5 m | 4 Servings

Ingredients:

- 1 cup Arborio rice
- 1 cup of coconut milk
- 3 tbsp. almonds, sliced and toasted
- 2 tbsp. shredded coconut

- 2 cups almond milk
- 1/2 tsp vanilla
- 1/3 cup coconut sugar

Directions:

1. Add coconut and almond milk in instant pot and set the pot on sauté mode.
2. Once the milk begins to boil then add rice and stir well.
3. Seal pot with lid and cook on manual high pressure for 5 minutes.
4. Once done then allow to release pressure naturally then open the lid.
5. Add remaining ingredients and stir well.
6. Serve and enjoy.

Nutrition:

Calories 425 Fat 20.6 g Carbohydrates 53.7 g Sugar 9.6 g Protein 6.8 g Cholesterol 0 mg

87. Creamy Polenta
⏱ Prep Time 10 m | ⏱ Cooking Time 5 m | 3 Servings

Ingredients:

- 1/2 cup polenta
- 1 cup of coconut milk
- 1 cup of water

- 1/2 tbsp. butter
- 1/4 tsp salt

Directions:

1. Set instant pot on sauté mode.
2. Add milk, water, and salt in a pot and stir well.
3. Once milk mixture begins to boil then add polenta and stir to combine.
4. Seal pot with lid and cook on high pressure for 5 minutes.
5. Once done then allow to release pressure naturally then open the lid.
6. Stir and serve.

Nutrition:

Calories 293 Fat 21.2 g Carbohydrates 24.7 g Sugar 2.9 g Protein 3.8 g Cholesterol 5 mg

88. Sweet Cherry Chocolate Oat
⏱ Prep Time 10 m | ⏱ Cooking Time 15 m | 4 Servings

Ingredients:

- 2 cups steel cuts oats
- 3 tbsp. honey
- 2 cups of water
- 2 cups of milk
- 3 tbsp. chocolate chips
- 1 1/2 cups cherries
- 1/4 tsp cinnamon
- Pinch of salt

Directions:

1. Spray instant pot from inside with cooking spray.
2. Add all ingredients into the pot and stir everything well.
3. Seal pot with lid and cook on high pressure for 15 minutes.
4. Once done then allow to release pressure naturally then open the lid.
5. Stir well and serve.

Nutrition:
Calories 503 Fat 10.9 g Carbohydrates 85.5 g Sugar 22.5 g Protein 16.8 g Cholesterol 12 mg

89. Coconut Lime Breakfast Quinoa
⏱ Prep Time 10 m | ⏱ Cooking Time 1 m | 5 Servings

Ingredients:

- 1 cup quinoa, rinsed
- 1/2 tsp coconut extract
- 1 lime juice
- 1 lime zest
- 2 cups of coconut milk
- 1 cup of water

Directions:

1. Add all ingredients into the instant pot and stir well.
2. Seal pot with lid and cook on manual high pressure for 1 minute.
3. Once done then allow to release pressure naturally for 10 minutes then release using the quick-release method. Open the lid.
4. Stir well and serve.

Nutrition:
Calories 350 Fat 25 g Carbohydrates 28.1 g Sugar 3.5 g Protein 7.1 g Cholesterol 0 mg

90. Quick & Easy Farro
⏱ Prep Time 5 m | ⏱ Cooking Time 10 m | 4 Servings

Ingredients:

- 1 cup pearl farro
- 1 tsp olive oil
- 2 cups vegetable broth
- 1/4 tsp salt

Directions:

1. Add all ingredients into the instant pot and stir well.
2. Seal pot with lid and cook on manual mode for 10 minutes.
3. Once done then allow to release pressure naturally for 5 minutes then release using the quick-release method. Open the lid.
4. Stir well and serve.

Nutrition:
Calories 169 Fat 1.9 g Carbohydrates 30.5 g Sugar 0.4 g Protein 8.4 g Cholesterol 0 mg

91. Chicken Spinach Casserole
⏱ Prep Time 10 m | ⏱ Cooking Time 25 m | 4 Servings

Ingredients:

- 1-pound chicken meat, ground
- One tablespoon olive oil
- ½ tablespoon sweet paprika
- 12 eggs, whisked
- 1 cup baby spinach
- Salt and black pepper to taste

Directions:

1. Beat eggs with paprika, salt, and pepper in a large bowl. Stir in spinach and chicken. Pour the egg spinach mixture into a small casserole dish and place it inside the Instant Pot. Put on the Instant Air Fryer lid and cook on Bake mode for 25 minutes at 350 degrees F. Once done, remove the cover and serve warm.

Nutrition:
Calories: 270 Protein: 7g Carbs: 14g Fat: 1g

92. Cheese Sausage Quiche
⏱ Prep Time 10 m | ⏱ Cooking Time 20 m | 6 Servings

Ingredients:

- Four bacon slices, cooked and crumbled
- A drizzle olive oil
- 2 cups of coconut milk
- 2½ cups cheddar cheese, shredded
- 1-pound breakfast sausage, chopped
- Two eggs
- Salt and black pepper to taste
- Three tablespoon cilantro, chopped

Directions:

1. Beat eggs with cheese, milk, salt, cilantro, and pepper in a suitable bowl. Pour eggs into the Instant Pot and top it with sausage and bacon. Put on the Instant Air Fryer lid and cook on Bake mode for 20 minutes at 350 degrees F. Once done, remove the lid and serve warm.

Nutrition:
Calories: 244 Protein: 9g Carbs: 15g Fat: 11g

93. Salsa Chicken Burrito

⏱ Prep Time 10 m | ⏱ Cooking Time 14 m | 4 Servings

Ingredients:

- Four chicken breast slices, cooked and shredded
- One green bell pepper, sliced
- Two eggs whisked
- One avocado, peeled, pitted and sliced

- Two tablespoons mild salsa
- Salt and black pepper to taste
- Two tablespoon cheddar cheese, grated
- Two tortillas

Directions:

1. Take a pan, small enough to fit the Instant. Whisk eggs with salt and pepper, pour it into the pan.
2. Transfer this pan in the Instant Pot. Put on the Instant Air Fryer lid and cook on Bake mode for 5 minutes at 400 degrees F. Once done, remove the lid and serve warm.
3. Cook for exactly 5 minutes at 400 degrees F. Crumble the cooked egg and toss it with

chicken, avocado, bell peppers and cheese in a bowl. Spread the tortillas on the working surface and divide the egg mixture. Roll the tortillas to make the burritos. Layer the air fryer basket with a foil sheet and place the burritos in the basket. Put on the Instant Air Fryer lid and cook on Air Fry mode for 4 minutes at 400 degrees F. Once done, remove the lid and serve warm.

Nutrition:

Calories: 329 Protein: 8g Carbs: 20g Fat: 13g

94. Morning Oats Casserole

⏱ Prep Time 10 m | ⏱ Cooking Time 20 m | 4 Servings

Ingredients:

- 2 cups old fashioned oats
- One tablespoon baking powder
- 1/3 Cup of sugar
- One tablespoon cinnamon powder
- 1 cup blueberries
- One banana, peeled and mashed

- 2 cups of milk
- Two eggs whisked
- Two tablespoon butter
- One tablespoon vanilla extract
- Cooking spray

Directions:

1. Beat eggs with sugar, cinnamon, baking powder, blueberries, banana, and vanilla in a suitable bowl. Pour it into the Instant Pot and top it with oats. Put on the Instant Air

Fryer lid and cook on Bake mode for 20 minutes at 320 degrees F. Once done, remove the lid and serve warm.

Nutrition:

Calories: 260 Protein: 10g Carbs: 9g Fat: 4g

95. Cheesy Bread Bake

⏱ Prep Time 10 m | ⏱ Cooking Time 30 m | 6 Servings

Ingredients:

- 1-pound white bread, cubed
- 1-pound smoked bacon, cooked and chopped
- ¼ cup avocado oil
- One red onion, chopped
- 30 oz. canned tomatoes, chopped
- ½ pound cheddar cheese, shredded

- Two tablespoon chives, chopped
- ½ pound Monterey jack cheese, shredded
- Two tablespoon chicken stock
- Salt and black pepper to taste
- Eight eggs whisked

Directions:

1. Grease the baking pan with oil. Add everything to this pan except the chives. Place the pan in the Instant Pot and Put on

the Instant Air Fryer lid and cook on Bake mode for 30 minutes at 350 degrees F. Once done, remove the lid and serve warm.

Nutrition:

Calories: 211 Protein: 3g Carbs: 14g Fat: 8g

96. Cream Cheese Omelet

⏱ Prep Time 10 m | ⏱ Cooking Time 20 m | 6 Servings

Ingredients:

- 1½ pounds hash browns
- 1 cup almond milk
- Olive oil a drizzle
- Six bacon slices, chopped
- 8 oz. cream cheese, softened

- One yellow onion, chopped
- 1 cup cheddar cheese, shredded
- Six spring onions, chopped
- Salt and black pepper to taste
- Six eggs

Directions:

1. Whisk everything in a bowl except the spring onions. Pour this mixture into the Instant Pot. Put on the Instant Air Fryer lid and

cook on Bake mode for 20 minutes at 350 degrees F. Once done, remove the lid and garnish with spring onions. Serve fresh.

Nutrition:

Calories: 231 Protein: 12g Carbs: 8g Fat: 9g

97. Roasted Peppers Frittata

⏱ Prep Time 10 m | ⏱ Cooking Time 20 m | 6 Servings

Ingredients:

- 6 oz. jarred roasted red bell peppers, chopped
- 12 eggs, whisked
- ½ cup parmesan cheese, grated
- Three garlic cloves, minced
- Two tablespoon parsley, chopped
- Salt and black pepper to taste
- Two tablespoon chives, chopped
- Six tablespoon ricotta cheese
- A drizzle olive oil

Directions:

1. Whisk eggs with bell peppers, parsley, garlic, pepper, salt, ricotta and chives in a suitable bowl.
2. Transfer the egg mixture into the pan and drizzle the parmesan on top. Place this pan in the Instant Pot. Put on the Instant Air Fryer lid and cook on Bake mode for 20 minutes at 350 degrees F. Once done, remove the lid and serve warm.

Nutrition: Calories: 262 Protein: 8g Carbs: 18g Fat: 6g

98. Blackberries Cornflakes Bowl

⏱ Prep Time 10 m | ⏱ Cooking Time 10 m | 4 Servings

Ingredients:

- 3 cups of milk
- One tablespoon sugar
- Two eggs whisked
- ¼ tablespoon nutmeg, a ground
- ¼ cup blackberries
- Four tablespoon cream cheese, whipped
- 1½ cups of corn flakes

Directions:

1. Add everything to a suitably sized bowl and stir well. Add this prepared mixture to the Instant Pot. Put on the Instant Air Fryer lid and cook on Air Fryer mode for 10 minutes at 350 degrees F. Once done, remove the lid and serve warm.

Nutrition: Calories: 180 Protein: 5 Carbs: 12g Fat: 5g

99. Egg Paprika Scramble

⏱ Prep Time 10 m | ⏱ Cooking Time 10 m | 6 Servings

Ingredients:

- Four eggs whisked
- A drizzle olive oil
- Salt and black pepper to taste
- One red onion, chopped
- Two teaspoons sweet paprika

Directions:

1. Add everything to a suitably sized bowl and stir well. Add this prepared mixture to the Instant Pot. Put on the Instant Air Fryer lid and cook on Bake mode for 10 minutes at 200 degrees F. Once done, remove the lid and serve warm.

Nutrition: Calories: 190 Protein: 4g Carbs: 12g Fat: 7g

100. White Mushroom Pie

⏱ Prep Time 10 m | ⏱ Cooking Time 20 m | 6 Servings

Ingredients:

- One tablespoon olive oil
- 9inch pie dough
- Six white mushrooms, chopped
- Two tablespoon bacon cooked and crumbled
- Three eggs
- One red onion, chopped
- ½ cup heavy cream
- Salt and black pepper to taste
- ½ tablespoon thyme, a dried
- ¼ cup cheddar cheese, grated

Directions:

1. Grease a pie pan with oil, suitable to fit the Instant Pot. Spread the dough in the pie pan. Beat everything in a bowl except the cheese. Pour this mixture over the dough and drizzle cheese on top. Put on the Instant Air Fryer lid and cook on Bake mode for 10 minutes at 400 degrees F. Once done, remove the lid and serve warm.

Nutrition: Calories: 192 Protein: 7g Carbs: 14g Fat: 6g

101. Morning Cauliflower Bake

⏱ Prep Time 10 m | ⏱ Cooking Time 10 m | 4 Servings

Ingredients:

- One cauliflower head stems removed, florets separated and steamed
- Three carrots, chopped and steamed
- 2 oz. cheddar cheese, grated
- Three eggs
- 2 oz. milk
- Two teaspoon cilantro, chopped
- Salt and black pepper to taste

Directions:

1. Beat eggs with salt, pepper, parsley, and milk in a bowl. Spread the carrots and cauliflower in the Instant Pot. Pour the egg mixture over them. Put on the Instant Air Fryer lid and cook on Bake mode for 20 minutes at 350 degrees F. Once done, remove the lid and serve warm.

Nutrition: Calories: 194 Protein: 6g Carbs: 11g Fat: 4g

102. Cheese Bread Pizza
⏱ Prep Time 8 m | ⏱ Cooking Time 14 m | 4 Servings

Ingredients:

- Six bread slices
- Five tablespoon butter, melted
- Three garlic cloves, minced
- Six teaspoon basil and tomato pesto
- 1 cup mozzarella cheese, grated

Directions:

1. Spread the bread slices on the working surface. Whisk butter with garlic and pesto in a bowl. Spread this mixture over the slices. Set the air fryer basket in the Instant Pot and place the pizza slices in the Air fryer basket and drizzle half of the cheese over them. Put on the Instant Air Fryer lid and cook on Air Fry mode for 8minutes at 350 degrees F. Once done, remove the cover and serve warm.

Nutrition:
Calories: 187 Protein: 5 g Carbs: 13g Fat: 6g

103. Cherry Tomato Omelet
⏱ Prep Time 11 m | ⏱ Cooking Time 15 m | 4 Servings

Ingredients:

- One sausage link, sliced
- Two eggs whisked
- Four cherry tomatoes halved
- One tablespoon cilantro, chopped
- One tablespoon olive oil
- One tablespoon cheddar cheese, grated
- Salt and black pepper to taste

Directions:

1. Add sausage and tomatoes to the Instant Pot. Put on the Instant Air Fryer lid and cook on Bake mode for 5 minutes at 350 degrees F. Once done, remove the cover and serve warm. Take a pan, suitable to fit the Instant Pot. Add the sausage and tomatoes to the pan. Whisk remaining things in a bowl and pour it over the vegetables. Place this pan in the Instant pot and put on the Instant Air Fryer lid and cook on Bake mode for 6minutes at 360 degrees F. Once done, remove the lid and serve warm.

Nutrition:
Calories: 270 Protein: 16g Carbs: 23g Fat: 14g

104. Polenta Bites
⏱ Prep Time 10 m | ⏱ Cooking Time 15 m | 4 Servings

Ingredients:

- 1 cup cornmeal
- 3 cups of water
- Salt and black pepper to taste
- One tablespoon butter softened
- ¼ cup potato starch
- A drizzle vegetable oil
- Maple syrup for serving

Directions:

1. Add water and cornmeal to a pot and cook for 10 minutes on medium heat. Stir in butter and mix well, then put off the heat. Once the cornmeal is cooled, make small balls out of it. Place them in a greased baking pan and flatten them with a press of your hand. Drizzle oil over them then places the container in the Instant Pot. Put on the Instant Air Fryer lid and cook on Bake mode for 15 minutes at 380 degrees F. Once done, remove the cover and allow the bites to cool. Garnish with maple syrup and serve.

Nutrition:
Calories: 170 Protein: 4g Carbs: 12g Fat: 2g

105. Sweet Vanilla Toast
⏱ Prep Time 5 m | ⏱ Cooking Time 10 m | 6 Servings

Ingredients:

- One stick butter softened
- 12 bread slices
- ½ cup brown sugar
- Two teaspoon vanilla extract

Directions:

1. Beat butter with vanilla and sugar in a bowl. Place the bread slices on the working surface and spread the butter mixture over them. Place all the slices in the Air fryer basket inside the Instant Pot. Put on the Instant Air Fryer lid and cook on Air Fry mode for 5 minutes at 400 degrees F. Once done, remove the lid and serve fresh.

Nutrition:
Calories: 170 Protein: 2g Carbs: 11g Fat: 6g

106. Farro Breakfast Risotto

☉ Prep Time 10 m | ☉ Cooking Time 12 m | 4 Servings

Ingredients:

- 1 cup farro
- 1 tsp Italian seasoning
- 1/2 cup parmesan cheese, grated
- 1/2 cup mozzarella cheese, grated
- 2 tbsp. heavy whipping cream
- 2 cups vegetable stock
- 1 tbsp. butter

Directions:

1. Add butter into the instant pot and set the pot on sauté mode.
2. Add farro and cook for 2 minutes. Add stock and stir everything well.
3. Seal pot with lid and cook on manual high pressure for 10 minutes.
4. Once done then allow to release pressure naturally for 10 minutes then release using the quick-release method. Open the lid.
5. Add remaining ingredients and stir well.
6. Serve and enjoy.

Nutrition:

Calories 206 Fat 13.7 g Carbohydrates 13.4 g Sugar 1.8 g Protein 9.9 g Cholesterol 37 mg

107. Tapioca Pudding

☉ Prep Time 10 m | ☉ Cooking Time 7 m | 4 Servings

Ingredients:

- 1/2 cup tapioca
- 2 cups of water
- 2 egg yolks
- 1/2 tsp vanilla
- 1/2 cup sugar
- 1/2 cup milk

Directions:

1. Add water and tapioca into the instant pot and stir well.
2. Seal pot with lid and cook on high pressure for 5 minutes.
3. Once done then release pressure using the quick-release method than open the lid.
4. Set pot on sauté mode. In a small bowl, whisk together milk and egg yolks
5. Slowly pour egg mixture into the pot and stir constantly.
6. Add vanilla and sugar and stir until sugar is dissolved.
7. Transfer pudding to a bowl and let it cool completely.
8. Place in refrigerator until pudding thickens.
9. Serve and enjoy.

Nutrition:

Calories 206 Fat 2.9 g Carbohydrates 43.7 g Sugar 27.1g Protein 2.4g Cholesterol 107 mg

108. Sweetened Breakfast Oats

☉ Prep Time 10 m | ☉ Cooking Time 7 m | 4 Servings

Ingredients:

- 1 cup steel-cut oats
- 3/4 cup shredded coconut
- 1/4 tsp ground ginger
- 1/4 tsp ground nutmeg
- 1/2 tsp ground cinnamon
- 1/4 cup raisins
- 1 large apple, chopped
- 2 large carrots, grated
- 1 cup of coconut milk
- 3 cups of water

Directions:

1. Add oats, nutmeg, ginger, cinnamon, raisins, apple, carrots, milk, and water into the instant pot and stir to combine.
2. Seal pot with lid and cook on manual mode for 4 minutes.
3. Once done then allow to release pressure naturally for 20 minutes then release using the quick-release method. Open the lid.
4. Top with coconut and serve.

Nutrition:

Calories 341 Fat 20.8 g Carbohydrates 38.2 g Sugar 16.1 g Protein 5.3 g Cholesterol 0 mg

109. Cauliflower Mash

☉ Prep Time 10 m | ☉ Cooking Time 3 m | 6 Servings

Ingredients:

- 1 large cauliflower head, cut into florets
- 1/2 cup parmesan cheese, shredded
- 1/2 tsp garlic powder
- 2 tbsp. butter
- 2 cups vegetable stock
- 1/4 tsp salt

Directions:

1. Pour the stock into the instant pot then place a steamer basket into the pot.
2. Add cauliflower florets into the steamer basket.
3. Seal pot with lid and cook on high pressure for 3 minutes.
4. Once done then release pressure using the quick-release method than open the lid.
5. Transfer cauliflower into the food processor along with remaining ingredients and blend until smooth.
6. Serve and enjoy.

Nutrition:

Calories 102 Fat 6 g Carbohydrates 8.2 g Sugar 3.7 g Protein 6 g Cholesterol 17 mg

110. Chia Oatmeal

Ingredients:

- 1 cup steel-cut oatmeal
- 1/2 tsp vanilla
- 2 tbsp. chia seeds
- 1 1/2 cups coconut milk
- 1 1/2 cup water
- 1/4 tsp sea salt

Directions:

1. Spray instant pot from inside with cooking spray.
2. Add all ingredients into the instant pot and stir well.
3. Seal pot with lid and cook on porridge mode for 15 minutes.
4. Once done then allow to release pressure naturally for 10 minutes then release using the quick-release method. Open the lid.
5. Stir well and serve.

Nutrition:
Calories 210 Fat 17.7 g Carbohydrates 11.8 g Sugar 2 g Protein 3.8 g Cholesterol 0 mg

111. Blueberry Lemon Oatmeal

Ingredients:

- 1 cup steel-cut oats
- 1/4 cup chia seeds
- 1 cup blueberries
- 1/2 tbsp. lemon zest
- 2 tbsp. sugar
- 1/2 cup half and half
- 3 cups of water
- 1 tbsp. butter
- Salt

Directions:

1. Add butter into the instant pot and set the pot on sauté mode.
2. Add oats into the pot and stir well.
3. Add remaining ingredients and stir everything well.
4. Seal pot with lid and cook on manual high pressure for 10 minutes.
5. Once done then allow to release pressure naturally then open the lid.
6. Stir well and serve.

Nutrition:
Calories 130 Fat 5.6 g Carbohydrates 18.2 g Sugar 6.6 g Protein 2.8 g Cholesterol 13 mg

112. Breakfast Cobbler

Ingredients:

- 2 tbsp. sunflower seeds
- 1/4 cup pecan
- 1/4 cup shredded coconut
- 1/2 tsp cinnamon
- 2 1/2 tbsp. coconut oil
- 2 tbsp. honey
- 1 plum, diced
- 1 apple, diced
- 1 pear, diced

Directions:

1. Add fruits, cinnamon, coconut oil, and honey into the instant pot and stir well.
2. Seal pot with a lid and select steam mode and set timer for 10 minutes.
3. Once done then release pressure using the quick-release method than open the lid.
4. Transfer fruit mixture into the serving bowl.
8.
5. Add sunflower seeds, pecans, and coconut into the pot and cook on sauté mode for 5 minutes.
6. Pour sunflower seed, pecans and coconut mixture on top of fruit mixture.
7. Serve and enjoy.

Nutrition:
Calories 426 Fat 27.2 g Carbohydrates 50.9 g Sugar 40.1 g Protein 2.6 g Cholesterol 0 mg

113. Tomato Corn Risotto

Ingredients:

- 1 1/2 cups Arborio rice
- 1 cup cherry tomatoes, halved
- 1/4 cup basil, chopped
- 1/4 cup parmesan cheese, grated
- 1/4 cup half and half
- 32 oz. vegetable broth
- 1 cup sweet corn
- 3 garlic cloves, minced
- 1/2 cup onion, chopped
- 2 tbsp. olive oil
- 4 tbsp. butter
- 1 tsp salt

Directions:

1. Add butter into the instant pot and set the pot on sauté mode.
2. Add garlic and onion and sauté for 5 minutes.
3. Add rice and cook for 2-3 minutes.
4. Add broth, corn, pepper, and salt and stir well.
5. Seal pot with lid and cook on high pressure for 6 minutes.
6. Once done then release pressure using the quick-release method than open the lid.
7. Stir in cherry tomatoes, basil, parmesan, and a half and half.

Nutrition: Calories 548 Fat 24 g Carbohydrates 69.6 g Sugar 3.8 g Protein 14.1 g Cholesterol 41 mg

114. Pancetta & Spinach Frittata
⏲ Prep Time 15 m | ⏱ Cooking Time 16 m | 2 Servings

Ingredients:

- ¼ cup pancetta
- ½ of tomato, cubed
- ¼ cup fresh baby spinach
-

- 3 eggs
- Salt and ground black pepper, as required
- ¼ cup parmesan cheese, grated

Directions:

1. Heat a nonstick skillet over medium heat and cook the pancetta for about 5 minutes.
2. Add the tomato and spinach cook for about 2-3 minutes.
3. Remove from the heat and drain the grease from skillet.
4. Set aside to cool slightly.
5. Meanwhile, in a small bowl, add the eggs, salt and black pepper and beat well.
6. In the bottom of a greased baking pan, place the pancetta mixture and top with the eggs, followed by the cheese.
7. Press "power button" of air fry oven and turn the dial to select the "air fry" mode.
8. Press the time button and again turn the dial to set the cooking time to 8 minutes.
9. Now push the temp button and rotate the dial to set the temperature at 355 degrees f.
10. Press "start/pause" button to start.
11. When the unit beeps to show that it is preheated, open the lid.
12. Arrange pan over the "wire rack" and insert in the oven.
13. Cut into equal-sized wedges and serve.

Nutrition:

Calories 287 Fat 20.8g Cholesterol 285 mg Carbs 1.7 g Fiber 0.3 g Protein 23.1 g

115. Bacon, Mushroom & Tomato Frittata
⏲ Prep Time 15 m | ⏱ Cooking Time 16 m | 2 Servings

Ingredients:

- 1 cooked bacon slice, chopped
- 6 cherry tomatoes, halved
- 6 fresh mushrooms, sliced
- Salt and ground black pepper, as required

- 3 eggs
- 1 tablespoon fresh parsley, chopped
- ¼ cup parmesan cheese, grated

Directions:

1. In a baking pan, add the bacon, tomatoes, mushrooms, salt, and black pepper and mix well.
2. Press "power button" of air fry oven and turn the dial to select the "air fry" mode.
3. Press the time button and again turn the dial to set the cooking time to 16 minutes.
4. Now push the temp button and rotate the dial to set the temperature at 320 degrees f.
5. Press "start/pause" button to start.
6. When the unit beeps to show that it is preheated, open the lid.
7. Arrange pan over the "wire rack" and insert in the oven.
8. Meanwhile, in a bowl, add the eggs and beat well.
9. Add the parsley and cheese and mix well.
10. After 6 minutes of cooking, top the bacon mixture with egg mixture evenly.
11. Cut into equal-sized wedges and serve.

Nutrition:

Calories228 Fat15.5g Cholesterol270mg Sodium608mg Carbs3.5g Fiber0.9g Protein19.8g

116. Sausage, Spinach & Broccoli Frittata
⏲ Prep Time 15 m | ⏱ Cooking Time 30 m | 4 Servings

Ingredients:

- 1 teaspoon butter
- 6 turkey sausage links, cut into small pieces
- 1 cup broccoli florets, cut into small pieces
- ½ cup fresh spinach, chopped up
- 6 eggs

- 1/8 teaspoon hot sauce
- 2 tablespoons half-and-half
- 1/8 teaspoon garlic salt
- Salt and ground black pepper, as required
- ¾ cup cheddar cheese, shredded

Directions:

1. In a skillet, melt the butter over medium heat and cook the sausage for about 7-8 minutes or until browned.
2. Add the broccoli and cook for about 3-4 minutes.
3. Add the spinach and cook for about 2-3 minutes.
4. Remove from the heat and set aside to cool slightly.
5. Meanwhile, in a bowl, add the eggs, half-and-half, hot sauce, garlic salt, salt and black pepper and beat until well combined.
6. Add the cheese and stir to combine.
7. In the bottom of a lightly greased pan, place the broccoli mixture and to with the egg mixture.
8. Press "power button" of air fry oven and turn the dial to select the "air bake" mode.
9. Press the time button and again turn the dial to set the cooking time to 15 minutes.
10. Now push the temp button and rotate the dial to set the temperature at 400 degrees.
11. Press "start/pause" button to start.
12. When the unit beeps to show that it is preheated, open the lid.
13. Arrange pan over the "wire rack" and insert in the oven.
14. Cut into equal-sized wedges and serve hot.

Nutrition:

Calories 339 Fat 27.4g Cholesterol 229 mg Carbs 3.7 g Fiber 0.7 g Protein 19.6 g

117. Grilled Cheese Sandwich

⏱ Prep Time 5 m | ⏱ Cooking Time 5 m | 2 Servings

Ingredients
- 2 slices of bread, softened
- 1 tsp. butter
- 2 slices of cheddar cheese

Directions
1. Set the air fryer at a temperature of 350°F.
2. Apply 1/2 teaspoon of the softened butter to one side of the slice of bread. Repeat for the remaining bread.
3. Create the sandwich by putting the cheese in between the non-buttered sides of bread.
4. Transfer to the hot air fryer and set for 5 minutes. Flip the sandwich at the halfway point and remove it.
5. Serve immediately and enjoy it.

Nutrition
Calories 235 | Fat 13 g | Fiber 27 g| Carbs 37 g | Protein 40 g

118. Italian Meatballs

⏱ Prep Time 15 m | ⏱ Cooking Time 20 m | 4 Servings

Ingredients
- One egg, large
- Ground beef - 16 oz.
- Pepper - 1/8 tsp.
- Oregano seasoning - 1/2 tsp.
- Bread crumbs - 1 1/4 cup
- Garlic - 1/2 clove, chopped
- Parsley - 1 oz., chopped
- Salt - 1/4 tsp.
- Parmigiano-Reggiano cheese - 1 oz. cup, grated
- Cooking spray (avocado oil)

Directions
1. Whisk the oregano, breadcrumbs, chopped garlic, salt, chopped parsley, pepper, and grated Parmigiano-Reggiano cheese until combined.
2. Blend the ground beef and egg into the mixture using your hands. Incorporate the ingredients thoroughly.
3. Divide the meat into 12 sections and roll into rounds.
4. Coat the inside of the basket with avocado oil spray to grease.
5. Adjust the temperature to 350°F and heat for approximately 12 minutes.
6. Roll the meatballs over and steam for another 4 minutes and remove to a serving plate.
7. Enjoy as-is or combine with your favorite pasta or sauce.

Nutrition
Calories 321| Fat 3 g | Fiber 8 g | Carbs 22 g | Protein 16 g

119. Loaded Baked Potatoes

⏱ Prep Time 10 m | ⏱ Cooking Time 15 m | 3 Servings

Ingredients
- 1/3 cup milk
- 2 oz. sour cream
- 1/3 cup white cheddar, grated
- 2 oz. Parmesan cheese, grated
- 1/8 tsp. garlic salt
- 6 oz. ham, diced
- 2 medium russet potatoes
- 4 oz. sharp cheddar, shredded
- 1/8 cup. green onion, diced

Directions
1. Puncture the potatoes deeply with a fork a few times and microwave for approximately 5 minutes. Flip them to the other side and nuke for an additional 5 minutes. The potatoes should be soft.
2. Use oven mitts to remove from the microwave and cut them in halves.
3. Spoon out the insides of the potatoes to about a quarter-inch from the skins and distribute the potato flesh to a glass bowl.
4. Combine the parmesan, garlic salt, sour cream, and white cheddar cheese to the potato dish and incorporate fully.
5. Distribute the mixture back to the emptied potato skins. Create a small hollow in the middle by pressing with a spoon.
6. Divide the ham evenly between the potatoes and place the ham inside the hollow.
7. Position the potatoes in the fryer and set the air fryer to the temperature of 300°F.
8. Heat for 8 minutes and then sprinkle the cheddar cheese on top of each potato.
9. Melt the cheese for two more minutes than serve with diced onions on top.

Nutrition
Calories 143 | Fat 22 g | Fiber 14 g | Carbs 18 g | Protein 29 g

120. Pepperoni Pizza

⏱ Prep Time 5 m | ⏱ Cooking Time 5 m | 7 Servings

Ingredients
- 1 mini naan flatbread
- 2 tbsp. pizza sauce
- 7 slices mini pepperoni
- 1 tbsp. olive oil
- 2 tbsp. mozzarella cheese, shredded

Directions
1. Prepare the naan flatbread by brushed the olive oil on the top.
2. Layer the naan with pizza sauce, mozzarella cheese, and pepperoni.
3. Transfer to the frying basket and set the air fryer to the temperature of 375°F.
4. Heat for approximately 6 minutes and enjoy immediately.

Nutrition
Calories 430 | Fat 4 g | Fiber 9 g | Carbs 11 g | Protein 10 g

121. Southern Style Fried Chicken

⏱ Prep Time 10 m | ⏱ Cooking Time 15 m | 8 Servings

Ingredients

- Italian seasoning - 1 tsp.
- Chicken legs or breasts - 2 lbs.
- Buttermilk - 2 tbsp.
- Paprika seasoning - 1 1/2tsp.
- Cornstarch - 2 oz.
- Onion powder - 1 tsp.
- Hot sauce - 3 tsp.
- Pepper - 1 1/2 tsp.
- 2 large eggs
- 1 cup self-rising flour
- 2 tsp. salt
- Cooking spray (olive oil)
- 1/4 cup water
- Garlic powder - 1 1/2tsp.

Directions

1. Clean the chicken by washing thoroughly and pat dry with paper towels.
2. Use a glass dish to blend the pepper, paprika, garlic powder, onion powder, salt, and Italian seasoning.
3. Rub approximately 1 tablespoon of the spices into the pieces of chicken to cover entirely.
4. Blend the cornstarch, flour, and spices by shaking in a large ziplock bag.
5. In a separate dish, combine the eggs, hot sauce, water, and milk until integrated.
6. Completely cover the spiced chicken in the flour and then immerse in the eggs.
7. Coat in the flour for a second time and set on a tray for approximately 15 minutes.
8. Before transferring the chicken to the air fryer, spray liberally with olive oil and space the pieces out, frying a separate batch if required.
9. Adjust the temperature to 350° F for approximately 18 minutes.
10. Bring the chicken out and put on a plate. Wait about 5 minutes before serving.

Nutrition

Calories 230 | Fat 10 g | Fiber 19 g | Carbs 13 g | Protein 12 g

122. Tuna Patties

⏱ Prep Time 5 m | ⏱ Cooking Time 15 m | 2 Servings

Ingredients

- Garlic powder - 1 tsp.
- Tuna - 2 cans, in water
- Dill seasoning - 1 tsp.
- All-purpose flour - 4 tsp.
- Salt - 1/4 tsp.
- Mayonnaise - 4 tsp.
- Lemon juice - 2 tbsp.
- Onion powder - 1/2 tsp.
- Pepper - 1/4 tsp.

Directions

1. Set the temperature of the air fryer to 400°F.
2. Combine the almond flour, mayonnaise, salt, onion powder, dill, garlic powder, and pepper using a food blender for approximately 30 seconds until incorporated.
3. Empty the canned tuna and lemon juice into the blender and pulse for an additional 30 seconds until integrated fully.
4. Divide evenly into 4 sections and create patties by hand.
5. Transfer to the fryer basket in a single layer and heat for approximately 12 minutes.

Nutrition

Calories 286 | Fat 3 g | Fiber 6 g | Carbs 22 g | Protein 16 g

123. Stuffed Bell Peppers

⏱ Prep Time 15 m | ⏱ Cooking Time 15 m | 9 Servings

Ingredients

- Medium onion - 1/2, chopped
- Cheddar cheese - 4 oz., shredded
- Pepper - 1/2 tsp.
- Ground beef - 8 oz.
- Olive oil - 1 tsp.
- Tomato sauce - 4 oz.
- Worcestershire sauce - 1 tsp.
- Medium green peppers - 2, stems and seeds discarded
- Salt - 1 tsp., separated
- Water - 4 cups
- Garlic - 1 clove, minced

Directions

1. Boil the water in pot steam the green peppers with the tops and seeds removed with 1/2 teaspoon of the salt. Move from the burner after approximately 3 minutes and drain.
2. Pat the peppers with paper towels to properly dry.
3. In a hot frying pan, melt the olive oil and toss the garlic and onion for approximately 2 minutes until browned. Drain thoroughly.
4. Set the air fryer temperature to 400°F to warm up.
5. Using a glass dish, blend the beef along with Worcestershire sauce, 2 ounces of tomato sauce, salt, vegetables, 2 ounces of cheddar cheese, and pepper until fully incorporated.
6. Spoon the mixture evenly into the peppers and drizzle the remaining 2 ounces of tomato sauce on top. Then dust with the remaining 2 ounces of cheddar cheese.
7. Assemble the peppers in the basket of the air fryer and heat fully for approximately 18 minutes. The meat should be fully cooked before removing it.
8. Place on a platter and serve immediately.

Nutrition

Calories 120 | Fat 9 g | Fiber 2 g | Carbs 17 g | Protein 28 g

124. Easy Hot Dogs

⏱ Prep Time 10 m | ⏱ Cooking Time 7 m | 2 Servings

Ingredients

- 2 hot dog buns
- 2 hot dogs
- 1 tablespoon Dijon mustard
- 2 tablespoons cheddar cheese, grated

Directions

1. Put hot dogs in the preheated air fryer and cook them at 390 degrees F for 5 minutes.
2. Divide hot dogs into hot dog buns, spread mustard and cheese, return everything to your air fryer and cook for 2 minutes more at 390 degrees F.
3. Serve for lunch. Enjoy!

Nutrition: Calories 211 | Fat 3 g | Fiber 8 g | Carbs 12 g | Protein 4 g

125. Ham and Cheese Sandwich

⏱ Prep Time 15 m | ⏱ Cooking Time 20 m | 2 Servings

Ingredients

- 2 eggs
- 4 slices of bread of choice
- 4 slices turkey
- 4 slices ham
- 6 tbsp. half and half cream
- 2 tsp. melted butter
- 4 slices Swiss cheese
- ¼ tsp. pure vanilla extract
- Powdered sugar and raspberry jam for serving

Directions

1. Mix the eggs, vanilla, and cream in a bowl and set aside.
2. Make a sandwich with the bread layered with cheese slice, turkey, ham, cheese slice, and the top slice of bread to make two sandwiches. Gently press on the sandwiches to somewhat flatten them.
3. Set your air fryer toast oven to 350 degrees F.
4. Spread out kitchen aluminum foil and cut it about the same size as the sandwich and spread the melted butter on the surface of the foil.
5. Dip the sandwich in the egg mixture and let it soak for about 20 seconds on each side. Repeat this for the other sandwich. Place the soaked sandwiches on the prepared foil sheets then place them on the basket in your fryer.
6. Cook for 12 minutes then flip the sandwiches and brush with the remaining butter and cook for another 5 minutes or until well browned.
7. Place the sandwich on a plate and top with the powdered sugar and serve with a small bowl of raspberry jam.

Nutrition

Calories 170 | Fat 22 g | Fiber 10 g | Carbs 12 g | Protein 20 g

126. Japanese Chicken Mix

⏱ Prep Time 10 m | ⏱ Cooking Time 8 m | 2 Servings

Ingredients

- 2 chicken thighs, skinless and boneless
- 2 ginger slices, chopped
- 3 garlic cloves, minced
- ¼ cup soy sauce
- ¼ cup mirin
- 1/8 cup sake
- ½ teaspoon sesame oil
- 1/8 cup water
- 2 tablespoons sugar
- 1 tablespoon cornstarch mixed with 2 tablespoons water
- Sesame seeds for serving

Directions

1. In a bowl, mix chicken thighs with ginger, garlic, soy sauce, mirin, sake, oil, water, sugar, and cornstarch, toss well, transfer to preheated air fryer and cook at 360 degrees F for 8 minutes.
2. Divide among plates, sprinkle sesame seeds on top and serve with a side salad for lunch.

Nutrition

Calories 300 | Fat 7 g | Fiber 9 g | Carbs 17 g | Protein 10 g

127. Prosciutto Sandwich

⏱ Prep Time 10 m | ⏱ Cooking Time 5 m | 1 Servings

Ingredients

- 2 bread slices
- 2 mozzarella slices
- 2 tomato slices
- 2 prosciutto slices
- 2 basil leaves
- 1 teaspoon olive oil
- A pinch of salt and black pepper

Directions

1. Arrange mozzarella and prosciutto on a bread slice.
2. Season with salt and pepper, place in your air fryer and cook at 400 degrees F for 5 minutes.
3. Drizzle oil over prosciutto, add tomato and basil, cover with the other bread slice, cut the sandwich in half, and serve.

Nutrition

Calories 172 | Fat 3 g | Fiber 7 g | Carbs 9 g | Protein 5

128. Lentils Fritters

⏱ Prep Time 10 m | ⏱ Cooking Time 10 m | 2 Servings

Ingredients

- 1 cup yellow lentils, soaked in water for 1 hour and drained
- 1 hot chili pepper, chopped
- 1-inch ginger piece, grated
- ½ teaspoon turmeric powder
- 1 teaspoon garam masala
- 1 teaspoon baking powder
- Salt and black pepper to the taste
- 2 teaspoons olive oil
- 1/3 cup water
- ½ cup cilantro, chopped
- 1 and ½ cup spinach, chopped
- 4 garlic cloves, minced
- ¾ cup red onion, chopped
- Mint chutney for serving

Directions

1. In your blender, mix lentils with chili pepper, ginger, turmeric, garam masala, baking powder, salt, pepper, olive oil, water, cilantro, spinach, onion, and garlic, blend well and shape medium balls out of this mix.
2. Place them all in your preheated air fryer at 400 degrees F and cook for 10 minutes.
3. Serve your veggie fritters with a side salad for lunch.

Nutrition:

Calories 142 | Fat 2 g | Fiber 8 g | Carbs 12 g | Protein 4 g

129. Lunch Potato Salad

⏱ Prep Time 10 m | ⏱ Cooking Time 25 m | 4 Servings

Ingredients

- 2-pound red potatoes, halved
- 2 tablespoons olive oil
- Salt and black pepper to the taste
- 2 green onions, chopped
- 1 red bell pepper, chopped
- 1/3 cup lemon juice
- 3 tablespoons mustard

Directions

1. On your air fryer's basket, mix potatoes with half of the olive oil, salt, and pepper and cook at 350 degrees F for 25 minutes shaking the fryer once.
2. In a bowl, mix onions with bell pepper and roasted potatoes and toss.
3. In a small bowl, mix lemon juice with the rest of the oil and mustard and whisk really well.
4. Add this to potato salad, toss well and serve for lunch.

Nutrition

Calories 211 | Fat 6 g | Fiber 8 g | Carbs 12 g | Protein 4 g

130. Corn Casserole

⏱ Prep Time 10 m | ⏱ Cooking Time 15 m | 4 Servings

Ingredients

- 2 cups corn
- 3 tablespoons flour
- 1 egg
- ¼ cup milk
- ½ cup light cream
- ½ cup Swiss cheese, grated
- 2 tablespoons butter
- Salt and black pepper to the taste
- Cooking spray

Directions

1. In a bowl, mix the corn with flour, egg, milk, light cream, cheese, salt, pepper, and butter and stir well.
2. Grease your air fryer's pan with cooking spray, pour the cream mix, spread, and cook at 320 degrees F for 15 minutes.
3. Serve warm for lunch.

Nutrition:

Calories 281 | Fat 7 g | Fiber 8 g | Carbs 9 g | Protein 6 g

131. Bacon and Garlic Pizzas

⏱ Prep Time 10 m | ⏱ Cooking Time 10 m | 4 Servings

Ingredients

- 4 dinner rolls, frozen
- 4 garlic cloves minced
- ½ teaspoon oregano dried
- ½ teaspoon garlic powder
- 1 cup tomato sauce
- 8 bacon slices, cooked and chopped
- 1 and ¼ cups cheddar cheese, grated
- Cooking spray

Directions

1. Place dinner rolls on a working surface and press them to obtain 4 ovals.
2. Spray each oval with cooking spray, transfer them to your air fryer and cook them at 370 degrees F for 2 minutes.
3. Spread tomato sauce on each oval, divide garlic, sprinkle oregano, and garlic powder, and top with bacon and cheese.
4. Return pizzas to your heated air fryer and cook them at 370 degrees F for 8 minutes more.
5. Serve them warm for lunch.

Nutrition

Calories 217 | Fat 5 g | Fiber 8 g | Carbs 12 g | Protein 4 g

132. Sweet and Sour Sausage Mix

⏱ Prep Time 10 m | ⏱ Cooking Time 10 m | 4 Servings

Ingredients

- 1 pound sausages, sliced
- 1 red bell pepper, cut into strips
- ½ cup yellow onion, chopped
- 3 tablespoons brown sugar
- 1/3 cup ketchup
- 2 tablespoons mustard
- 2 tablespoons apple cider vinegar
- ½ cup chicken stock

Directions

1. In a bowl, mix sugar with ketchup, mustard, stock, and vinegar and whisk well.
2. In your air fryer's pan, mix sausage slices with bell pepper, onion, and sweet and sour mix, toss and cook at 350 degrees F for 10 minutes.
3. Divide into bowls and serve for lunch.

Nutrition

Calories 162 | Fat 6 g | Fiber 9 g | Carbs 12 g | Protein 6 g

133. Meatballs and Tomato Sauce
⏱ Prep Time 10 m | ⏱ Cooking Time 15 m | 4 Servings

Ingredients

- 1 pound lean beef, ground
- 3 green onions, chopped
- 2 garlic cloves, minced
- 1 egg yolk
- ¼ cup bread crumbs
- Salt and black pepper to the taste
- 1 tablespoon olive oil
- 16 ounces' tomato sauce
- 2 tablespoons mustard

Directions

1. In a bowl, mix beef with onion, garlic, egg yolk, bread crumbs, salt, and pepper, stir well, and shape medium meatballs out of this mix.
2. Grease meatballs with the oil, place them in your air fryer, and cook them at 400 degrees F for 10 minutes.
3. In a bowl, mix tomato sauce with mustard, whisk, add over meatballs, toss them and cook at 400 degrees F for 5 minutes more.
4. Divide meatballs and sauce among plates and serve for lunch.

Nutrition

Calories 300 | Fat 8 g | Fiber 9 g | Carbs 16 g | Protein 5 g

134. Stuffed Meatballs
⏱ Prep Time 10 m | ⏱ Cooking Time 10 m | 4 Servings

Ingredients

- 1/3 cup bread crumbs
- 3 tablespoons milk
- 1 tablespoon ketchup
- 1 egg
- ½ teaspoon marjoram, dried
- Salt and black pepper to the taste
- 1 pound lean beef, ground
- 20 cheddar cheese cubes
- 1 tablespoon olive oil

Directions

1. In a bowl, mix bread crumbs with ketchup, milk, marjoram, salt, pepper, and the egg and whisk well.
2. Add beef, stir and shape 20 meatballs out of this mix.
3. Shape each meatball around a cheese cube, drizzle the oil over them and rub.
4. Place all meatballs in your preheated air fryer and cook at 390 degrees F for 10 minutes.
5. Serve them for lunch with a side salad.

Nutrition

Calories 200 | Fat 5 g | Fiber 8 g | Carbs 12 g | Protein 5 g

135. Steaks and Cabbage
⏱ Prep Time 10 m | ⏱ Cooking Time 10 m | 4 Servings

Ingredients

- ½ pound sirloin steak, cut into strips
- 2 teaspoons cornstarch
- 1 tablespoon peanut oil
- 2 cups green cabbage, chopped
- 1 yellow bell pepper, chopped
- 2 green onions, chopped
- 2 garlic cloves, minced
- Salt and black pepper to the taste

Directions

1. In a bowl, mix cabbage with salt, pepper, and peanut oil, toss, transfer to air fryer's basket, cook at 370 degrees F for 4 minutes and transfer to a bowl.
2. Add steak strips to your air fryer, also add green onions, bell pepper, garlic, salt and pepper, toss, and cook for 5 minutes.
3. Add over cabbage, toss, divide among plates, and serve for lunch. Enjoy!

Nutrition

Calories 282 | Fat 6 g | Fiber 8 g | Carbs 14 g | Protein 6 g

136. Succulent Lunch Turkey Breast
⏱ Prep Time 10 m | ⏱ Cooking Time 47 m | 4 Servings

Ingredients

- 1 big turkey breast
- 2 teaspoons olive oil
- ½ teaspoon smoked paprika
- 1 teaspoon thyme, dried
- ½ teaspoon sage, dried
- Salt and black pepper to the taste
- 2 tablespoons mustard
- ¼ cup maple syrup
- 1 tablespoon butter, soft

Directions

1. Brush turkey breast with olive oil, season with salt, pepper, thyme, paprika, and sage. Rub, place in your air fryer's basket and fry at 350 degrees F for 25 minutes.
2. Flip turkey, cook for 10 minutes more, flip one more time, and cook for another 10 minutes.
3. Meanwhile, heat up a pan with the butter over medium heat, add mustard and maple syrup, stir well, cook for a couple of minutes and take off the heat.
4. Slice the turkey breast, divide among plates and serve with the maple glaze drizzled on top.

Nutrition

Calories 280 | Fat 2 g | Fiber 7 g | Carbs 16 g | Protein 14 g

137. Italian Eggplant Sandwich

☺ Prep Time 10 m | ☺ Cooking Time 16 m | 2 Servings

Ingredients

- 1 eggplant, sliced
- 2 teaspoons parsley, dried
- Salt and black pepper to the taste
- ½ cup breadcrumbs
- ½ teaspoon Italian seasoning
- ½ teaspoon garlic powder
- ½ teaspoon onion powder

- 2 tablespoons milk
- 4 bread slices
- Cooking spray
- ½ cup mayonnaise
- ¾ cup tomato sauce
- 2 cups mozzarella cheese, grated

Directions

1. Season eggplant slices with salt and pepper, leave aside for 10 minutes, and then pat dry them well.
2. In a bowl, mix parsley with breadcrumbs, Italian seasoning, onion and garlic powder, salt and black pepper and stir.
3. In another bowl, mix milk with mayo and whisk well.
4. Brush eggplant slices with mayo mix, dip them in breadcrumbs, place them in your air fryer's basket, spray with cooking oil and cook them at 400 degrees F for 15 minutes, flipping them after 8 minutes.

5. Brush each bread slice with olive oil and arrange 2 on a working surface.
6. Add mozzarella and parmesan on each, add baked eggplant slices, spread tomato sauce and basil and top with the other bread slices, greased side down.
7. Divide sandwiches among plates, cut them in halves, and serve for lunch.

Nutrition

Calories 324 | Fat 16 g | Fiber 4 g | Carbs 39 g | Protein 12 g

138. Creamy Chicken Stew

☺ Prep Time 10 m | ☺ Cooking Time 25 m | 4 Servings

Ingredients

- 1 and ½ cups canned cream of celery soup
- 6 chicken tenders
- Salt and black pepper to the taste
- 2 potatoes, chopped
- 1 bay leaf

- 1 thyme spring, chopped
- 1 tablespoon milk
- 1 egg yolk
- ½ cup heavy cream

Directions

1. In a bowl, mix chicken with cream of celery, potatoes, heavy cream, bay leaf, thyme, salt and pepper, toss, pour into your air fryer's pan, and cook at 320 degrees F for 25 minutes.

2. Leave your stew to cool down a bit, discard bay leaf, divide among plates, and serve right away.

Nutrition

Calories 300 | Fat 11 g | Fiber 2 g | Carbs 23 g | Protein 14 g

139. Lunch Pork and Potatoes

☺ Prep Time 10 m | ☺ Cooking Time 25 m | 2 Servings

Ingredients

- 2 pounds' pork loin
- Salt and black pepper to the taste
- 2 red potatoes, cut into medium wedges
- ½ teaspoon garlic powder

- ½ teaspoon red pepper flakes
- 1 teaspoon parsley, dried
- A drizzle of balsamic vinegar

Directions

1. In your air fryer's pan, mix pork with potatoes, salt, pepper, garlic powder, pepper flakes, parsley, and vinegar, toss and cook at 390 degrees F for 25 minutes.

2. Slice pork, divide it, divide the potatoes among plates, and serve for lunch.

Nutrition

Calories 400 | Fat 15 g | Fiber 7 g | Carbs 27 g | Protein 20 g

140. Bacon Cheddar Chicken Fingers

☺ Prep Time 8 m | ☺ Cooking Time 12 m | 8 Servings

Ingredients

For the chicken fingers:

- 1 lb. chicken tenders, about 8 pieces
- Cooking spray (canola oil)
- Cheddar cheese - 1 cup, shredded
- Two eggs, large
- 1/3 cup bacon bits
- 2 tbsp. water

For the breading:

- 1 tsp. of onion powder
- Panko bread crumbs - 2 cups
- Black pepper - 1 tsp., freshly ground
- Paprika - 2 tbsp.
- Garlic powder - 1 tsp.
- Salt - 2 tsp.

Directions

1. Set the air fryer to the temperature of 360°F.
2. In a glass dish, whip the water and eggs until combined.
3. Use a zip lock bag, shake the garlic powder, salt, breadcrumbs, cayenne, onion powder, and pepper together.
4. Immerse the chicken into the eggs and shake in the ziplock bag until fully covered.
5. Dip again in the mixture of egg and back into the seasonings until a thick coating is present.

6. Remove the tenders from the bag and set in the frying pan in the basket. Do them in batches if you need to not overpack the pan.
7. Apply the canola oil spray to the top of the tenders and heat for 6 minutes.
8. Flip the tenders to the other side. Steam for another 4 m.
9. Blend the bacon bits and shredded cheese in a dish.
10. Evenly dust the bacon and cheese onto the hot tenders and fry for 2 more minutes.
11. Remove and serve while hot.

Nutrition:

Calories 320 | Fat 25 g | Fiber 17 g | Carbs 37 g | Protein 40 g

141. Battered Cod

⏱ Prep Time 16 m | ⏱ Cooking Time 14 m | 2 Servings

Ingredients

- Cod - 20 oz.
- Salt - 1/4 tsp.
- All-purpose flour - 8 oz.
- Parsley seasoning - 1 tbsp.
- Cornstarch - 3 tsp.
- Garlic powder - 1/2 tsp.
- Two eggs, preferably large
- Onion powder - 1/2 tsp.

Directions

1. Whip the eggs in a glass dish until smooth and set to the side.
2. In a separate dish, blend the cornstarch, salt, almond flour, garlic powder, parsley, and onion powder, whisking to remove any lumpiness.
3. Immerse the pieces of cod into the egg and then into the spiced flour, covering completely.
4. Transfer to the fryer basket in a single layer.
5. Heat the fish for 7 minutes at a temperature of 350°F. Turn the cod over and steam for an additional 7 minutes.

Nutrition

Calories 254 | Fat 4 g | Fiber 10 g | Carbs 17 g | Protein 12 g

142. Beef Kabobs

⏱ Prep Time 10 m | ⏱ Cooking Time 12 m | 3 Servings

Ingredients

- Low-fat sour cream - 1/3 cup
- One bell pepper
- 16 oz. of beef chuck ribs, boneless
- Soy sauce - 2 tbsp.
- 6-inch skewers - 8
- Pepper - 1/4 tsp.
- Medium onion - 1/2

Directions

1. Slice the ribs into sections about 1-inch wide
2. In a lidded tub, combine the soy sauce, ribs, and sour cream, making sure the meat is fully covered.
3. Refrigerate for half an hour, at least, if not overnight.
4. Immerse the wooden skewers for approximately 10 minutes in water.
5. Set the temperature of the air fryer oven to 400°F.
6. Slice the onion and bell pepper in 1-inch sections.
7. Remove the meat from the marinade, draining well.
8. Layer the onions, beef, and bell peppers on the skewers and dust with pepper.
9. Heat for 10 minutes, ensuring you spin the skewers 5 minutes into cooking time.
10. Serve while hot and enjoy.

Nutrition

Calories 312 | Fat 10 g | Fiber 8 g | Carbs 29 g | Protein 30 g

143. Cheese Dogs

⏱ Prep Time 3 m | ⏱ Cooking Time 10 m | 7 Servings

Ingredients

- 4 hotdogs
- 1/4 cup your choice of cheese, grated
- 4 hotdog buns

Directions

1. Adjust the air fryer to heat at a temperature of 390°F for approximately 5 minutes.
2. Set the hot dogs in the basket and broil for 5 minutes.
3. Remove and create the hot dog with the bun and cheese as desired and move back to the basket for another 2 minutes.
4. Remove and enjoy while hot.

Nutrition

Calories 200 | Fat 5 g | Fiber 10 g | Carbs 17 g | Protein 18 g

144. Cheeseburger Patties

⏱ Prep Time 10 m | ⏱ Cooking Time 13 m | 4 Servings

Ingredients

- Garlic - 1/2 clove, minced
- Ground beef - 1 1/3 cup
- Onion - 4 oz., diced
- Worcestershire sauce - 2 tbsp.
- One egg, large
- Panko breadcrumbs - 2 oz.
- Cayenne pepper - 1/8 tsp.
- Cooking spray (olive oil)
- Salt - 1/4 tsp.
- 4 slices of cheese of your choice
- 1/8 tsp. pepper

Directions

1. Using a big glass dish, combine the diced onion, pepper, minced garlic, cayenne pepper, breadcrumbs, and salt until incorporated.
2. Blend the ground beef, Worcestershire sauce, and egg and integrate thoroughly by hand.
3. Form the meat into 4 individual patties and move to the air fryer basket.
4. Coat the patties with cooking spray.
5. Adjust the temperature for 375°F and heat for 8 minutes.
6. Turn the burgers over and steam for an additional 2 minutes.
7. Cover with a slice of cheese and continue cooking for approximately 3 minutes.
8. Enjoy or place on a bun with your favorite toppings.

Nutrition

Calories 287 | Fat 6 g | Fiber 12 g | Carbs 11 g | Protein 21 g

145. Chicken Cordon Bleu

⏱ Prep Time 15 m | ⏱ Cooking Time 20 m | 2 Servings

Ingredients

- Pepper - 1/4 tsp.
- Chicken paillards - 4
- Salt - 1/4 tsp.
- Swiss cheese - 8 slices
- All-purpose flour - 1/2 cup
- Parmesan cheese - 2/3 cup, grated
- Panko breadcrumbs - 1 1/2 cup
- Ham - 8 slices
- Two eggs, large
- Dijon mustard - 2 tbsp.
- 8 toothpicks
- Grapeseed oil spray

Directions

1. On a section of baking lining, brush the Dijon mustard on each chicken paillard and sprinkle with pepper and salt.
2. Layer 1 cheese, 2 slices of the ham, and then the additional slice of cheese on each of the pieces of chicken.
3. Rotate the chicken beginning with the longer side to create a roll. Fasten in place with two toothpicks.
4. Whip the egg in one dish, empty the flour into a second dish and blend the parmesan cheese and breadcrumbs into a third.
5. Immerse one chicken first in flour, secondly immerse in the egg and then roll the chicken completely in the breadcrumbs. Press the cheese and breadcrumbs into the chicken to secure and place onto a plate.
6. Repeat for the other pieces of chicken.
7. Apply the grapeseed oil spray to each section of chicken and transfer to the air fryer basket after 5 minutes.
8. Set the air fryer temperature to heat at 350°.
9. Grill for 8 minutes and carefully turn the chicken to the other side—heat for an additional 8 minutes.
10. Remove to a serving dish and wait approximately 5 minutes before serving hot.

Nutrition

Calories 176 | Fat 22 g | Fiber 20 g | Carbs 33 g | Protein 12 g

146. Quinoa and Spinach Cakes

⏱ Prep Time 5 m | ⏱ Cooking Time 8 m | 4 Servings | Intermediate Recipe

Ingredients:

- 2 c. cooked quinoa
- 1 c. chopped baby spinach
- 1 egg
- 2 tbsps. Minced parsley
- 1 teaspoon minced garlic
- 1 carrot, peeled and shredded
- 1 chopped onion
- ¼ c. oat milk
- ¼ c. parmesan cheese, grated
- 1 c. breadcrumbs
- Sea salt
- Ground black

Directions:

1. In a mixing bowl, mix all ingredients. Season with salt and pepper to taste.
2. Preheat your Air Fryer to 390°F.
3. Scoop ¼ cup of quinoa and spinach mixture and place in the Air Fryer cooking basket. Cook in batches until browned for about 8 minutes.
4. Serve and enjoy!

Nutrition:

Calories 188 | Fat 4.4 g | Carbs 31.2g | Protein 8.1g.

147. Spinach in Cheese Envelopes

⏱ Prep Time 5 m | ⏱ Cooking Time 12 m | 8 Servings | Intermediate Recipe

Ingredients:

- 1½ c. almond flour
- 3 egg yolks
- 2 eggs
- ½ c. cheddar cheese
- 2 c. steamed spinach
- ¼ teaspoon salt
- ½ teaspoon pepper
- 3 c. cream cheese
- ¼ c. chopped onion

Directions:

1. Place cream cheese in a mixing bowl then whisks until soft and fluffy.
2. Add egg yolks to the mixing bowl then continue whisking until incorporated.
3. Stir in coconut flour to the cheese mixture then mix until becoming a soft dough.
4. Place the dough on a flat surface then roll until thin.
5. Cut the thin dough into 8 squares then keep.
6. Crash the eggs then place in a bowl.
7. Season with salt, pepper, and grated cheese, then mix well.
8. Add chopped spinach and onion to the egg mixture, then stir until combined.
9. Put spinach filling on a square dough then fold until becoming an envelope. Repeat with the remaining spinach filling and dough. Glue with water.
10. Preheat an Air Fryer to 425°F (218°C).
11. Arrange the spinach envelopes in the Air Fryer then cook for 12 minutes or until lightly golden brown.
12. Remove from the Air Fryer then serve warm. Enjoy!

Nutrition:

Calories 365 | Fat 34.6g | Protein 10.4g | Carbs 4.4g

148. Avocado Sticks

⏰ Prep Time 5 m | ⏰ Cooking Time 8 m | 6 Servings | Basic Recipe

Ingredients:

- 2 avocados
- 1 c. coconut flour
- 2 teaspoon Black pepper
- 3 egg yolks
- 1½ tbsps. Water
- ¼ teaspoon salt
- 1 c.vegan butter
- 2 teaspoon Minced garlic
- ¼ c. chopped parsley
- 1 tablespoon lemon juice

Directions:

1. Place butter in a mixing bowl then adds minced garlic, chopped parsley, and lemon juice to the bowl.
2. Using an electric mixer mix until smooth and fluffy.
3. Transfer the garlic butter to a container with a lid then store in the fridge.
4. Peel the avocados then cut into wedges. Set aside.
5. Put the egg yolks in a mixing bowl then pour water into it.
6. Season with salt and black pepper, then stir until incorporated.
7. Take an avocado wedge then roll in the coconut flour.
8. Dip in the egg mixture then returns back to the coconut flour. Roll until the avocado wedge is completely coated. Repeat with the remaining avocado wedges.
9. Preheat an Air Fryer to 400°F (204°C).
10. Arrange the coated avocado wedges in the Air Fryer basket then cook for 8 minutes or until golden.
11. Remove from the Air Fryer then arrange on a serving dish.
12. Serve with garlic butter then enjoy right away.

Nutrition:

Calories 340| Fat 33.8g |Protein 4.5g |Carbs 8.5g

149. Chili Roasted Eggplant Soba

⏰ Prep Time 10 m | ⏰ Cooking Time 15 m | 4 Servings |Basic Recipe

Ingredients:

- 200g eggplants
- Kosher salt
- Ground black pepper
- Noodles:
- 8 oz. soba noodles
- 1 c. sliced button mushrooms
- 2 tbsps. Peanut oil
- 2 tbsps. Light soy sauce
- 1 Tablespoon rice vinegar
- 2 tbsps. Chopped cilantro
- 2 chopped red chili pepper
- 1 teaspoon sesame oil

Directions:

1. In a mixing bowl, mix together ingredients for the marinade.
2. Wash eggplants and then slice into ¼-inch thick cuts. Season with salt and pepper, to taste.
3. Preheat your Air Fryer to 390°F.
4. Place eggplants in the Air Fryer cooking basket. Cook for 10 minutes.
5. Meanwhile, cook the soba noodles according to packaging directions. Drain the noodles.
6. In a large mixing bowl, combine the peanut oil, soy sauce, rice vinegar, cilantro, chili, and sesame oil. Mix well.
7. Add the cooked soba noodles, mushrooms, and roasted eggplants; toss to coat.
8. Transfer mixture into the Air Fryer cooking basket. Cook for another 5 minutes.
9. Serve and enjoy!

Nutrition:

Calories 318| Fat 8.2g | Carbs 54g| Protein 11.3g.

150. Broccoli Popcorn

⏰ Prep Time 5 m | ⏰ Cooking Time 6 m | 4 Servings |Basic Recipe

Ingredients:

- 2 c. broccoli florets
- 2 c. almond flour
- 4 egg yolks
- ½ teaspoon salt
- ½ teaspoon pepper

Directions:

1. Soak the broccoli florets in salty water to remove all the insects inside.
2. Wash and rinse the broccoli florets then pat them dry.
3. Crack the eggs. Add almond flour to the liquid then season with salt and pepper. Mix until incorporated.
4. Preheat an Air Fryer to 400°F (204°C).
5. Dip a broccoli floret in the coconut flour mixture then place in the Air Fryer. Repeat with the remaining broccoli florets.
6. Cook the broccoli florets 6 minutes. You may do this in several batches.
7. Once it is done, remove the fried broccoli popcorn from the Air Fryer then place on a serving dish.
8. Serve and enjoy immediately.

Nutrition: Calories 202 |Fat 17.5g |Protein 5.1g |Carbs 7.8g

151. Marinated Portabello Mushroom

🕐 Prep Time 30 m | 🕐 Cooking Time 15-20 m | 4 Servings | Basic Recipe

Ingredients:

- 4 pcs. Portabello mushrooms
- 1 chopped shallot
- 1 teaspoon minced garlic
- 2 tbsps. Olive oil
- 2 tbsps. Balsamic vinegar
- Ground black pepper

Directions:

1. Clean and wash portabello mushrooms and remove stems. Set aside.
2. In a bowl, mix together the shallot, garlic, olive oil, and balsamic vinegar. Season with pepper, to taste.
3. Arrange portabello mushrooms, cap side up and brush with balsamic vinegar mixture. Let it stand for at least 30 minutes.
4. Preheat your Air Fryer to 360°F.
5. Place marinated portabello mushroom on Air Fryer cooking basket. Cook for about 15-20 minutes or until mushrooms are tender.
6. Serve and enjoy!

Nutrition:

Calories 96 | Fat 7.9g | Carbs 7.5g | Protein 3.6g.

152. Fettuccini with Roasted Vegetables in Tomato Sauce

🕐 Prep Time 10 m | 🕐 Cooking Time 25 m | 4 Servings | Intermediate Recipe

Ingredients:

- 10 oz. spaghetti, cooked
- 1 eggplant, chopped
- 1 chopped bell pepper
- 1 zucchini, chopped
- 4 oz. halved grape tomatoes
- 1 teaspoon minced garlic
- 4 tbsps. Divided olive oil
- Kosher salt
- Ground black pepper
- 12 oz. can diced tomatoes
- ½ teaspoon dried basil
- ½ teaspoon dried oregano
- 1 teaspoon Spanish paprika
- 1 teaspoon brown sugar

Directions:

1. In a mixing bowl, combine together eggplant, red bell pepper, zucchini, grape tomatoes, garlic, and 2 tablespoons olive oil. Add some salt and pepper, to taste.
2. Preheat your Air Fryer to 390°F.
3. Place vegetable mixture in the Air Fryer cooking basket and cook for about 10-12 minutes, or until vegetables are tender. Meanwhile, you can start preparing the tomato sauce.
4. In a saucepan, heat remaining 2 tablespoons olive oil. Stir fry garlic for 2 minutes. Add diced tomatoes and simmer for 3 minutes.
5. Stir in basil, oregano, paprika, and brown sugar. Season with salt and pepper, to taste. Let it cook for another 5-7 minutes. Once cooked, transfer the vegetables from Air Fryer to a mixing bowl.
6. Add the cooked spaghetti and prepared a sauce. Toss to combine well.
7. Divide among 4 serving plates.
8. Serve and enjoy!

Nutrition:

Calories 330 | Fat 12.4g | Carbs 45.3g | Protein 9.9g.

153. Air Fried Tofu with Peanut Dipping Sauce

🕐 Prep Time 5 m | 🕐 Cooking Time 8 m | 6 Servings | Basic Recipe

Ingredients:

- 16 oz. cubed firm tofu
- 185g all-purpose flour
- ½ teaspoon Himalayan salt
- ½ teaspoon ground black pepper
- Olive oil spray
- For the dipping sauce:
- 1/3 c. smooth low-sodium peanut butter
- 1 teaspoon minced garlic
- 2 tbsps. Light soy sauce
- 1 tablespoon fresh lime juice
- 1 teaspoon brown sugar
- 1/3 c. water
- 2 tbsps. Chopped roasted

Directions:

1. In a bowl, mix all dipping sauce ingredients. Cover it with plastic wrap and keep refrigerated until ready to serve.
2. To make the fried tofu, season all-purpose flour with salt and pepper.
3. Coat the tofu cubes with the flour mixture. Spray with oil.
4. Preheat your Air Fryer to 390°F.
5. Place coated tofu in the cooking basket. Careful not to overcrowd them.
6. Cook until browned for approximately 8 minutes.
7. Serve with prepared peanut dipping sauce.
8. Enjoy!

Nutrition:

Calories 256 | Fat 14.1g | Carbs 21.2g | Protein 12.4 g

154. Air Fryer Baked Garlic Parsley Potatoes

Prep Time 15 m | Cooking Time 35 m | 4 Servings | Basic Recipe

Ingredients:

- 3 russet potatoes
- 2 tbsps. Olive oil
- 1 tablespoon salt
- 1 tablespoon garlic powder
- 1 teaspoon parsley

Directions:

1. Rinse the potatoes under running water and pierce with a fork in several places.
2. Season with salt and garlic and drizzle with olive oil. Rub the seasonings with your hands, so the potatoes are evenly coated.
3. Put the potatoes in the basket of your air fryer and slide it into the air fryer.
4. Set the temperature of 400 °F and the timer for 35 minutes and turn the button On Check the doneness and once the potatoes are fork tender remove from the fryer.
5. Serve the potatoes garnished with chopped fresh parsley and topped with a dollop of sour cream.

Nutrition:

Calories 147 | Fat 3.7g | Carbs 26.7g | Protein 3g.

155. Zucchini Parmesan Bites

Prep Time 2 m | Cooking Time 10 m | 4 Servings | Basic Recipe

Ingredients:

- 4 medium zucchinis
- 1 c. grated coconuts
- 1-tablespoon Italian seasoning
- ¼ c. chopped parsley
- ½ c. grated Parmesan cheese
- 1 egg

Directions:

1. Peel the zucchinis then cut into halves.
2. Discard the seeds then grate the zucchinis. Place in a bowl.
3. Add grated coconuts, parsley, Italian seasoning, egg, and Parmesan cheese to the bowl. Mix well.
4. Shape the zucchini mixture into small balls forms then set aside.
5. Preheat an Air Fryer to 400°F (204°C).
6. Place a rack in the Air Fryer then arrange the zucchini balls on it.
7. Cook the zucchini balls for 10 minutes then remove from heat.
8. Serve and enjoy.

Nutrition:

Calories 225 | Fat 17.9g | Protein 9g | Carbs 10.6g

156. Cauliflower Florets in Tomato Puree

Prep Time 30 m | Cooking Time 20 m | 2 Servings | Basic Recipe

Ingredients:

- 2 c. cauliflower florets
- 3 teaspoon Granulated garlic
- ½ teaspoon salt
- ½ teaspoon coriander
- 2 c. water
- 3 eggs
- ½ teaspoon pepper
- ¼ c. grated Mozzarella cheese
- 3 tbsps. Tomato pure

Directions:

1. Place garlic, salt, and coriander in a container then pour water into it. Stir until the seasoning is completely dissolved.
2. Add the cauliflower florets to the brine then submerge for at least 30 minutes.
3. After 30 minutes, remove the cauliflower florets from the brine, then wash and rinse them. Pat them dry.
4. Preheat an Air Fryer to 400°F (204°C).
5. Crash the eggs and place in a bowl.
6. Season with pepper then whisks until incorporated.
7. Dip a cauliflower floret in the egg then place in the air fryer. Repeat with the remaining cauliflower florets and egg.
8. Cook the cauliflower florets for 12 minutes or until lightly golden and the egg is curly.
9. Sprinkle grated Mozzarella cheese then drizzle tomato puree on top.
10. Cook the cauliflower florets again for another 5 minutes then remove from the Air Fryer.
11. Transfer to a serving dish then serve. Enjoy warm.

Nutrition:

Calories 276 | Fat 21.8g | Protein 13.8g | Carbs 5.4g

157. Fried Green Beans Garlic

Prep Time 5 m | Cooking Time 5 m | 2 Servings | Basic Recipe

Ingredients:

- ¾ c. chopped green beans
- 2 teaspoon Granulated garlic
- 2 tbsps. Rosemary
- ½ teaspoon salt
- 1 tablespoon vegan butter

Directions:

1. Preheat an Air Fryer to 390°F (200°C). Place the chopped green beans in the Air Fryer then brush with butter. Sprinkle salt, garlic, and rosemary over the green beans, then cook for 5 minutes.
2. Once the green beans are done, remove from the Air Fryer then place on a serving dish. Serve and enjoy warm.

Nutrition:

Calories 72 | Fat 6.3g | Protein 0.7g | Carbs 4.5g

158. Tender Potato Pancakes

⏱ Prep Time 5 m | ⏱ Cooking Time 12 m | 4 Servings |Basic Recipe

Ingredients:

- 4 potatoes, peeled and cleaned
- 1 chopped onion
- 1 beaten egg
- ¼ c. oat milk
- 2 tbsps. Vegan butter
- ½ teaspoon garlic powder
- ¼ teaspoon salt
- 3 tbsps. All-purpose flour
- Pepper

Directions:

1. Peel your potatoes and shred them up.
2. Soak the shredded potatoes under cold water to remove starch.
3. Drain the potatoes.
4. Take a bowl and add eggs, milk, butter, garlic powder, salt, and pepper.
5. Add in flour.
6. Mix well.
7. Add the shredded potatoes.
8. Pre-heat your air fryer to 390 degrees F.
9. Add ¼ cup of the potato pancake batter to your cooking basket and cook for 12 minutes until the golden brown texture is seen.
10. Enjoy!

Nutrition:

Calories 248| Fat 11g |Carbs 33g |Protein 6g.

159. Brussels Sprout and Cheese

⏱ Prep Time 5 m | ⏱ Cooking Time 20 m | 2 Servings |Basic Recipe

Ingredients:

- ¾ c. Brussels sprouts
- 1 tablespoon extra-virgin olive oil
- ¼ teaspoon salt
- Freshly ground black pepper
- ¼ c. grated Mozzarella cheese

Directions:

1. Cut the Brussels sprouts into halves then place in a bowl.
2. Drizzle extra virgin olive oil over the Brussels sprouts then sprinkle salt on top. Toss to combine.
3. Preheat an Air Fryer to 375°F (191°C).
4. Transfer the seasoned Brussels sprouts to the Air Fryer then cook for 15 minutes.
5. After 15 minutes, open the Air Fryer and sprinkle grated Mozzarella cheese over the cooked Brussels sprouts.
6. Cook the Brussels sprouts in the Air Fryer for 5 minutes or until the Mozzarella cheese is melted.
7. Once it is done, remove from the Air Fryer then transfer to a serving dish.
8. Serve and enjoy.

Nutrition:

Calories 224 |Fat 18.1g| Protein 10.1g| Carbs 4.5g

160. Zucchini, Tomato and Mozzarella Pie

⏱ Prep Time 10 m | ⏱ Cooking Time 25 m | 4 Servings |Intermediate Recipe

Ingredients:

- 3 medium zucchinis
- Sea salt
- 5 minced cloves garlic
- Freshly ground pepper
- Olive oil
- 8 oz. sliced mozzarella
- 3 sliced vine-ripe or heirloom tomatoes
- Freshly chopped basil

Directions:

1. Preheat the air fryer to 400 °F.
2. Halve the zucchini and thinly cut lengthwise into strips
3. Apply pepper and salt for seasoning and allow to sit in a colander for 9-10 minutes.
4. Transfer to paper towels to drain.
5. In an even layer, arrange the zucchini in a small baking dish and sprinkle with the minced garlic and pepper.
6. Sprinkle with olive oil and top with the mozzarella slices, followed by the tomato slices.
7. Sprinkle with the chopped basil, sea salt, and pepper.
8. Place the pan in the basket and bake at 400 °F for 25 minutes, until the cheese has melted.
9. Remove from the air fryer and let it sit for 10 minutes.
10. Serve warm and enjoy.

Nutrition:

Calories 195 |Fat 10.4g |Carbs 9.6g |Protein 18.2g.

161. Air fryer Cauliflower Rice

⏱ Prep Time 5 m | ⏱ Cooking Time 20 m | 4 Servings | Basic Recipe

Ingredients:

Round 1:

- Teaspoon Turmeric
- 1 c. Diced carrot
- ½ c. Diced onion
- 2 tablespoon Low-sodium soy sauce
- ½ block of extra firm tofu

Round 2:

- ½ c. Frozen peas

- 2 minced garlic cloves
- ½ c. Chopped broccoli
- 1 tablespoon Minced ginger
- 1 tablespoon Rice vinegar
- 1 ½ teaspoon Toasted sesame oil
- 2 tablespoon Reduced-sodium soy sauce
- 3 c. Riced cauliflower

Directions:

1. Crumble tofu in a large bowl and toss with all the round one ingredient.
2. Preheat the air fryer oven to 370 degrees, place the baking dish in the air fryer oven cooking basket, set temperature to 370°f, and set

time to 10 minutes and cook 10 minutes, making sure to shake once.

3. In another bowl, toss ingredients from round 2 together.
4. Add round 2 mixture to air fryer and cook another 10 minutes, ensuring to shake 5 minutes in.

Nutrition:

Calories 67 | Fat 8g | Protein 3g

162. Air Fried Carrots, Yellow Squash & Zucchini

⏱ Prep Time 5 m | ⏱ Cooking Time 35 m | 4 Servings | Intermediate Recipe

Ingredients:

- 1 tablespoon Chopped tarragon leaves
- ½ teaspoon White pepper
- 1 teaspoon Salt
- 1 pound yellow squash

- 1 pound zucchini
- 6 teaspoon Olive oil
- ½ pound carrots

Directions:

1. Stem and root the end of squash and zucchini and cut in ¾-inch half-moons. Peel and cut carrots into 1-inch cubes. Combine carrot cubes with 2 teaspoons of olive oil, tossing to combine.
2. Pour into the air fryer oven basket, set temperature to 400°f, and set time to 5 minutes. As carrots cook, drizzle remaining olive oil

over squash and zucchini pieces, then season with pepper and salt. Toss well to coat.

3. Add squash and zucchini when the timer for carrots goes off. Cook 30 minutes, making sure to toss 2-3 times during the cooking process. Once done, take out veggies and toss with tarragon. Serve up warm.

Nutrition:

Calories 122 | Fat 9g | Protein 6g

163. Brown Rice, Spinach and Tofu Frittata

⏱ Prep Time 5 m | ⏱ Cooking Time 55 m | 4 Servings | Intermediate Recipe

Ingredients:

- ½ cup baby spinach, chopped
- ½ cup kale, chopped
- ½ onion, chopped
- ½ teaspoon turmeric
- 1 ¾ cups brown rice, cooked
- 1 flax egg (1 tablespoon flaxseed meal + 3 tablespoon cold water) 1 package firm tofu
- 1 tablespoon olive oil
- 1 yellow pepper, chopped

- 2 tablespoons soy sauce
- 2 teaspoons arrowroot powder
- 2 teaspoons Dijon mustard
- 2/3 cup almond milk
- 3 big mushrooms, chopped
- 3 tablespoons nutritional yeast
- 4 cloves garlic, crushed
- 4 spring onions, chopped
- A handful of basil leaves, chopped

Directions:

1. Preheat the air fryer oven to 375°f. Grease a pan that will fit inside the air fryer oven.
2. Prepare the frittata crust by mixing the brown rice and flax egg. Press the rice onto the baking dish until you form a crust. Brush with a little oil and cook for 10 minutes.
3. Meanwhile, heat olive oil in a skillet over medium flame and sauté the garlic and onions for 2 minutes.
4. Add the pepper and mushroom and continue stirring for 3 minutes.

5. Stir in the kale, spinach, spring onions, and basil. Remove from the pan and set aside.
6. In a food processor, pulse together the tofu, mustard, turmeric, soy sauce, nutritional yeast, vegan milk and arrowroot powder. Pour in a mixing bowl and stir in the sautéed vegetables.
7. Pour the vegan frittata mixture over the rice crust and cook in the air fryer oven for 40 minutes.

Nutrition:

Calories 226 | Fat 8.5g | Protein 10.6g

164. Instant Brussels sprouts With Balsamic Oil

⏰ Prep Time 5 m | ⏱ Cooking Time 15 m | 4 Servings | Basic Recipe

Ingredients:

- ¼ teaspoon salt
- 1 tablespoon balsamic vinegar
- 2 cups Brussels sprouts, halved
- Tablespoons olive oil

Directions:

1. Preheat the air fryer oven for 5 minutes.
2. Mix all ingredients in a bowl until the zucchini fries are well coated.
3. Place in the air fryer oven basket.
4. Close and cook for 15 minutes for 350°f.

Nutrition:

Calories 82 | Fat 6.8g| Protein 1.5g

165. Cheesy Cauliflower Fritters

⏰ Prep Time 10 m | ⏱ Cooking Time 7 m | 8 Servings | Basic Recipe

Ingredients:

- ½ c. Chopped parsley
- 1 c. Italian breadcrumbs
- 1/3 c. Shredded mozzarella cheese
- 1/3 c. Shredded sharp cheddar cheese
- 1 egg
- 2 minced garlic cloves
- 3 chopped scallions
- 1 head of cauliflower

Directions:

1. Cut cauliflower up into florets. Wash well and pat dry. Place into a food processor and pulse 20-30 seconds till it looks like rice. Place cauliflower rice in a bowl and mix with pepper, salt, egg, cheeses, breadcrumbs, garlic, and scallions.
2. With hands, form 15 patties of the mixture. Add more breadcrumbs if needed. With olive oil, spritz patties, and place into your air fryer oven basket in a single layer. Set temperature to 390°f, and set time to 7 minutes, flipping after 7 minutes.

Nutrition:

Calories 209 | Fat 17g | Protein 6g | Sugar 0.5

166. Delicious Buttered Carrot-Zucchini with Mayo

⏰ Prep Time 10 m | ⏱ Cooking Time 25 m | 4 Servings | Basic Recipe

Ingredients:

- 1 tablespoon grated onion
- 2 tablespoons butter, melted
- 1/2-pound carrots, sliced
- 1-1/2 zucchinis, sliced
- 1/4 cup water
- 1/4 cup mayonnaise
- 1/4 teaspoon prepared horseradish
- 1/4 teaspoon salt
- 1/4 teaspoon ground black pepper
- 1/4 cup Italian bread crumbs

Directions:

1. Lightly grease baking pan of air fryer with cooking spray. Add carrots. For 8 minutes, cook on 360°f.
2. Add zucchini and continue cooking for another 5 minutes. Meanwhile, in a bowl whisk well pepper, salt, horseradish, onion, mayonnaise, and water. Pour into pan of veggies. Toss well to coat.
3. In a small bowl mix melted butter and bread crumbs. Sprinkle over veggies.
4. Pour into the oven rack/basket. Place the rack on the middle-shelf of the air fryer oven.
5. Set temperature to 490°f, and set time to 10 minutes until tops are lightly browned.
6. Serve and enjoy.

Nutrition:

Calories 223 | Fat 17g | Protein 2.7g | Sugar 0.5

167. Yummy Cheddar, Squash and Zucchini Casserole

⏰ Prep Time 5 m | ⏱ Cooking Time 30 m | 4 Servings | Intermediate Recipe

Ingredients:

- 1 egg
- 5 saltine crackers, or as needed, crushed
- 2 tablespoons bread crumbs
- 1/2-pound yellow squash, sliced
- 1/2-pound zucchini, sliced
- 1/2 cup shredded cheddar cheese
- 1-1/2 teaspoons white sugar
- 1/2 teaspoon salt
- 1/4 onion, diced
- 1/4 cup biscuit baking mix
- 1/4 cup butter

Directions:

1. Lightly grease baking pan of air fryer with cooking spray.
2. Add onion, zucchini, and yellow squash.
3. Cover pan with foil and for 15 minutes, cook on 360° f or until tender.
4. Stir in salt, sugar, egg, butter, baking mix, and cheddar cheese.
5. Mix well. Fold in crushed crackers. Top with bread crumbs.
6. Cook for 15 minutes at 390° f until tops are lightly browned.
7. Serve and enjoy.

Nutrition:

Calories 285 | Fat 20.5g | Protein 8.6g

168. Zucchini Parmesan Chips

⏱ Prep Time 10 m | ⏱ Cooking Time 8 m | 10 Servings | Basic Recipe

Ingredients:

- ½ teaspoon Paprika
- ½ c. Grated parmesan cheese
- ½ c. Italian breadcrumbs
- 1 lightly beaten egg
- 2 thinly sliced zucchinis

Directions:

1. Use a very sharp knife or mandolin slicer to slice zucchini as thinly as you can. Pat off extra moisture.
2. Beat egg with a pinch of pepper and salt and a bit of water.
3. Combine paprika, cheese, and breadcrumbs in a bowl.
4. Dip slices of zucchini into the egg mixture and then into breadcrumb mixture. Press gently to coat.
5. With olive oil cooking spray, mist coated zucchini slices. Place into your air fryer oven basket in a single layer. Set temperature to 350°f, and set time to 8 minutes.
6. Sprinkle with salt and serve with salsa.

Nutrition:

Calories 211 | Fat 16g | Protein 8g | Sugar 0g

169. Jalapeño Cheese Balls

⏱ Prep Time 10 m | ⏱ Cooking Time 8 m | 12 Servings | Basic Recipe

Ingredients:

- 4 ounces cream cheese
- 1/3 Cup shredded mozzarella cheese
- 1/3 Cup shredded cheddar cheese
- 2 jalapeños, finely chopped
- ½ cup bread crumbs
- 2 eggs
- ½ cup all-purpose flour
- Salt
- Pepper
- Cooking oil

Directions:

1. In a medium bowl, combine the cream cheese, mozzarella, cheddar, and jalapeños. Mix well.
2. Form the cheese mixture into balls about an inch thick. Using a small ice cream scoop works well.
3. Arrange the cheese balls on a sheet pan and place in the freezer for 15 minutes. This will help the cheese balls maintain their shape while frying.
4. Spray the air fryer oven basket with cooking oil. Place the bread crumbs in a small bowl. In another small bowl, beat the eggs. In a third small bowl, combine the flour with salt and pepper to taste, and mix well. Remove the cheese balls from the freezer. Dip the cheese balls in the flour, then the eggs, and then the bread crumbs.
5. Place the cheese balls in the air fryer. Spray with cooking oil. Set temperature to 360°f. Cook for 8 minutes.
6. Open the air fryer oven and flip the cheese balls. I recommend flipping them instead of shaking so the balls maintain their form. Cook an additional 4 minutes. Cool before serving.

Nutrition:

Calories 96 | Fat 6g | Protein 4g | Sugar 0g

170. Crispy Roasted Broccoli

⏱ Prep Time 10 m | ⏱ Cooking Time 8 m | 2 Servings | Basic Recipe

Ingredients:

- ¼ teaspoon Masala
- ½ teaspoon Red chili powder
- ½ teaspoon Salt
- ¼ teaspoon Turmeric powder
- 1 tablespoon Chickpea flour
- 2 tablespoon Yogurt
- 1 pound broccoli

Directions:

1. Cut broccoli up into florets. Soak in a bowl of water with 2 teaspoons of salt for at least half an hour to remove impurities.
2. Take out broccoli florets from water and let drain. Wipe down thoroughly.
3. Mix all other ingredients together to create a marinade.
4. Toss broccoli florets in the marinade. Cover and chill 15-30 minutes.
5. Preheat the air fryer oven to 390 degrees.
6. Place marinated broccoli florets into the fryer basket, set temperature to 350°f, and set time to 10 minutes.
7. Florets will be crispy when done.

Nutrition:

Calories 96 | Fat 1.3g | Protein 7g | Sugar 4.5g

171. Coconut Battered Cauliflower Bites

⏰ Prep Time 5 m | ⏰ Cooking Time 20 m | 4 Servings |Basic Recipe

Ingredients:

- Salt and pepper to taste
- 1 flax egg (1 tablespoon flaxseed meal + 3 tablespoon water) 1 small cauliflower, cut into florets
- 1 teaspoon mixed spice
- ½ teaspoon mustard powder
- 2 tablespoons maple syrup

- 1 clove of garlic, minced
- 2 tablespoonssoy sauce
- 1/3 cupoatsflour
- 1/3 cup plain flour
- 1/3 cup desiccated coconut

Directions:

1. Preheat the air fryer oven to 400°f. In a mixing bowl, mix together oats, flour, and desiccated coconut. Season with salt and pepper to taste. Set aside.
2. In another bowl, place the flax egg and add a pinch of salt to taste. Set aside. Season the cauliflower with mixed spice and mustard powder. Dredge the florets in the flax egg first then in the flour mixture. Place inside the air fryer oven and cook for 15 minutes.

Meanwhile, place the maple syrup, garlic, and soy sauce in a sauce pan and heat over medium flame. Bring to a boil and adjust the heat to low until the sauce thickens. After 15 minutes, take out the florets from the air fryer and place them in the saucepan. Toss to coat the florets and place inside the air fryer and cook for another 5 minutes.

Nutrition: Calories 154| Fat 2.3g |Protein 4.69g

172. Creamy and Cheese Broccoli Bake

⏰ Prep Time 5 m | ⏰ Cooking Time 30 m | 2 Servings |Intermediate Recipe

Ingredients:

- 1-pound fresh broccoli, coarsely chopped
- 2 tablespoons all-purpose flour
- Salt to taste
- 1 tablespoon dry bread crumbs, or to taste
- 1/2 large onion, coarsely chopped

- 1/2 (14 ounce) can evaporated milk, divided
- 1/2 cup cubed sharp cheddar cheese
- 1-1/2 teaspoons butter, or to taste
- 1/4 cup water

Directions:

1. Lightly grease baking pan of air fryer with cooking spray.
2. Mix in half of the milk and flour in pan and for 5 minutes, cook on 360°f.
3. Halfway through cooking time, mix well.
4. Add broccoli and remaining milk.
5. Mix well and cook for another 5 minutes.
6. Stir in cheese and mix well until melted.
7. In a small bowl mix well, butter and bread crumbs.
8. Sprinkle on top of broccoli.
9. Place the baking pan in the air fryer oven. Cook for 20 minutes at 360°f until tops are lightly browned.

Nutrition: Calories 444| Fat 22.3g|Protein 23g

173. Crispy Jalapeno Coins

⏰ Prep Time 10 m | ⏰ Cooking Time 5 m | 2 Servings |Basic Recipe

Ingredients:

- 1 egg
- 2-3 tablespoon Coconut flour
- 1 sliced and seeded jalapeno
- Pinch of garlic powder

- Pinch of onion powder
- Pinch of Cajun seasoning (optional)
- Pinch of pepper and salt

Directions:

1. Ensure your air fryer oven is preheated to 400 degrees.
2. Mix together all dry ingredients.
3. Pat jalapeno slices dry. Dip coins into egg wash and then into dry mixture. Toss to thoroughly coat.
4. Add coated jalapeno slices to air fryer basket in a singular layer. Spray with olive oil.
5. Set temperature to 350°f, and set time to 5 minutes. Cook just till crispy.

Nutrition: Calories 128| Fat 8g |Protein 7g | Sugar 0g

174. Buffalo Cauliflower

⏰ Prep Time 5 m | ⏰ Cooking Time 15 m | 2 Servings |Basic Recipe

Ingredients:

- Cauliflower:
- 1 c. Panko breadcrumbs
- 1 teaspoon Salt
- 4 c. Cauliflower florets

- Buffalo coating:
- ¼ c. Vegan buffalo sauce
- ¼ c. Melted vegan butter

Directions:

1. Melt butter in microwave and whisk in buffalo sauce.
2. Dip each cauliflower floret into buffalo mixture, ensuring it gets coated well.
3. Hold over a bowl till floret is done dripping.
4. Mix breadcrumbs with salt.
5. Dredge dipped florets into breadcrumbs and place into air fryer basket.
6. Set temperature to 350°f, and set time to 15 minutes. When slightly browned, they are ready to eat!
7. Serve with your favorite keto dipping sauce.

Nutrition: Calories 194| Fat 17g | Protein 10g | Sugar 3

175. Smoked Beef Burgers

⏰ Prep Time 10 m | ⏱ Cooking Time 10 m | 4 Servings | Basic Recipe

Ingredients:

- 1 ¼ pounds lean ground beef
- 1 tablespoon soy sauce
- 1 teaspoon Dijon mustard
- A few dashes of liquid smoke
- 1 teaspoon shallot powder
- 1 clove garlic, minced
- 1/2 teaspoon cumin powder
- 1/4 cup scallions, minced
- 1/3 teaspoon sea salt flakes
- 1/3 teaspoon freshly cracked mixed peppercorns
- 1 teaspoon celery seeds
- 1 teaspoon parsley flakes

Directions:

1. Mix all of the above ingredients in a bowl; knead until everything is well incorporated.
2. Shape the mixture into four patties. Next, make a shallow dip in the center of each patty to prevent them puffing up during air-frying.
3. Spritz the patties on all sides using a non-stick cooking spray. Cook approximately 12 minutes at 360 degrees F.
4. Check for doneness – an instant read thermometer should read 160 degrees F. Bon appétit!

Nutrition:

167 Calories | 5.5g Fat | 1.4g Carbs | 26.4g Protein | 0g Sugars | 0.4g Fiber

176. Spicy Holiday Roast Beef

⏰ Prep Time 15 m | ⏱ Cooking Time 45 m | 2 Servings | Basic Recipe

Ingredients:

- 2 pounds roast beef, at room temperature
- 2 tablespoons extra-virgin olive oil
- 1 teaspoon sea salt flakes
- 1 teaspoon black pepper, preferably freshly ground
- 1 teaspoon smoked paprika
- A few dashes of liquid smoke
- 2 jalapeño peppers, thinly sliced

Directions:

1. Start by preheating the Air Fryer to 330 degrees F. Then, pat the roast dry using kitchen towels. Rub with extra-virgin olive oil and all seasonings along with liquid smoke.
2. Roast for 30 minutes in the preheated Air Fryer; then, pause the machine and turn the roast over; roast for additional 15 minutes.
3. Check for doneness using a meat thermometer and serve sprinkled with sliced jalapeños. Bon appétit!

Nutrition:

243 Calories | 10.6g Fat | 0.4g Carbs | 34.5g Protein

177. Rich Beef and Sausage Meatloaf

⏰ Prep Time 15 m | ⏱ Cooking Time 25 m | 4 Servings | Basic Recipe

Ingredients:

- 3/4 pound ground chuck
- 1/4 pound ground pork sausage
- 1 cup shallot, finely chopped
- 2 eggs, well beaten
- 3 tablespoons plain milk
- 1 tablespoon oyster sauce
- 1 teaspoon porcini mushrooms
- 1/2 teaspoon cumin powder
- 1 teaspoon garlic paste
- 1 tablespoon fresh parsley
- Seasoned salt and crushed red pepper flakes, to taste
- 1 cup parmesan cheese, grated

Directions:

1. Simply place all ingredients in a large-sized mixing dish; mix until everything is thoroughly combined.
2. Press the meatloaf mixture into the Air Fryer baking dish; set your Air Fryer to cook at 360 degrees F for 25 minutes. Press the power button and cook until heated through.
3. Check for doneness and serve with your favorite wine!

Nutrition:

206 Calories | 7.9g Fat | 15.9g Carbs | 17.6g Protein | 0.8g Sugars | 0.4g Fiber

178. Japanese Miso Steak

⏰ Prep Time 1 h | ⏱ Cooking Time 15 m | 4 Servings | Intermediate Recipe

Ingredients:

- 1 ¼ pounds flank steak
- 1 ½ tablespoons sake
- 1 tablespoon brown miso paste
- 2 garlic cloves, pressed
- 1 tablespoon olive oil

Directions:

1. Place all the ingredients in a sealable food bag; shake until completely coated and place in your refrigerator for at least 1 hour.
2. Then, spritz the steak with a non-stick cooking spray; make sure to coat on all sides. Place the steak in the Air Fryer baking pan.
3. Set your Air Fryer to cook at 400 degrees F. Roast for 12 minutes, flipping twice. Serve immediately.

Nutrition:

367 Calories | 15.1g Fat | 6.4g Carbs | 48.6g Protein | 3.4g Sugars | 0.3g Fiber

179. Classic Keto Cheeseburgers

⏰ Prep Time 10 m | ⏰ Cooking Time 15 m | 4 Servings | Basic Recipe

Ingredients:

- 1 ½ pounds ground chuck
- 1 envelope onion soup mix
- Kosher salt and freshly ground black pepper, to taste
- 1 teaspoon paprika
- 4 slices Monterey-Jack cheese

Directions:

1. In a mixing dish, thoroughly combine ground chuck, onion soup mix, salt, black pepper, and paprika.
2. Then, set your Air Fryer to cook at 385 degrees F. Shape the mixture into 4 patties. Air-fry them for 10 minutes.
3. Next step, place the slices of cheese on the top of the warm burgers. Air-fry for one minute more.
4. Serve with mustard and pickled salad of choice. Bon appétit!

Nutrition:

271 Calories | 13.3g Fat | 21.9g Carbs | 15.3g Protein | 2.9g Sugars | 0.2g Fiber

180. Beef Steaks with Mediterranean Herbs

⏰ Prep Time 5 m | ⏰ Cooking Time 25 m | 4 Servings | Intermediate Recipe

Ingredients:

- 2 tablespoons soy sauce
- 3 heaping tablespoons fresh chives
- 2 tablespoons olive oil
- 3 tablespoons dry white wine
- 4 small-sized beef steaks
- 2 teaspoons smoked cayenne pepper
- 1/2 teaspoon dried basil
- 1/2 teaspoon dried rosemary
- 1 teaspoon freshly ground pepper
- 1 teaspoon sea salt, or more to taste

Directions:

1. Firstly, coat the steaks with the cayenne pepper, black pepper, salt, basil, and rosemary.
2. Drizzle the steaks with olive oil, white wine, soy sauce, and honey.
3. Finally, roast in an Air Fryer basket for 20 minutes at 335 degrees F. Serve garnished with fresh chives. Bon appétit!

Nutrition:

445 Calories | 23.7g Fat | 11.3g Carbs | 51.1g Protein | 10.3g Sugars | 0.7g Fiber

181. Japanese Beef with Broccoli

⏰ Prep Time 40 m | ⏰ Cooking Time 15 m | 4 Servings | Intermediate Recipe

Ingredients:

- ½ had broccoli, broken into florets
- 1/3 cup keto teriyaki marinade
- Fine sea salt and ground black pepper, to taste
- ½ pound rump steak
- 2 red capsicums, sliced
- 1 ½ teaspoons sesame oil

Directions:

1. Add rump roast and teriyaki marinade to a mixing dish; stir to coat. Let it marinate for about 40 minutes.
2. Then, roast in the preheated Air Fryer for 13 minutes at 395 degrees F. Stir halfway through cooking time.
3. Meanwhile, sauté the broccoli in the hot sesame oil along with sliced capsicum; cook until tender and season with salt and pepper to savor.
4. Place the prepared rump steak on a serving platter and serve garnished with sautéed broccoli. Bon appétit!

Nutrition:

220 Calories | 12.4g Fat | 8.3g Carbs | 19.8g Protein | 4.4g Sugars | 1.4g Fiber

182. The Best Minute Steaks

⏰ Prep Time 3 h | ⏰ Cooking Time 15 m | 4 Servings | Intermediate Recipe

Ingredients:

- 1 1/2 tablespoons extra-virgin olive oil
- 1/2 cup herb vinegar
- 1/3 teaspoon celery seed
- 4 minute steaks
- 1 teaspoon salt
- 2 teaspoons cayenne pepper
- 1/3 teaspoon ground black pepper, or to taste

Directions:

1. Toss all ingredients in a mixing dish. Cover the dish and marinate the steaks in the refrigerator for about 3 hours.
2. Finally, cook minute steaks for 13 minutes at 355 degrees F. Eat warm with your favorite salad and French fries. Bon appétit!

Nutrition:

296 Calories | 14g Fat | 6.7g Carbs | 36.5g Protein | 0.6g Sugars | 0.3g Fiber

183. Almond and Caraway Crust Steak
Prep Time 10 m | Cooking Time 10 m | 4 Servings | Intermediate Recipe

Ingredients:
- 1/3 cup almond flour
- 2 eggs
- 2 teaspoons caraway seeds
- 4 beef steaks
- 2 teaspoons garlic powder
- 1 tablespoon melted butter
- Fine sea salt and cayenne pepper, to taste

Directions:
1. Generously coat steaks with garlic powder, caraway seeds, salt, and cayenne pepper.
2. In a mixing dish, thoroughly combine melted butter with seasoned crumbs. In another bowl, beat the eggs until they're well whisked.
3. First, coat steaks with the beaten egg; then, coat beef steaks with the buttered crumb mixture.
4. Place the steaks in the Air Fryer cooking basket; cook for 10 minutes at 355 degrees F. Bon appétit!

Nutrition:
474 Calories | 22.1g Fat | 8.7g Carbs | 54.7g Protein | 1.6g Sugars | 0.6g Fiber

184. Spicy Mexican Beef with Cotija Cheese
Prep Time 15 m | Cooking Time 15 m | 6 Servings | Intermediate Recipe

Ingredients:
- 3 eggs, whisked
- 1/3 cup finely grated cotija cheese
- 1 cup parmesan cheese
- 6 minute steaks
- 2 tablespoons Mexican spice blend
- 1 ½ tablespoons olive oil
- Fine sea salt and ground black pepper, to taste

Directions:
1. Begin by sprinkling minute steaks with Mexican spice blend, salt and pepper.
2. Take a mixing dish and thoroughly combine the oil, cotija cheese, and parmesan cheese. In a separate mixing dish, beat the eggs.
3. Firstly, dip minute steaks in the egg; then, dip them in the cheese mixture.
4. Air-fry for 15 minutes at 345 degrees F; work in batches. Bon appétit!

Nutrition:
397 Calories | 23g Fat | 3.5g Carbs | 41.2g Protein | 0.4g Sugars | 0g Fiber

185. Top Chuck with Mustard and Herbs
Prep Time 10 m | Cooking Time 50 m | 3 Servings | Basic Recipe

Ingredients:
- 1 ½ pounds top chuck
- 2 teaspoons olive oil
- 1 tablespoon Dijon mustard
- Sea salt and ground black pepper, to taste
- 1 teaspoon dried marjoram
- 1 teaspoon dried thyme
- 1/2 teaspoon fennel seeds

Directions:
1. Start by preheating your Air Fryer to 380 degrees F
2. Add all ingredients in a Ziploc bag; shake to mix well. Next, spritz the bottom of the Air Fryer basket with cooking spray.
3. Place the beef in the cooking basket and cook for 50 minutes, turning every 10 to 15 minutes.
4. Let it rest for 5 to 7 minutes before slicing and serving. Enjoy!

Nutrition:
406 Calories | 24.1g Fat | 0.3g Carbs | 44.1g Protein

186. Mediterranean Herbed Beef with Zucchini
Prep Time 6 m | Cooking Time 12 m | 4 Servings | Intermediate Recipe

Ingredients:
- 1 ½ pounds beef steak
- 1 pound zucchini
- 1 teaspoon dried rosemary
- 1 teaspoon dried basil
- 1 teaspoon dried oregano
- 2 tablespoons extra-virgin olive oil
- 2 tablespoons fresh chives, chopped

Directions:
1. Start by preheating your Air Fryer to 400 degrees F.
2. Toss the steak and zucchini with the spices and olive oil. Transfer to the cooking basket and cook for 6 minutes.
3. Now, shale the basket and cook another 6 minutes. Serve immediately garnished with fresh chives. Enjoy!

Nutrition:
396 Calories | 20.4g Fat | 3.5g Carbs | 47.8g Protein | 0.1g Sugars | 1.5g Fiber

187. Italian Peperonata with a Twist

⏲ Prep Time 15 m | ⏲ Cooking Time 30 m | 4 Servings | Intermediate Recipe

Ingredients:

- 2 teaspoons canola oil
- 2 bell peppers, sliced
- 1 green bell pepper, sliced
- 1 Serrano pepper, sliced
- 1 shallot, sliced
- Sea salt and pepper, to taste

- 1/2 dried thyme
- 1 teaspoon dried rosemary
- 1/2 teaspoon mustard seeds
- 1 teaspoon fennel seeds
- 2 pounds thin beef parboiled sausage

Directions:

1. Brush the sides and bottom of the cooking basket with 1 teaspoon of canola oil. Add the peppers and shallot to the cooking basket.
2. Toss them with the spices and cook at 390 degrees F for 15 minutes, shaking the basket occasionally. Reserve.
3. Turn the temperature to 380 degrees F
4. Then, add the remaining 1 teaspoon of oil. Once hot, add the sausage and cook in the preheated Air Frye for 15 minutes, flipping them halfway through the cooking time.
5. Serve with reserved pepper mixture. Bon appétit!

Nutrition:

563 Calories | 41.5g Fat | 10.6g Carbs | 35.6g Protein | 7.9g Sugars | 1g Fiber

188. Duo Crisp Chicken Wings

⏲ Prep Time 10 m | ⏲ Cooking Time 18 m | 6 Servings

Ingredients:

- 12 chicken vignettes
- 1/2 cup chicken broth

- Salt and black pepper to taste
- 1/4 cup melted butter

Directions:

1. Set a metal rack in the Instant Pot Duo Crisp and pour broth into it.
2. Place the wingettes on the metal rack then put on its pressure-cooking lid.
3. Hit the "Pressure Button" and select 8 minutes of cooking time, then press "Start."
4. Once the Instant Pot Duo beeps, do a quick release and remove its lid.
5. Transfer the pressure cooked wingettes to a plate.
6. Empty the pot and set an Air Fryer Basket in the Instant Pot Duo
7. Toss the wingettes with butter and seasoning.
8. Spread the seasoned wingettes in the Air Fryer Basket.
9. Put on the Air Fryer lid and hit the Air fryer Button, then set the time to 10 minutes.
10. Remove the lid and serve.
11. Enjoy!

Nutrition:

Calories 246 Fat 18.9g Cholesterol 115mg Carbo 0g Fiber 0g Sugars 0g Protein 20.2g

189. Italian Whole Chicken

⏲ Prep Time 10 m | ⏲ Cooking Time 35 m | 4 Servings

Ingredients:

- 1 whole chicken
- 2 tablespoon or spray of oil of choice
- 1 teaspoon garlic powder
- 1 teaspoon onion powder

- 1 teaspoon paprika
- 1 teaspoon Italian seasoning 2 tablespoon Montreal steak seasoning 1.5 cup chicken broth

Directions:

1. Whisk all the seasoning in a bowl and rub it on the chicken.
2. Set a metal rack in the Instant Pot Duo Crisp and pour broth into it.
3. Place the chicken on the metal rack then put on its pressure-cooking lid.
4. Hit the "Pressure Button" and select 25 minutes of cooking time, then press "Start."
5. Once the Instant Pot Duo beeps, do a natural release and remove its lid.
6. Transfer the pressure-cooked chicken to a plate.
7. Empty the pot and set an Air Fryer Basket in the Instant Pot Duo.
8. Toss the chicken pieces with oil to coat well.
9. Spread the seasoned chicken in the air Fryer Basket.
10. Put on the Air Fryer lid and hit the Air fryer Button, then set the time to 10 minutes.
11. Remove the lid and serve.
12. Enjoy!

Nutrition:

Calories 163 Fat 10.7g Cholesterol 33mg Sodium 1439mg Carbo 1.8g Fiber 0.3g Protein 12.6g

190. Chicken Pot Pie

⏲ Prep Time 10 m | ⏲ Cooking Time 17 m | 6 Servings

Ingredients:

- 2 tbsp. olive oil
- 1-pound chicken breast cubed
- 1 tbsp. garlic powder
- 1 tbsp. thyme
- 1 tbsp. pepper
- 1 cup chicken broth

- 12 oz. bag frozen mixed vegetables
- 4 large potatoes cubed
- 10 oz. Can cream of chicken soup
- 1 cup heavy cream
- 1 pie crust
- 1 egg 1 tbsp. water

Directions:

1. Hit Sauté on the Instant Pot Duo Crispy and add chicken and olive oil.
2. Sauté chicken for 5 minutes then stir in spices.
3. Pour in the broth along with vegetables and cream of chicken soup
4. Put on the pressure-cooking lid and seal it.
5. Hit the "Pressure Button" and select 10 minutes of cooking time, then press "Start."
6. Once the Instant Pot Duo beeps, do a quick release and remove its lid.
7. Remove the lid and stir in cream.
8. Hit sauté and cook for 2 minutes.
9. Enjoy!

Nutrition:

Calories 568 Fat 31.1g Cholesterol 95mg Sodium 1111mg Carbo 50.8g Fiber 3.9g Protein 23.4g

191. Chicken Casserole

⏲ Prep Time 10 m | ⏲ Cooking Time 9 m | 6 Servings

Ingredients:

- 3 cup chicken, shredded
- 12 oz. bag egg noodles
- 1/2 large onion
- 1/2 cup chopped carrots
- 1/4 cup frozen peas
- 1/4 cup frozen broccoli pieces
- 2 stalks celery chopped

- 5 cup chicken broth
- 1 teaspoon garlic powder
- Salt and pepper to taste
- 1 cup cheddar cheese, shredded
- 1 package French's onions
- 1/4 c sour cream
- 1 can cream of chicken and mushroom soup

Directions:

1. Add chicken, broth, black pepper, salt, garlic powder, vegetables, and egg noodles to the Instant Pot Duo.
2. Put on the pressure-cooking lid and seal it.
3. Hit the "Pressure Button" and select 4 minutes of cooking time, then press "Start."
4. Once the Instant Pot Duo beeps, do a quick release and remove its lid.
5. Stir in cheese, 1/3 of French's onions, can of soup and sour cream.
6. Mix well and spread the remaining onion top.
7. Put on the Air Fryer lid and seal it.
8. Hit the "Air fryer Button" and select 5 minutes of cooking time, then press "Start."
9. Once the Instant Pot Duo beeps, remove its lid.
10. Serve.

Nutrition:

Calories 494 Fat 19.1g Cholesterol 142mg Sodium 1233mg Carbo 29g Fiber 2.6g Protein 48.9g

192. Ranch Chicken Wings

⏲ Prep Time 10 m | ⏲ Cooking Time 35 m | 6 Servings

Ingredients:

- 12 chicken wings
- 1 tablespoon olive oil
- 1 cup chicken broth
- 1/4 cup butter
- 1/2 cup Red Hot Sauce
- 1/4 teaspoon Worcestershire sauce

- 1 tablespoon white vinegar
- 1/4 teaspoon cayenne pepper
- 1/8 teaspoon garlic powder
- Seasoned salt to taste
- Ranch dressing for dipping Celery for garnish

Directions:

1. Set the Air Fryer Basket in the Instant Pot Duo and pour the broth in it.
2. Spread the chicken wings in the basket and put on the pressure-cooking lid.
3. Hit the "Pressure Button" and select 10 minutes of cooking time, then press "Start."
4. Meanwhile, Preparation are the sauce and add butter, vinegar, cayenne pepper, garlic powder, Worcestershire sauce, and hot sauce in a small saucepan.
5. Stir cook this sauce for 5 minutes on medium heat until it thickens.
6. Once the Instant Pot Duo beeps, do a quick release and remove its lid.
7. Remove the wings and empty the Instant Pot Duo.
8. Toss the wings with oil, salt, and black pepper.
9. Set the Air Fryer Basket in the Instant Pot Duo and arrange the wings in it.
10. Put on the Air Fryer lid and seal it.
11. Hit the "Air Fryer Button" and select 20 minutes of cooking time, then press "Start."
12. Once the Instant Pot Duo beeps, remove its lid.
13. Transfer the wings to the sauce and mix well.
14. Serve.

Nutrition:

Calories 414 Fat 31.6g Cholesterol 98mg Sodium 568mg Carbo 11.2g Fiber 0.3g Protein 20.4g

193. Chicken Mac and Cheese
Prep Time 10 m | Cooking Time 9 m | 6 Servings

Ingredients:

- 2 1/2 cup macaroni
- 2 cup chicken stock
- 1 cup cooked chicken, shredded
- 1 1/4 cup heavy cream
- 8 tablespoon butter
- 2 2/3 cups cheddar cheese, shredded
- 1/3 cup parmesan cheese, shredded
- 1 bag Ritz crackers
- 1/4 teaspoon garlic powder
- Salt and pepper to taste

Directions:

1. Add chicken stock, heavy cream, chicken, 4 tablespoon butter, and macaroni to the Instant Pot Duo.
2. Put on the pressure-cooking lid and seal it.
3. Hit the "Pressure Button" and select 4 minutes of cooking time, then press "Start."
4. Crush the crackers and mix them well with 4 tablespoons melted butter.
5. Once the Instant Pot Duo beeps, do a quick release and remove its lid.
6. Put on the Air Fryer lid and seal it.
7. Hit the "Air Fryer Button" and select 5 minutes of cooking time, then press "Start."
8. Once the Instant Pot Duo beeps, remove its lid.
9. Serve.

Nutrition: Calories 611 Fat 43.6g Cholesterol 147mg Sodium 739mg Carbo 29.5g Fiber 1.2g Protein 25.4g

194. Broccoli Chicken Casserole
Prep Time 10 m | Cooking Time 22 m | 6 Servings

Ingredients:

- 1 1/2 lbs. chicken, cubed
- 2 teaspoon chopped garlic
- 2 tablespoon butter
- 1 1/2 cups chicken broth
- 1 1/2 cups long-grain rice
- 1 (10.75 oz.) can cream of chicken soup
- 2 cups broccoli florets
- 1 cup crushed Ritz cracker
- 2 tablespoon melted butter
- 2 cups shredded cheddar cheese

Directions:

1. Add 1 cup water to the Instant Pot Dup and place a basket in it.
2. Place the broccoli in the basket evenly.
3. Put on the pressure-cooking lid and seal it.
4. Hit the "Pressure Button" and select 1 minute of cooking time, then press "Start."
5. Once the Instant Pot Duo beeps, do a quick release and remove its lid.
6. Remove the broccoli and empty the Instant Pot Duo.
7. Hit the sauté button then add 2 tablespoon butter.
8. Toss in chicken and stir cook for 5 minutes, then add garlic and sauté for 30 seconds.
9. Stir in rice, chicken broth, and cream of chicken soup.
10. Put on the pressure-cooking lid and seal it.
11. Hit the "Pressure Button" and select 12 minutes of cooking time, then press "Start."
12. Once the Instant Pot Duo beeps, do a quick release and remove its lid.
13. Add cheese and broccoli, then mix well gently.
14. Toss the cracker with 2 tablespoon butter in a bowl and spread over the chicken in the Pot.
15. Put on the Air Fryer lid and seal it.
16. Hit the "Air Fryer Button" and select 4 minutes of cooking time, then press "Start."
17. Once the Instant Pot Duo beeps, remove its lid.
18. Serve.

Nutrition: Calories 609 Fat 24.4g Cholesterol 142mg Sodium 924mg Carbo.5g Fiber 1.4g Protein 49.2g

195. Chicken Tikka Kebab
Prep Time 10 m | Cooking Time 17 m | 4 Servings

Ingredients:

- 1 lb. Chicken thighs boneless skinless, cubed
- 1 tablespoon oil
- 1/2 cup red onion, cubed
- 1/2 cup green bell pepper, cubed
- 1/2 cup red bell pepper, cubed
- Lime wedges to garnish
- Onion rounds to garnish

For marinade:

- 1/2 cup yogurt Greek
- 3/4 tablespoon ginger, grated
- 3/4 tablespoon garlic, minced
- 1 tablespoon lime juice
- 2 teaspoon red chili powder mild
- 1/2 teaspoon ground turmeric
- 1 teaspoon garam masala
- 1 teaspoon coriander powder
- 1/2 tablespoon dried fenugreek leaves
- 1 teaspoon salt

Directions:

1. Prepare the marinade by mixing yogurt with all its **Ingredients:** in a bowl.
2. Fold in chicken, then mix well to coat and refrigerate for 8 hours.
3. Add bell pepper, onions, and oil to the marinade and mix well.
4. Thread the chicken, peppers, and onions on the skewers.
5. Set the Air Fryer Basket in the Instant Pot Duo.
6. Put on the Air Fryer lid and seal it.
7. Hit the "Air Fry Button" and select 10 minutes of cooking time, then press "Start."
8. Once the Instant Pot Duo beeps, and remove its lid.
9. Flip the skewers and continue Air frying for 7 minutes.

Nutrition:
Calories 241 Fat 14.2g Cholesterol 92mg Sodium 695mg Carbo 8.5g Fiber 1.6g Protein 21.8g

196. Bacon Cheddar Chicken Fingers
⏱ Prep Time 10 m | ⏱ Cooking Time 20 m | 4 Servings

Ingredients

For the chicken fingers:
- 1 lb. chicken tenders, about 8 pieces
- Cooking spray (canola oil)
- Cheddar cheese - 1 cup, shredded
- Two eggs, large
- 1/3 cup bacon bits
- 2 tbsp. water

For the breading:
- 1 tsp. of onion powder
- Panko breadcrumbs - 2 cups
- Black pepper - 1 tsp., freshly ground
- Paprika - 2 tbsp.
- Garlic powder - 1 tsp.
- Salt - 2 tsp.

Directions:
1. Set the air fryer to the temperature of 360°F.
2. In a glass dish, whip the water and eggs until combined.
3. Use a zip lock bag, shake the garlic powder, salt, breadcrumbs, cayenne, onion powder, and pepper together.
4. Immerse the chicken into the eggs and shake in the Ziploc bag until fully covered.
5. Dip again in the egg mixture and back into the seasonings until a thick coating is present.
6. Remove the tenders from the bag and set in the frying pan in the basket. Do them in batches if need to not over pack the pan.
7. Apply the canola oil spray to the top of the tenders and heat for 6 minutes.
8. Flip the tenders to the other side. Steam for another 4 minutes.
9. Blend the bacon bits and shredded cheese in a dish.
10. Evenly dust the bacon and cheese onto the hot tenders and fry for 2 more minutes.
11. Remove and serve while hot.

Nutrition: Calories: 341 Fat: 11g Cholesterol: 31.5g Fiber:1g Sodium:297mg Protein:28g

197. Battered Cod
⏱ Prep Time 10 m | ⏱ Cooking Time 30 m | 4 Servings

Ingredients
- Cod - 20 oz.
- Salt - 1/4 tsp.
- All-purpose flour - 8 oz.
- Parsley seasoning - 1 tbsp.
- Cornstarch - 3 tsp.
- Garlic powder - 1/2 tsp.
- Two eggs, preferably large
- Onion powder - 1/2 tsp.

Directions:
1. Whip the eggs in a glass dish until smooth and set to the side.
2. In a separate dish, blend the cornstarch, salt, almond flour, garlic powder, parsley, and onion powder, whisking to remove any lumpiness.
3. Immerse the pieces of cods into the egg and then into the spiced flour, covering completely.
4. Transfer to the fryer basket in a single layer.
5. Heat the fish for 7 minutes at a temperature of 350°F. Turn the cod over and steam for an additional 7 minutes.

Nutrition: Calories 245 Fat 11g Cholesterol: 31.5g Fiber: 1g Sodium: 297mg Protein: 28g

198. Beef Kabobs
⏱ Prep Time 10 m | ⏱ Cooking Time 30 m |Marinating Time 1 h |4 Kabos

Ingredients
- Low-fat sour cream - 1/3 cup
- One bell pepper
- 16 oz. of beef chuck ribs, boneless
- Soy sauce - 2 tbsp.
- 6-inch skewers - 8
- Pepper - 1/4 tsp.
- Medium onion - 1/2

Directions:
1. Slice the ribs into sections about 1-inch wide
2. In a lidded tub, combine the soy sauce, ribs and sour cream making sure the meat is fully covered.
3. Refrigerate for half an hour at least, if not overnight.
4. Immerse the wooden skewers for approximately 10 minutes in water.
5. Set the temperature of the air fryer to 400°F.
6. Slice the onion and bell pepper in 1-inch sections.
7. Remove the meat from the marinade, draining well.
8. Layer the onions, beef and bell peppers on the skewers and dust with pepper.
9. Heat for 10 minutes, ensuring you spin the skewers 5 minutes into cooking time.
10. Serve while hot and enjoy.

Nutrition: Calories: 261 Fat: 11g Cholesterol: 31.5g Fiber: 1g Sodium: 297mg Protein: 28g

199. Cheese Dogs
⏱ Prep Time 10 m | ⏱ Cooking Time 15 m | 4 Hot Dogs

Ingredients
- 4 hotdogs
- 1/4 cup your choice of cheese, grated
- 4 hotdog buns

Directions:
1. Adjust the air fryer to heat at a temperature of 390°F for approximately 5 minutes.
2. Set the hot dogs in the basket and broil for 5 minutes.
3. Remove and create the hot dog with the bun and cheese as desired and move back to the basket for another 2 minutes.
4. Remove and enjoy while hot.

Nutrition: Calories: 432 Fat: 11g Cholesterol: 31.5g Fiber: 1g Sodium: 297mg Protein: 28g

200. Cheeseburger Patties

⏱ Prep Time 10 m | ⏱ Cooking Time 20 m | 4 Servings

Ingredients

- Garlic - 1/2 clove, minced
- Ground beef - 1 1/3 cup
- Onion - 4 oz., diced
- Worcestershire sauce - 2 tbsp.
- One egg, large
- Panko breadcrumbs - 2 oz.
- Cayenne pepper - 1/8 tsp.
- Cooking spray (olive oil)
- Salt - 1/4 tsp.
- 4 slices of cheese of your choice
- 1/8 tsp. pepper

Directions:

1. Using a big glass dish, combine the diced onion, pepper, minced garlic, cayenne pepper, breadcrumbs, and salt until incorporated.
2. Blend the ground beef, Worcestershire sauce, and egg and integrate thoroughly by hand.
3. Form the meat into 4 individual patties and move to the air fryer basket.
4. Coat the patties with cooking spray.
5. Adjust the temperature for 375°F and heat for 8 minutes.
6. Turn the burgers over and steam for an additional 2 minutes.
7. Cover with a slice of cheese and continue cooking for approximately 3 minutes.
8. Enjoy as is or place on a bun with your favorite toppings.

Nutrition:

Calories: 367 Fat: 11g Cholesterol: 31.5g Fiber: 1g Sodium: 297mg Protein: 28g

201. Chicken Cordon Bleu

⏱ Prep Time 10 m | ⏱ Cooking Time 35 m | 4 Servings

Ingredients

- Pepper - 1/4 tsp.
- Chicken pail lards - 4
- Salt - 1/4 tsp.
- Swiss cheese - 8 slices
- All-purpose flour - 1/2 cup
- Parmesan cheese - 2/3 cup, grated
- Panko breadcrumbs - 1 1/2 cup
- Ham - 8 slices
- Two eggs, large
- Dijon mustard - 2 tbsp.
- 8 toothpicks
- Grapeseed oil spray

Directions:

1. On a section of baking lining, brush the Dijon mustard on each chicken pail lard and sprinkle with pepper and salt
2. Layer 1 cheese, 2 slices of the ham and then the additional slice of cheese on each of the pieces of chicken.
3. Rotate the chicken beginning with the longer side to create a roll. Fasten in place with two toothpicks.
4. Whip the egg in one dish, empty the flour into a second dish and blend the parmesan cheese and breadcrumbs into a third.
5. Immerse one chicken first in flour, secondly immerse in the egg and then roll the chicken completely in the breadcrumbs. Press the cheese and breadcrumbs into the chicken to secure and place onto a plate.
6. Repeat for the other pieces of chicken.
7. Apply the grape seed oil spray to each section of chicken and transfer to the air fryer basket after 5 minutes.
8. Set the air fryer temperature to heat at 350°.
9. Grill for 8 minutes and carefully turn the chicken to the other side. Heat for an additional 8 minutes.
10. Remove to a serving dish and wait approximately 5 minutes before serving hot.

Nutrition:

Calories: 548 Fat: 11g Cholesterol: 31.5g Fiber: 1g Sodium: 297mg Protein: 28g

202. Grilled Cheese Sandwich

⏱ Prep Time 10 m | ⏱ Cooking Time 10 m | 1 Servings

Ingredients

- 2 slices bread, softened
- 1 tsp. butter
- 2 slices cheddar cheese

Directions:

1. Set the air fryer at a temperature of 350°F.
2. Apply 1/2 teaspoon of the softened butter to one side of the slice of bread. Repeat for the remaining bread.
3. Create the sandwich by putting the cheese in between the non-buttered sides of bread.
4. Transfer to the hot air fryer and set for 5 minutes. Flip the sandwich at the halfway point and remove.
5. Serve immediately and enjoy.

Nutrition:

Calories: 378 Fat: 11g Cholesterol: 31.5g Fiber: 1g Sodium: 297mg Protein: 28g

203. Italian Meatballs

⏱ Prep Time 10 m | ⏱ Cooking Time 35 m | 3 Servings

Ingredients

- One egg, large
- Ground beef - 16 oz.
- Pepper - 1/8 tsp.
- Oregano seasoning - 1/2 tsp.
- Breadcrumbs - 1 1/4 cup
- Garlic - 1/2 clove, chopped
- Parsley - 1 oz., chopped
- Salt - 1/4 tsp.
- Parmigiano-Reggiano cheese - 1 oz. Cup, grated
- Cooking spray (avocado oil)

Directions:

1. Whisk the oregano, breadcrumbs, chopped garlic, and salt, chopped parsley, pepper, and grated Parmigiano-Reggiano cheese until combined.
2. Blend the ground beef and egg into the mixture using your hands. Incorporate the ingredients thoroughly.
3. Divide the meat into 12 sections and roll into rounds.
4. Coat the inside of the basket with avocado oil spray to grease.
5. Adjust the temperature to 350°F and heat for approximately 12 minutes.
6. Roll the meatballs over and steam for another 4 minutes and remove to a serving plate.
7. Enjoy as is or combine with your favorite pasta or sauce.

Nutrition:

Calories: 432 Fat: 11g Cholesterol: 31.5g Fiber: 1g Sodium: 297mg Protein: 28g

204. Loaded Baked Potatoes

⏱ Prep Time 10 m | ⏱ Cooking Time 25 m | 4 Servings

Ingredients

- 1/3 cup milk
- 2 oz. sour cream
- 1/3 cup white cheddar, grated
- 2 oz. Parmesan cheese, grated
- 1/8 tsp. garlic salt
- 6 oz. ham, diced
- 2 medium russet potatoes
- 4 oz. sharp cheddar, shredded
- 1/8 cup. Green onion, diced

Directions:

1. Puncture the potatoes deeply with a fork a few time and microwave for approximately 5 minutes. Flip them to the other side and nuke for an additional 5 minutes. The potatoes should be soft.
2. Use oven mitts to remove from the microwave and cut them in halves.
3. Spoon out the insides of the potatoes to about a quarter inch from the skins and distribute the potato flesh to a glass bowl.
4. Combine the parmesan, garlic salt, sour cream, and white cheddar cheese to the potato dish and incorporate fully.
5. Distribute the mixture back to the emptied potato skins. Create a small hollow in the middle by pressing with a spoon.
6. Divide the ham evenly between the potatoes and place the ham inside the hollow.
7. Position the potatoes in the fryer and set the air fryer to the temperature of 300°F.
8. Heat for 8 minutes and then sprinkle the cheddar cheese on top of each potato.
9. Melt the cheese for two more minutes than serve with diced onions on top.

Nutrition: Calories: 253 Fat: 32g Cholesterol: 31.5g Fiber: 1g Sodium: 297mg Protein: 28g

205. Pepperoni Pizza

⏱ Prep Time 10 m | ⏱ Cooking Time 10 m | 1 Pizza

Ingredients

- 1 mini naan flatbread
- 2 tbsp. pizza sauce
- 7 slices mini pepperoni
- 1 tbsp. olive oil
- 2 tbsp. mozzarella cheese, shredded

Directions:

1. Prepare the naan flatbread by brushed the olive oil on the top.
2. Layer the naan with pizza sauce, mozzarella cheese, and pepperoni.
3. Transfer to the frying basket and set the air fryer to the temperature of 375°F.
4. Heat for approximately 6 minutes and enjoy immediately.

Nutrition:

Calories: 270 Fat: 11g Cholesterol: 31.5g Fiber: 1g Sodium: 297mg Protein: 28g

206. Buttered Corn
🕐 Prep Time 5 m | 🕐 Cooking Time 20 m | 2 Servings

Ingredients

- 2 corn on the cob
- Salt and freshly ground black pepper, as needed
- 2 tablespoons butter, softened and divided

Directions

1. Sprinkle the cobs evenly with salt and black pepper.
2. Then, rub with 1 tablespoon of butter.
3. With 1 piece of foil, wrap each cob.
4. Press the "Power Button" of Air Fry Oven and turn the dial to select the "Air Fry" mode.
5. Press the Time button and again turn the dial to set the cooking time to 20 minutes.
6. Now push the Temp button and rotate the dial to set the temperature at 320 degrees F.
7. Press the "Start/Pause" button to start.
8. When the unit beeps to show that it is preheated, open the lid.
9. Arrange the cobs in "Air Fry Basket" and insert them in the oven.
10. Serve warm.

Nutrition

Calories 186 | Fat 12.2g | Saturated Fat 7.4g | Cholesterol 31mg | Sodium 163mg | Carbs 20.1g | Fiber 2.5g | Sugar 3.2g | Protein 2.9g

207. Bread Sticks
🕐 Prep Time 15 m | 🕐 Cooking Time 6 m | 6 Servings

Ingredients

- 1 egg 1/8 teaspoon ground cinnamon
- Salt, to taste
- 2 bread slices
- Pinch of nutmeg Pinch of ground cloves
- 1 tablespoon butter, softened
- Nonstick cooking spray
- 1 tablespoon icing sugar

Directions

1. In a bowl, add the eggs, cinnamon, nutmeg, cloves, and salt and beat until well combined.
2. Spread the butter over both sides of the slices evenly.
3. Cut each bread slice into strips.
4. Dip bread strips into egg mixture evenly.
5. Press the "Power Button" of Air Fry Oven and turn the dial to select the "Air Fry" mode.
6. Press the Time button and again turn the dial to set the cooking time to 6 minutes.
7. Now push the Temp button and rotate the dial to set the temperature at 355 degrees F.
8. Press the "Start/Pause" button to start.
9. When the unit beeps to show that it is preheated, open the lid.
10. Arrange the breadsticks in "Air Fry Basket" and insert it in the oven.
11. After 2 minutes of cooking, spray both sides of the bread strips with cooking spray.
12. Serve immediately with the topping of icing sugar.

Nutrition

Calories 41 | Fat 2.8g | Saturated Fat 1.5g | Cholesterol 32mg | Sodium 72mg | Carbs 3g | Fiber 0.1g | Sugar 1.5g | Protein 1.2g

208. Polenta Sticks
🕐 Prep Time 15 m | 🕐 Cooking Time 6 m | 4 Servings

Ingredients

- 1 tablespoon oil
- 2½ cups cooked polenta
- Salt, to taste
- ¼ cup Parmesan cheese

Directions

1. Place the polenta in a lightly greased baking pan.
2. With a plastic wrap, cover, and refrigerate for about 1 hour or until set.
3. Remove from the refrigerator and cut into desired sized slices.
4. Sprinkle with salt.
5. Press the "Power Button" of Air Fry Oven and turn the dial to select the "Air Fry" mode.
6. Press the Time button and again turn the dial to set the cooking time to 6 minutes.
7. Now push the Temp button and rotate the dial to set the temperature at 350 degrees F.
8. Press the "Start/Pause" button to start.
9. When the unit beeps to show that it is preheated, open the lid.
10. Arrange the pan over the "Wire Rack" and insert it in the oven.
11. Top with cheese and serve.

Nutrition

Calories 397 | Fat 5.6g | Saturated Fat 1.3g | Cholesterol 4mg | Sodium 127mg | Carbs 76.2g | Fiber 2.5g | Sugar 1g | Protein 9.1g

209. Crispy Eggplant Slices
🕐 Prep Time 15 m | 🕐 Cooking Time 8 m | 4 Servings

Ingredients

- 1 medium eggplant, shredded and cut into ½-inch round slices
- Salt, as required
- ½ cup all-purpose flour
- 2 eggs, beaten
- 1 cup Italian-style breadcrumbs
- ¼ cup olive oil

Directions

1. In a colander, add the eggplant slices and sprinkle with salt. Set aside for about 45 minutes.
2. With paper towels, pat dries the eggplant slices.
3. In a shallow dish, place the flour.
4. Crack the eggs in a second dish and beat well.
5. In a third dish, mix together the oil and breadcrumbs.
6. Coat each eggplant slice with flour, then dip into beaten eggs, and finally, coat with the breadcrumbs mixture.
7. Press the "Power Button" of Air Fry Oven and turn the dial to select the "Air Fry" mode.
8. Press the Time button and again turn the dial to set the cooking time to 8 minutes.
9. Now push the Temp button and rotate the dial to set the temperature at 390 degrees F.
10. Press the "Start/Pause" button to start.
11. When the unit beeps to show that it is preheated, open the lid.
12. Arrange the eggplant slices in "Air Fry Basket" and insert it in the oven.
13. Serve warm.

Nutrition

Calories 332 | Fat 16.6g | Saturated Fat 2.8g | Cholesterol 82 mg | Sodium 270mg | Carbs 38.3g | Fiber 5.7g | Sugar 5.3g | Protein 9.1g

210. Simple Cauliflower Poppers

⏱ Prep Time 10 m | ⏱ Cooking Time 8 m | 4 Servings

Ingredients

- ½ large head cauliflower, cut into bite-sized florets
- One tablespoon olive oil
- Salt and ground black pepper, as required

Directions

1. In a large bowl, add all the ingredients and toss to coat well.
2. Press the "Power Button" of Air Fry Oven and turn the dial to select the "Air Fry" mode.
3. Press the Time button and again turn the dial to set the cooking time to 8 minutes.
4. Now push the Temp button and rotate the dial to set the temperature at 390 degrees F.
5. Press the "Start/Pause" button to start.
6. When the unit beeps to show that it is preheated, open the lid.
7. Arrange the cauliflower florets in "Air Fry Basket" and insert it in the oven.
8. Toss the cauliflower florets once halfway through.
9. Serve warm.

Nutrition

Calories 138 | Fat 23.5g | Saturated Fat 0.5g | Cholesterol 0mg | Sodium 49mg | Carbs 1.8g | Fiber 0.8g | Sugar 0.8g | Protein 0.7g

211. Crispy Cauliflower Poppers

⏱ Prep Time 10 m | ⏱ Cooking Time 20 m | 4 Servings

Ingredients

- 1 egg white
- 1½ tablespoons ketchup
- 1 tablespoon hot sauce
- 1/3 cup panko breadcrumbs
- 2 cups cauliflower florets

Directions

1. In an open bowl, mix together the egg white, ketchup, and hot sauce.
2. In another bowl, place the breadcrumbs.
3. Dip the cauliflower florets in ketchup mixture and then coat with the breadcrumbs.
4. Press the "Power Button" of Air Fry Oven and turn the dial to select the "Air Fry" mode.
5. Press the Time button and again turn the dial to set the cooking time to 20 minutes.
6. Now push the Temp button and rotate the dial to set the temperature at 320 degrees F.
7. Press the "Start/Pause" button to start.
8. When the unit beeps to show that it is preheated, open the lid.
9. Arrange the cauliflower florets in "Air Fry Basket" and insert it in the oven.
10. Toss the cauliflower florets once halfway through.
11. Serve warm.

Nutrition

Calories 55 | Fat 0.7g | Saturated Fat 0.3g | Cholesterol 0mg | Sodium 181mg | Carbs 5.6g | Fiber 1.3g | Sugar 2.6g | Protein 2.3g

212. Broccoli Poppers

⏱ Prep Time 15 m | ⏱ Cooking Time 10 m | 4 Servings

Ingredients

- 2 tablespoons plain yogurt
- ½ teaspoon red chili powder
- ¼ teaspoon ground cumin
- ¼ teaspoon ground turmeric
- Salt, to taste
- 1 lb. broccoli, cut into small florets
- 2 tablespoons chickpea flour

Directions

1. In an open bowl, mix together the yogurt, and spices.
2. Add the broccoli and coat with marinade generously.
3. Refrigerate for about 20 minutes.
4. Press the "Power Button" of Air Fry Oven and turn the dial to select the "Air Fry" mode.
5. Press the Time button and again turn the dial to set the cooking time to 10 minutes.
6. Now push the Temp button and rotate the dial to set the temperature at 400 degrees F.
7. Press the "Start/Pause" button to start.
8. When the unit beeps to show that it is preheated, open the lid.
9. Arrange the broccoli florets in "Air Fry Basket" and insert it in the oven.
10. Toss the broccoli florets once halfway through.
11. Serve warm.

Nutrition

Calories 69 | Fat 0.9g | Saturated Fat 0.1g | Cholesterol 0mg | Sodium 87mg | Carbs 12.2 g | Fiber 4.2g | Sugar 3.2g | Protein 4.9g

213. Cheesy Broccoli Bites

⏱ Prep Time 15 m | ⏱ Cooking Time 12 m | 5 Servings

Ingredients

- 1 cup broccoli florets
- 1 egg, beaten
- ¾ cup cheddar cheese, grated
- 2 tablespoons Parmesan cheese, grated
- ¾ cup panko breadcrumbs
- Salt and freshly ground black pepper, as needed

Directions

1. In a food processor, add the broccoli and pulse until finely crumbled.
2. In a large bowl, mix together the broccoli and remaining ingredients.
3. Make small equal-sized balls from the mixture.
4. Press the "Power Button" of Air Fry Oven and turn the dial to select the "Air Fry" mode.
5. Press the Time button and again turn the dial to set the cooking time to 12 minutes.
6. Now push the Temp button and rotate the dial to set the temperature at 350 degrees F.
7. Press the "Start/Pause" button to start.
8. When the unit beeps to show that it is preheated, open the lid.
9. Arrange the broccoli balls in "Air Fry Basket" and insert them in the oven.
10. Serve warm.

Nutrition

Calories 153 | Fat 8.2 g | Fat 4.5g | Cholesterol 52mg | Sodium 172mg | Carbs 4g | Fiber 0.5g | Sugar 0.5g | Protein 7.1g

214. Mixed Veggie Bites

Prep Time 15 m | Cooking Time 10 m | 5 Servings

Ingredients

- ¾ lb. fresh spinach, blanched, drained, and chopped
- ¼ of onion, chopped
- ½ of carrot, peeled and chopped
- 1 garlic clove, minced
- 1 American cheese slice, cut into tiny pieces
- 1 bread slice, toasted and processed into breadcrumbs
- ½ tablespoon cornflour
- ½ teaspoon red chili flakes
- Salt, as required

Directions

1. Place all ingredients in a bowl, except breadcrumbs, and mix until well combined.
2. Add the breadcrumbs and gently stir to combine.
3. Make 10 equal-sized balls from the mixture.
4. Press the "Power Button" of Air Fry Oven and turn the dial to select the "Air Fry" mode.
5. Press the Time button and again turn the dial to set the cooking time to 10 minutes.
6. Now push the Temp button and rotate the dial to set the temperature at 355 degrees F.
7. Press the "Start/Pause" button to start.
8. When the unit beeps to show that it is preheated, open the lid.
9. Arrange the veggie balls in "Air Fry Basket" and insert them in the oven.
10. Serve warm.

Nutrition

Calories 43 | Fat 1.4g | Saturated Fat 0.7g | Cholesterol 3mg | Sodium 155mg | Carbs 5.6g | Fiber 1.9g | Sugar 1.2g | Protein 3.1g

215. Risotto Bites

Prep Time 15 m | Cooking Time 10 m | 4 Servings

Ingredients

- 1½ cups cooked risotto
- 3 tablespoons Parmesan cheese, grated
- ½ egg, beaten
- 1½ oz. mozzarella cheese, cubed
- 1/3 cup breadcrumbs

Directions

1. In a bowl, add the risotto, Parmesan, and egg and mix until well combined.
2. Make 20 equal-sized balls from the mixture.
3. Insert a mozzarella cube in the center of each ball.
4. With your fingers, smooth the risotto mixture to cover the ball.
5. In a shallow dish, place the breadcrumbs.
6. Coat the balls with the breadcrumbs evenly.
7. Press the "Power Button" of Air Fry Oven and turn the dial to select the "Air Fry" mode.
8. Press the Time button and again turn the dial to set the cooking time to 10 minutes.
9. Now push the Temp button and rotate the dial to set the temperature at 390 degrees F.
10. Press the "Start/Pause" button to start.
11. When the unit beeps to show that it is preheated, open the lid.
12. Arrange the balls in "Air Fry Basket" and insert them in the oven.
13. Serve warm.

Nutrition

Calories 340 | Fat 4.3g | Saturated Fat 2g | Cholesterol 29mg | Sodium 173mg | Carbs 62.4g | Fiber 1.3g | Sugar 0.7g | Protein 11.3g

216. Rice Flour Bites

Prep Time 15 m | Cooking Time 12 m | 4 Servings

Ingredients

- 6 tablespoons milk
- ½ teaspoon vegetable oil
- ¾ cup of rice flour
- 1 oz. Parmesan cheese, shredded

Directions

1. In a bowl, add milk, flour, oil, and cheese and mix until a smooth dough forms.
2. Make small equal-sized balls from the dough.
3. Press the "Power Button" of Air Fry Oven and turn the dial to select the "Air Fry" mode.
4. Press the Time button and again turn the dial to set the cooking time to 12 minutes.
5. Now push the Temp button and rotate the dial to set the temperature at 300 degrees F.
6. Press the "Start/Pause" button to start.
7. When the unit beeps to show that it is preheated, open the lid.
8. Arrange the balls in "Air Fry Basket" and insert them in the oven.
9. Serve warm.

Nutrition

Calories 148 | Fat 3g | Saturated Fat 1.5g | Cholesterol 7mg | Sodium 77mg | Carbs 25.1g | Fiber 0.7g | Sugar 1.1g | Protein 4.8g

217. Lemon Parmesan and Peas Risotto

Prep Time 10 m | Cooking Time 17 m | 6 Servings

Ingredients

- 2 tablespoons butter
- 1½ cup of rice
- 1 yellow onion, peeled and chopped
- 1 tablespoon extra-virgin olive oil
- 1 teaspoon lemon zest, grated
- 3½ cups chicken stock
- 2 tablespoons lemon juice
- 2 tablespoons parsley, diced
- 2 tablespoons Parmesan cheese, finely grated
- Salt and ground black pepper, to taste
- 1½ cup peas

Directions

1. Put the Instant Pot in the sauté mode, add 1 tablespoon of butter and oil, and heat them. Add the onion, mix, and cook for 5 minutes.
2. Add the rice, mix, and cook for another 3 minutes. Add 3 cups of broth and lemon juice, mix, cover, and cook for 5 minutes on rice.
3. Release the pressure, put the fryer in manual mode, add the peas and the rest of the broth, stir and cook for 2 minutes.
4. Add the cheese, parsley, remaining butter, lemon zest, salt, and pepper to taste and mix. Divide between plates and serve.

Nutrition

Calories 140 | Fat 1.5 g | Fiber 1 g | Carbohydrate 27 g | Proteins 5 g

71

218. Spinach and Goat Cheese Risotto

⏱ Prep Time 10 m | ⏱ Cooking Time 10 m | 6 Servings

Ingredients

- ¾ cup yellow onion, chopped
- 1½ cups Arborio rice
- 12 ounces' spinach, chopped
- 3½ cups hot vegetable stock
- ½ cup white wine
- 2 garlic cloves, peeled and minced
- 2 tablespoons extra virgin olive oil
- Salt and ground black pepper, to taste
- ⅓ cup pecans, toasted and chopped
- 4 ounces' goat cheese, soft and crumbled
- 2 tablespoons lemon juice

Directions

1. Put the Instant Pot in the sauté mode, add the oil and heat. Add garlic and onion, mix and cook for 5 minutes.
2. Add the rice, mix, and cook for 1 minute. Add wine, stir and cook until it is absorbed. Add 3 cups of stock, cover the Instant Pot, and cook the rice for 4 minutes.
3. Release the pressure, uncover the Instant Pot, add the spinach, stir and cook for 3 minutes in Manual mode. Add salt, pepper, the rest of the stock, lemon juice, and goat cheese and mix. Divide between plates, decorate with nuts and serve.

Nutrition

Calories 340 | Fat 23 g | Fiber 4.5 g | Carbohydrate 24 g | Proteins 18.9 g

219. Rice and Artichokes

⏱ Prep Time 10 m | ⏱ Cooking Time 20 m | 4 Servings

Ingredients

- 2 garlic cloves, peeled and crushed
- 1¼ cups chicken broth
- 1 tablespoon extra-virgin olive oil
- 5 ounces Arborio rice
- 1 tablespoon white wine
- 15 ounces canned artichoke hearts, chopped
- 16 ounces' cream cheese
- 1 tablespoon grated Parmesan cheese
- 1½ tablespoons fresh thyme, chopped
- Salt and ground black pepper, to taste
- 6 ounces' graham cracker crumbs
- 1¼ cups water

Directions

1. Put the Instant Pot in the sauté mode, add the oil, heat, add the rice, and cook for 2 minutes. Add the garlic, mix, and cook for 1 minute.
2. Transfer to a heat-resistant plate. Add the stock, crumbs, salt, pepper, and wine, mix and cover the plate with aluminum foil.
3. Place the dish in the basket to cook the Instant Pot, add water, cover, and cook for 8 minutes on rice. Release the pressure, remove the dish, uncover, add cream cheese, parmesan, artichoke hearts, and thyme.
4. Mix well and serve.

Nutrition

Calories 240 | Fat 7.2 g | Fiber 5.1 g | Carbohydrate 34 g | Proteins 6 g

220. Potatoes Au Gratin

⏱ Prep Time 10 m | ⏱ Cooking Time 17 m | 6 Servings

Ingredients

- ½ cup yellow onion, chopped
- 2 tablespoons butter
- 1 cup chicken stock
- 6 potatoes, peeled and sliced
- ½ cup sour cream
- Salt and ground black pepper, to taste
- 1 cup Monterey jack cheese, shredded
- For the topping:
- 3 tablespoons melted butter
- 1 cup breadcrumbs

Directions

1. Put the Instant Pot in Saute mode, add the butter and melt. Add the onion, mix, and cook for 5 minutes. Add the stock, salt, and pepper and put the steamer basket in the Instant Pot also.
2. Add the potatoes, cover the Instant Pot, and cook for 5 minutes in the Manual setting. In a bowl, mix 3 tablespoons of butter with breadcrumbs and mix well. Relieve the pressure of the Instant Pot, remove the steam basket, and transfer the potatoes to a pan.
3. Pour the cream and cheese into the instant pot and mix. Add the potatoes and mix gently.
4. Spread breadcrumbs, mix everywhere, place on a preheated grill, and cook for 7 minutes. Let cool for more minutes and serve.

Nutrition

Calories 340 | Fat 22 g | Fiber 2 g | Carbohydrate 32 g | Proteins 11 g

221. Easy Hot Dogs

⏱ Prep Time 10 m | ⏱ Cooking Time 7 m | 2 Servings

Ingredients:

- 2 hot dog buns
- 2 hot dogs
- 1 tablespoon Dijon mustard
- 2 tablespoons cheddar cheese, grated

Directions:

1. Put hot dogs in preheated air fryer and cook them at 390 degrees F for 5 minutes.
2. Divide hot dogs into hot dog buns, spread mustard and cheese, return everything to your air fryer and cook for 2 minutes more at 390 degrees F.
3. Serve for lunch.
4. Enjoy!

Nutrition:

Calories 211 | Fat 3 | Fiber 8 | Carbs 12 | Protein 4

222. Japanese Chicken Mix

⏱ Prep Time 10 m | ⏱ Cooking Time 8 m | 2 Servings

Ingredients:

- 2 chicken thighs, skinless and boneless
- 2 ginger slices, chopped
- 3 garlic cloves, minced
- ¼ cup soy sauce
- ¼ cup mirin
- 1/8 cup sake
- ½ teaspoon sesame oil
- 1/8 cup water
- 2 tablespoons sugar
- 1 tablespoon cornstarch mixed with 2 tablespoons water
- Sesame seeds for serving

Directions:

1. In a bowl, mix chicken thighs with ginger, garlic, soy sauce, mirin, sake, oil, water, sugar and cornstarch, toss well, transfer to preheated air fryer and cook at 360 degrees F for 8 minutes.
2. Divide among plates, sprinkle sesame seeds on top and serve with a side salad for lunch.
3. Enjoy!

Nutrition:

Calories 300| Fat 7 |Fiber 9 | Carbs 17 |Protein 10

223. Prosciutto Sandwich

⏱ Prep Time 10 m | ⏱ Cooking Time 5 m | 1 Servings

Ingredients:

- 2 bread slices
- 2 mozzarella slices
- 2 tomato slices
- 2 prosciutto slices
- 2 basil leaves
- 1 teaspoon olive oil
- A pinch of salt and black pepper

Directions:

1. Arrange mozzarella and prosciutto on a bread slice.
2. Season with salt and pepper, place in your air fryer and cook at 400 degrees F for 5 minutes.
3. Drizzle oil over prosciutto, add tomato and basil, cover with the other bread slice, cut sandwich in half and serve.
4. Enjoy!

Nutrition:

Calories 172 | Fat 3 |Fiber 7| Carbs 9 | Protein 5

224. Lentils Fritters

⏱ Prep Time 10 m | ⏱ Cooking Time 10 m | 2 Servings

Ingredients:

- 1 cup yellow lentils, soaked in water for 1 hour and drained
- 1 hot chili pepper, chopped
- 1 inch ginger piece, grated
- ½ teaspoon turmeric powder
- 1 teaspoon gram masala
- 1 teaspoon baking powder
- Salt and black pepper to the taste
- 2 teaspoons olive oil
- 1/3 cup water
- ½ cup cilantro, chopped
- 1 and ½ cup spinach, chopped
- 4 garlic cloves, minced
- ¾ cup red onion, chopped
- Mint chutney for serving

Directions:

1. In your blender, mix lentils with chili pepper, ginger, turmeric, gram masala, baking powder, salt, pepper, olive oil, water, cilantro, spinach, onion and garlic, blend well and shape medium balls out of this mix.
2. Place them all in your preheated air fryer at 400 degrees F and cook for 10 minutes.
3. Serve your veggie fritters with a side salad for lunch.
4. Enjoy!

Nutrition:

Calories 142|Fat 2| Fiber 8 |Carbs 12 |Protein 4

225. Lunch Potato Salad

⏱ Prep Time 10 m | ⏱ Cooking Time 25 m | 4 Servings

Ingredients:

- 2 pound red potatoes, halved
- 2 tablespoons olive oil
- Salt and black pepper to the taste
- 2 green onions, chopped
- 1 red bell pepper, chopped
- 1/3 cup lemon juice
- 3 tablespoons mustard

Directions:

1. On your air fryer's basket, mix potatoes with half of the olive oil, salt and pepper and cook at 350 degrees F for 25 minutes shaking the fryer once.
2. In a bowl, mix onions with bell pepper and roasted potatoes and toss.
3. In a small bowl, mix lemon juice with the rest of the oil and mustard and whisk really well.
4. Add this to potato salad, toss well and serve for lunch.
5. Enjoy!

Nutrition:

Calories 211| Fat 6| Fiber 8 |Carbs 12 |Protein 4

226. Corn Casserole

🕛 Prep Time 10 m | 🕛 Cooking Time 15 m | 4 Servings

Ingredients:

- 2 cups corn
- 3 tablespoons flour
- 1 egg
- ¼ cup milk
- ½ cup light cream
- ½ cup Swiss cheese, grated
- 2 tablespoons butter
- Salt and black pepper to the taste
- Cooking spray

Directions:

1. In a bowl, mix corn with flour, egg, milk, light cream, cheese, salt, pepper and butter and stir well.
2. Grease your air fryer's pan with cooking spray, pour cream mix, spread and cook at 320 degrees F for 15 minutes.
3. Serve warm for lunch.
4. Enjoy!

Nutrition:

Calories 281| Fat 7 |Fiber 8 |Carbs 9| Protein 6

227. Bacon and Garlic Pizzas

🕛 Prep Time 10 m | 🕛 Cooking Time 10 m | 4 Servings

Ingredients:

- 4 dinner rolls, frozen
- 4 garlic cloves minced
- ½ teaspoon oregano dried
- ½ teaspoon garlic powder
- 1 cup tomato sauce
- 8 bacon slices, cooked and chopped
- 1 and ¼ cups cheddar cheese, grated
- Cooking spray

Directions:

1. Place dinner rolls on a working surface and press them to obtain 4 ovals.
2. Spray each oval with cooking spray, transfer them to your air fryer and cook them at 370 degrees F for 2 minutes.
3. Spread tomato sauce on each oval, divide garlic, sprinkle oregano and garlic powder and top with bacon and cheese.
4. Return pizzas to your heated air fryer and cook them at 370 degrees F for 8 minutes more.
5. Serve them warm for lunch.
6. Enjoy!

Nutrition:

Calories 217 |Fat 5| Fiber 8 |Carbs 12 |Protein 4

228. Sweet and Sour Sausage Mix

🕛 Prep Time 10 m | 🕛 Cooking Time 10 m | 4 Servings

Ingredients:

- 1 pound sausages, sliced
- 1 red bell pepper, cut into strips
- ½ cup yellow onion, chopped
- 3 tablespoons brown sugar
- 1/3 cup ketchup
- 2 tablespoons mustard
- 2 tablespoons apple cider vinegar
- ½ cup chicken stock

Directions:

1. In a bowl, mix sugar with ketchup, mustard, stock and vinegar and whisk well.
2. In your air fryer's pan, mix sausage slices with bell pepper, onion and sweet and sour mix, toss and cook at 350 degrees F for 10 minutes.
3. Divide into bowls and serve for lunch.
4. Enjoy!

Nutrition: Calories 162 |Fat 6| Fiber 9| Carbs 12 |Protein 6

229. Meatballs and Tomato Sauce

🕛 Prep Time 10 m | 🕛 Cooking Time 15 m | 4 Servings

Ingredients:

- 1 pound lean beef, ground
- 3 green onions, chopped
- 2 garlic cloves, minced
- 1 egg yolk
- ¼ cup bread crumbs
- Salt and black pepper to the taste
- 1 tablespoon olive oil
- 16 ounces tomato sauce
- 2 tablespoons mustard

Directions:

1. In a bowl, mix beef with onion, garlic, egg yolk, bread crumbs, salt and pepper, stir well and shape medium meatballs out of this mix.
2. Grease meatballs with the oil, place them in your air fryer and cook them at 400 degrees F for 10 minutes.
3. In a bowl, mix tomato sauce with mustard, whisk, add over meatballs, toss them and cook at 400 degrees F for 5 minutes more.
4. Divide meatballs and sauce on plates and serve for lunch.
5. Enjoy!

Nutrition:

Calories 300 |Fat 8 |Fiber 9 |Carbs 16 |Protein 5

230. Stuffed Meatballs

⏰ Prep Time 10 m | ⏱ Cooking Time 10 m | 4 Servings

Ingredients:

- 1/3 cup bread crumbs
- 3 tablespoons milk
- 1 tablespoon ketchup
- 1 egg
- ½ teaspoon marjoram, dried
- Salt and black pepper to the taste
- 1 pound lean beef, ground
- 20 cheddar cheese cubes
- 1 tablespoon olive oil

Directions:

1. In a bowl, mix bread crumbs with ketchup, milk, marjoram, salt, pepper and egg and whisk well.
2. Add beef, stir and shape 20 meatballs out of this mix.
3. Shape each meatball around a cheese cube, drizzle the oil over them and rub.
4. Place all meatballs in your preheated air fryer and cook at 390 degrees F for 10 minutes.
5. Serve them for lunch with a side salad.
6. Enjoy!

Nutrition:

Calories 200 | Fat 5 | Fiber 8 | Carbs 12 | Protein 5

231. Steaks and Cabbage

⏰ Prep Time 10 m | ⏱ Cooking Time 10 m | 4 Servings

Ingredients:

- ½ pound sirloin steak, cut into strips
- 2 teaspoons cornstarch
- 1 tablespoon peanut oil
- 2 cups green cabbage, chopped
- 1 yellow bell pepper, chopped
- 2 green onions, chopped
- 2 garlic cloves, minced
- Salt and black pepper to the taste

Directions:

1. In a bowl, mix cabbage with salt, pepper and peanut oil, toss, transfer to air fryer's basket, cook at 370 degrees F for 4 minutes and transfer to a bowl.
2. Add steak strips to your air fryer, also add green onions, bell pepper, garlic, salt and pepper, toss and cook for 5 minutes.
3. Add over cabbage, toss, divide among plates and serve for lunch.
4. Enjoy!

Nutrition:

Calories 282 | Fat 6 | Fiber 8 | Carbs 14 | Protein 6

232. Succulent Lunch Turkey Breast

⏰ Prep Time 10 m | ⏱ Cooking Time 47 m | 4 Servings

Ingredients:

- 1 big turkey breast
- 2 teaspoons olive oil
- ½ teaspoon smoked paprika
- 1 teaspoon thyme, dried
- ½ teaspoon sage, dried
- Salt and black pepper to the taste
- 2 tablespoons mustard
- ¼ cup maple syrup
- 1 tablespoon butter, soft

Directions:

1. Brush turkey breast with the olive oil, season with salt, pepper, thyme, paprika and sage, rub, place in your air fryer's basket and fry at 350 degrees F for 25 minutes.
2. Flip turkey, cook for 10 minutes more, flip one more time and cook for another 10 minutes.
3. Meanwhile, heat up a pan with the butter over medium heat, add mustard and maple syrup, stir well, and cook for a couple of minutes and take off heat.
4. Slice turkey breast, divide among plates and serve with the maple glaze drizzled on top.
5. Enjoy!

Nutrition:

Calories 280 | Fat 2 | Fiber 7 | Carbs 16 | Protein 14

233. Creamy Chicken Stew

⏰ Prep Time 10 m | ⏱ Cooking Time 25 m | 4 Servings

Ingredients:

- 1 and ½ cups canned cream of celery soup
- 6 chicken tenders
- Salt and black pepper to the taste
- 2 potatoes, chopped
- 1 bay leaf
- 1 thyme spring, chopped
- 1 tablespoon milk
- 1 egg yolk
- ½ cup heavy cream

Directions:

1. In a bowl, mix chicken with cream of celery, potatoes, heavy cream, bay leaf, thyme, salt and pepper, toss, pour into your air fryer's pan and cook at 320 degrees F for 25 minutes.
2. Leave your stew to cool down a bit, discard bay leaf, divide among plates and serve right away.

Nutrition:

Calories 300 | Fat 11 | Fiber 2 | Carbs 23 | Protein 14

234. Italian Eggplant Sandwich

⏰ Prep Time 10 m | ⏰ Cooking Time 16 m | 2 Servings

Ingredients:

- 1 eggplant, sliced
- 2 teaspoons parsley, dried
- Salt and black pepper to the taste
- ½ cup breadcrumbs
- ½ teaspoon Italian seasoning
- ½ teaspoon garlic powder
- ½ teaspoon onion powder
- 2 tablespoons milk
- 4 bread slices
- Cooking spray
- ½ cup mayonnaise
- ¾ cup tomato sauce
- 2 cups mozzarella cheese, grated

Directions:

1. Season eggplant slices with salt and pepper, leave aside for 10 minutes and then pat dry them well.
2. In a bowl, mix parsley with breadcrumbs, Italian seasoning, onion and garlic powder, salt and black pepper and stir.
3. In another bowl, mix milk with mayo and whisk well.
4. Brush eggplant slices with mayo mix, dip them in breadcrumbs, place them in your air fryer's basket, spray with cooking oil and cook them at 400 degrees F for 15 minutes, flipping them after 8 minutes.
5. Brush each bread slice with olive oil and arrange 2 on a working surface.
6. Add mozzarella and parmesan on each, add baked eggplant slices, spread tomato sauce and basil and top with the other bread slices, greased side down.
7. Divide sandwiches on plates, cut them in halves and serve for lunch.
8. Enjoy!

Nutrition:

Calories 324| Fat 16| Fiber 4 |Carbs 39| Protein 12

235. Lunch Pork and Potatoes

⏰ Prep Time 10 m | ⏰ Cooking Time 25 m | 2 Servings

Ingredients:

- 2 pounds pork loin
- Salt and black pepper to the taste
- 2 red potatoes, cut into medium wedges
- ½ teaspoon garlic powder
- ½ teaspoon red pepper flakes
- 1 teaspoon parsley, dried
- A drizzle of balsamic vinegar

Directions:

1. In your air fryer's pan, mix pork with potatoes, salt, pepper, garlic powder, pepper flakes, parsley and vinegar, toss and cook at 390 degrees F for 25 minutes.
2. Slice pork, divide it and potatoes on plates and serve for lunch.
3. Enjoy!

Nutrition:

Calories 400 |Fat 15| Fiber 7 |Carbs 27 |Protein 20

236. Grilled Cheese Sandwich

⏰ Prep Time 5 m | ⏰ Cooking Time 5 m | 2 Servings

Ingredients:

- 2 slices bread, softened
- 1 tsp. butter
- 2 slices cheddar cheese

Directions:

1. Set the air fryer at a temperature of 350°F.
2. Apply 1/2 teaspoon of the softened butter to one side of the slice of bread. Repeat for the remaining bread.
3. Create the sandwich by putting the cheese in between the non-buttered sides of bread.
4. Transfer to the hot air fryer and set for 5 minutes. Flip the sandwich at the halfway point and remove.
5. Serve immediately and enjoy.

Nutrition: Calories 235| Fat 13| Fiber 27| Carbs 37 |Protein 40

237. Italian Meatballs

⏰ Prep Time 15 m | ⏰ Cooking Time 20 m | 4 Servings

Ingredients:

- One egg, large
- Ground beef - 16 oz.
- Pepper - 1/8 tsp.
- Oregano seasoning - 1/2 tsp.
- Bread crumbs - 1 1/4 cup
- Garlic - 1/2 clove, chopped
- Parsley - 1 oz., chopped
- Salt - 1/4 tsp.
- Parmigiano-Reggiano cheese - 1 oz. cup, grated
- Cooking spray (avocado oil)

Directions:

1. Whisk the oregano, breadcrumbs, chopped garlic, and salt, chopped parsley, pepper, and grated Parmigiano-Reggiano cheese until combined.
2. Blend the ground beef and egg into the mixture using your hands. Incorporate the ingredients thoroughly.
3. Divide the meat into 12 sections and roll into rounds.
4. Coat the inside of the basket with avocado oil spray to grease.
5. Adjust the temperature to 350°F and heat for approximately 12 minutes.
6. Roll the meatballs over and steam for another 4 minutes and remove to a serving plate.
7. Enjoy as is or combine with your favorite pasta or sauce.

Nutrition: Calories 321 |Fat 3 |Fiber 8 |Carbs 22 |Protein 16

238. Pepperoni Pizza

⏱ Prep Time 5 m | ⏱ Cooking Time 5 m | 7 Servings

Ingredients:

- 1 mini naan flatbread
- 2 tbsp. pizza sauce
- 7 slices mini pepperoni
- 1 tbsp. olive oil
- 2 tbsp. mozzarella cheese, shredded

Directions:

1. Prepare the naan flatbread by brushed the olive oil on the top.
2. Layer the naan with pizza sauce, mozzarella cheese, and pepperoni.
3. Transfer to the frying basket and set the air fryer to the temperature of 375°F.
4. Heat for approximately 6 minutes and enjoy immediately.

Nutrition:

Calories 430 | Fat 4 | Fiber 9 | Carbs 11 | Protein 10

239. Loaded Baked Potatoes

⏱ Prep Time 10 m | ⏱ Cooking Time 15 m | 3 Servings

Ingredients:

- 1/3 cup milk
- 2 oz. sour cream
- 1/3 cup white cheddar, grated
- 2 oz. Parmesan cheese, grated
- 1/8 tsp. garlic salt
- 6 oz. ham, diced
- 2 medium russet potatoes
- 4 oz. sharp cheddar, shredded
- 1/8 cup. Green onion, diced

Directions:

1. Puncture the potatoes deeply with a fork a few time and microwave for approximately 5 minutes. Flip them to the other side and nuke for an additional 5 minutes. The potatoes should be soft.
2. Use oven mitts to remove from the microwave and cut them in halves.
3. Spoon out the insides of the potatoes to about a quarter-inch from the skins and distribute the potato flesh to a glass bowl.
4. Combine the parmesan, garlic salt, sour cream, and white cheddar cheese to the potato dish and incorporate fully.
5. Distribute the mixture back to the emptied potato skins. Create a small hollow in the middle by pressing with a spoon.
6. Divide the ham evenly between the potatoes and place the ham inside the hollow.
7. Position the potatoes in the fryer and set the air fryer to the temperature of 300°F.
8. Heat for 8 minutes and then sprinkle the cheddar cheese on top of each potato.
9. Melt the cheese for two more minutes than serve with diced onions on top.

Nutrition:

Calories 143 | Fat 22 | Fiber 14 | Carbs 18 | Protein 29

240. Southern Style Fried Chicken

⏱ Prep Time 10 m | ⏱ Cooking Time 15 m | 8 Servings

Ingredients:

- Italian seasoning - 1 tsp.
- Chicken legs or breasts - 2 lbs.
- Buttermilk - 2 tbsp.
- Paprika seasoning - 1 1/2tsp.
- Cornstarch - 2 oz.
- Onion powder - 1 tsp.
- Hot sauce - 3 tsp.
- Pepper - 1 1/2 tsp.
- 2 large eggs
- 1 cup self-rising flour
- 2 tsp. salt
- Cooking spray (olive oil)
- 1/4 cup water
- Garlic powder - 1 1/2tsp.

Directions:

1. Clean the chicken by washing thoroughly and pat dry with paper towels.
2. Use a glass dish to blend the pepper, paprika, garlic powder, onion powder, salt, and Italian seasoning.
3. Rub approximately 1 tablespoon of the spices into the pieces of chicken to cover entirely.
4. Blend the cornstarch, flour, and spices by shaking in a large zip lock bag.
5. In a separate dish, combine the eggs, hot sauce, water, and milk until integrated.
6. Completely cover the spiced chicken in the flour and then immerse in the eggs.
7. Coat in the flour for a second time and set on a tray for approximately 15 minutes.
8. Before transferring the chicken to the air fryer, spray liberally with olive oil and space the pieces out, frying a separate batch if required.
9. Adjust the temperature to 350° F for approximately 18 minutes.
10. Bring the chicken out and put on a plate. Wait about 5 minutes before serving.

Nutrition:

Calories 230 | Fat 10 | Fiber 19 | Carbs 13 | Protein 12

241. Tuna Patties

⏱ Prep Time 5 m | ⏱ Cooking Time 15 m | 2 Servings

Ingredients:

- Garlic powder - 1 tsp.
- Tuna - 2 cans, in water
- Dill seasoning - 1 tsp.
- All-purpose flour - 4 tsp.
- Salt - 1/4 tsp.

- Mayonnaise - 4 tsp.
- Lemon juice - 2 tbsp.
- Onion powder - 1/2 tsp.
- Pepper - 1/4 tsp.

Directions:

1. Set the temperature of the air fryer to 400°F.
2. Combine the almond flour, mayonnaise, salt, onion powder, dill, garlic powder and pepper using a food blender for approximately 30 seconds until incorporated.
3. Empty the canned tuna and lemon juice into the blender and pulse for an additional 30 seconds until integrated fully.
4. Divide evenly into 4 sections and create patties by hand.
5. Transfer to the fryer basket in a single layer and heat for approximately 12 minutes.

Nutrition:

Calories 286| Fat 3 |Fiber 6 |Carbs 22 |Protein 16

242. Stuffed Bell Peppers

⏱ Prep Time 15 m | ⏱ Cooking Time 15 m | 9 Servings

Ingredients:

- Medium onion - 1/2, chopped
- Cheddar cheese - 4 oz., shredded
- Pepper - 1/2 tsp.
- Ground beef - 8 oz.
- Olive oil - 1 tsp.
- Tomato sauce - 4 oz.

- Worcestershire sauce - 1 tsp.
- Medium green peppers - 2, stems and seeds discarded
- Salt - 1 tsp., separated
- Water - 4 cups
- Garlic - 1 clove, minced

Directions:

1. Boil the water in pot steam the green peppers with the tops and seeds removed with 1/2 teaspoon of the salt. Move from the burner after approximately 3 minutes and drain.
2. Pat the peppers with paper towels to properly dry.
3. In a hot frying pan, melt the olive oil and toss the garlic and onion for approximately 2 minutes until browned. Drain thoroughly.
4. Set the air fryer temperature to 400°F to warm up.
5. Using a glass dish, blend the beef along with Worcestershire sauce, 2 ounces of tomato sauce, salt, vegetables, 2 ounces of cheddar cheese and pepper until fully incorporated.
6. Spoon the mixture evenly into the peppers and drizzle the remaining 2 ounces of tomato sauce on top. Then dust with the remaining 2 ounces of cheddar cheese.
7. Assemble the peppers in the basket of the air fryer and heat fully for approximately 18 minutes. The meat should be fully cooked before removing.
8. Place on a platter and serve immediately.

Nutrition:

Calories 120 | Fat 9 |Fiber 2 |Carbs 17 |Protein 28

243. Ham and Cheese sandwich

⏱ Prep Time 15 m | ⏱ Cooking Time 20 m | 2 Servings

Ingredients:

- 2 eggs
- 4 slices of bread of choice
- 4 slices turkey
- 4 slices ham
- 6 tbsp. half and half cream

- 2 tsp. melted butter
- 4 slices Swiss cheese
- ¼ tsp. pure vanilla extract
- Powdered sugar and raspberry jam for serving

Directions:

1. Mix the eggs, vanilla and cream in a bowl and set aside.
2. Make a sandwich with the bread layered with cheese slice, turkey, ham, cheese slice and the top slice of bread to make two sandwiches. Gently press on the sandwiches to somewhat flatten them.
3. Set your air fryer toast oven to 350 degrees F.
4. Spread out kitchen aluminum foil and cut it about the same size as the sandwich and spread the melted butter on the surface of the foil.
5. Dip the sandwich in the egg mixture and let it soak for about 20 seconds on each side. Repeat this for the other sandwich. Place the soaked sandwiches on the prepared foil sheets then place on the basket in your fryer.
6. Cook for 12 minutes then flip the sandwiches and brush with the remaining butter and cook for another 5 minutes or until well browned.
7. Place the cooked sandwiched on a plate and top with the powdered sugar and serve with a small bowl of raspberry jam.
8. Enjoy!

Nutrition:

Calories 170| Fat 22 |Fiber 10|Carbs 12 |Protein 20

244. Mexican Style Cauliflower Bake

🕐 Prep Time 25 m | 🕐 Cooking Time 20-30 m | 4 Servings

Ingredients:

- Two cups cauliflower florets; roughly chopped.
- One red chili pepper; chopped.
- Two tomatoes; cubed
- One avocado, peeled, pitted and sliced
- Four garlic cloves; minced
- 1 tbsp. Coriander; chopped.
- 1 tbsp. Lime juice
- 1 tbsp. Olive oil
- 1 tsp. Cumin powder
- ½ tsp. Chili powder
- Salt and black pepper to taste.

Directions:

1. In a pan that fits the air fryer, combine the cauliflower with the other ingredients except for the coriander, avocado and lime juice, toss, introduce the pan in the machine and cook at 380°f for 20 minutes
2. Divide between plates, top each serving with coriander, avocado and lime juice and serve as a side dish.

Nutrition:

Calories: 187; Fat: 8g; Fiber: 2g; Carbs: 5g; Protein: 7g

245. Curry Cabbage

🕐 Prep Time 25 m | 🕐 Cooking Time 20 m | 4 Servings

Ingredients:

- 30 oz. Green cabbage; shredded
- 3 tbsp. Coconut oil; melted
- 1 tbsp. Red curry paste
- A pinch of salt and black pepper

Directions:

1. In a pan that fits the air fryer, combine the cabbage with the rest of the ingredients, toss, introduce the pan in the machine and cook at 380°f for 20 minutes
2. Divide between plates and serve as a side dish.

Nutrition:

Calories: 180; Fat: 14g; Fiber: 4g; Carbs: 6g; Protein: 8g

246. Brussels Sprouts

🕐 Prep Time 15 m | 🕐 Cooking Time 20-30 m | 4 Servings

Ingredients:

- 1 lb. Brussels sprouts
- 1 tbsp. Unsalted butter; melted.
- 1 tbsp. Coconut oil

Directions:

1. Remove all loose leaves from Brussels sprouts and cut each in half.
2. Drizzle sprouts with coconut oil and place into the air fryer basket
3. Adjust the temperature to 400 degrees f and set the timer for 10 minutes.
4. You may want to gently stir halfway through the cooking time, depending on how they are beginning to brown
5. When thoroughly cooked, they should be tender with darker caramelized spots.
6. Remove from fryer basket and drizzle with melted butter.
7. Serve immediately.

Nutrition: Calories: 90; Protein: 2.9g; Fiber: 3.2g; Fat: 6.1g; Carbs: 7.5g

247. Kale and Walnuts

🕐 Prep Time 20 m | 🕐 Cooking Time 25 m | 4 Servings

Ingredients:

- 3 garlic cloves
- 10 cups kale; roughly chopped.
- 1/3 cup parmesan; grated
- ½ cup almond milk
- ¼ cup walnuts; chopped.
- 1 tbsp. Butter; melted
- ¼ tsp. Nutmeg, ground
- Salt and black pepper to taste.

Directions:

1. In a pan that fits the air fryer, combine all the ingredients, toss, introduce the pan in the machine and cook at 360°f for 15 minutes
2. Divide between plates and serve.

Nutrition: Calories: 160; Fat: 7g; Fiber: 2g; Carbs: 4g; Protein: 5g

248. Pesto Zucchini Pasta

🕐 Prep Time 20 m | 🕐 Cooking Time 25 m | 4 Servings

Ingredients:

- 4 oz. Mozzarella; shredded
- 2 cups zucchinis, cut with a spiralizer
- ½ cup coconut cream
- ¼ cup basil pesto
- 1 tbsp. Olive oil
- Salt and black pepper to taste.

Directions:

1. In a pan that fits your air fryer, mix the zucchini noodles with the pesto and the rest of the ingredients, toss, introduce the pan in the fryer and cook at 370°f for 15 minutes
2. Divide between plates and serve as a side dish.

Nutrition: Calories: 200; Fat: 8g; Fiber: 2g; Carbs: 4g; Protein: 10g

249. Kale and Cauliflower Mash

⏱ Prep Time 25 m | ⏱ Cooking Time 20-30 m | 4 Servings

Ingredients:

- One cauliflower head, florets separated
- Four garlic cloves; minced
- Three cups kale; chopped.
- Two scallions; chopped.

- 1/3 cup coconut cream
- 1 tbsp. Parsley; chopped.
- 4 tsp. Butter; melted
- A pinch of salt and black pepper

Directions:

1. In a pan that fits the air fryer, combine the cauliflower with the butter, garlic, scallions, salt, pepper and the cream, toss, introduce the pan in the machine and cook at 380°f for 20 minutes

2. Mash the mix well, add the remaining ingredients, whisk, divide between plates and serve.

Nutrition: Calories: 198; Fat: 9g; Fiber: 2g; Carbs: 6g; Protein: 8g

250. Zucchini Gratin

⏱ Prep Time 30 m | ⏱ Cooking Time 20-30 m | 4 Servings

Ingredients:

- 4 cups zucchinis; sliced
- 1 ½ cups mozzarella; shredded
- ½ cup coconut cream

- ½ tbsp. Parsley; chopped.
- 2 tbsp. Butter; melted
- ½ tsp. Garlic powder

Directions:

1. In a baking pan that fits the air fryer, mix all the ingredients except the mozzarella and the parsley and toss.

2. Sprinkle the mozzarella and parsley, introduce in the air fryer and cook at 370°f for 25 minutes.

3. Divide between plates and serve as a side dish

Nutrition: Calories: 220; Fat: 14g; Fiber: 2g; Carbs: 5g; Protein: 9g

251. Spiced Cauliflower

⏱ Prep Time 20 m | ⏱ Cooking Time 20-30 m | 4 Servings

Ingredients:

- One cauliflower head, florets separated
- 1 tbsp. Olive oil
- 1 tbsp. Butter; melted
- ¼ tsp. Cinnamon powder

- ¼ tsp. Cloves, ground
- ¼ tsp. Turmeric powder
- ½ tsp. Cumin, ground
- A pinch of salt and black pepper

Directions:

1. Take a bowl and mix cauliflower florets with the rest of the ingredients and toss.
2. Put the cauliflower in your air fryer's basket and cook at 390°f for 15 minutes

3. Divide between plates and serve as a side dish.

Nutrition: Calories: 182; Fat: 8g; Fiber: 2g; Carbs: 4g; Protein: 8g

252. Roasted Tomatoes

⏱ Prep Time 20 m | ⏱ Cooking Time 25 m | 4 Servings

Ingredients:

- Four tomatoes; halved
- ½ cup parmesan; grated
- 1 tbsp. Basil; chopped.
- ½ tsp. Onion powder

- ½ tsp. Oregano; dried
- ½ tsp. Smoked paprika
- ½ tsp. Garlic powder
- Cooking spray

Directions:

1. Take a bowl and mix all the ingredients except the cooking spray and the parmesan.

2. Arrange the tomatoes in your air fryer's pan, sprinkle the parmesan on top and grease with cooking spray
3. Cook at 370°f for 15 minutes, divide between plates and serve.

Nutrition: Calories: 200; Fat: 7g; Fiber: 2g; Carbs: 4g; Protein: 6g

253. Cauliflower and Artichokes

⏱ Prep Time 25 m | ⏱ Cooking Time 20-30 m | 4 Servings

Ingredients:

- Two garlic cloves; minced
- ½ cup chicken stock
- 1 cup cauliflower florets
- 15 oz. canned artichoke hearts; chopped.

- 1 ½ tbsp. Parsley; chopped.
- 1 tbsp. Olive oil
- 1 tbsp. Parmesan; grated
- Salt and black pepper to taste.

Directions:

1. In a pan that fits your air fryer, mix all the ingredients except the parmesan and toss.
2. Sprinkle the parmesan on top, introduce the pan in the air fryer and cook at 380°f for 20 minutes

3. Divide between plates and serve as a side dish.

Nutrition: Calories: 195; Fat: 6g; Fiber: 2g; Carbs: 4g; Protein: 8g

254. Zucchini Noodles and Sauce

⏲ Prep Time 20 m | ⏲ Cooking Time 20-30 m | 4 Servings

Ingredients:

- Four zucchinis, cut with **a** spiralizer
- 1 ½ cups tomatoes, crushed
- Four garlic cloves; minced
- ¼ cup green onions; chopped.
- 1 tbsp. Olive oil
- 1 tbsp. Basil; chopped.
- Salt and black pepper to taste.

Directions:

1. In **a** pan that fits your air fryer, mix zucchini noodles with the other ingredients, toss, introduce in the fryer and cook at 380°f for 15 minutes.

2. Divide between plates and serve as **a** side dish

Nutrition:
Calories: 194; Fat: 7g; Fiber: 2g; Carbs: 4g; Protein: 9g

255. Broccoli Mash

⏲ Prep Time 20 m | ⏲ Cooking Time 20-30 m | 4 Servings

Ingredients:

- 20 oz. Broccoli florets
- 3 oz. Butter; melted
- One garlic clove; minced
- 4 tbsp. Basil; chopped.
- A drizzle of olive oil
- A pinch of salt and black pepper

Directions:

1. Take **a** bowl and mix the broccoli with the oil, salt and pepper, toss and transfer to your air fryer's basket.
2. Cook at 380°f for 20 minutes, cool the broccoli down and put it in **a** blender

3. Add the rest of the ingredients, pulse, divide the mash between plates and serve as **a** side dish.

Nutrition:
Calories: 200; Fat: 14g; Fiber: 3g; Carbs: 6g; Protein: 7g

256. Cream Cheese Zucchini

⏲ Prep Time 20 m | ⏲ Cooking Time 20-30 m | 4 Servings

Ingredients:

- 1 lb. Zucchinis; cut into wedges
- 1 green onion; sliced
- 1 cup cream cheese, soft
- 1 tbsp. Butter; melted
- 2 tbsp. Basil; chopped.
- 1 tsp. Garlic powder
- A pinch of salt and black pepper

Directions:

1. In **a** pan that fits your air fryer, mix the zucchinis with all the other ingredients, toss, introduce in the air fryer and cook at 370°f for 15 minutes

2. Divide between plates and serve as **a** side dish.

Nutrition:
Calories: 129; Fat: 6g; Fiber: 2g; Carbs: 5g; Protein: 8g

257. Parmesan Zucchini Rounds

⏲ Prep Time 25 m | ⏲ Cooking Time 20-30 m | 4 Servings

Ingredients:

- Four zucchinis; sliced
- 1 ½ cups parmesan; grated
- ¼ cup parsley; chopped.
- One egg; whisked
- One egg white; whisked
- ½ tsp. Garlic powder
- Cooking spray

Directions:

1. Take **a** bowl and mix the egg with egg whites, parmesan, parsley and garlic powder and whisk.
2. Dredge each zucchini slice in this mix, place them all in your air fryer's basket, grease them with cooking spray and cook at 370°f for 20 minutes
3. Divide between plates and serve as **a** side dish.

Nutrition: Calories: 183; Fat: 6g; Fiber: 2g; Carbs: 3g; Protein: 8g

258. Zucchini Spaghetti

⏲ Prep Time 20 m | ⏲ Cooking Time 20-30 m | 4 Servings

Ingredients:

- 1 lb. Zucchinis, cut with **a** spiralizer
- 1 cup parmesan; grated
- ¼ cup parsley; chopped.
- ¼ cup olive oil
- 6 garlic cloves; minced
- ½ tsp. Red pepper flakes
- Salt and black pepper to taste.

Directions:

1. In **a** pan that fits your air fryer, mix all the ingredients, toss, introduce in the fryer and cook at 370°f for 15 minutes

2. Divide between plates and serve as **a** side dish.

Nutrition: Calories: 200; Fat: 6g; Fiber: 3g; Carbs: 4g; Protein: 5g

259. Roasted Eggplant

🕙 Prep Time 30 m | 🕙 Cooking Time 20-30 m | 4 Servings

Ingredients:

- 1 large eggplant
- 2 tbsp. Olive oil
- ½ tsp. Garlic powder.
- ¼ tsp. Salt

Directions:

1. Remove top and bottom from eggplant. Slice eggplant into ¼-inch-thick round slices.
2. Brush slices with olive oil. Sprinkle with salt and garlic powder
3. Place eggplant slices into the air fryer basket. Adjust the temperature to 390 degrees f and set the timer for 15 minutes. Serve immediately.

Nutrition:

Calories: 91; Protein: 1.3g; Fiber: 3.7g; Fat: 6.7g; Carbs: 7.5g

260. Crispy Brussels Sprouts

🕙 Prep Time 20 m | 🕙 Cooking Time 20-30 m | 4 Servings

Ingredients:

- 1 lb. Brussels sprouts; trimmed and shredded
- ¼ cup almonds, toasted and chopped.
- ½ cup olive oil
- Juice of 1 lemon
- Zest of 1 lemon; grated
- 1 tsp. Chili paste
- ½ tsp. Cumin, crushed
- A pinch of salt and black pepper

Directions:

1. In a pan that fits the air fryer, combine the brussels sprouts with all the other ingredients, toss, put the pan in the fryer and cook at 390°f for 15 minutes
2. Divide between plates and serve as a side dish.

Nutrition:

Calories: 200; Fat: 9g; Fiber: 2g; Carbs: 6g; Protein: 9g

261. Coated Avocado Tacos

🕙 Prep Time 10 m | 🕙 Cooking Time 20 m | 12 Servings

Ingredients:

- 1 avocado
- Tortillas and toppings
- ½ cup panko breadcrumbs
- 1 egg
- Salt

Directions:

1. Scoop out the meat from each avocado shell and slice them into wedges.
2. Beat the egg in a shallow bowl and put the breadcrumbs in another bowl.
3. Dip the avocado wedges in the beaten egg and coat with breadcrumbs. Sprinkle them with a bit of salt. Arrange them in the cooking basket in a single layer.
4. Cook for 15 minutes at 392 degrees. The basket should shake halfway through the cooking process.
5. Put the cooked avocado wedges in tortillas and add your preferred toppings.

Nutrition:

Calories: 179 Fat: 6.07g Carbs: 26.29g Protein: 4.94g

262. Cheeseburger Egg Rolls
Prep Time 10 m | Cooking Time 7 m | 6 Servings

Ingredients
- 6 egg roll wrappers
- 6 chopped dill pickle chips
- 1 tbsp. yellow mustard
- 3 tbsp. cream cheese
- 3 tbsp. shredded cheddar cheese
- ½ C. chopped onion
- ½ C. chopped bell pepper
- ¼ tsp. onion powder
- ¼ tsp. garlic powder
- 8 ounces of raw lean ground beef

Directions
1. In a skillet, add the spices, meat, onion, and bell pepper. Stir and mash the meat until it is fully cooked and the vegetables are soft.
2. Remove skillet from heat and add cream cheese, mustard, and cheddar cheese, stirring until melted.
3. Pour the meat mixture into a bowl and add the pickles.
4. Place egg wrappers and spoon 1/6 of the meat mixture into each. Dampen the edges of the egg roll with water. Fold the sides in half and seal with water.
5. Repeat with all the other egg rolls.
6. Place the rolls in a deep fryer, one batch at a time.
7. Pour into the Oven rack/basket. Place the air fryer Rack on the middle-shelf of the Smart Air Fryer Oven. Set temperature to 391°F, and set time to 7 minutes.

Nutrition
Calories 153 | Fat 4 g | Protein 12 g | Sugar 3 g

263. Air Fried Grilled Steak
Prep Time 5 m | Cooking Time 45 m | 2 Servings

Ingredients
- Top sirloin steaks
- Tablespoons butter, melted
- 3 tablespoons olive oil
- Salt and pepper to taste

Directions
1. Preheat the Smart Air Fryer for 5 minutes.
2. Season the sirloin steaks with olive oil, salt, and pepper.
3. Place the beef in the air fryer oven basket.
4. Cook for 45 minutes at 350°F.
5. Once cooked, serve with butter.

Nutrition
Calories 1536 | Fat 123.7 g | Protein 103.4 g

264. Juicy Cheeseburgers
Prep Time 5 m | Cooking Time 15 m | 4 Servings

Ingredients
- 1 pound 93% lean ground beef
- 1 teaspoon Worcestershire sauce
- 1 tablespoon burger seasoning
- Salt
- Pepper
- Cooking oil
- Slices cheese
- Buns

Directions
1. In a large bowl, combine the ground beef, Worcestershire, hamburger seasoning, and salt and pepper to taste until well combined. Spray the fryer basket with cooking oil. You will only need a quick spray because hamburgers produce oil while they cook. Form 4 patties with the mixture. Place the burgers in the deep fryer. Burgers should fit without having to be stacked, but stacking is fine if necessary.
2. Place on the oven rack/basket. Place the rack on the middle shelf of the Smart Air Fryer. Set the temperature to 375 ° F and set the time to 8 minutes. Cook for 8 minutes. Open the fryer and flip the patties—Cook for 3 to 4 more minutes. Check the inside of the patties to see if they have finished cooking. You can stick a knife or fork in the center to examine the color.
3. Fill each burger with a slice of cheese. Cook for one more minute or until cheese is melted. Serve on buns with any additional toppings of your choice.

Nutrition
Calories 566 | Fat 39 g | Protein 29 g | Fiber 1 g

265. Spicy Thai Beef Stir-Fry
Prep Time 15 m | Cooking Time 9 m | 4 Servings

Ingredients
- 1 pound sirloin steaks, thinly sliced
- Tablespoons lime juice, divided
- ⅓ cup crunchy peanut butter
- ½ cup beef broth
- 1 tablespoon olive oil
- 1½ cups broccoli florets
- Cloves garlic, sliced
- 1 to 2 red chile peppers, sliced

Directions
1. In a medium bowl, combine the steak with 1 tablespoon of the lime juice. Set aside.
2. Combine the peanut butter and beef broth in a small bowl and mix well. Drain the beef and add the juice from the bowl into the peanut butter mixture.
3. In a 6-inch metal bowl, combine the olive oil, steak, and broccoli.
4. Pour into the Oven rack/basket. Place the air fryer Rack on the middle-shelf of the Smart Air Fryer Oven. Set temperature to 375°F, and set time to 4 minutes. Cook for 4 more minutes or until the steak is almost cooked and the broccoli is crisp and tender, shaking the basket once during cooking time.
5. Add the garlic, chile peppers, and the peanut butter mixture and stir.
6. Cook for 5 more minutes or until the sauce is bubbling and the broccoli is tender.
7. Serve over hot rice.

Nutrition
Calories 387 | Fat 22 g | Protein 42 g | Fiber 2 g

266. Beef Brisket Recipe from Texas

⏱ Prep Time 15 m | ⏱ Cooking Time 1 h 30 m | 8 Servings

Ingredients

- 1 ½ cup beef stock
- 1 bay leaf
- 1 tablespoon garlic powder
- 1 tablespoon onion powder
- Pounds beef brisket, trimmed

- 2 tablespoons chili powder
- 2 teaspoons dry mustard
- Tablespoons olive oil
- Salt and pepper to taste

Directions

1. Preheat the Air Fryer Oven for 5 minutes. Place all ingredients in a deep baking dish that will fit in the air fryer.

2. Bake for 1 hour and 30 minutes at 400°F.
3. Stir the beef every after 30 minutes to soak in the sauce.

Nutrition

Calories 306 | Fat 24.1 g | Protein 18.3 g

267. Copycat Taco Bell Crunch Wraps

⏱ Prep Time 10 m | ⏱ Cooking Time 2 m | 6 Servings

Ingredients

- Wheat tostadas
- C. sour cream
- 2 C. Mexican blend cheese
- 2 C. shredded lettuce
- 12 ounces low-sodium nacho cheese

- Roma tomatoes
- 12-inch wheat tortillas
- 1 1/3 C. water
- 2 packets low-sodium taco seasoning
- 2 pounds of lean ground beef

Directions

1. Ensure your air fryer is preheated to 400 degrees.
2. Make beef according to taco seasoning packets.
3. Place 2/3 C. prepared beef, 4 tbsp. cheese, 1 tostada, 1/3 C. sour cream, 1/3 C. lettuce, 1/6th of tomatoes, and 1/3 C. cheese on each tortilla.

4. Fold up tortillas edges and repeat with remaining ingredients. Lay the folded sides of tortillas down into the air fryer and spray with olive oil.
5. Set temperature to 400°F, and set time to 2 minutes. Cook 2 minutes until browned.

Nutrition

Calories 311 | Fat 9g | Protein 22g | Sugar 2g

268. Steak and Mushroom Gravy

⏱ Prep Time 15 m | ⏱ Cooking Time 15 m | 4 Servings

Ingredients

- Cubed steaks
- 2 large eggs
- 1/2 dozen mushrooms
- Tablespoons unsalted butter
- Tablespoons black pepper
- 2 tablespoons salt
- 1/2 teaspoon onion powder

- 1/2 teaspoon garlic powder
- 1/4 teaspoon cayenne powder
- 1 1/4 teaspoons paprika
- 1 1/2 cups whole milk
- 1/3 cup flour
- Tablespoons vegetable oil

Directions

1. Mix 1/2 flour and a pinch of black pepper in a shallow bowl or on a plate.
2. Beat 2 eggs in a bowl and mix with a pinch of salt and pepper.
3. In another shallow bowl, mix the other half of the flour with pepper to taste, garlic powder, paprika, cayenne, and onion powder.
4. Chop the mushrooms and reserve.
5. Squeeze the fillet into the first bowl of flour, then dip it into the egg and then press the fillet into the second bowl of flour until completely covered.

6. Place on the oven rack/basket. Place the rack on the middle shelf of the Smart Air Fryer. Set the temperature to 360 ° F and set the time to 15 minutes by turning it halfway.
7. While the steak is cooking, heat the butter over medium heat and add the mushrooms to the stir-fry.
8. Add 4 tablespoons of flour and pepper to the skillet and mix until there are no lumps of flour.
9. Mix in whole milk and simmer.

Nutrition

Calories 442 | Fat 27 g | Protein 32 g | Fiber 2.3 g

269. Air Fryer Beef Casserole

⏱ Prep Time 5 m | ⏱ Cooking Time 30 m | 4 Servings

Ingredients

- 1 green bell pepper, seeded and chopped
- 1 onion, chopped
- 1-pound ground beef
- Cloves of garlic, minced

- Tablespoons olive oil
- Cups eggs, beaten
- Salt and pepper to taste

Directions

1. Preheat the Smart Air Fryer oven for 5 minutes.
2. In a skillet that will fit in the deep fryer, combine the ground beef, onion, garlic, olive oil, and pepper. Season with salt and pepper to taste.
3. Add the beaten eggs and mix well.

4. Place the plate with the meat and egg mixture in the deep fryer.
5. Place on the oven rack/basket. Place the rack on the middle shelf of the Smart Air Fryer. Set the temperature to 325 ° F and set the time to 30 minutes. Bake for 30 minutes.

Nutrition

Calories 1520 | Fat 125.11 g | Protein 87.9 g

270. Country Fried Steak

Ingredients

- 1 tsp. pepper
- C. almond milk
- 2 tbsp. almond flour
- Ounces ground sausage meat
- 1 tsp. pepper
- 1 tsp. salt

- 1 tsp. garlic powder
- 1 tsp. onion powder
- 1 C. panko breadcrumbs
- 1 C. almond flour
- Beaten eggs
- Ounces sirloin steak, pounded till thin

Directions

1. Season panko breadcrumbs with spices.
2. Dredge steak in flour, then egg, and then seasoned panko mixture.
3. Place into the air fryer basket.
4. Set temperature to 370°F, and set time to 12 minutes.

5. To make sausage gravy, cook sausage and drain off fat, but reserve 2 tablespoons.
6. Add flour to sausage and mix until incorporated. Gradually mix in milk over medium to high heat until it becomes thick.
7. Season mixture with pepper and cook 3 minutes longer.

Nutrition

Calories 395 | Fat 11 g | Protein 39 g | Sugar 5 g

271. Meat Lovers' Pizza

Prep Time 10 m | Cooking Time 12 m | 2 Servings

Ingredients

- 1 pre-prepared 7-inch pizza pie crust, defrosted if necessary
- 1/3 cup of marinara sauce.
- ounces of grilled steak, sliced into bite-sized pieces
- 2 ounces of salami, sliced fine

- 2 ounces of pepperoni, sliced fine
- ¼ cup of American cheese
- ¼ cup of shredded mozzarella cheese

Directions

1. Preheat the Smart Air Fryer Oven to 350 degrees. Lay the pizza dough flat on a sheet of parchment paper or tin foil, cut large enough to hold the entire pie crust, but small enough that it will leave the edges of the air frying basket uncovered to allow for air circulation.
2. Using a fork, stab the pizza dough several times across the surface – piercing the pie crust will allow air to circulate throughout the crust and ensure even cooking.
3. With a deep soup spoon, scoop the marinara sauce onto the pizza dough, and spread evenly in expanding circles over the surface of the pie-crust. Be sure to leave at least ½ inch of bare dough around the edges, to ensure that extra-crispy crunchy first bite of the crust!

4. Distribute the pieces of steak and the slices of salami and pepperoni evenly over the sauce-covered dough, then sprinkle the cheese in an even layer on top.
5. Set the air fryer timer to 12 minutes, and place the pizza with foil or paper on the fryer's basket surface. Again, be sure to leave the edges of the basket uncovered to allow for proper air circulation, and don't let your bare fingers touch the hot surface.
6. After 12 minutes, when the Smart Air Fryer Oven shuts off, the cheese should be perfectly melted and lightly crisped, and the pie crust should be golden brown. Using a spatula – or two, if necessary, remove the pizza from the air fryer basket and set on a serving plate.
7. Wait a few minutes until the pie is cool enough to handle, then cut into slices and serve.

Nutrition

Calories 342 | Fat 17 g | Protein 12 g | Fiber 4.3 g

272. Chimichurri Skirt Steak

Prep Time 10 m | Cooking Time 8 m | 2 Servings

Ingredients

- x 8 oz. Skirt Steak
- 1 cup finely chopped parsley
- ¼ cup finely chopped mint
- 2 tbsp. fresh oregano (washed & finely chopped)
- Finely chopped cloves of garlic
- 1 tsp red pepper flakes (Crushed)
- 1 tbsp. ground cumin

- 1 tsp cayenne pepper
- 2 tsp smoked paprika
- 1 tsp salt
- ¼ tsp pepper
- ¾ cup oil
- Tbsp. red wine vinegar

Directions

1. Throw all the ingredients in a bowl (besides the steak) and mix well.
2. Put ¼ cup of the mixture in a plastic baggie with the steak and leave in the fridge overnight (2–24hrs).
3. Leave the bag out at room temperature for at least 30 min before popping into the air fryer. Preheat for a minute or two to 390° F before

cooking until med–rare (8–10 min). Pour into the oven rack/basket. Place the air fryer Rack on the middle-shelf of the Smart Air Fryer Oven. Set temperature to 390°F, and set time to 10 minutes.
4. Put 2 tablespoons of the chimichurri mix on top of each steak before serving.

Nutrition

Calories 272 | Fat 3 g | Protein 32 g | Fiber 2.8 g

273. Warming Winter Beef with Celery
⏱ Prep Time 5 m | ⏱ Cooking Time 12 m | 4 Servings

Ingredients

- 9 ounces tender beef, chopped
- 1/2 cup leeks, chopped
- 1/2 cup celery stalks, chopped
- Cloves garlic, smashed
- Tablespoons red cooking wine
- 3/4 cup cream of celery soup
- 2 sprigs rosemary, chopped
- 1/4 teaspoon smoked paprika
- 3/4 teaspoons salt
- Salt and 1/4 teaspoon black pepper to taste

Directions

1. Add the beef, leeks, celery, and garlic to the baking dish; cook for about 5 minutes at 390 degrees F.
2. Once the meat is starting to tender, pour in the wine and soup. Season with rosemary, smoked paprika, salt, and black pepper. Now, cook an additional 7 minutes.

Nutrition Calories 312 | Fat 17 g | Protein 22 g | Fiber 32 g

274. Creamy Burger & Potato Bake
⏱ Prep Time 5 m | ⏱ Cooking Time 55 m | 3 Servings

Ingredients

- Salt to taste
- Freshly ground pepper, to taste
- 1/2 (10.75 ounces) can of condensed cream of mushroom soup
- 1/2-pound lean ground beef
- 1-1/2 cups peeled and thinly sliced potatoes
- 1/2 cup shredded cheddar cheese
- 1/4 cup chopped onion
- 1/4 cup and 2 tablespoons milk

Directions

1. Lightly grease baking pan of the air fryer with cooking spray. Add ground beef. For 10 minutes, cook on 360°F. Stir and crumble halfway through cooking time.
2. Meanwhile, in a bowl, whisk well pepper, salt, milk, onion, and mushroom soup. Mix well.
3. Drain fat off ground beef and transfer beef to a plate.
4. In the same air fryer baking pan, layer ½ of potatoes on the bottom, then ½ of soup mixture, and then ½ of beef. Repeat process.
5. Cover pan with foil.
6. Cook for 30 minutes. Remove the aluminum foil and cook for another 15 minutes or until potatoes are tender.
7. Serve and enjoy.

Nutrition
Calories 399 | Fat 26.9 g | Protein 22.1 g

275. Beefy 'n Cheesy Spanish Rice Casserole
⏱ Prep Time 10 m | ⏱ Cooking Time 50 m | 3 Servings

Ingredients

- Tablespoons chopped green bell pepper
- 1 tablespoon chopped fresh cilantro
- 1/2-pound lean ground beef
- 1/2 cup water
- 1/2 teaspoon salt
- 1/2 teaspoon brown sugar
- 1/2 pinch ground black pepper
- 1/3 cup uncooked long-grain rice
- 1/4 cup finely chopped onion
- 1/4 cup chile sauce
- 1/4 teaspoon ground cumin
- 1/4 teaspoon Worcestershire sauce
- 1/4 cup shredded Cheddar cheese
- 1/2 (14.5 ounces) can canned tomatoes

Directions

1. Lightly grease baking pan of the air fryer with cooking spray. Add ground beef.
2. For 10 minutes, cook on 360°F. Halfway through cooking time, stir and crumble beef. Discard excess fat.
3. Stir in pepper, Worcestershire sauce, cumin, brown sugar, salt, chile sauce, rice, water, tomatoes, green bell pepper, and onion. Mix well. Cover pan with foil and cook for 25 minutes. Stirring occasionally.
4. Give it one last good stir, press down firmly, and sprinkle cheese on top.
5. Cook uncovered for 15 minutes at 390°F until tops are lightly browned.
6. Serve and enjoy with chopped cilantro.

Nutrition
Calories 346 | Fat: 19.1 g | Protein 18.5 g

276. Beef & Veggie Spring Rolls
⏱ Prep Time 5 m | ⏱ Cooking Time 12 m | 10 Servings

Ingredients

- 2-ounce Asian rice noodles
- 1 tablespoon sesame oil
- 7-ounce ground beef
- 1 small onion, chopped
- garlic cloves, crushed
- 1 cup of fresh mixed vegetables
- 1 teaspoon soy sauce
- 1 packet spring roll skins
- Tablespoons water
- Olive oil, as required

Directions

1. Soak the noodles in warm water till it becomes soft.
2. Drain and cut into small lengths. In a pan heat the oil and add the onion and garlic and sauté for about 4-5 minutes.
3. Add beef and cook for about 4-5 minutes.
4. Add vegetables and cook for about 5-7 minutes or till cooked through.
5. Stir in soy sauce and remove from the heat.
6. Immediately, stir in the noodles and keep aside till all the juices have been absorbed.
7. Preheat the Smart Air Fryer Oven to 350 degrees F.
8. Place the spring rolls skin onto a smooth surface.
9. Add a line of the filling diagonally across.
10. Fold the top point over the filling and then fold in both sides.
11. On the final point brush it with water before rolling to seal.
12. Brush the spring rolls with oil.
13. Arrange the rolls in batches in the air fryer and cook for about 8 minutes.
14. Repeat with remaining rolls. Now, place spring rolls onto a baking sheet.
15. Bake for about 6 minutes per side.

Nutrition
Calories 532 | Fat 8 g | Protein 31 g | Fiber 12.3 g

277. Garlic and Rosemary Lamb Cutlets

⏱ Prep Time 30 m | ⏱ Cooking Time 25 m | 2 Servings

Ingredients

- 2 lamb racks (with 3 cutlets per rack)
- 2 cloves garlic, peeled and thinly sliced into slivers
- 2 long sprigs of fresh rosemary, leaves removed

Directions

1. Trim fat from racks and cut slits with a sharp knife in the top of the lamb. Insert slices of the garlic and rosemary leaves in the slits and set the lamb aside.
2. Make the marinade by whisking the mustard, honey, and mint sauce together and brush over the lamb racks. Let the marinade in a cool area for 20 minutes.

Nutrition

Calories 309 | Fat 2 g | Protein 33 g | Fiber 16 g

- 2 tablespoons wholegrain mustard
- 1 tablespoon honey
- 2 tablespoons mint sauce (I use mint jelly)

3. Preheat the air fryer to 360 degrees for about 5 minutes.
4. Spray the basket using cooking spray and place the lamb rack or racks into the basket, propping them up however you can get them in to fit.
5. Cook 10 minutes, open and turn the racks and cook 10 more minutes.
6. Place on a platter and cover with foil to let sit 10 minutes before slicing and serving.

278. Asian Inspired Sichuan Lamb

⏱ Prep Time 5 m | ⏱ Cooking Time 10 m | 4 Servings

Ingredients

- 1 ½ tablespoons cumin seed (do not use ground cumin)
- 1 teaspoon Sichuan peppers or ½ teaspoon cayenne
- 2 tablespoons vegetable oil
- 1 tablespoon garlic, peeled and minced
- 1 tablespoon light soy sauce
- 2 red chili peppers, seeded and chopped (use gloves)

Directions

1. Turn on the burner to medium-high on the stove and heat up a dry skillet. Pour in the cumin seed and Sichuan peppers or cayenne and toast until fragrant. Turn off the burner and set aside until they are cool. Grind them in a grinder or mortar and pestle.
2. In a large bowl that will contain the marinade and the lamb, combine the vegetable oil, garlic, soy sauce, chili peppers, granulated sugar, and salt. Pour in the cumin/pepper combination and mix well.
3. Using a fork, poke holes in the lamb all over the top and bottom. Place the lamb in the marinade, cover, and refrigerate. You can also use a closeable plastic bag.

Nutrition

Calories 142 | Fat 7 g | Protein 17 g | Fiber 4 g

- ¼ teaspoon granulated sugar
- ½ teaspoon salt
- 1 pound lamb shoulder, cut in ½ to 1-inch pieces
- 2 green onions, chopped
- 1 handful fresh cilantro, chopped

4. Preheat the air fryer to 360 degrees for 5 minutes.
5. Spray the basket with cooking spray.
6. Remove the lamb pieces from the marinade with tongs or slotted spoon and place them in the basket of the air fryer in a single layer. You may need to do more than 1 batch.
7. Cook for 10 minutes, flipping over 1 halfway through. Make sure the lamb's internal temperature is 145 degrees F with a meat thermometer. Put on a serving platter and repeat with the rest of the lamb.
8. Sprinkle the chopped green onions and cilantro over top, stir and serve.

279. Garlic Sauced Lamb Chops

⏱ Prep Time 15 m | ⏱ Cooking Time 25 m | 4 Servings

Ingredients

- 1 garlic bulb
- 1 teaspoon + 3 tablespoons olive oil
- 1 tablespoon fresh oregano, chopped fine

Directions

1. Preheat the air fryer to 400 degrees F 5 minutes and while it is preheating take the excess paper from the garlic bulb.
2. Coat the garlic bulb with the 1 teaspoon of olive oil and drop it in the basket that has been treated with cooking spray. Roast for 12 minutes.
3. Combine the 3 tablespoons of olive oil, oregano, salt, and pepper and lightly coat the lamb chops on both with the resulting oil. Let them sit at room temperature for 5 minutes.
4. Remove the garlic bulb from the basket and if it is cool, preheat again to 400 degrees for 3 minutes.

Nutrition

Calories 194 | Fat 11 g | Protein 29 g | Fiber 13 g

- ¼ teaspoon ground pepper
- ½ teaspoon sea salt
- 8 lamb chops

5. Spray the air fryer basket with cooking oil and place 4 chops in cooking at 400 degrees F for 5 minutes. Place them on a platter and cover to keep them warm while you do the other chops.
6. Squeeze each garlic clove between the thumb and index finger into a small bowl.
7. Taste and add salt and pepper and mix. Serve along with the chops like serving ketchup.

280. Herb Encrusted Lamb Chops

⏱ Prep Time 5 m | ⏱ Cooking Time 15 m | 2 Servings

Ingredients

- 1 teaspoon oregano
- 1 teaspoon coriander
- 1 teaspoon thyme
- 1 teaspoon rosemary
- ½ teaspoon salt

Directions

1. In a closeable bag, combine the oregano, coriander, thyme, rosemary, salt, pepper, lemon juice, and olive oil and shake well so it mixes.
2. Place the chops in the bag and squish around so the mixture is on them. Refrigerate 1 hour.
3. Preheat the air fryer to 390 degrees F for 5 minutes.

Nutrition Calories 321 | Fat 34g | Protein 18 g | Fiber 15 g

- ¼ teaspoon pepper
- 2 tablespoons lemon juice
- 2 tablespoons olive oil
- 1 pound lamb chops

4. Place the chops in the basket that has been sprayed with cooking spray.
5. Cook for 3 minutes and pause. Flip the chops to the other side and cook for another 4 minutes for medium rare. If you want them more well done, cook 4 minutes, pause, turn and cook 5 more minutes.

281. Herbed Rack of Lamb

⏱ Prep Time 15 m | ⏱ Cooking Time 35 m | 2 Servings

Ingredients

- 1 tablespoon olive oil
- 1 clove garlic, peeled and minced
- 1 ½ teaspoons fresh ground pepper
- 1 tablespoon fresh rosemary, chopped
- 1 tablespoon fresh thyme, chopped
- ¾ cup breadcrumbs
- 1 egg
- 1 to 2 pounds rack of lamb

Directions

1. Place the olive oil in a small dish and add the garlic. Mix well.
2. Brush the garlic on the rack of lamb and season with pepper.
3. In one bowl combine the rosemary, thyme, and breadcrumbs and break the egg and whisk in another bowl.
4. Preheat air fryer 350 degrees F for 5 minutes. Spray with cooking spray.
5. Dip the rack in the egg and then place in the breadcrumb mixture and coat the rack.
6. Place rack in the air fryer basket and cook 20 minutes.
7. Raise the temperature to 400 degrees F and set for 5 more minutes.
8. Tear a piece of aluminum foil that will fit to wrap the rack. Take it out of the basket with tongs and put it in the middle of the foil. Carefully wrap and let sit about 10 minutes. Unwrap and serve.

Nutrition

Calories 282 | Fat 23 g | Protein 26 g | Fiber 23 g

282. Lamb Roast with Root Vegetables

⏱ Prep Time 35 m | ⏱ Cooking Time 1 h 15 m | 6 Servings

Ingredients

- 4 cloves garlic, peeled and sliced thin, divided
- 2 springs fresh rosemary, leaves pulled off, divided
- 3 pounds leg of lamb
- salt and pepper to taste, divided
- 2 medium-sized sweet potatoes, peeled and cut into wedges
- 2 tablespoon oil, divided
- 2 cups baby carrots
- 1 teaspoon butter
- 4 large red potatoes, cubed

Directions

1. Slice the garlic and take the leaves of the rosemary.
2. Cut about 5 to 6 slits in the top of the lamb and insert slices of garlic and some rosemary in each. Salt and pepper the roast to your taste and set aside to cook after the vegetables are done.
3. Coat the sweet potatoes in 1 tablespoon of olive oil and season with salt and pepper.
4. Spray the basket of the air fryer with cooking spray and put it in the wedges. You may have to do two batches. Set for 400 degrees F and air fry 8 minutes, shake and cook another 8 minutes or so. Dump into a bowl and cover with foil.
5. Place the carrots in some foil to cover and put the butter on top of them. Enclose them in the foil and place them in the air fryer. Set for 400 degrees for 20 minutes. Remove from the air fryer.
6. Coat the basket with cooking spray. Mix the red potatoes with the other tablespoon of oil and salt and pepper to taste. Place in the air fryer oven and cook at 400 degrees F for 20 minutes, shaking after 10 minutes have elapsed.
7. Use a foil tray or baking dish that fits into the air fryer and coat with cooking spray. Place the leftover garlic and rosemary in the bottom and place the lamb on top.
8. Set for 380 degrees F and cook 1 hour, checking after 30 minutes and 45 minutes to make sure it isn't getting too done. Increase the air fryer oven heat to 400 degrees F and cook for 10 to 15 minutes.
9. Remove the roast from the air fryer and set on a platter. Cover with foil and rest 10 minutes while you dump all the vegetables back in the basket and cooking at 350 degrees F for 8 to 10 minutes or until heated through.
10. Serve all together.

Nutrition

Calories 398 | Fat 5 g | Protein 18 g | Fiber 30.3 g

283. Lemon and Cumin Coated Rack of Lamb

⏱ Prep Time 15 m | ⏱ Cooking Time 200 m | 4 Servings

Ingredients

- 1 ½ to 1 ¾ pound Frenched rack of lamb
- Salt and pepper to taste
- ½ cup breadcrumbs
- 1 teaspoon cumin seed
- 1 teaspoon ground cumin
- ½ teaspoon salt
- 1 teaspoon garlic, peeled and grated
- Lemon zest (1/4 of a lemon)
- 1 teaspoon vegetable or olive oil
- 1 egg, beaten

Directions

1. Season the lamb rack with pepper and salt to taste and set it aside.
2. In a large bowl, combine the breadcrumbs, cumin seed, ground cumin, salt, garlic, lemon zest, and oil and set aside.
3. In another bowl, beat the egg.
4. Preheat to air fryer to 250 degrees F for 5 minutes
5. Dip the rack in the egg to coat and then into the breadcrumb mixture. Make sure it is well coated.
6. Spray the basket of the air fryer using cooking spray and put the rack in. You may have to bend it a little to get it to fit.
7. Set for 250 degrees and cook 25 minutes.
8. Increase temperature to 400 degrees F and cook another 5 minutes. Check internal temperature to make sure it is 145 degrees for medium-rare or more.
9. Remove rack when done and cover with foil for 10 minutes before separating ribs into individual servings.

Nutrition

Calories 276 | Fat 24 g | Protein 33 g | Fiber 12.3 g

284. Macadamia Rack of Lamb
Prep Time 20 m | Cooking Time 32 m | 4 Servings

Ingredients
- 1 tablespoon olive oil
- 1 clove garlic, peeled and minced
- 1 ½ to 1 ¾ pound rack of lamb
- Salt and pepper to taste
- ¾ cup unsalted macadamia nuts
- 1 tablespoon fresh rosemary, chopped
- 1 tablespoon breadcrumbs
- 1 egg, beaten

Directions
1. Mix together the olive oil and garlic and brush it all over the rack of lamb. Season with salt and pepper.
2. Preheat the air fryer 250 degrees F for 8 minutes.
3. Chop the macadamia nuts as fine as possible and put them in a bowl.
4. Mix in the rosemary and breadcrumbs and set it aside.
5. Beat the egg in another bowl.
6. Dip the rack in the egg mixture to coat completely.
7. Place the rack in the breadcrumb mixture and coat well.
8. Spray the basket of the air fryer using cooking spray and place the rack inside.
9. Cook at 250 degrees for 25 minutes and then increase to 400 and cook another 5 to 10 minutes or until done.
10. Cover with foil paper for 10 minutes, uncover and separate into chops and serve.

Nutrition
Calories 321 | Fat 9 g | Protein 12 g | Fiber 8.3 g

285. Perfect Lamb Burgers
Prep Time 10 m | Cooking Time 20 m | 4 Servings

Ingredients
For the Moroccan spice mix:
- 1 teaspoon ground ginger
- 1 teaspoon ground cumin
- 1 teaspoon sea salt
- ¾ teaspoon ground black pepper
- ½ teaspoon ground coriander
- ½ teaspoon ground allspice
- ½ teaspoon ground cloves
- ½ teaspoon ground cinnamon
- ½ teaspoon cayenne

For burgers and dip:
- 1 ½ pound ground lamb
- 1 teaspoon Harissa paste
- 2 tablespoons Moroccan spice mix, divided
- 2 teaspoons garlic, peeled and minced
- ¼ teaspoon fresh chopped oregano
- 3 tablespoons plain Greek yogurt
- 1 small lemon, juiced

Directions
Moroccan Spice Mix:
1. Whisk the ginger, cumin, salt, pepper, coriander, allspice, cloves, cinnamon, and cayenne in a small bowl and set aside.

Burgers and dip:
1. Place the lamb in a large bowl and add the Harissa sauce, 1 tablespoon of the homemade Moroccan spice mix, and the garlic. Mix in everything with the hands and form 4 patties.
2. Preheat the air fryer to 360 degrees for 5 minutes while making the patties.
3. Spray the basket of the air fryer using cooking spray and place two of the burgers in.
4. Cook a total of 12 minutes, flipping after 6 minutes.
5. Repeat with the other two burgers.
6. While burgers cook, make the dip by chopping the fresh oregano and placing it in a bowl with the yogurt, 1 teaspoon of the Moroccan spice mix, and the juice of the lemon. Whisk this with a fork and divide it into small containers to serve with the burgers when they are done.

Nutrition
Calories 534 | Fat 8 g | Protein 21 g | Fiber 8.7 g

286. Tandoori Lamb
Prep Time 10 m | Cooking Time 20 m | 4 Servings

Ingredients
- ½ onion, peeled and quartered
- 5 cloves garlic, peeled
- 4 slices fresh ginger, peeled
- 1 teaspoon ground fennel
- 1 teaspoon Garam Masala
- 1 teaspoon ground cinnamon
- ½ teaspoon ground cardamom
- ½ teaspoon cayenne
- 1 teaspoon salt
- 1 pound boneless lamb sirloin steaks

Directions
1. Place the onion, garlic, ginger, fennel, Garam Masala, cinnamon, cardamom, cayenne, and salt in a blender and pulse 4 to 6 times until ground.
2. Place the lamb steaks in a large bowl and slash the meat so the spices will permeate into it.
3. Pour the spice mix over top and rub it on both sides. Let sit room temperature 30 minutes or cover and refrigerate overnight.
4. Preheat the air fryer to 350 degrees F for 10 minutes.
5. Spray the basket using cooking spray and place lamb steaks in without letting them overlap much. You may have to do this in batches.
6. Cook 7 minutes, turn and cook another 8 minutes.
7. Test with the meat thermometer to make sure they are done. The medium-well will be 150 degrees F.

Nutrition
Calories 232 | Fat 20 g | Protein 42 g | Fiber 5 g

287. Simple Yet Tasty Lamb Chops

⏱ Prep Time 15 m | ⏱ Cooking Time 30 m | 4 Servings

Ingredients
- 1 clove of garlic separated from the head of garlic (maybe 2)
- 1 ½ tablespoons olive oil
- 4 lamb chops

- ½ tablespoon fresh oregano, chopped
- Salt and pepper to taste

Directions
1. Preheat the air fryer oven to 400 degrees F for 6 minutes.
2. Take a little of the olive oil and coat the garlic clove(s). Place in the basket of the air fryer and roast 12 minutes.
3. While the garlic is cooking, mix the oregano, salt, and pepper in a small bowl. Add all the remaining olive oil and mix well.
4. Spread a thin coating of the oregano mixture on both sides of the lamb chops and reserve the rest.
5. Remove the clove(s) of garlic from the basket of the air fryer with rubber-tipped tongs. Be careful because the cloves will be very soft and you don't want them to break open quite yet.
6. Spray the basket of the air fryer using cooking spray and place the lamb chops in, 2 at a time in 2 batches. Cook 5 minutes, turn and cook another 4 minutes.
7. When chops are done, squeeze the garlic out of the papery shell into the rest of the oregano mixture and mix it in. Serve this on the side like ketchup.

Nutrition
Calories 542 | Fat 4 g | Protein 23 g | Fiber 6 g

288. Barbecue Flavored Pork Ribs

⏱ Prep Time 5 m | ⏱ Cooking Time 15 m | 6 Servings

Ingredients
- ¼ cup honey, divided
- ¾ cup BBQ sauce
- 2 tablespoons tomato ketchup
- 1 tablespoon Worcestershire sauce

- 1 tablespoon soy sauce
- ½ teaspoon garlic powder
- Freshly ground white pepper, to taste
- 1¾ pound pork ribs

Directions
1. In a large bowl, mix together 3 tablespoons of honey and remaining ingredients except for the pork ribs.
2. Refrigerate to marinate for about 20 minutes.
3. Preheat the Air fryer oven to 355 degrees F.
4. Place the ribs in an Air fryer rack/basket.
5. Cook for about 13 minutes.
6. Remove the ribs from the Air fryer oven and coat with remaining honey.
7. Serve hot.

Nutrition
Calories 376 | Fat 20 g | Protein 32 g | Fiber 12 g

289. Rustic Pork Ribs

⏱ Prep Time 5 m | ⏱ Cooking Time 15 m | 4 Servings

Ingredients
- 1 rack of pork ribs
- 3 tablespoons dry red wine
- 1 tablespoon soy sauce
- 1/2 teaspoon dried thyme
- 1/2 teaspoon onion powder

- 1/2 teaspoon garlic powder
- 1/2 teaspoon ground black pepper
- 1 teaspoon smoked salt
- 1 tablespoon cornstarch
- 1/2 teaspoon olive oil

Directions
1. Begin by preheating your Air fryer oven to 390 degrees F. Place all ingredients in a mixing bowl and let them marinate at least 1 hour.

Air Frying:
2. Cook the marinated ribs approximately 25 minutes at 390 degrees F.
3. Serve hot.

Nutrition
Calories 326 | Fat 14 g | Protein 23 g | Fiber 13 g

290. Italian Parmesan Breaded Pork Chops

⏱ Prep Time 5 m | ⏱ Cooking Time 25 m | 5 Servings

Ingredients
- 5 (3½- to 5-ounce) pork chops (bone-in or boneless)
- 1 teaspoon Italian seasoning
- Seasoning salt
- Pepper

- ¼ cup all-purpose flour
- 2 tablespoons Italian bread crumbs
- 3 tablespoons finely grated Parmesan cheese
- Cooking oil

Directions
1. Season the pork chops with the Italian seasoning and seasoning salt and pepper to taste.
2. Sprinkle the flour on each side of the pork chops, then coat both sides with the bread crumbs and Parmesan cheese.
3. Place the pork chops in the air fryer oven. Stacking them is okay. Spray the pork chops with cooking oil. Set temperature to 360°F. Cook for 6 minutes.
4. Open the air fryer oven and flip the pork chops. Cook for an additional 6 minutes.
5. Cool before serving. Instead of seasoning salt, you can use either chicken or pork rub for additional flavor. You can find these rubs in the spice aisle of the grocery store.

Nutrition
Calories 334 | Fat 7 g | Protein 34 g | Fiber 0 g

291. Crispy Breaded Pork Chops

Prep Time 10 m | Cooking Time 15 m | 8 Servings

Ingredients
- 1/8 tsp. pepper
- ¼ tsp. chili powder
- ½ tsp. onion powder
- ½ tsp. garlic powder
- 1 ¼ tsp. sweet paprika
- tbsp. grated parmesan cheese
- 1/3 C. crushed cornflake crumbs
- ½ C. panko breadcrumbs
- 1 beaten egg
- 6 center-cut boneless pork chops

Directions
1. Ensure that your air fryer is preheated to 400 degrees. Spray the basket with olive oil.
2. With ½ teaspoon salt and pepper, season both sides of pork chops.
3. Combine ¾ teaspoon salt with pepper, chili powder, onion powder, garlic powder, paprika, cornflake crumbs, panko breadcrumbs, and parmesan cheese.
4. Beat egg in another bowl.
5. Dip the pork chops into the egg and then crumb mixture.
6. Add pork chops to air fryer and spritz with olive oil.

Air Frying:
1. Set temperature to 400°F, and set time to 12 minutes. Cook 12 minutes, making sure to flip over halfway through the cooking process.
2. Only add 3 chops in at a time and repeat the process with remaining pork chops.

Nutrition
Calories 378 | Fat 13 g | Protein 33 g | Sugar 1 g

292. Caramelized Pork Shoulder

Prep Time 10 m | Cooking Time 20 m | 8 Servings

Ingredients
- 1/3 cup soy sauce
- tablespoons sugar
- 1 tablespoon honey
- 2 pounds pork shoulder, cut into 1½-inch thick slices

Directions
1. In a bowl, mix all the ingredients except pork.
2. Add pork and coat with marinade generously.
3. Cover and refrigerate o marinate for about 2-8 hours.
4. Preheat the Air fryer oven to 335 degrees F.
5. Place the pork in an Air fryer rack/basket.
6. Cook for about 10 minutes.
7. Now, set the Air fryer oven to 390 degrees F. Cook for about 10 minutes.

Nutrition
Calories 268 | Fat 10 g | Protein 23 g | Sugar 5 g

293. Roasted Pork Tenderloin

Prep Time 5 m | Cooking Time 1 h | 4 Servings

Ingredients
- 1 (3-pound) pork tenderloin
- tablespoons extra-virgin olive oil
- 2 garlic cloves, minced
- 1 teaspoon dried basil
- 1 teaspoon dried oregano
- 1 teaspoon dried thyme
- Salt
- Pepper

Directions
1. Dip the pork fillet in olive oil.
2. Grate the garlic, basil, oregano, thyme, and salt and pepper to taste throughout the steak.
3. Place the steak in the oven of the deep fryer. Cook for 45 minutes.
4. Use a meat thermometer to check for politeness
5. Open the Air Fryer and flip the pork fillet. Cook for 15 more minutes.
6. Take the cooked pork out of the deep fryer and let it rest for 10 minutes before slicing it.

Nutrition
Calories 283 | Fat 10 g | Protein 48 g

294. Bacon-Wrapped Pork Tenderloin

Prep Time 5 m | Cooking Time 15 m | 4 Servings

Ingredients
Pork:
- 1-2 tbsp. Dijon mustard
- 3-4 strips of bacon
- 1 pork tenderloin

Apple Gravy:
- ½ - 1 tsp. Dijon mustard
- 1 tbsp. almond flour
- tbsp. ghee
- 1 chopped onion
- 2-3 Granny Smith apples
- 1 C. vegetable broth

Directions
1. Spread Dijon mustard all over the tenderloin and wrap the meat with strips of bacon.
2. Place into the Air fryer oven, set the temperature to 360°F, and set time to 15 minutes, and cook 10-15 minutes at 360 degrees.
3. To make sauce, heat ghee in a pan and add shallots. Cook 1-2 minutes.
4. Then add apples, cooking 3-5 minutes until softened.
5. Add flour and ghee to make a roux. Add broth and mustard, stirring well to combine.
6. When the sauce starts to bubble, add 1 cup of sautéed apples, cooking till sauce thickens.
7. Once the pork tenderloin is cooked, let it sit 5-10 minutes to rest before slicing.
8. Serve topped with apple gravy.

Nutrition
Calories 552 | Fat 25 g | Protein 29 g | Sugar 6 g

295. Dijon Garlic Pork Tenderloin

Prep Time 5 m | Cooking Time 10 m | 6 Servings

Ingredients

- 1 C. breadcrumbs
- Pinch of cayenne pepper
- Crushed garlic cloves
- 2 tbsp. ground ginger
- 2 tbsp. Dijon mustard

- 2 tbsp. raw honey
- tbsp. water
- 2 tsp. salt
- 1 pound pork tenderloin, sliced into 1-inch rounds

Directions

1. With pepper and salt, season all sides of the tenderloin.
2. Combine cayenne pepper, garlic, ginger, mustard, honey, and water until smooth.
3. Dip pork rounds into the honey mixture and then into breadcrumbs, ensuring they all get coated well.
4. Place coated pork rounds into your Air fryer oven.
5. Set temperature to 400°F, and set time to 10 minutes. Cook 10 minutes at 400 degrees. Flip and then cook an additional 5 minutes until golden in color.

Nutrition

Calories 423 | Fat 18 g | Protein 31 g | Sugar 3 g

296. Pork Neck with Salad

Prep Time 10 m | Cooking Time 12 m | 2 Servings

Ingredients

For Pork:
- 1 tablespoon soy sauce
- 1 tablespoon fish sauce
- ½ tablespoon oyster sauce
- ½ pound pork neck

For Salad:
- 1 ripe tomato, sliced tickly
- 8-10 Thai shallots, sliced
- 1 scallion, chopped
- 1 bunch fresh basil leaves
- 1 bunch fresh cilantro leaves

For Dressing:
- Tablespoons fish sauce
- 2 tablespoons olive oil
- 1 teaspoon apple cider vinegar
- 1 tablespoon palm sugar
- 2 bird's eye chili
- 1 tablespoon garlic, minced

Directions

For the pork:
1. In a bowl, mix all the ingredients except the pork.
2. Add the pork neck and marinade layer evenly. Refrigerate for about 2-3 hours.
3. Preheat the deep fryer oven to 340 degrees F.
4. Air fry. Place the pork neck in a grill pan. Cook for about 12 minutes.
5. Meanwhile, in a large bowl, combine all of the salad ingredients.
6. In a bowl, add all the dressing ingredients and beat until well combined.
7. Remove the pork neck from the fryer and cut it into the desired slices.
8. Place the pork slices on top of the salad.

Nutrition

Calories 296 | Fat: 20 g | Protein 24 g | Sugar 8 g

297. Chinese Braised Pork Belly

Prep Time 5 m | Cooking Time 20 m | 8 Servings

Ingredients

- 1 lb. pork belly, sliced
- 1 tbsp. oyster sauce
- 1 tbsp. sugar
- Red fermented bean curds
- 1 tbsp. red fermented bean curd paste

- 1 tbsp. cooking wine
- 1/2 tbsp. soy sauce
- 1 tsp sesame oil
- 1 cup all-purpose flour

Directions

1. Preheat the Air fryer oven to 390 degrees.
2. In a small bowl, mix up the ingredients together and rub the pork thoroughly with this mixture
3. Set aside to marinate for at least 30 minutes or preferably overnight for the flavors to permeate the meat
4. Coat each marinated pork belly slice in flour and place in the Air fryer oven tray
5. Cook for 20 minutes until crispy and tender.

Nutrition

Calories 409 | Fat 14 g | Protein 19 g | Sugar 9 g

298. Juicy Pork Ribs Ole

Prep Time 10 m | Cooking Time 25 m | 4 Servings

Ingredients

- 1 rack of pork ribs
- 1/2 cup low-fat milk
- 1 tablespoon envelope taco seasoning mix
- 1 can tomato sauce

- 1/2 teaspoon ground black pepper
- 1 teaspoon seasoned salt
- 1 tablespoon cornstarch
- 1 teaspoon canola oil

Directions

1. Place all ingredients in a mixing dish; let them marinate for 1 hour.
2. Cook the marinated ribs approximately 25 minutes at 390 degrees F
3. Work with batches. Enjoy.

Nutrition

Calories 218 | Fat 8 g | Protein 11 g | Sugar 1 g

299. Air Fryer Sweet and Sour Pork

⏱ Prep Time 10 m | ⏱ Cooking Time 12 m | 6 Servings

Ingredients

- Tbsp. olive oil
- 1/16 tsp. Chinese five-spice
- ¼ tsp. pepper
- ½ tsp. sea salt
- 1 tsp. pure sesame oil
- 2 eggs
- 1 C. almond flour
- 2 pounds pork, sliced into chunks

Sweet and Sour sauce:

- ¼ tsp. sea salt
- ½ tsp. garlic powder
- 1 tbsp. low-sodium soy sauce
- ½ C. rice vinegar
- tbsp. tomato paste
- 1/8 tsp. water
- ½ C. sweetener of choice

Directions

1. To make the dipping sauce, whisk all sauce ingredients together over medium heat, stirring 5 minutes. Simmer uncovered 5 minutes till thickened.
2. Meanwhile, combine almond flour, five-spice, pepper, and salt.
3. In another bowl, mix eggs with sesame oil.
4. Dredge pork in flour mixture and then in the egg mixture. Shake any excess off before adding to the air fryer rack/basket.
5. Set temperature to 340°F, and set time to 12 minutes.
6. Serve with sweet and sour dipping sauce!

Nutrition

Calories 371 | Fat 17 g | Protein 27 g | Sugar 1 g

300. Teriyaki Pork Rolls

⏱ Prep Time 10 m | ⏱ Cooking Time 8 m | 6 Servings

Ingredients

- 1 tsp. almond flour
- tbsp. low-sodium soy sauce
- tbsp. mirin
- tbsp. brown sugar
- Thumb-sized amount of ginger, chopped
- Pork belly slices
- Enoki mushrooms

Directions

1. Mix brown sugar, mirin, soy sauce, almond flour, and ginger until brown sugar dissolves.
2. Take pork belly slices and wrap around a bundle of mushrooms. Brush each roll with teriyaki sauce. Chill half an hour.
3. Preheat your Air fryer oven to 350 degrees and add marinated pork rolls.
4. Set temperature to 350°F, and set time to 8 minutes.

Nutrition

Calories 412 | Fat 9 g | Protein 19 g | Sugar 4 g

301. Garlic Herb Rib-Eye Steak

⏱ Prep Time 8 m | ⏱ Cooking Time 12 m | 3 Servings

Ingredients

- 8 oz. ribeye steak
- 1 tsp Worcestershire sauce
- 2 tsp garlic, minced
- 2 tbsp. parsley, chopped
- 1 stick grass-fed butter, softened
- 1/2 tsp salt

Directions

1. In a bowl, mix together parsley, butter, garlic, Worcestershire sauce, and salt.
2. Rub the butter mixture all over the steak and place it in the refrigerator for 1 hour.
3. Preheat the air fryer to 400 F/204 C.
4. Place marinated steak in the air fryer basket and cook for 12 minutes.
5. Serve and enjoy.

Nutrition

Calories 203 | Carbohydrates 10g | Protein 13g | Fat 2g

302. Tasty Beef Patties

⏱ Prep Time 10 m | ⏱ Cooking Time 10 m | 5 Servings

Ingredients

- 1 lb. ground beef
- 1 tsp dried parsley
- 1/2 tsp dried oregano
- 1/2 tsp onion powder
- 1 tbsp. Worcestershire sauce
- 1/2 tsp salt
- 1/2 tsp garlic powder
- 1/2 tsp black pepper

Directions

1. Preheat the air fryer to 176 C/ 350 F.
2. In a small bowl, mix together all ingredients except meat.
3. Add ground meat into the large mixing bowl. Add seasoning mixture into the ground meat and mix until well combined.
4. Make four burger shape patties from the mixture.
5. Place patties in the air fryer basket and cook for 10 minutes.
6. Serve and enjoy.

Nutrition

Calories 250 | Carbohydrates 11g | Protein 40g | Fat 9g

303. Saucy beef bake

⏱ Prep Time 10 m | ⏱ Cooking Time 36 m | 6 Servings

Ingredients

- tablespoons olive oil
- 1 large onion, diced
- lbs. (907.185g) Ground beef
- teaspoons salt
- cloves garlic, chopped
- 1/2 cup red wine
- cloves garlic, chopped
- teaspoons ground cinnamon
- teaspoons ground cumin
- teaspoons dried oregano
- 1 teaspoon black pepper
- 1 can 28 oz. Crushed tomatoes
- 1 tablespoon tomato paste

Directions:

1 Put a suitable wok over moderate heat and add oil to heat.
2 Toss in onion, salt, and beef meat then stir cook for 12 minutes.
3 Stir in red wine and cook for 2 minutes.
4 Add cinnamon, garlic, oregano, cumin, and pepper, then stir cook for 2 minutes.
5 Add tomato paste and tomatoes and cook for 20 minutes on a simmer.
6 Spread this mixture in a casserole dish.
7 Press "power button" of air fry oven and turn the dial to select the "bake" mode.
8 Press the time button and again turn the dial to set the cooking time to 30 minutes.
9 Now push the temp button and rotate the dial to set the temperature at 350 degrees f.
10 Once preheated, place casserole dish in the oven and close its lid.
11 Serve warm.

Nutrition:

Calories 405 | Fat 22.7 g | Cholesterol 4 mg | Sodium 227 mg | Carbs 26.1 g | Fiber 1.4 g | Protein 45.2 g

304. Parmesan meatballs

⏱ Prep Time 10 m | ⏱ Cooking Time 20 m | 6 Servings

Ingredients

- lbs. (907.185g) Ground beef
- eggs
- 1 cup ricotta cheese
- 1/4 cup parmesan cheese shredded
- 1/2 cup panko breadcrumbs
- 1/4 cup basil chopped
- 1/4 cup parsley chopped
- 1 tablespoon fresh oregano chopped
- teaspoon kosher salt
- 1 teaspoon ground fennel
- 1/2 teaspoon red pepper flakes
- 32 oz. spaghetti sauce, to serve

Directions:

1 Thoroughly mix the beef with all other ingredients for meatballs in a bowl.
2 Make small meatballs out of this mixture then place them in the air fryer basket.
3 Press "power button" of air fry oven and turn the dial to select the "bake" mode.
4 Press the time button and again turn the dial to set the cooking time to 20 minutes.
5 Now push the temp button and rotate the dial to set the temperature at 400 degrees f.
6 Once preheated, place meatballs basket in the oven and close its lid.
7 Flip the meatballs when cooked halfway through then resume cooking.
8 Pour spaghetti sauce on top.
9 Serve warm.

Nutrition:

Calories 545 | Total fat 36.4 g | Saturated fat 10.1 g | Protein 42.5 g

305. Tricolor beef skewers

⏱ Prep Time 10 m | ⏱ Cooking Time 25 m | 4 Servings

Ingredients

- garlic cloves, minced
- tablespoon rapeseed oil
- 1 cup cottage cheese, cubed
- cherry tomatoes
- tablespoon cider vinegar
- Large bunch thyme
- 1 ¼ lb. (566.99g) Boneless beef, diced

Directions:

1. Toss beef with all its thyme, oil, vinegar, and garlic.
2. Marinate the thyme beef for 2 hours in a closed container in the refrigerator.
3. Thread the marinated beef, cheese, and tomatoes on the skewers.
4. Place these skewers in an air fryer basket.
5. Press "power button" of air fry oven and turn the dial to select the "air fry" mode.
6. Press the time button and again turn the dial to set the cooking time to 25 minutes.
7. Now push the temp button and rotate the dial to set the temperature at 350 degrees f.
8. Once preheated, place the air fryer basket in the oven and close its lid.
9. Flip the skewers when cooked halfway through then resume cooking.
10. Serve warm.

Nutrition:

Calories 695 | Total fat 17.5 g | Saturated fat 4.8 g | Protein 117.4 g

306. Yogurt beef kebabs

⏲ Prep Time 10 m | ⏲ Cooking Time 25 m | 4 Servings

Ingredients

- ½ cup yogurt
- 1½ tablespoon mint
- 1 teaspoon ground cumin

- 1 cup eggplant, diced
- oz. Lean beef, diced
- ½ small onion, cubed

Directions:

1. Whisk yogurt with mint and cumin in a suitable bowl.
2. Toss in beef cubes and mix well to coat. Marinate for 30 minutes.
3. Alternatively, thread the beef, onion, and eggplant on the skewers.
4. Place these beef skewers in the air fry basket.
5. Press "power button" of air fry oven and turn the dial to select the "air fryer" mode.
6. Press the time button and again turn the dial to set the cooking time to 25 minutes.
7. Now push the temp button and rotate the dial to set the temperature at 370 degrees f.
8. Once preheated, place the air fryer basket in the oven and close its lid.
9. Flip the skewers when cooked halfway through then resume cooking.
10. Serve warm.

Nutrition:

Calories 301 |Total fat 8.9 g| Saturated fat 4.5 g | Protein 15.3 g

307. Agave beef kebabs

⏲ Prep Time 10 m | ⏲ Cooking Time 20 m | 6 Servings

Ingredients

- lbs. (907.185g) Beef steaks, cubed
- tablespoon jerk seasoning
- Zest and juice of 1 lime

- 1 tablespoon agave syrup
- ½ teaspoon thyme leaves, chopped

Directions:

1. Mix beef with jerk seasoning, lime juice, zest, agave and thyme.
2. Toss well to coat then marinate for 30 minutes.
3. Alternatively, thread the beef on the skewers.
4. Place these beef skewers in the air fry basket.
5. Press "power button" of air fry oven and turn the dial to select the "air fryer" mode.
6. Press the time button and again turn the dial to set the cooking time to 20 minutes.
7. Now push the temp button and rotate the dial to set the temperature at 360 degrees f.
8. Once preheated, place the air fryer basket in the oven and close its lid.
9. Flip the skewers when cooked halfway through then resume cooking.
10. Serve warm.

Nutrition:

Calories 548|Fat 22.9 g|Cholesterol 105 mg|Sodium 350mg|Carbs 17.5g|Fiber 6.3g|Protein 40.1 g

308. Beef skewers with potato salad

⏲ Prep Time 10 m | ⏲ Cooking Time 25 m | 4 Servings

Ingredients

- Juice ½ lemon
- tablespoon olive oil
- 1 garlic clove, crushed
- 1 ¼ lb. (566.99g) Diced beef
- For the salad
- potatoes, boiled, peeled and diced

- large tomatoes, chopped
- 1 cucumber, chopped
- 1 handful black olives, chopped
- oz. Pack feta cheese, crumbled
- 1 bunch of mint, chopped

Directions:

1. Whisk lemon juice with garlic and olive oil in a bowl.
2. Toss in beef cubes and mix well to coat. Marinate for 30 minutes.
3. Alternatively, thread the beef on the skewers.
4. Place these beef skewers in the air fry basket.
5. Press "power button" of air fry oven and turn the dial to select the "air fryer" mode.
6. Press the time button and again turn the dial to set the cooking time to 25 minutes.
7. Now push the temp button and rotate the dial to set the temperature at 360 degrees f.
8. Once preheated, place the air fryer basket in the oven and close its lid.
9. Flip the skewers when cooked halfway through then resume cooking.
10. Meanwhile, whisk all the salad ingredients in a salad bowl.
11. Serve the skewers with prepared salad.

Nutrition:

Calories 609|Fat 50.5 g|Cholesterol 58 mg|Sodium 463 mg|Carbs 9.9 g|Fiber 1.5 g|Protein 29.3 g

309. Classic souvlaki kebobs

☉ Prep Time 10 m | ☉ Cooking Time 20 m | 6 Servings

Ingredients

- lbs. (907.185g) Beef shoulder fat trimmed, cut into chunks
- 1/3 cup olive oil
- ½ cup red wine
- teaspoon dried oregano
- ½ cup of orange juice
- 1 teaspoon orange zest
- garlic cloves, crushed

Directions:

1. Whisk olive oil, red wine, oregano, oranges juice, zest, and garlic in a suitable bowl.
2. Toss in beef cubes and mix well to coat. Marinate for 30 minutes.
3. Alternatively, thread the beef, onion, and bread on the skewers.
4. Place these beef skewers in the air fry basket.
5. Press "power button" of air fry oven and turn the dial to select the "air fryer" mode.
6. Press the time button and again turn the dial to set the cooking time to 20 minutes.
7. Now push the temp button and rotate the dial to set the temperature at 370 degrees f.
8. Once preheated, place the air fryer basket in the oven and close its lid.
9. Flip the skewers when cooked halfway through then resume cooking.
10. Serve warm.

Nutrition:
Calories 537 | Fat 19.8 g | Cholesterol 10 mg | Sodium 719 mg | Carbs 25.1 g | Fiber 0.9g | Protein 37.8 g

310. Harissa dipped beef skewers

☉ Prep Time 10 m | ☉ Cooking Time 16 m | 6 Servings

Ingredients

- 1 lb. (453.592g) Beef mince
- tablespoon harissa
- oz. Feta cheese
- 1 large red onion, shredded
- 1 handful parsley, chopped
- 1 handful mint, chopped
- 1 tablespoon olive oil
- Juice 1 lemon

Directions:

1. Whisk beef mince with harissa, onion, feta, and seasoning in a bowl.
2. Make 12 sausages out of this mixture then thread them on the skewers.
3. Place these beef skewers in the air fry basket.
4. Press "power button" of air fry oven and turn the dial to select the "bake" mode.
5. Press the time button and again turn the dial to set the cooking time to 16 minutes.
6. Now push the temp button and rotate the dial to set the temperature at 370 degrees f.
7. Once preheated, place the air fryer basket in the oven and close its lid.
8. Flip the skewers when cooked halfway through then resume cooking.
9. Toss the remaining salad ingredients in a salad bowl.

Nutrition: Calories 452 | Total fat 4 g | Saturated fat 2 g | Cholesterol 65 mg

311. Onion pepper beef kebobs

☉ Prep Time 10 m | ☉ Cooking Time 20 m | 4 Servings

Ingredients

- tablespoon pesto paste
- 2/3 lb. (303.9g) Beefsteak, diced
- red peppers, cut into chunks
- red onions, cut into wedges
- 1 tablespoon olive oil

Directions:

1. Toss in beef cubes with harissa and oil, then mix well to coat. Marinate for 30 minutes.
2. Alternatively, thread the beef, onion, and peppers on the skewers.
3. Place these beef skewers in the air fry basket.
4. Press "power button" of air fry oven and turn the dial to select the "air fryer" mode.
5. Press the time button and again turn the dial to set the cooking time to 20 minutes.
6. Now push the temp button and rotate the dial to set the temperature at 370 degrees f.
7. Once preheated, place the air fryer basket in the oven and close its lid.
8. Flip the skewers when cooked halfway through then resume cooking.
9. Serve warm.

Nutrition:
Calories 301 | Total fat 15.8 g | Saturated fat 2.7 g | Cholesterol 75 mg

312. Mayo spiced kebobs

⏱ Prep Time 10 m | ⏲ Cooking Time 10 m | 4 Servings

Ingredients

- tablespoon cumin seed
- tablespoon coriander seed
- tablespoon fennel seed
- 1 tablespoon paprika

- tablespoon garlic mayonnaise
- garlic cloves, finely minced
- ½ teaspoon ground cinnamon
- 1 ½ lb. (680.389g) Lean minced beef

Directions:

1. Blend all the spices and seeds with garlic, cream, and cinnamon in a blender.
2. Add this cream paste to the minced beef then mix well.
3. Make 8 sausages and thread each on the skewers.
4. Place these beef skewers in the air fry basket.
5. Press "power button" of air fry oven and turn the dial to select the "air fryer" mode.
6. Press the time button and again turn the dial to set the cooking time to 10 minutes.
7. Now push the temp button and rotate the dial to set the temperature at 370 degrees f.
8. Once preheated, place the air fryer basket in the oven and close its lid.
9. Flip the skewers when cooked halfway through then resume cooking.
10. Serve warm.

Nutrition:

Calories 308| Total fat 20.5 g | Saturated fat 3 g | Cholesterol 42 mg

313. Beef with orzo salad

⏱ Prep Time 10 m | ⏲ Cooking Time 27 m | 4 Servings

Ingredients

- 2/3 lbs. Beef shoulder, cubed
- 1 teaspoon ground cumin
- ½ teaspoon cayenne pepper
- 1 teaspoon sweet smoked paprika
- 1 tablespoon olive oil
- 24 cherry tomatoes
- Salad:

- ½ cup orzo, boiled
- ½ cup frozen pea
- 1 large carrot, grated
- Small pack coriander, chopped
- Small pack mint, chopped
- Juice 1 lemon
- tablespoon olive oil

Directions:

1. Toss tomatoes and beef with oil, paprika, pepper, and cumin in a bowl.
2. Alternatively, thread the beef and tomatoes on the skewers.
3. Place these beef skewers in the air fry basket.
4. Press "power button" of air fry oven and turn the dial to select the "air fryer" mode.
5. Press the time button and again turn the dial to set the cooking time to 25 minutes.
6. Now push the temp button and rotate the dial to set the temperature at 370 degrees f.
7. Once preheated, place the air fryer basket in the oven and close its lid.
8. Flip the skewers when cooked halfway through then resume cooking.
9. Meanwhile, sauté carrots and peas with olive oil in a pan for 2 minutes.
10. Stir in mint, lemon juice, coriander, and cooked couscous.
11. Serve skewers with the couscous salad.

Nutrition:

Calories 231 | Fat 20.1 g | Cholesterol 110 mg | Sodium 941mg | Carbs 20.1g | Fiber 0.9g | Protein 14.6 g

314. Beef zucchini shashliks

⏱ Prep Time 10 m | ⏲ Cooking Time 25 m | 4 Servings

Ingredients

- 1lb. (453.592g) Beef, boned and diced
- 1 lime, juiced and chopped
- tablespoon olive oil
- 20 garlic cloves, chopped

- 1 handful rosemary, chopped
- green peppers, cubed
- zucchinis, cubed
- red onions, cut into wedges

Directions:

1. Toss the beef with the rest of the skewer's ingredients in a bowl.
2. Thread the beef, peppers, zucchini, and onion on the skewers.
3. Place these beef skewers in the air fry basket.
4. Press "power button" of air fry oven and turn the dial to select the "air fryer" mode.
5. Press the time button and again turn the dial to set the cooking time to 25 minutes.
6. Now push the temp button and rotate the dial to set the temperature at 370 degrees f.
7. Once preheated, place the air fryer basket in the oven and close its lid.
8. Flip the skewers when cooked halfway through then resume cooking.
9. Serve warm.

Nutrition:

Calories 472 | Fat 11.1 g | Cholesterol 610mg | Sodium 749 mg | Carbs 19.9g | Fiber 0.2g | Protein 13.5 g

315. Spiced beef skewers
Prep Time 10 m | Cooking Time 18 m | 4 Servings

Ingredients
- teaspoons ground cumin
- teaspoons ground coriander
- 1/4 teaspoon ground cinnamon
- 1/8 teaspoon ground smoked paprika
- teaspoons lime zest

- 1/2 teaspoon salt
- 1/2 teaspoon black pepper
- 1 tablespoon lemon juice
- teaspoons olive oil
- 1 1/2 lbs. Lean beef, cubed

Directions:
1. Toss beef with the rest of the skewer's ingredients in a bowl.
2. Thread the beef and veggies on the skewers alternately.
3. Place these beef skewers in the air fry basket.
4. Press "power button" of air fry oven and turn the dial to select the "air fryer" mode.
5. Press the time button and again turn the dial to set the cooking time to 18 minutes.
6. Now push the temp button and rotate the dial to set the temperature at 370 degrees f.
7. Once preheated, place the air fryer basket in the oven and close its lid.
8. Flip the skewers when cooked halfway through then resume cooking.
9. Serve warm.

Nutrition:
Calories 327 | Fat 3.5 g | Cholesterol 162 mg | Sodium 142 mg | Carbs 33.6 g | Protein 24.5 g

316. Beef sausage with cucumber sauce
Prep Time 10 m | Cooking Time 15 m | 6 Servings

Ingredients
- Beef kabobs
- 1 lb. (453.592g) Ground beef
- 1/2 an onion, finely diced
- garlic cloves, finely minced
- teaspoons cumin
- teaspoons coriander
- 1 ½ teaspoons salt

- tablespoons chopped mint
- Yogurt sauce:
- 1 cup Greek yogurt
- tablespoons cucumber, chopped
- garlic cloves, minced
- 1/4 teaspoon salt

Directions:
1. Toss beef with the rest of the kebob ingredients in a bowl.
2. Make 6 sausages out of this mince and thread them on the skewers.
3. Place these beef skewers in the air fry basket.
4. Press "power button" of air fry oven and turn the dial to select the "air fryer" mode.
5. Press the time button and again turn the dial to set the cooking time to 15 minutes.
6. Now push the temp button and rotate the dial to set the temperature at 370 degrees f.
7. Once preheated, place the air fryer basket in the oven and close its lid.
8. Flip the skewers when cooked halfway through then resume cooking.
9. Meanwhile, prepare the cucumber sauce by whisking all its ingredients in a bowl.

Nutrition:
Calories 353 | Fat 7.5 g | Cholesterol 20 mg | Sodium 297 mg | Carbs 10.4 g | Fiber 0.2 g | Protein 13.1 g

317. Beef eggplant medley
Prep Time 10 m | Cooking Time 20 m | 4 Servings

Ingredients
- cloves of garlic
- 1 teaspoon dried oregano
- Olive oil
- beef steaks, diced

- eggplant, cubed
- fresh bay leaves
- lemons, juiced
- A few sprigs parsley, chopped

Directions:
1. Toss beef with the rest of the skewer's ingredients in a bowl.
2. Thread the beef and veggies on the skewers alternately.
3. Place these beef skewers in the air fry basket.
4. Press "power button" of air fry oven and turn the dial to select the "air fryer" mode.
5. Press the time button and again turn the dial to set the cooking time to 20 minutes.
6. Now push the temp button and rotate the dial to set the temperature at 370 degrees f.
7. Once preheated, place the air fryer basket in the oven and close its lid.
8. Flip the skewers when cooked halfway through then resume cooking.
9. Serve warm.

Nutrition:
Calories 248 | Fat 13 g | Cholesterol 387 mg | Sodium 353 mg | Carbs 1 g | Fiber 0.4 g | Protein 29 g

318. Glazed beef kebobs

⏱ Prep Time 10 m | ⏱ Cooking Time 20 m | 6 Servings

Ingredients

- lb. (453.592g) Beef, cubed
- 1/2 cup olive oil
- 1 lemon, juice only
- cloves garlic, minced
- 1 onion, sliced
- 1 teaspoon oregano, dried
- 1/4 teaspoon dried thyme,
- 1 teaspoon salt
- 1/4 teaspoon black pepper
- 1 tablespoon parsley, chopped
- 1 cup Worcestershire sauce

Directions:

1. Toss beef with the rest of the kebab ingredients in a bowl.
2. Cover the beef and marinate it for 30 minutes.
3. Thread the beef and veggies on the skewers alternately.
4. Place these beef skewers in the air fry basket. Brush the skewers with the Worcestershire sauce.
5. Press "power button" of air fry oven and turn the dial to select the "air fryer" mode.
6. Press the time button and again turn the dial to set the cooking time to 20 minutes.
7. Now push the temp button and rotate the dial to set the temperature at 370 degrees f.
8. Once preheated, place the air fryer basket in the oven and close its lid.
9. Flip the skewers when cooked halfway through then resume cooking.
10. Serve warm.

Nutrition:

Calories 457 | Fat 19.1 g | Cholesterol 262 mg | Sodium 557mg | Carbs 18.9g | Fiber 1.7g | Protein 32.5 g

319. Asian beef skewers

⏱ Prep Time 10 m | ⏱ Cooking Time 15 m | 4 Servings

Ingredients

- tablespoons hoisin sauce
- tablespoons sherry
- 1/4 cup soy sauce
- 1 teaspoon barbeque sauce
- green onions, chopped
- cloves garlic, minced
- 1 tablespoon minced fresh ginger root
- 1 1/2 lbs. (453.592g) Flank steak, cubed

Directions:

1. Toss steak cubes with sherry, all the sauces and other ingredients in a bowl.
2. Marinate the saucy spiced skewers for 30 minutes.
3. Place these beef skewers in the air fry basket.
4. Press "power button" of air fry oven and turn the dial to select the "air fryer" mode.
5. Press the time button and again turn the dial to set the cooking time to 15 minutes.
6. Now push the temp button and rotate the dial to set the temperature at 350 degrees f.
7. Once preheated, place the air fryer basket in the oven and close its lid.
8. Flip the skewers when cooked halfway through then resume cooking.
9. Serve warm.

Nutrition:

Calories 321 | Total fat 7.4 g | Saturated fat 4.6 g | Cholesterol 105 mg

320. Beef kebobs with cream dip

⏱ Prep Time 10 m | ⏱ Cooking Time 20 m | 6 Servings

Ingredients

- Beef kebabs
- lbs. (453.592g) Beef, diced
- 1 large onion, squares
- Salt
- For the dressing
- 1 tablespoon mayonnaise
- 1 tablespoon olive oil
- tablespoons lemon juice
- 1 teaspoon yellow mustard
- 1/4 teaspoon salt
- 1/8 teaspoon black pepper

Directions:

1. Toss beef and onion with salt in a bowl to season them.
2. Thread the beef and onion on the skewers alternately.
3. Place these beef skewers in the air fry basket.
4. Press "power button" of air fry oven and turn the dial to select the "air fryer" mode.
5. Press the time button and again turn the dial to set the cooking time to 20 minutes.
6. Now push the temp button and rotate the dial to set the temperature at 370 degrees f.
7. Once preheated, place the air fryer basket in the oven and close its lid.
8. Flip the skewers when cooked halfway through then resume cooking.
9. Prepare the cream dip by mixing its ingredients in a bowl.
10. Serve skewers with cream dip.

Nutrition:

Calories 392 | Fat 16.1 g | Cholesterol 231 mg | Sodium 466 mg | Carbs 3.9 g | Fiber 0.9 g | Protein 48 g

321. Korean bbq skewers
⏱ Prep Time 10 m | ⏱ Cooking Time 15 m | 4 Servings

Ingredients

- oz. Lean sirloin steaks, cubed
- 1 small onion, finely diced
- 1/3 cup low sodium soy sauce
- 1/3 cup brown sugar
- 1 tablespoon sesame seeds
- teaspoons sesame oil
- cloves garlic, diced
- 1 tablespoon ginger, grated
- 1 teaspoon Sirach
- tablespoons honey
- Salt and pepper

Directions:

1 Toss steak cubes with sauces and other ingredients in a bowl.
2 Marinate the saucy spiced skewers for 30 minutes.
3 Place these beef skewers in the air fry basket.
4 Press "power button" of air fry oven and turn the dial to select the "air fryer" mode.
5 Press the time button and again turn the dial to set the cooking time to 15 minutes.
6 Now push the temp button and rotate the dial to set the temperature at 350 degrees f.
7 Once preheated, place the air fryer basket in the oven and close its lid.
8 Flip the skewers when cooked halfway through then resume cooking.
9 Serve warm.

Nutrition:

Calories 248| Total fat 15.7 g |Saturated fat 2.7 g | Cholesterol 75 mg

322. Pork Rinds
⏱ Prep Time 10 m | ⏱ Cooking Time 7 m | 8 Servings

Ingredients

- 1 teaspoon chili flakes
- ½ teaspoon salt
- ½ teaspoon ground black pepper
- 1-pound pork rinds
- 1 teaspoon olive oil

Directions:

1 Heat up the air fryer to 365 F.
2 Sprinkle the air fryer basket with the inside olive oil.
3 Then place the pork rinds on the tray of the fryer.
4 Sprinkle salt and chili flakes with pork rinds and black ground pepper.
5 Mix them gently. Balance them gently.
6 Cook the pork rinds for 7 minutes after that.
7 When the time is done, shake the pork carefully.
8 Move the platter to the broad serving plate and allow 1-2 minutes to chill.
9 Serve and eat!

Nutrition:

Calories 329 |Fat 20.8 |Fiber 0| Carbs 0.1 |Protein 36.5

323. Asian Inspired Sichuan Lamb
⏱ Prep Time 5 m | ⏱ Cooking Time 10 m | 4 Servings

Ingredients:

- 1 ½ tablespoons cumin seed (do not use ground cumin)
- 1 teaspoon Sichuan peppers or ½ teaspoon cayenne
- 2 tablespoons vegetable oil
- 1 tablespoon garlic, peeled and minced
- 1 tablespoon light soy sauce
- 2 red chili peppers, seeded and chopped (use gloves)
- ¼ teaspoon granulated sugar
- ½ teaspoon salt
- 1 pound lamb shoulder, cut in ½ to 1-inch pieces
- 2 green onions, chopped
- 1 handful fresh cilantro, chopped

Directions:

1. Turn on the burner to medium high on the stove and heat up a dry skillet. Pour in the cumin seed and Sichuan peppers or cayenne and toast until fragrant. Turn off the burner and set aside until they are cool. Grind them in a grinder or mortar and pestle.
2. In a large bowl that will contain the marinade and the lamb, combine the vegetable oil, garlic, soy sauce, chili peppers, granulated sugar and salt. Pour in the cumin/pepper combination and mix well.
3. Using a fork, poke holes in the lamb all over the top and bottom. Place the lamb in the marinade, cover and refrigerate. You can also use a closeable plastic bag.
4. Preheat the air fryer to 360 degrees for 5 minutes.
5. Spray the basket with cooking spray.
6. Remove the lamb pieces from the marinade with tongs or slotted spoon and place in basket of the air fryer in a single layer. You may need to do more than 1 batch.
7. Cook for 10 minutes, flipping over 1 half way through. Make sure the lamb's internal temperature is 145 degrees F with a meat thermometer. Put on a serving platter and repeat with rest of the lamb.
8. Sprinkle the chopped green onions and cilantro over top, stir and serve.

Nutrition:

Calories: 142| Fat: 7g |Protein: 17g| Fiber: 4g

324. Garlic and Rosemary Lamb Cutlets

⏱ Prep Time 30 m | ⏱ Cooking Time 25 m | 2 Servings

Ingredients:

- 2 lamb racks (with 3 cutlets per rack)
- 2 cloves garlic, peeled and thinly sliced into slivers
- 2 long sprigs of fresh rosemary, leaves removed
- 2 tablespoon wholegrain mustard
- 1 tablespoon honey
- 2 tablespoons mint sauce (I use mint jelly)

Directions:

1. Trim fat from racks and cut slits with a sharp knife in the top of the lamb. Insert slices of the garlic and rosemary leaves in the slits and set the lamb aside.
2. Make the marinade by whisking the mustard, honey and mint sauce together and brush over the lamb racks. Let marinade in a cool area for 20 minutes.
3. Preheat the air fryer to 360 degrees for about 5 minutes.
4. Spray the basket using cooking spray and place the lamb rack or racks into the basket, propping them up however you can get them in to fit.
5. Cook 10 minutes, open and turn the racks and cook 10 more minutes.
6. Place on a platter and cover with foil to let sit 10 minutes before slicing and serving.

Nutrition:

Calories: 309| Fat: 2g |Protein: 33g| Fiber: 16g

325. Garlic Sauced Lamb Chops

⏱ Prep Time 15 m | ⏱ Cooking Time 25 m | 4 Servings

Ingredients:

- 1 garlic bulb
- 1 teaspoon + 3 tablespoons olive oil
- 1 tablespoon fresh oregano, chopped fine
- ¼ teaspoon ground pepper
- ½ teaspoon sea salt
- 8 lamb chops

Directions:

1. Preheat the air fryer to 400 degrees F 5 minutes and while it is preheating take excess paper from the garlic bulb.
2. Coat the garlic bulb with the 1 teaspoon of olive oil and drop it in the basket that has treated with cooking spray. Roast for 12 minutes.
3. Combine the 3 tablespoons of olive oil, oregano, salt and pepper and lightly coat the lamb chops on both with the resulting oil. Let them sit at room temperature for 5 minutes.
4. Remove the garlic bulb from the basket and if it is cool, preheat again to 400 degrees for 3 minutes.
5. Spray the air fryer basket with cooking oil and place 4 chops in cooking at 400 degrees F for 5 minutes. Place them on a platter and cover to keep them warm while you do the other chops.
6. Squeeze each garlic clove between the thumb and index finger into a small bowl.
7. Taste and add salt and pepper and mix. Serve along the chops like serving ketchup.

Nutrition: Calories: 194| Fat: 11g| Protein: 29g| Fiber: 13g

326. Herb Encrusted Lamb Chops

⏱ Prep Time 5 m | ⏱ Cooking Time 15 m | 2 Servings

Ingredients:

- 1 teaspoon oregano
- 1 teaspoon coriander
- 1 teaspoon thyme
- 1 teaspoon rosemary
- ½ teaspoon salt
- ¼ teaspoon pepper
- 2 tablespoons lemon juice
- 2 tablespoons olive oil
- 1 pound lamb chops

Directions:

1. In a closeable bag, combine the oregano, coriander, thyme, rosemary, salt, pepper, lemon juice and olive oil and shake well so it mixes.
2. Place the chops in the bag and squish around so the mixture is on them. Refrigerate 1 hour.
3. Preheat the air fryer to 390 degrees F for 5 minutes.
4. Place the chops in the basket that has been sprayed with cooking spray.
5. Cook for 3 minutes and pause. Flip the chops to the other side and cook for another 4 minutes for medium rare. If you want them better done cook 4 minutes, pause, turn and cook 5 more minutes.

Nutrition:

Calories: 321|Fat: 34g| Protein: 18g |Fiber: 15g

327. Herbed Rack of Lamb
Prep Time 15 m | Cooking Time 35 m | 2 Servings

Ingredients:

- 1 tablespoon olive oil
- 1 clove garlic, peeled and minced
- 1 ½ teaspoons fresh ground pepper
- 1 tablespoon fresh rosemary, chopped
- 1 tablespoon fresh thyme, chopped
- ¾ cup breadcrumbs
- 1 egg
- 1 to 2 pound rack of lamb

Directions:

1. Place the olive oil in a small dish and add the garlic. Mix well.
2. Brush the garlic on the rack of lamb and season with pepper.
3. In one bowl combine the rosemary, thyme and breadcrumbs and break the egg and whisk in another bowl.
4. Preheat air fryer 350 degrees F for 5 minutes. Spray with cooking spray.
5. Dip the rack in the egg and then place in the breadcrumb mixture and coat the rack.
6. Place rack in air fryer basket and cook 20 minutes.
7. Raise the temperature to 400 degrees F and set for 5 more minutes.
8. Tear a piece of aluminum foil that will fit to wrap the rack. Take it out of the basket with tongs and put it in the middle of the foil. Carefully wrap and let sit about 10 minutes. Unwrap and serve.

Nutrition:

Calories: 282 |Fat: 23g |Protein: 26g| Fiber: 23g

328. Macadamia Rack of Lamb
Prep Time 20 m | Cooking Time 32 m | 4 Servings

Ingredients:

- 1 tablespoon olive oil
- 1 clove garlic, peeled and minced
- 1 ½ to 1 ¾ pound rack of lamb
- Salt and pepper to taste
- ¾ cup unsalted macadamia nuts
- 1 tablespoon fresh rosemary, chopped
- 1 tablespoon breadcrumbs
- 1 egg, beaten

Directions:

1. Mix together the olive oil and garlic and brush it all over the rack of lamb. Season with salt and pepper.
2. Preheat the air fryer 250 degrees F for 8 minutes.
3. Chop the macadamia nuts as fine as possible and put them in a bowl.
4. Mix in the rosemary and breadcrumbs and set it aside.
5. Beat the egg in another bowl.
6. Dip the rack in the egg mixture to coat completely.
7. Place the rack in the breadcrumb mixture and coat well.
8. Spray the basket of the air fryer using cooking spray and place the rack inside.
9. Cook at 250 degrees for 25 minutes and then increase to 400 and cook another 5 to 10 minutes or until done.
10. Cover with foil paper for 10 minutes, uncover and separate into chops and serve.

Nutrition:

Calories: 321 |Fat: 9g| Protein: 12g| Fiber: 8.3g

329. Lamb Roast with Root Vegetables
Prep Time 35 m | Cooking Time 1 h 15 m | 6 Servings

Ingredients:

- 4 cloves garlic, peeled and sliced thin, divided
- 2 springs fresh rosemary, leaves pulled off, divided
- 3 pound leg of lamb
- Salt and pepper to taste, divided
- 2 medium sized sweet potatoes, peeled and cut into wedges
- 2 tablespoon oil, divided
- 2 cups baby carrots
- 1 teaspoon butter
- 4 large red potatoes, cubed

Directions:

1. Slice the garlic and take the leaves of the rosemary.
2. Cut about 5 to 6 slits in the top of the lamb and insert slices of garlic and some rosemary in each. Salt and pepper the roast to your taste and set aside to cook after the vegetables are done.
3. Coat the sweet potatoes in 1 tablespoon of olive oil and season with salt and pepper.
4. Spray the basket of the air fryer with cooking spray and put in the wedges. You may have to do two batches. Set for 400 degrees F and air fry 8 minutes, shake and cook another 8 minutes or so. Dump into a bowl and cover with foil.
5. Place the carrots in some foil to cover and put the butter on top of them. Enclose them in the foil and place them in the air fryer. Set for 400 degrees for 20 minutes. Remove from the air fryer.
6. Coat the basket with cooking spray. Mix the red potatoes with the other tablespoon of oil and salt and pepper to taste. Place in the air fryer oven and cook at 400 degrees F for 20 minutes, shaking after 10 minutes have elapsed.
7. Use a foil tray or baking dish that fits into the air fryer and coat with cooking spray. Place the left over garlic and rosemary in the bottom and place the lamb on top.
8. Set for 380 degrees F and cook 1 hour, checking after 30 minutes and 45 minutes to make sure it isn't getting too done. Increase the air fryer oven heat to 400 degrees F and cook for 10 to 15 minutes.
9. Remove the roast from the air fryer and set on a platter. Cover with foil and rest 10 minutes while you dump all the vegetables back in the basket and cooking at 350 degrees F for 8 to 10 minutes or until heated through.
10. Serve all together.

Nutrition:

Calories: 398| Fat: 5g |Protein: 18g| Fiber: 30.3g

330. Lemon and Cumin Coated Rack of Lamb

⏱ Prep Time 15 m | ⏱ Cooking Time 200 m | 4 Servings

Ingredients:

- 1 ½ to 1 ¾ pound Frenched rack of lamb
- Salt and pepper to taste
- ½ cup breadcrumbs
- 1 teaspoon cumin seed
- 1 teaspoon ground cumin
- ½ teaspoon salt
- 1 teaspoon garlic, peeled and grated
- Lemon zest (1/4 of a lemon)
- 1 teaspoon vegetable or olive oil
- 1 egg, beaten

Directions:

1. Season the lamb rack with pepper and salt to taste and set it aside.
2. In a large bowl, combine the breadcrumbs, cumin seed, ground cumin, salt, garlic, lemon zest and oil and set aside.
3. In another bowl, beat the egg.
4. Preheat to air fryer to 250 degrees F for 5 minutes
5. Dip the rack in the egg to coat and then into the breadcrumb mixture. Make sure it is well coated.
6. Spray the basket of the air fryer using cooking spray and put the rack in. You may have to bend it a little to get it to fit.
7. Set for 250 degrees and cook 25 minutes.
8. Increase temperature to 400 degrees F and cook another 5 minutes. Check internal temperature to make sure it is 145 degrees for medium rare or more.
9. Remove rack when done and cover with foil for 10 minutes before separating ribs into individual servings.

Nutrition:

Calories: 276 | Fat: 24g| Protein: 33g | Fiber: 12.3g

331. Perfect Lamb Burgers

⏱ Prep Time 10 m | ⏱ Cooking Time 20 m | 4 Servings

Ingredients:

- For Moroccan Spice Mix:
- 1 teaspoon ground ginger
- 1 teaspoon ground cumin
- 1 teaspoon sea salt
- ¾ teaspoon ground black pepper
- ½ teaspoon ground coriander
- ½ teaspoon ground allspice
- ½ teaspoon ground cloves
- ½ teaspoon ground cinnamon
- ½ teaspoon cayenne
- For Burgers and Dip:
- 1 ½ pound ground lamb
- 1 teaspoon Harissa paste
- 2 tablespoons Moroccan spice mix, divided
- 2 teaspoons garlic, peeled and minced
- ¼ teaspoon fresh chopped oregano
- 3 tablespoons plain Greek yogurt
- 1 small lemon, juiced

Directions:

1. Moroccan Spice Mix:
2. Whisk the ginger, cumin, salt, pepper, coriander, allspice, cloves, cinnamon and cayenne in a small bowl and set aside.
3. Burgers and Dip:
4. Place the lamb in a large bowl and add the Harissa sauce, 1 tablespoon of the homemade Moroccan spice mix, and the garlic. Mix in everything with the hands and form 4 patties.
5. Preheat the air fryer to 360 degrees for 5 minutes while making the patties.
6. Spray the basket of the air fryer using cooking spray and place two of the burgers in.
7. Cook a total of 12 minutes, flipping after 6 minutes.
8. Repeat with the other two burgers.
9. While burgers cook, make the dip by chopping the fresh oregano and placing it in a bowl with the yogurt, 1 teaspoon of the Moroccan spice mix and the juice of the lemon. Whisk this with a fork and divide into small containers to serve with the burgers when they are done.
10.

Nutrition:

Calories: 534 | Fat: 8g| Protein: 21g| Fiber: 8.7g

332. Simple yet Tasty Lamb Chops

⏱ Prep Time 15 m | ⏱ Cooking Time 30 m | 4 Servings

Ingredients:

- 1 clove of garlic separated from the head of garlic (maybe 2)
- 1 ½ tablespoons olive oil
- 4 lamb chops
- ½ tablespoon fresh oregano, chopped
- Salt and pepper to taste

Directions:

1. Preheat the air fryer oven to 400 degrees F for 6 minutes.
2. Take a little of the olive oil and coat the garlic clove(s). Place in the basket of the air fryer and roast 12 minutes.
3. While the garlic is cooking, mix the oregano, salt and pepper in a small bowl. Add the all the remaining olive oil and mix well.
4. Spread a thin coating of the oregano mixture on both sides of the lamb chops and reserve the rest.
5. Remove the clove(s) of garlic from the basket of the air fryer with rubber tipped tongs. Be careful because the cloves will be very soft and you don't want them to break open quite yet.
6. Spray the basket of the air fryer using cooking spray and place the lamb chops in, 2 at a time in 2 batches. Cook 5 minutes, turn and cook another 4 minutes.
7. When chops are done, squeeze the garlic out of the papery shell into the rest of the oregano mixture and mix it in. Serve this on the side like ketchup.

Nutrition:

Calories: 542 | Fat: 4g | Protein: 23g | Fiber: 6g

333. Tandoori Lamb
Prep Time 10 m | Cooking Time 20 m | 4 Servings

Ingredients:

- ½ onion, peeled and quartered
- 5 cloves garlic, peeled
- 4 slices fresh ginger, peeled
- 1 teaspoon ground fennel
- 1 teaspoon Garam Masala
- 1 teaspoon ground cinnamon
- ½ teaspoon ground cardamom
- ½ teaspoon cayenne
- 1 teaspoon salt
- 1 pound boneless lamb sirloin steaks

Directions:

1. Place the onion, garlic, ginger, fennel, Garam Masala, cinnamon, cardamom, cayenne and salt in a blender and pulse 4 to 6 times until ground.
2. Place the lamb steaks in a large bowl and slash the meat so the spices will permeate into it.
3. Pour the spice mix over top and rub in both sides. Let sit room temperature 30 minutes or cover and refrigerate overnight.
4. Preheat the air fryer to 350 degrees F for 10 minutes.
5. Spray the basket using cooking spray and place lamb steaks in without letting them overlap much. You may have to do this in batches.
6. Cook 7 minutes, turn and cook another 8 minutes.
7. Test with meat thermometer to make sure they are done. Medium well will be 150 degrees F.

Nutrition:

Calories: 232| Fat: 20g |Protein: 42g | Fiber: 5g

Pork Recipes

334. Barbecue Flavored Pork Ribs
Prep Time 5 m | Cooking Time 15 m | 6 Servings

Ingredients:

- ¼ cup honey, divided
- ¾ cup BBQ sauce
- 2 tablespoons tomato ketchup
- 1 tablespoon Worcestershire sauce
- 1 tablespoon soy sauce
- ½ teaspoon garlic powder
- Freshly ground white pepper, to taste
- 1¾ pound pork ribs

Directions:

1. Preparing the Ingredients. In a large bowl, mix together 3 tablespoons of honey and remaining ingredients except pork ribs.
2. Refrigerate to marinate for about 20 minutes.
3. Preheat the Air fryer oven to 355 degrees F.
4. Place the ribs in an Air fryer rack/basket.
5. Air Frying. Cook for about 13 minutes.
6. Remove the ribs from the Air fryer oven and coat with remaining honey.
7. Serve hot.

Nutrition:

Calories: 376|Fat: 20g |Protein: 32g| Fiber: 12g

335. Rustic Pork Ribs
Prep Time 5 m | Cooking Time 15 m | 4 Servings

Ingredients:

- 1 rack of pork ribs
- 3 tablespoons dry red wine
- 1 tablespoon soy sauce
- 1/2 teaspoon dried thyme
- 1/2 teaspoon onion powder
- 1/2 teaspoon garlic powder
- 1/2 teaspoon ground black pepper
- 1 teaspoon smoke salt
- 1 tablespoon cornstarch
- 1/2 teaspoon olive oil

Directions:

1. Preparing the Ingredients. Begin by preheating your Air fryer oven to 390 degrees F. Place all ingredients in a mixing bowl and let them marinate at least 1 hour.
2. Air Frying. Cook the marinated ribs approximately 25 minutes at 390 degrees F.
3. Serve hot.

Nutrition:

Calories: 326 |Fat: 14g |Protein: 23g| Fiber: 13g

336. Italian Parmesan Breaded Pork Chops
Prep Time 5 m | Cooking Time 25 m | 6 Servings

Ingredients:

- 5 (3½- to 5-ounce) pork chops (bone-in or boneless)
- 1 teaspoon Italian seasoning
- Seasoning salt
- Pepper
- ¼ cup all-purpose flour
- 2 tablespoons Italian bread crumbs
- 3 tablespoons finely grated Parmesan cheese
- Cooking oil

Directions:

1. Preparing the Ingredients. Season the pork chops with the Italian seasoning and seasoning salt and pepper to taste.
2. Sprinkle the flour on each sides of the pork chops, then coat both sides with the bread crumbs and Parmesan cheese.
3. Air Frying. Place the pork chops in the Air fryer oven. Stacking them is okay. Spray the pork chops with cooking oil. Set temperature to 360°F. Cook for 6 minutes.
4. Open the Air fryer oven and flip the pork chops. Cook for an additional 6 minutes.
5. Cool before serving. Instead of seasoning salt, you can use either chicken or pork rub for additional flavor. You can find these rubs in the spice aisle of the grocery store.

Nutrition: Calories: 334| Fat: 7g |Protein: 34g | Fiber: 0g

337. Crispy Breaded Pork Chops

⏱ Prep Time 10 m | ⏱ Cooking Time 15 m | 8 Servings

Ingredients:

- 1/8 tsp. pepper
- ¼ tsp. chili powder
- ½ tsp. onion powder
- ½ tsp. garlic powder
- 1 ¼ tsp. sweet paprika
- Tbsp. grated parmesan cheese
- 1/3 C. crushed cornflake crumbs
- ½ C. panko breadcrumbs
- 1 beaten egg
- 6 center-cut boneless pork chops

Directions:

1. Preparing the Ingredients. Ensure that your air fryer is preheated to 400 degrees. Spray the basket with olive oil.
2. With ½ teaspoon salt and pepper, season both sides of pork chops.
3. Combine ¾ teaspoon salt with pepper, chili powder, onion powder, garlic powder, paprika, cornflake crumbs, panko breadcrumbs, and parmesan cheese.
4. Beat egg in another bowl.
5. Dip the pork chops into the egg and then crumb mixture.
6. Add pork chops to air fryer and spritz with olive oil.
7. Air Frying. Set temperature to 400°F, and set time to 12 minutes. Cook 12 minutes, making sure to flip over halfway through the cooking process.
8. Only add 3 chops in at a time and repeat the process with remaining pork chops.

Nutrition:

Calories: 378| Fat: 13g | Protein: 33g |Sugar: 1

338. Caramelized Pork Shoulder

⏱ Prep Time 10 m | ⏱ Cooking Time20 m | 8 Servings

Ingredients:

- 1/3 cup soy sauce
- Tablespoons sugar
- 1 tablespoon honey
- 2 pound pork shoulder, cut into 1½-inch thick slices

Directions:

1. Preparing the Ingredients. In a bowl, mix all the ingredients except pork.
2. Add pork and coat with marinade generously.
3. Cover and refrigerate o marinate for about 2-8 hours.
4. Preheat the Air fryer oven to 335 degrees F.
5. Air Frying. Place the pork in an Air fryer rack/basket.
6. Cook for about 10 minutes.
7. Now, set the Air fryer oven to 390 degrees F. Cook for about 10 minutes.

Nutrition:

Calories: 268| Fat: 10g |Protein: 23g |Sugar: 5

339. Roasted Pork Tenderloin

⏱ Prep Time 5 m | ⏱ Cooking Time 1 h | 4 Servings

Ingredients:

- 1 (3-pound) pork tenderloin
- Tablespoons extra-virgin olive oil
- 2 garlic cloves, minced
- 1 teaspoon dried basil
- 1 teaspoon dried oregano
- 1 teaspoon dried thyme
- Salt
- Pepper

Directions:

1. Preparation of ingredients. Dip the pork fillet in olive oil.
2. Grate the garlic, basil, oregano, thyme, and salt and pepper to taste throughout the steak.
3. Air fry. Place the steak in the oven of the deep fryer. Cook for 45 minutes.
4. Use a meat thermometer to check for politeness
5. Open the Air Fryer and flip the pork fillet. Cook for 15 more minutes.
6. Take the cooked pork out of the deep fryer and let it rest for 10 minutes before slicing it.

Nutrition:

Calories: 283| Fat: 10g| Protein: 48

340. Dijon Garlic Pork Tenderloin

⏱ Prep Time 5 m | ⏱ Cooking Time 10 m | 6 Servings

Ingredients:

- 1 C. breadcrumbs
- Pinch of cayenne pepper
- Crushed garlic cloves
- 2 tbsp. ground ginger
- 2 tbsp. Dijon mustard
- 2 tbsp. raw honey
- Tbsp. water
- 2 tsp. salt
- 1 pound pork tenderloin, sliced into 1-inch rounds

Directions:

1. Preparing the Ingredients. With pepper and salt, season all sides of tenderloin.
2. Combine cayenne pepper, garlic, ginger, mustard, honey, and water until smooth.
3. Dip pork rounds into the honey mixture and then into breadcrumbs, ensuring they all get coated well.
4. Place coated pork rounds into your Air fryer oven.
5. Air Frying. Set temperature to 400°F, and set time to 10 minutes. Cook 10 minutes at 400 degrees. Flip and then cook an additional 5 minutes until golden in color.

Nutrition: Calories: 423 |Fat: 18g |Protein: 31g |Sugar: 3g

341. Bacon Wrapped Pork Tenderloin
ⓣ Prep Time 5 m | ⓣ Cooking Time 15 m | 4 Servings

Ingredients:

Pork:

- 1-2 tbsp. Dijon mustard
- 3-4 strips of bacon
- 1 pork tenderloin

Apple Gravy:

- ½ - 1 tsp. Dijon mustard
- 1 tbsp. almond flour
- Tbsp. ghee
- 1 chopped onion
- 2-3 Granny Smith apples
- 1 C. vegetable broth

Directions:

1. Preparing the Ingredients. Spread Dijon mustard all over tenderloin and wrap the meat with strips of bacon.
2. Air Frying. Place into the Air fryer oven, set temperature to 360°F, and set time to 15 minutes and cook 10-15 minutes at 360 degrees.
3. To make sauce, heat ghee in a pan and add shallots. Cook 1-2 minutes.
4. Then add apples, cooking 3-5 minutes until softened.
5. Add flour and ghee to make a roux. Add broth and mustard, stirring well to combine.
6. When the sauce starts to bubble, add 1 cup of sautéed apples, cooking till sauce thickens.
7. Once pork tenderloin I cook, allow to sit 5-10 minutes to rest before slicing.
8. Serve topped with apple gravy.

Nutrition:

Calories: 552| Fat: 25g| Protein: 29g |Sugar: 6g

342. Pork Neck with Salad
ⓣ Prep Time 10 m | ⓣ Cooking Time 12 m | 2 Servings

Ingredients:

For Pork:

- 1 tablespoon soy sauce
- 1 tablespoon fish sauce
- ½ tablespoon oyster sauce
- ½ pound pork neck

For Salad:

- 1 ripe tomato, sliced tickly
- 8-10 Thai shallots, sliced
- 1 scallion, chopped
- 1 bunch fresh basil leaves
- 1 bunch fresh cilantro leaves

For Dressing:

- Tablespoons fish sauce
- 2 tablespoons olive oil
- 1 teaspoon apple cider vinegar
- 1 tablespoon palm sugar
- 2 bird eye chili
- 1 tablespoon garlic, minced

Directions:

1. Preparation of ingredients. For the pork in a bowl, mix all the ingredients except the pork.
2. Add the pork neck and marinade layer evenly. Refrigerate for about 2-3 hours.
3. Preheat the deep fryer oven to 340 degrees F.
4. Air fry. Place the pork neck in a grill pan. Cook for about 12 minutes.
5. Meanwhile, in a large bowl, combine all of the salad ingredients.
6. In a bowl, add all the dressing ingredients and beat until well combined.
7. Remove the pork neck from the fryer and cut it into the desired slices.
8. Place the pork slices on top of the salad.

Nutrition:

Calories: 296 |Fat: 20g |Protein: 24g |Sugar: 8

343. Chinese Braised Pork Belly
ⓣ Prep Time 5 m | ⓣ Cooking Time 20 m | 8 Servings

Ingredients:

- 1 lb. Pork Belly, sliced
- 1 Tbsp. Oyster Sauce
- 1 Tbsp. Sugar
- Red Fermented Bean Curds
- 1 Tbsp. Red Fermented Bean Curd Paste

- 1 Tbsp. Cooking Wine
- 1/2 Tbsp. Soy Sauce
- 1 Tsp Sesame Oil
- 1 Cup All Purpose Flour

Directions:

1. Preparing the Ingredients. Preheat the Air fryer oven to 390 degrees.
2. In a small bowl, mix up the ingredients together and rub the pork thoroughly with this mixture
3. Set aside to marinate for at least 30 minutes or preferably overnight for the flavors to permeate the meat
4. Coat each marinated pork belly slice in flour and place in the Air fryer oven tray
5. Air Frying. Cook for 20 minutes until crispy and tender.

Nutrition:

Calories: 409 |Fat: 14g |Protein: 19g| Sugar: 9

344. Air Fryer Sweet and Sour Pork
Prep Time 10 m | Cooking Time 12 m | 6 Servings

Ingredients:

- Tbsp. olive oil
- 1/16 tsp. Chinese Five Spice
- ¼ tsp. pepper
- ½ tsp. sea salt
- 1 tsp. pure sesame oil
- 2 eggs
- 1 C. almond flour
- 2 pounds pork, sliced into chunks

- Sweet and Sour Sauce:
- ¼ tsp. sea salt
- ½ tsp. garlic powder
- 1 tbsp. low-sodium soy sauce
- ½ C. rice vinegar
- Tbsp. tomato paste
- 1/8 tsp. water
- ½ C. sweetener of choice

Directions:

1. Preparing the Ingredients. To make the dipping sauce, whisk all sauce ingredients together over medium heat, stirring 5 minutes. Simmer uncovered 5 minutes till thickened.
2. Meanwhile, combine almond flour, five spice, pepper, and salt.
3. In another bowl, mix eggs with sesame oil.
4. Dredge pork in flour mixture and then in egg mixture. Shake any excess off before adding to air fryer rack/basket.
5. Air Frying. Set temperature to 340°F, and set time to 12 minutes.
6. Serve with sweet and sour dipping sauce!

Nutrition:
Calories: 371 |Fat: 17g |Protein: 27g| Sugar: 1g

345. Juicy Pork Ribs Ole
Prep Time 10 m | Cooking Time 25 m | 4 Servings

Ingredients:

- 1 rack of pork ribs
- 1/2 cup low-fat milk
- 1 tablespoon envelope taco seasoning mix
- 1 can tomato sauce

- 1/2 teaspoon ground black pepper
- 1 teaspoon seasoned salt
- 1 tablespoon cornstarch
- 1 teaspoon canola oil

Directions:

1. Preparing the Ingredients. Place all ingredients in a mixing dish; let them marinate for 1 hour.
2. Air Frying. Cook the marinated ribs approximately 25 minutes at 390 degrees F
3. Work with batches. Enjoy.

Nutrition:
Calories: 218 |Fat: 8g |Protein: 11g| Sugar: 1

346. Teriyaki Pork Rolls
Prep Time 10 m | Cooking Time 8 m | 6 Servings

Ingredients:

- 1 tsp. almond flour
- Tbsp. low-sodium soy sauce
- Tbsp. mirin
- Tbsp. brown sugar

- Thumb-sized amount of ginger, chopped
- Pork belly slices
- Enki mushrooms

Directions:

1. Preparing the Ingredients. Mix brown sugar, mirin, soy sauce, almond flour, and ginger until brown sugar dissolves.
2. Take pork belly slices and wrap around a bundle of mushrooms. Brush each roll with teriyaki sauce. Chill half an hour.
3. Preheat your Air fryer oven to 350 degrees and add marinated pork rolls.
4. Air Frying. Set temperature to 350°F, and set time to 8 minutes.

Nutrition: Calories: 412| Fat: 9g |Protein: 19g

347. Air Fried Spicy Lamb Sirloin Steak
Prep Time 40 m | Cooking Time 15 m | 4 Servings

Ingredients:

- ½ onion
- 4 ginger cubes
- 5 garlic cloves
- 1 teaspoon of garam masala
- 1 teaspoon fennel, ground

- 1 teaspoon cinnamon, ground
- ½ teaspoon cayenne powder
- 1 teaspoon salt
- 1 pound lamb sirloin, boneless steaks

Directions:

1. Wash the lamb and pat dry.
2. Adding all the ingredients in a blender except for the lamb chops and blend it into a fine paste.
3. Make strips over the lamb chops to ensure the marinating reaches within the meat.
4. Rub the paste on to the chops and mix them well.
5. Let the marinade mixture rest for 30 minutes or overnight in the refrigerator, as preferred.
6. Place the lamb steaks in the air fryer basket and put it in the inner pot.
7. Close the crisp lid.
8. Select the smart option ROAST under AIR FRY mode for 15 minutes. Select the temperature to 380°F. It will automatically select temperature to 380°F by default.
9. Press START to begin the cooking.
10. Halfway through the cooking, open the crisp lid and flip the lamb for even cooking.
11. Close the crisp lid to resume cooking for the remaining period. Serve hot.

Nutrition: Calories: 171 Fat: 2.1g Carbs: 4g Protein: 24g

348. Air Fried Herb Rack of Lamb

⏰ Prep Time 5 m | ⏲ Cooking Time 20 m | 2 Servings

Ingredients:
- 1-pound whole rack of lamb
- 2 tablespoons rosemary, dried
- 1 tablespoon thyme, dried
- 2 teaspoons garlic, minced
- ½ teaspoon salt
- ½ teaspoon pepper
- 4 tablespoons olive oil

Directions:
1. Wash the lamb and pat dry.
2. In a mixing bowl, mix all the herbs along with olive oil and keep it aside.
3. Rub the herb mixture over the lamb rack and coat it thoroughly.
4. Place the lamb in the air fryer basket and put it in the inner pot of Instant Pot Air Fryer.
5. Close the crisp lid and set the temperature at 360° F in the AIR FRY mode.
6. Set the timer for 10 minutes.
7. Press START to begin the cooking.
8. Halfway through the cooking, open the crisp lid and flip the lamb for even cooking.
9. After flipping, close the crisp lid, so that the appliance can automatically resume cooking for the remaining period.
10. Once done, remove it from the air fryer and serve hot.

Nutrition:
Calories: 614 Fat: 46.7g Carbs: 3g Protein: 47g

349. Air Fryer Italian Pork Chops for Two

⏰ Prep Time 10 m | ⏲ Cooking Time 35 m | 2 Servings

Ingredients:
- 2 tablespoons all-purpose flour
- 1 egg, medium
- ¼ teaspoon kosher salt
- ¼ cup panko breadcrumbs
- 3 tablespoons parmesan cheese, grated
- 8 ounces (2 Nos.) pork loin chops, boneless

Directions:
1. Wash pork and pat dry.
2. Place a parchment paper at the bottom of the air fryer to avoid grease and ensure easy cleaning.
3. Beat egg with salt in a shallow bowl.
4. Put the all-purpose flour in another medium shallow bowl.
5. Combine breadcrumbs and grated parmesan cheese in a large bowl thoroughly.
6. Dredge the pork one by one in the flour mix, then dip in the egg mix and lastly dredge in the breadcrumb mix and press it gently to have proper bread coating.
7. Place these in the parchment paper on the air fryer basket.
8. Place the air fryer basket in the inner pot of the Instant Pot Air Fryer.
9. Close the crisp lid.
10. Under the AIR FRY mode, change the temperature to 325°F and the timer to 10 minutes.
11. Press START button to begin the cooking.
12. Open the crisp lid after 5 minutes and flip the meat.
13. Close the crisp lid to resume the remaining portion of the cooking.
14. Once the cooking over, serve the dish hot.

Nutrition:
Calories 330 Carbohydrates: 17g Fat 15g Protein: 33g

350. Air Fryer Meatloaf

⏰ Prep Time 10 m | ⏲ Cooking Time 25 m | 4 Servings

Ingredients:
- 1-pound lean beef
- 1 egg, medium, lightly beaten
- 3 tablespoons breadcrumbs
- 1 onion, small, finely chopped
- 1 tablespoon fresh thyme, chopped
- 1 teaspoon kosher salt
- ½ teaspoon ground black pepper
- 2 mushrooms, medium, sliced
- 1 tablespoon olive oil

Directions:
1. Wash beef and pat dry.
2. In a medium-large bowl, combine beef, egg, breadcrumbs, salt, thyme, onion, and pepper. Knead and mix the ingredients well.
3. Transfer this mix into a baking pan and place the mushroom on top of the mix.
4. Coat this mix with olive oil and place the pan in the air fryer basket.
5. Now put the air fryer basket in the inner pot of Instant Pot Air Fryer.
6. Close the crisp cover.
7. Under the ROAST mode, set the timer for 25 minutes and let the meatloaf roast. The smart ROAST option will automatically select the temperature to 380°F.
8. Press the START button to resume the cooking.
9. After cooking, allow the meatloaf to settle down the heat before you can slice and serve it.
10. Slice it into small portions and serve.

Nutrition:
Calories 297 Carbohydrates: 5.9g Fat 18.8g Protein: 24.8g

351. Air Fryer Pork Chops
Prep Time 5 m | Cooking Time 20 m | 4 Servings

Ingredients:
- 4 pork chops, boneless
- 7 tablespoons shredded parmesan cheese
- 1 teaspoon kosher salt
- 1 teaspoon paprika
- 1 teaspoon garlic powder
- 1 teaspoon onion powder
- ½ teaspoon ground black pepper
- 2 tablespoons extra-virgin olive oil

Directions:
1. Remove excess fat if anything on the pork chop, wash, and dry with paper towels.
2. Make both sides of the meat will coat with olive oil.
3. Take a medium bowl and combine the parmesan with all the spices thoroughly.
4. Marinate this mixture evenly on both sides of the meat.
5. Place the air fryer basket in the inner pot of the Instant Pot Air Fryer.
6. Put the marinated pork chops in the air fryer basket.
7. Close the crisp cover.
8. Under AIR FRYER, select the smart option ROAST and set the timer to 20 minutes. The default temperature with smart option ROAST is 380°F.
9. Press START to begin the cooking.
10. After 10 minutes of cooking, open the crisp lid and flip the chop for even cooking.
11. Close the crisp cover to resume for the remaining period.
12. Once the cooking over, you can serve the pork chops hot.

Nutrition:
Calories: 400 Fat: 22.9g Carbs: 3g Protein: 43g

352. Air Fryer Roast Beef
Prep Time 5 m | Cooking Time 15 m | 6 Servings

Ingredients:
- 2½ pound beef
- 1 tablespoon Montreal steak seasoning
- 1 tablespoon olive oil

Directions:
1. Tie up the beef to make it compact enough to cook.
2. Rub some olive oil all over the beef roast
3. Sprinkle the seasoning over the meat.
4. Put the air fryer basket in the inner pot of the Instant Pot Air Fryer.
5. Place the separator in the air fryer basket and keep the beef on the separator.
6. Close the crisp cover.
7. Select the smart option ROAST under AIR FRYER and set the timer to 15 minutes.
8. Press the START button and let the meat cook well.
9. Open the crisp cover and flip it halfway through for even cooking.
10. After flipping close the crisp cover again to resume cooking for the remaining period.
11. Once done, allow it to rest for 5 minutes before you serve.

Nutrition:
Calories 276 Fat: 13g Carbs: 1g Protein: 39g

353. Air Fryer Steak
Prep Time 10 m | Cooking Time 35 m | 4 Servings

Ingredients:
- 2 pounds bone-in-rib eye
- 4 tablespoon butter, softened
- 2 garlic cloves, minced
- 2 teaspoon parsley, freshly chopped
- 1 teaspoon chives, freshly chopped
- 1 teaspoon thyme, freshly chopped
- 1 teaspoon rosemary, freshly chopped
- ½ teaspoon black pepper, freshly ground
- 1 teaspoon kosher salt

Directions:
1. Wash and pat dry the rib eye.
2. Using a mixing bowl, mix the butter and herbs thoroughly.
3. In a plastic wrap, place the butter-herb mix in the center and roll it like a log. Close both ends of the wrap to keep it airtight and refrigerate it until it hardens. It will take about 20 minutes to freeze.
4. Salt and pepper over the steak on both sides.
5. Transfer the steak in the air fryer basket and place it in the inner pot of the Instant Pot Air Fryer.
6. Close the crisp cover.
7. Under the AIR FRY mode, select the temperature to 400°F and select timer to 14 minutes.
8. Press START to begin the cooking.
9. Halfway through the cooking, open the crisp cover and flip the steak.
10. After flipping, close the crisp cover to resume the cooking.
11. Now take out the refrigerated herb mix and slice it. Serve and top it with the herb slice mix.

Nutrition:
Calories: 407 Fat: 22.1g Carbs: 1g Protein: 52g

354. Air Fryer Beef with Homemade Marinade
⏰ Prep Time 10 m | ⏱ Cooking Time 45 m | 3 Servings

Ingredients:

- 1-pound beef sirloin
- ½ cup red onion slices
- ½ cup green onion slices
- 1 yellow bell pepper, cut into strips
- 1 green pepper, cut into strips
- 1 red bell pepper, cut into strips
- 1½ pounds broccoli florets
- 1 tablespoon vegetable oil

- For the marinade:
- ¼ cup of water
- 1 teaspoon minced ginger
- 1 tablespoon soy sauce
- 1 tablespoon sesame oil
- 2 teaspoons finely grated garlic
- ¼ cup hoisin sauce

Directions:

1. Wash and pat dry the beef.
2. Cut the beef sirloin into 2-inch strips.
3. For making the marinade, add the hoisin sauce, garlic, sesame oil, soy sauce, finely grated ginger, and water in a bowl and mix thoroughly.
4. Add the meat in the marinade and mix to coat for perfect seasoning.
5. Cover the bowl and refrigerate for 20 minutes.
6. Put all the vegetables in a large bowl and add one teaspoon vegetable oil into it and mix thoroughly for even coating.
7. Transfer the oil-coated vegetables into the air fryer basket and place it in the inner pot of the Instant Pot Air Fryer.
8. Close the crisp lid.
9. In the AIR FRY mode, select temperature 200°F and set the timer to 5 minutes.
10. Press START to begin the cooking.
11. After the vegetables become soft, transfer it into a bowl.
12. Now place the marinated meat in the air fryer basket.
13. Close the crisp cover and set the temperature at 360°F on AIR FRY mod.
14. Set the timer to 40 minutes.
15. Press START to begin cooking.
16. After 20 minutes, open the air fryer and flip the meat.
17. To resume cooking for the remaining period, close the crisp cover.
18. Serve it with salad.

Nutrition:
Calories: 509 Fat: 28.9g Carbs: 24g Protein: 41g

355. Bourbon Bacon Burger in the Air Fryer
⏰ Prep Time 10 m | ⏱ Cooking Time 25 m | 2 Servings

Ingredients:

- ¾ pound minced beef
- 3 strips bacon, cut into half
- 2 Kaiser Rolls
- 4 tablespoons barbeque sauce
- ¼ teaspoon paprika
- 2 tablespoons mayonnaise
- 1 teaspoon ground black pepper, fresh

- 1 tablespoon bourbon
- 1 tablespoon onion, finely chopped
- 2 tablespoons brown sugar
- ½ teaspoon salt
- ½ lettuce, finely chopped (serving)
- 1 tomato, chopped (serving)

Directions:

1. In a mixing bowl, combine the bourbon and brown sugar.
2. Brush this mixture over the bacon strips on both sides.
3. Place the marinated bacon strips in the air fryer basket.
4. Put the air fryer basket in the inner pot of the Instant Pot Air Fryer.
5. Close the crisp cover.
6. In the AIR FRY mode, select the temperature to 390°F and set the timer to 10 minutes.
7. Press START to begin the cooking.
8. Halfway through the cooking, open the air fryer, and flip the bacon.
9. Sprinkle the bourbon mixture on the bacon, if required and cook for the remaining period.
10. While the cooking in progress, make the burger patties by combining the ground beef, BBQ sauce, onion, salt, and pepper in a large bowl.
11. Combine it thoroughly and make 2 patties out of the mixture.
12. Take out the cooked bacon into a bowl and start the cooking process for burger patties.
13. Place the patties in the air fryer basket and put in the inner pot of the Instant Pot Air Fryer.
14. Close the crisp cover.
15. In the AIR FRY mode, select temperature 370°F and set the timer for 20 minutes.
16. Press START to begin the cooking process.
17. Now let us make the burger sauce by mixing BBQ sauce, paprika, mayonnaise, and pepper in a bowl.
18. Once the patties cooked, top it with cheese and air fry for one more minute.
19. Spread the sauce in the Kaiser rolls, place these burgers on rolls and top with the bourbon bacon, tomato, and lettuce.
20. Serve it with additional sauces if needed.

Nutrition:
Calories 1020 Carbohydrates: 49g Fat 68g Protein: 44g

356. Crispy Air Fryer Bacon
Prep Time 5 m | Cooking Time 10 m | 8 Servings

Ingredients:
- ¾ pound bacon, thick-cut pieces

Directions:
1. Place the bacon strips in the air fryer basket, don't overlap them.
2. Put the air fryer basket in the inner pot of the Instant Pot Air Fryer.
3. Close the crisp lid.
4. Under the BROIL mode, set the timer for 10 minutes. The default temperature will read at 400°F.
5. Press START to begin the cooking.
6. Check the air fryer halfway to flip the bacon strips.
7. You can open the crisp lid (this will pause the cooking procedure) and close the crisp cover once you have flipped the meat. The cooking will resume as soon as you close the lid.
8. Once the bacon is ready, serve hot.

Nutrition:
Calories: 132 Fat: 12.6g Carbs: 3g Protein: 5g

357. Crisp Breaded Pork Chops in the Air Fryer
Prep Time 10 m | Cooking Time 12 m | 6 Servings

Ingredients:
- 6 pork chops, center cut, boneless
- 1 egg, large, beaten
- ½ cup panko bread crumbs
- 1/3 Cup corn flakes crumbs, crushed
- 2 tablespoons parmesan cheese, grated
- 1¼ teaspoon sweet paprika
- 1 ½ teaspoon garlic powder
- ¼ teaspoon chili powder
- ½ teaspoon onion powder
- ½ teaspoon ground black pepper
- 1 teaspoon kosher salt
- Olive oil cooking spray

Directions:
1. Cut and remove excess fat of the pork.
2. Wash and pat dry.
3. Spray the air fryer basket with cooking oil and place it in the inner pot of the Instant Pot Air Fryer.
4. Close the crisp cover.
5. Set the air fryer temperature to 400°F and preheat for 5 minutes in the AIR FRY mode.
6. Press START to begin the preheating.
7. In the meantime, season the pork chops by rubbing half teaspoon salt on both sides and keep aside.
8. In a large shallow bowl, combine panko breadcrumbs, cornflakes, cheese, salt, garlic powder, paprika, chili powder, onion powder, and pepper.
9. In a medium shallow bowl, beat the egg.
10. Now batch by batch, do the breading and seasoning.
11. First, dip the pork chops in the beaten egg and then dredge in the breadcrumbs mix and press it gently so that it will have good breadcrumb coating on all sides.
12. Once the preheat timer goes off, put the pork chops in the air fryer basket in batches and spritz some more cooking oil. Close the crisp cover.
13. In the AIR FRY mode, at 400°F, select the timer for 40 minutes.
14. Press START to begin the cooking.
15. Halfway through the cooking, open the air fryer, and flip the pork chop.
16. To complete the remaining portion of the cooking, close the crisp cover. The Instant Pot will automatically resume cooking, from the point you have interrupted.
17. Once done, keep it aside and repeat the process with the rest of the batch.

Nutrition:
Calories 376 Fat: 18.8g Carbs: 7g Protein: 42g

358. Easy Air Fryer Pork Chops
Prep Time 10 m | Cooking Time 20 m | 4 Servings

Ingredients:
- 5 ounces (4 pieces) pork chops, center-cut
- ½ cup parmesan cheese, grated
- 1 teaspoon parsley, dried
- 1 teaspoon ground paprika
- ½ teaspoon ground black pepper
- 1 teaspoon garlic powder
- 1 teaspoon salt
- 2 tablespoon olive oil, extra-virgin
- Olive cooking oil spray

Directions:
1. Wash pork chops and pat dry.
2. Using a mixing bowl, combine the parmesan cheese, pepper, parsley, salt, garlic powder, and paprika.
3. Coat the pork chops with the olive oil and then dredge them in the parmesan mixture one by one and place it on a plate.
4. Spritz cooking oil in the air fryer basket and place in the inner pot of the Instant Pot Air Fryer.
5. Place these chops in the air fryer basket in batches.
6. Close the crisp lid.
7. Under the ROAST mode, select the timer for 25 minutes. The temperature by default will remain at 400°F.
8. Press START to begin the cooking.
9. Flip it halfway through for even cooking.
10. Once the cooking over, transfer the pork chop on a cutting board and let it rest for about 5 minutes before you slice and serve.

Nutrition:
Calories 305 Carbohydrates: 1.5g Fat 16.6g Protein: 35.3g

359. Pork Tenderloin in the Air Fryer

⏱ Prep Time 20 m | ⏱ Cooking Time 18 m | 6 Servings

Ingredients:

- 1½ pound pork tenderloin
- 1 tablespoon olive oil
- ¼ teaspoon ground black pepper
- ¼ teaspoon garlic powder
- ¼ teaspoon salt

Directions:

1. Wash and pat dry the pork tenderloin.
2. In a small bowl, mix the olive oil, black pepper, and garlic powder well and add salt as needed.
3. Rub the seasoning mixture over the tenderloin.
4. Transfer the meat in the air fryer basket.
5. Place the air fryer basket in the inner pot of the Instant Pot Air Fryer.
6. Close the crisp cover.
7. In the ROAST mode, set the timer to 25 minutes. The default heat will show 400°F, which you cannot change in the smart cooking option.
8. Press START to begin the cooking.
9. Flip the tenderloin midway for even cooking.
10. After cooking, allow the meat to cool down before you can slice and serve.

Nutrition: Calories: 183 Fat: 6.2g Carbs: 0g Protein: 30g

360. Perfect Air Fryer Steak

⏱ Prep Time 5 m | ⏱ Cooking Time 12 m | 4 Servings

Ingredients:

- 2 pounds sirloin steak
- 3 tablespoon steak seasoning, as preferred
- Olive oil cooking spray

Directions:

1. Wash and pat dry the sirloin steak.
2. Spray some oil over the steak and sprinkle the choice of seasoning, liberally.
3. Sprinkle some cooking oil in the air fryer basket.
4. Put the air fryer basket in the inner pot of the Instant Pot Air Fryer.
5. Close the crisp lid.
6. Under the ROAST mode, select the timer for 25 minutes. By default, the temperature will remain at 400°F in the ROAST mode.
7. Press START to begin the cooking process.
8. Open the crisp cover and flip the steak halfway for even cooking.
9. For resuming the cooking, simply close the crisp cover. So that the appliance can continue with the cooking.
10. Once the cooking over, allow the meet to cool down before you can slice and serve.

Nutrition: Calories: 270 Fat: 5.9g Carbs: 4g Protein: 46g

361. Spicy Lamb Sirloin Steak in the Air Fryer

⏱ Prep Time 40 m | ⏱ Cooking Time 15 m | 4 Servings

Ingredients:

- 2 pounds lamb sirloin steaks, boneless
- 1 teaspoon salt
- ½ teaspoon cayenne powder
- ½ teaspoon cardamom powder
- 1 teaspoon cinnamon powder
- 1 teaspoon ground fennel
- 1 teaspoon garam masala
- 5 garlic cloves, minced
- 4 ginger cubes, finely grated
- ½ onion, medium size, coarsely chopped
- Olive oil cooking spray.

Directions:

1. Wash the lamb and pat dry.
2. Put it on a chopping board and create deep strips, so that the marinade can penetrate the meat deeply.
3. In a blender, combine all the ingredients except for the lamb chops into a fine paste.
4. Rub this paste on the meat and coat it thoroughly.
5. Let the meat rest with the marinade for 30 minutes or put in the refrigerator overnight for a better marinade effect.
6. Spritz some cooking oil in the air fryer basket.
7. Place the seasoned sirloin steak in the air fryer basket and spray some cooking oil on the steak.
8. Close the crisp cover.
9. In the AIR FRY section, select the temperature to 330°F and select the timer for 25 minutes.
10. Press START to begin the cooking.
11. Open the crisp cover and flip the meat halfway for even cooking.
12. For resuming the remaining portion of the cooking, simply close the crisp lid.
13. Serve it hot.

Nutrition: Calories: 323 Fat: 11.8g Carbs: 4g Protein: 47g

362. Air Fryer Pork Belly Bites

⏱ Prep Time 15 m | ⏱ Cooking Time 20 m | 4 Servings

Ingredients:

- 1 lb. pork belly, rinsed and patted dry
- 1 tablespoon Worcestershire sauce or soy sauce
- ½ teaspoon garlic powder
- Black pepper and salt to taste
- Optional: ¼ cup BBQ sauce

Directions:

1. Cleanse pork belly and remove the skin if any. Cut into ¾-inch cubes and place them in a bowl. Add seasonings and spread pork belly cubes in the air fryer basket.
2. Put the air fryer inside the instant pot duo crisp. Attach the air fryer lid and air fry at 400 degrees F for 10-18 minutes. Shake and flip the air fryer basket for even coating twice through the cooking process, depending on desired crispiness.
3. If you want it to be crispier, extend the cooking time up to 20 minutes.
4. Drizzle with BBQ sauce if desired.

Nutrition: Calories 313 Carbohydrates 2.35 g Fat 20.81 g Protein 29 g

363. Air Fryer Pork Chop Bites with Mushrooms
⏱ Prep Time 15 m | ⏱ Cooking Time 20 m | 4 Servings

Ingredients:
- 2 tablespoons melted butter or olive oil
- 1 pound pork chops, cleansed and pat dried
- 8 ounces mushrooms, cleansed, washed and halved
- ½ teaspoon garlic powder
- 1 teaspoon Worcestershire sauce or soy sauce
- Black pepper and salt to taste

Directions:
1. Chop pork into ¾-inch cubes and combine with mushrooms. Brush pork and mushrooms with melted butter and add seasonings.
2. Cut the pork chops into ¾-inch-sized cubes and combine with the mushrooms. Coat the pork and mushrooms with melted butter or oil. Season with garlic powder, Worcestershire sauce, salt, and pepper. Spread the pork and mushrooms in even layer in the air fryer basket.
3. Air fry at 400 degrees F for 10-18 minutes, shaking and flipping the pork belly 2 times through cooking process. Check the pork chops to see how well done it is cooked. If you want it crispier, cook for an additional 2-5 minutes.
4. Season with additional salt and pepper if desired.
5. Serve warm.

Nutrition:
Calories 473 Carbohydrates 44.42 g Fat 17.23 g Protein 35.09 g

364. Air Fryer Steak Bites & Mushrooms
⏱ Prep Time 10 m | ⏱ Cooking Time 20 m | 4 Servings

Ingredients:
- 8 ounces mushrooms, cleaned, washed and halved
- 1 lb. steaks, cut into 1-inch cubes and patted dry
- 2 tablespoons butter, melted
- ½ teaspoon garlic powder
- 1 teaspoon Worcestershire sauce
- A dash of minced parsley for garnish
- Optional: melted butter or chili flakes for finishing
- Black pepper and salt to taste

Directions:
1. Add steak cubes and mushrooms in a bowl and coat with melted butter. Season the dish with garlic powder, Worcestershire sauce, salt and pepper to taste.
2. Arrange mushrooms and steak cubes in the instant pot air fryer basket. Set to air fry at 400 degrees F for 10-18 minutes, flipping from time to time for even cooking.
3. If you desire your steaks to be crispier, cook for an additional 2-5 minutes.
4. Garnish with parsley and drizzle with melted butter or chili flakes if desired.
5. Serve warm.

Nutrition:
Calories 471 Carbohydrates 44.38g Fat 15.94 g Protein 37.52 g

365. Air Fryer Steak Tips
⏱ Prep Time 10 m | ⏱ Cooking Time 20 m | 4 Servings

Ingredients:
- ½ lb. potatoes, peeled and cut into half-inch pieces
- 1 lb. steaks, cut into half-inch cubes and pat dry
- 2 tablespoons Melted butter, oil for alternative
- 1 teaspoon Worcestershire sauce
- ½ teaspoon garlic powder
- Salt and black pepper to taste
- A pinch of minced parsley for garnish
- Optional: melted butter or chili flakes for finishing

Directions:
1. Add potatoes to the instant pot duo crisp and boil for about 5 minutes or until tender, using the pressure cooker lid. Drain and set aside.
2. In a mixing bowl, toss together potatoes and steak cubes with melted butter, garlic powder, and Worcestershire sauce. Season with salt and pepper to taste.
3. Spread steak cubes and potatoes in the air fryer basket. Using the air fryer lid, air-fry at 400 degrees F for 10-18 minutes, shaking and flipping potatoes halfway through cooking, depending on preferred crispness. If you want your steak cubes to be crispier, cook for another 2-5 minutes.
4. Garnish with parsley, and drizzle with melted butter if desired. You may also use chili flakes.
5. Serve warm.

Nutrition:
Calories 344 Carbohydrates 11.54 g Fat 18.39 g Protein 33 g

366. Air-fried Garlic-rosemary Lamb Chops
⏱ Prep Time 3 m | ⏱ Cooking Time 12 m | 2 Servings

Ingredients:
- 2 lamb chops
- 1 clove of garlic
- 2 teaspoons olive oil
- 2 teaspoons garlic puree
- A sprig of fresh rosemary
- Salt and pepper to taste

Directions:
1. Place lamb chops in a bowl and season with salt and pepper and brush or spray with olive oil.
2. Top each lamb chop with garlic puree.
3. Between each chops place fresh rosemary and unpeeled garlic.
4. Leave the bowl with the lamb chops in the refrigerator for about an hour to marinate.
5. Transfer the marinated lamb chops to the instant pot duo crisp air fryer basket and air-fry at 360 degrees F for 6 minutes.
6. Flip lamb chops for even cooking and cook for another 6 minutes without changing the cooking temperature.
7. Let it rest for 2 minutes.
8. Discard the fresh garlic and rosemary and serve.

Nutrition:
Calories 426 Carbohydrates 1g Fat 10g Protein 83g

367. Seasoned Pork with Couscous

⏰ Prep Time 15 m | ⏰ Cooking Time 45 m | 6 Servings

Ingredients:

- 2-1/2 lbs. of pork loin (boneless and trimmed)
- 2-1/4 teaspoon of Sage (dried)
- 3/4 cup of chicken stock -
- 1/2 tablespoon of sweet paprika
- 1/2 tablespoon of garlic powder
- 1/4 teaspoon of marjoram (dried)
- 1/4 teaspoon of rosemary (dried)
- 1 teaspoon of basil (dried)
- 2 tablespoon of olive oil
- 2 cup of couscous (cooked)
- 1 teaspoon of oregano (dried)
- Salt and black pepper to taste

Direction:

1. Mix oil with stock, paprika, garlic powder, sage, rosemary, thyme, marjoram, oregano in a bowl.
2. Then add salt and pepper to taste.
3. Whisk properly before adding pork loin, then toss well and keep it aside for about an hour.
4. Move all of it to **a** pan that fits perfectly into your air fryer and cook at a temperature of 370 °F for 35 minutes.
5. Cut all of it into different plates
6. Serve with couscous as a side dish.

Nutrition:

Calories: 310 Fat: 4 Carbs: 37 Protein: 34

368. Chopped Creamy Pork

⏰ Prep Time 15 m | ⏰ Cooking Time 30 m | 6 Servings

Ingredients:

- 2 lbs. of pork meat (boneless and cubed)
- 2 yellow onions (chopped)
- 2 tablespoon of Dill (chopped)
- Sweet paprika - 2 tablespoon of
- 1 tablespoon of olive oil
- 1 garlic clove (minced)
- 3 cup of chicken stock
- 2 tablespoon of white flour
- 1-1/2 cup of sour cream
- Salt and black pepper to taste

Direction:

1. Mix pork with salt, pepper and oil in **a** pan that fits into your air fryer.
2. Toss well to coat before moving to your air fryer and cook at a temperature of 360 °F, for 7 minutes.
3. Pour some onion, garlic, stock, paprika, flour, sour cream and dill.
4. Toss well to coat and cook at a temperature of 370 °F for another 15 minutes.
5. Divide among different plates and serve immediately.

Nutrition:

Calories: 300 Fat: 4 Carbs: 26 Protein: 34

369. Lamb Roast and Potatoes Mix

⏰ Prep Time 10 m | ⏰ Cooking Time 45 m | 6 Servings

Ingredients:

- 4 lbs. of lamb roast
- 4 bay leaves
- 3 garlic cloves (minced)
- 1 spring rosemary
- 6 Potatoes (halved)
- 1/2 cup of lamb stock
- Salt and black pepper to taste

Direction:

1. Pour potatoes in **a** dish that fits perfectly into your air fryer, add lamb, garlic, rosemary spring, salt, pepper, bay leaves and stock,
2. Toss well to coat; then, introduce to your air fryer and cook at a temperature of 360 °F for 45 minutes.
3. Slice lamb and divide into different plates
4. Serve along with some potatoes and cooking juices.

Nutrition:

Calories: 273 Fat: 4 Carbs: 25 Protein: 29

370. Chinese Steak and Broccoli Mix

⏰ Prep Time 15 m | ⏰ Cooking Time 50 m | 4 Servings

Ingredients:

- 3/4 lb. round steak (cut into strips)
- 1 lb. of broccoli florets
- 1 teaspoon of sugar
- 1/3 cup of Sherry
- 1/3 cup of oyster sauce
- 1 tablespoon of olive oil
- 1 garlic clove (minced)
- 2 teaspoon of sesame oil
- 1 teaspoon of soy sauce

Direction:

1. Mix sesame oil with oyster sauce, soy sauce, sherry and sugar in a bowl.
2. Stir gently, then add beef, toss and keep it aside for about 30 minutes.
3. Move beef to **a** pan that fits right into your air fryer.
4. Follow this by adding broccoli, garlic and oil.
5. Toss all of the mix and cook at a temperature of 380 °F for 12 minutes.
6. Divide into different plates and serve right away.

Nutrition:

Calories: 330 Fat: 12 Carbs: 23 Protein: 23

371. Beef Fillet and Garlic Mayo Mix

⏱ Prep Time 10 m | ⏱ Cooking Time 35 m | 4 Servings

Ingredients:

- 3 lbs. beef fillet
- 1 cup of Mayonnaise
- 1/3 cup of sour cream
- 2 tablespoon of Chives (chopped)
- 2 tablespoon of Mustard
- 2 tablespoon of Mustard
- 1/4 cup of Tarragon (chopped)
- 2 garlic cloves minced
- Salt and black pepper to taste

Direction:

1. Add salt and pepper to the beef; do this to allow it to taste.
2. Place in your air fryer and cook at a temperature of 370 °F for 20 minutes.
3. Move to a clean plate and keep it aside for some minutes.
4. Mix garlic with sour cream, chives, mayo, some salt and pepper in a bowl; then, whisk and keep it aside for a while.
5. Mix mustard with Dijon mustard and tarragon in another bowl, whisk, add beef, toss, return to your air fryer and cook at a temperature of 350 °F, for another 20 minutes.
6. Divide beef into different plates.
7. Spread garlic mayo on the plate as toppings and serve.

Nutrition:
Calories: 400 Fat: 12 Carbs: 27 Protein: 19

372. Seasoned Simple Braised Pork

⏱ Prep Time 15 m | ⏱ Cooking Time 1 h 10 m | 4 Servings

Ingredients:

- 2 lbs. pork loin roast (boneless and cubed)
- 4 tablespoon of Butter (melted)
- 2 cup of chicken stock
- 1/2 lb. red grapes
- 1 Bay leaf
- 1/2 yellow onion (chopped)
- 1/2 cup of dry white wine
- 2 garlic cloves (minced)
- 1 teaspoon of Thyme (chopped)
- 1 thyme sprig
- 2 tablespoon of White flour
- Salt and black pepper to taste

Direction:

1. Add salt and pepper to some pork cubes, then rub with 2 tablespoon of melted butter.
2. Place in your air fryer and cook at a temperature of 370 °F for 8 minutes.
3. Add medium-high heat to a pan that fits your air fryer; the pan should also contain 2 tablespoon of butter.
4. Follow this by adding garlic and onion; stir gently and cook for 2 minutes.
5. Add wine, stock, salt, pepper, thyme, flour and bay leaf.
6. Stir gently, before bringing to a simmer and remove the heat.
7. Add pork cubes and grapes, toss well to coat.
8. Move to your air fryer and cook at a temperature of 360 °F for another 30 minutes.
9. Divide everything into different plates and serve.

Nutrition: Calories: 320 Fat: 4 Carbs: 29 Protein: 38

373. Seasoned Lamb and Lemon Sauce Mix

⏱ Prep Time 10 m | ⏱ Cooking Time 30 m | 4 Servings

Ingredients:

- 2 lamb shanks
- 2 garlic cloves (minced)
- 4 tablespoon of Olive oil
- 1/2 cup of lemon juice
- 1/2 cup of lemon zest
- 1/2 teaspoon of oregano (dried)
- Salt and black pepper to taste

Direction:

1. Sprinkle some salt, pepper on the lamb; then rub with garlic.
2. Place this in your air fryer and cook at 350 °F. Do this for about 30 minutes.
3. Mix lemon juice with lemon zest, some salt and pepper, olive oil and oregano in a clean bowl and whisk properly.
4. Shred the lamb, remove the bone and divide into different plates.
5. Drizzle the lemon dressing all over on each of the plates and serve.

Nutrition: Calories: 260 Fat: 7 Carbs: 15 Protein: 12

374. Seasoned Provencal Pork

⏱ Prep Time 10 m | ⏱ Cooking Time 125 m | 2 Servings

Ingredients:

- 7 ounces pork tenderloin
- 1 red onion sliced
- 1 yellow bell pepper (cut into strips)
- 2 teaspoon of Provencal herbs
- 1/2 tablespoon of Mustard
- 1 tablespoon of olive oil
- 1 green bell pepper (cut into strips)
- Salt and black pepper to taste

Direction:

1. Mix yellow bell pepper with green bell pepper, onion, salt, pepper, Provencal herbs and half of the oil in a baking dish that fits right into your air fryer.
2. Toss well to coat
3. Add salt, pepper, mustard and the rest of the oil to the pork.
4. Then, toss well to ensure it is well coated before adding the veggies.
5. Move all of it into your air fryer,
6. Cook at a temperature of 370 °F for 15 minutes.
7. Divide into different plates and serve.

Nutrition: Calories: 300 Fat: 8 Carbs: 21 Protein: 23

375. Lemony Lamb Leg

⏱ Prep Time 15 m | ⏱ Cooking Time 1 h | 6 Servings

Ingredients:

- 4 lbs. lamb leg
- 2 tablespoon of olive oil
- 2 springs rosemary (chopped)
- 2 tablespoon of lemon juice
- 2 lbs. of baby potatoes
- 1 cup of beef stock
- 2 tablespoon of Parsley (chopped)
- 2 tablespoon of Oregano (chopped)
- 1 tablespoon of lemon rind (grated)
- 3 garlic cloves (minced)
- Salt and black pepper to taste

Directions:

1. Do some little cuts all over the lamb, then insert rosemary springs into the openings?
2. Add salt and pepper as seasoning.
3. Add 1 tablespoon of oil with oregano, parsley, garlic, lemon juice and rind together in a clean bowl.
4. Stir gently; then rub the lamb and mix together.
5. Add medium-high heat to a pan that fits right into your air fryer. The fryer should contain the remaining oil.
6. Then add potatoes; stir gently and cook for 3 minutes.
7. Add lamb and stock; stir gently and move to your air fryer.
8. Cook at 360 °F, for about an hour.
9. Divide all of it into different plates and serve.

Nutrition:

Calories: 264 Fat: 4 Carbs: 27 Protein: 32

376. Lasagna

⏱ Prep Time 15 m | ⏱ Cooking Time 40 m | 4 Servings

Ingredients:

- Meat Filling
- 1/2 cup yellow onion diced
- 1 Tablespoon olive oil
- 1 large clove fresh garlic minced
- 1/2 pound extra lean ground beef 97% lean
- 1/2 pound Italian sausage I used sweet Italian
- 1/4 cup chopped Italian parsley
- Cheese Filling
- 1 cup ricotta cheese I used whole milk
- 1 large egg
- 1/4 teaspoon sea salt
- 1/4 teaspoon black pepper
- 1 Tablespoon Italian parsley
- 1/4 cup Parmesan cheese finely grated
- 1 cup grated mozzarella cheese
- For Assembly
- 5 no-boil lasagna noodles broken into pieces
- 2 1/2 cups pasta sauce
- 1/2 cup grated mozzarella cheese

Directions:

1. Meat Filling, Press the "Sauté" button and wait for the display to say "Hot". Add the oil and the onions. Cook until softened, about 3 minutes, stirring occasionally to keep them from burning.
2. Add the garlic, stir for one minute. Add the ground beef and Italian sausage. Stir and cook until thoroughly cooked.
3. Remove the meat and drain. Place in a large bowl and stir in the Italian parsley. Set aside.
4. Cheese Filling. Mix the ricotta, egg, salt, pepper, and parsley together in a medium sized bowl.
5. Stir in the Parmesan and mozzarella cheese. Set aside.
6. To Assemble
7. Break apart noodles and lay them across the bottom of the pan. Pour 1 cup of sauce over the noodles, spread to cover.
8. Spread 1/2 of the meat filling over the sauce. Spread 1/2 of the cheese filling over the meat.
9. Add a second layer of noodles. Spread 1 cup of sauce over the noodles.
10. Add a second layer of the remaining beef filling, then a second layer of the remaining cheese filling.
11. Add an additional layer of noodles, top with 1/2 cup of sauce, and 1/2 cup of mozzarella cheese.
12. Pour 1 1/2 cups of water into the liner of your pressure cooker and add the steamer rack.
13. Carefully place the lasagna on top of the rack. Secure the lid and check to make sure the knob is in the "Sealing" position.
14. Press the "Manual" button and use the + and – buttons to set the time for 24 minutes on "High Pressure".
15. When the pressure cooker beeps, allow the pressure to release naturally for 15 minutes. Release any remaining pressure by turning the knob to "Venting".
16. Carefully remove the pan from the liner. I used a dish towel, but oven mitts would be thicker.
17. Place the pan on a baking sheet and broil until the cheese is bubbly and golden brown.
18. Remove the pan from the oven and allow it to rest for 10 minutes.
19. Release the lever on the pan and remove the ring. You may need to run a knife along the edge to separate the cheese from the sides of the pan. Carefully slide the lasagna onto a large plate. Slice and serve.

Nutrition:

Calories: 491 Carbohydrates: 26g Protein: 32g Fat: 28g

377. Beef and Broccoli
⏰ Prep Time 15 m | ⏱ Cooking Time 12 m | 4 Servings

Ingredients:

- 1-1/4 pounds boneless beef chuck roast or flank steak sliced thinly across the grain
- 1/8 teaspoon sea salt and 1/4 teaspoon black pepper or to taste
- 1/2 teaspoon sesame oil
- 2 cloves garlic minced
- 1/2 teaspoon fresh minced or grated ginger
- 3-1/2 cups broccoli florets
- For the Sauce
- 1/3 cup low sodium soy sauce use coconut amino for paleo or keto
- 2/3 cup low sodium beef broth
- 2 Tablespoons oyster sauce can also use vegetarian oyster sauce as needed
- 3 Tablespoons brown sugar coconut sugar or 2 drops of Stevia for paleo or low carb as needed
- 1-1/2 teaspoons sesame oil
- 1/4 - 1/2 teaspoon red pepper chili flake or Sriracha optional
- Cornstarch slurry
- 2-1/2 Tablespoons cornstarch plus 3 tablespoons water arrowroot starch for paleo

Directions:

1. Season beef with salt, pepper, and 1/2 teaspoon sesame oil. Add olive oil to the Instant Pot and press the "Sauté" button. Once the Instant Pot is hot, sear the beef for 1-2 minutes until brown (cook in batches as needed) then add garlic and ginger.
2. In a medium bowl, whisk together the beef broth, soy sauce, oyster sauce, brown sugar, 1 1/2 teaspoons sesame oil and chili flakes (if using). Pour over beef.
3. PRESS Cancel, then press "Manual" or "Pressure Cook" on "High". Set to 6 minutes and cover with a lid. Turn the heating valve to "Seal".
4. Meanwhile, place broccoli in a microwave-safe bowl with 1/4 cup water. Microwave 2 – 3 minutes until broccoli is tender.
5. Quick release the pressure of the Instant Pot after the beef is cooked and there is a beeping to tell you it's done.
6. Carefully open the lid and whisk together the cornstarch and water to create a slurry in a small bowl. Stir into the Instant Pot and press "Sauté". Add the broccoli and cook until sauce has thickened and broccoli is hot.
7. Adjust seasonings and sprinkle with sesame seeds, green onions. Serve hot with your favorite sides - rice, noodles, zoodles, cauliflower rice or quinoa.

Nutrition: Calories: 354 Fat: 18g Carbohydrates: 17g Protein: 31g

378. Vegetable Beef Soup
⏰ Prep Time 15 m | ⏱ Cooking Time 63 m | 8 Servings

Ingredients:

- 1 pound diced beef (package will often say stew meat)
- 1/2 teaspoon garlic powder (to season the beef - omit if using leftover pot roast)
- 1/2 medium yellow onion, diced
- 2 celery stalks, diced
- 1 cup diced carrots
- Cooking spray or olive oil
- 4 1/2 cups beef broth/ stock (OR I often used water, plus 1 Tablespoon Better Than Bouillon Beef Base)
- 1/2 teaspoon dried oregano
- Salt and pepper to taste
- 2 cups frozen corn kernels
- 1 cup frozen green beans
- 2 cups diced potatoes
- 1 can diced tomatoes (14.5 ounces)
- 1 bay leaf (remove after cooking is complete)

Directions:

1. Preheat the Instant Pot, and spray the pot with cooking spray (or olive oil, if preferred).
2. Add the meat to the pot with garlic powder; salt and pepper generously, and brown for about 3 to 4 minutes.*
3. Add the onions, celery and carrots, and cook for another 3 to 4 minutes.
4. Turn off the pot, and add all other ingredients.
5. Put on the lid, lock it and set to manual high pressure for 8 minutes. (It will take a while to come to pressure with such a full pot, FYI. Mine took 22 minutes.).
6. After the cooking time is complete, allow the pressure to release naturally (without using the quick release lever). Mine took about 25 minutes, FYI. If your pot is still pressurized at 25 minutes, go ahead and quick release any remaining pressure. Remove bay leaf, and serve.

Nutrition: Calories: 179 Fat: 3g Carbohydrates: 20g Protein: 18g

379. Mexican Beef Stew
⏰ Prep Time 15 m | ⏱ Cooking Time 30 m | 6 Servings

Ingredients:

- 2 tablespoons fat -I used lard but avocado oil, coconut oil, or butter would also work
- 1 large yellow onion diced
- 2 pounds stew meat thawed
- 2 teaspoons salt to taste
- 2 teaspoons cumin
- 1 teaspoon paprika
- 1 teaspoon dried oregano
- 1/2 teaspoon black pepper
- 1/2 teaspoon chipotle powder
- 1 cup bone broth
- 1-15oz. can fire-roasted tomatoes
- 1-6oz.can diced green chilies

Directions:

1. Press the "Sauté" button on the Instant Pot and add the fat to the pot.
2. Once melted, add the diced onion and sauté 2 to 3 minutes.
3. Add the remaining ingredients and stir to mix well.
4. Place the lid on the Instant Pot, and make sure the vent is closed.
5. Press the "Manual" or "Pressure Cook" button and adjust the time to 30 minutes on high pressure.
6. When it beeps, immediately release the pressure. Remove the lid and serve!

Nutrition: Calories: 393 Fat: 24g Carbohydrates: 4.5g Protein: 29g

380. Ground Beef Stew

Prep Time 15 m | Cooking Time 5 m | 6 Servings

Ingredients:

- 1 pound lean ground beef
- 1 sweet onion finely chopped
- 1 teaspoon salt
- 4 Yukon gold or red potatoes peeled and chopped into 1" pieces
- 1 pound bag carrots peeled and diced
- 1 can tomato sauce
- 1 can tomato paste (6 ounces)

- 1 can diced tomatoes
- 3 cups low-sodium beef broth
- 2 teaspoon minced garlic
- 1 teaspoon parsley flakes
- 2 teaspoon Italian seasoning
- 1 teaspoon salt if needed
- 1 cups frozen green peas

Directions:

1. Brown ground beef in the instant pot on the sauté setting.
2. Add the remaining ingredients and stir together.
3. Cover and set the valve to sealing.
4. Set the pressure to 5 minutes.
5. Do a quick release to remove the pressure.
6. Stir to combine and serve.

Nutrition:

Calories: 295 Fat: 5g Carbohydrates: 40g Protein: 26g

381. Pork Mushroom Bake

Prep Time 10 m | Cooking Time 30 m | 4 Servings

Ingredients:

2 tablespoons olive oil
1 onion, chopped
½ lb. (226.8g) Ground pork
4 fresh mushrooms, sliced
2 cups marinara sauce

1 teaspoon butter
4 teaspoons flour
1 cup milk
1 egg, beaten
1 cup cheddar cheese, grated

Directions:

1. Put a wok on moderate heat and add oil to heat.
2. Toss in onion and sauté until soft.
3. Stir in mushrooms and pork, then cook until meat is brown.
4. Add marinara sauce and cook it to a simmer.
5. Spread this mixture in a casserole dish.
6. Prepare the white sauce by melting butter in a saucepan over moderate heat.
7. Stir in flour and whisk well, pour in the milk.
8. Mix well and whisk ¼ cup sauce with egg then return it to the saucepan.
9. Stir cook for 1 minute then pour this sauce over the pork.
10. Drizzle cheese over the pork casserole.
11. Press "power button" of air fry oven and turn the dial to select the "bake" mode.
12. Press the time button and again turn the dial to set the cooking time to 30 minutes.
13. Now push the temp button and rotate the dial to set the temperature at 350 degrees f.
14. Once preheated, place casserole dish in the oven and close its lid.
15. Serve warm.

Nutrition:

Calories 361 Fat 16.3 g Cholesterol 114 mg Sodium 515 mg Carbs 19.3 g Fiber 0.1 g Protein 33.3 g

382. Cider Pork Skewers

Prep Time 10 m | Cooking Time 15 m | 4 Servings

Ingredients:

- 3 garlic cloves, minced
- 4 tablespoon rapeseed oil
- 2 tablespoon cider vinegar

- Large bunch thyme
- 1 ¼ lb. (566.99g) Boneless pork, diced

Directions:

1. Toss pork with all its thyme, oil, vinegar, and garlic.
2. Marinate the thyme pork for 2 hours in a closed container in the refrigerator.
3. Thread the marinated pork on the skewers.
4. Place these skewers in an air fryer basket.
5. Press "power button" of air fry oven and turn the dial to select the "air fry" mode.
6. Press the time button and again turn the dial to set the cooking time to 15 minutes.
7. Now push the temp button and rotate the dial to set the temperature at 350 degrees f.
8. Once preheated, place the air fryer basket in the oven and close its lid.
9. Flip the skewers when cooked halfway through then resume cooking.
10. Serve the skewers with salad.

Nutrition:

Calories 395 Fat 17.5 g Cholesterol 283 mg Sodium 355 mg Carbs 26.4 g Fiber 1.8 g Protein 17.4 g

383. Saucy Pork Mince

Prep Time 10 m | Cooking Time 60 m | 8 Servings

Ingredients:

- 2 tablespoons olive oil
- 1 large onion, diced
- 2 lbs. (907.185g) Ground pork
- 2 teaspoons salt
- 6 cloves garlic, chopped
- 1/2 cup red wine
- 6 cloves garlic, chopped

- 3 teaspoons ground cinnamon
- 2 teaspoons ground cumin
- 2 teaspoons dried oregano
- 1 teaspoon black pepper
- 1 can 28 oz. Crushed tomatoes
- 1 tablespoon tomato passata

Directions:

1. Put a suitable wok over moderate heat and add oil to heat.
2. Toss in onion, salt, and pork meat then stir cook for 12 minutes.
3. Stir in red wine and cook for 2 minutes.

4. Add cinnamon, garlic, oregano, cumin, and pepper, then stir cook for 2 minutes.
5. Add tomato passata and tomatoes and cook for 20 minutes on a simmer.
6. Spread this mixture in a casserole dish.
7. Press "power button" of air fry oven and turn the dial to select the "bake" mode.
8. Press the time button and again turn the dial to set the cooking time to 20 minutes.
9. Now push the temp button and rotate the dial to set the temperature at 350 degrees f.
10. Once preheated, place casserole dish in the oven and close its lid.
11. Serve warm.

Nutrition:
Calories 405 Fat 22.7 g Cholesterol 4 mg Sodium 227 mg Carbs 26.1 g Fiber 1.4 g Protein 45.2 g

384. Mint Pork Kebobs

⏱ Prep Time 10 m | ⏱ Cooking Time 15 m | 4 Servings

Ingredients:
- ½ cup cream
- 1½ tablespoon mint
- 1 teaspoon ground cumin
- oz. Diced pork
- ½ small onion, cubed
- 1 cup cottage cheese, cubed

Directions:
1. Whisk the cream with mint and cumin in a suitable bowl.
2. Toss in pork cubes and mix well to coat. Marinate for 30 minutes.
3. Alternatively, thread the pork, onion and cottage cheese on the skewers.
4. Place these pork skewers in the air fry basket.
5. Press "power button" of air fry oven and turn the dial to select the "air fryer" mode.
6. Press the time button and again turn the dial to set the cooking time to 15 minutes.
7. Now push the temp button and rotate the dial to set the temperature at 370 degrees f.
8. Once preheated, place the air fryer basket in the oven and close its lid.
9. Flip the skewers when cooked halfway through then resume cooking.
10. Serve warm.

Nutrition:
Calories 311 Fat 8.9 g Cholesterol 57 mg Sodium 340 mg Carbs 24.7 g Fiber 1.2 g Protein 15.3 g

385. Pork Squash Bake

⏱ Prep Time 10 m | ⏱ Cooking Time 50 m | 6 Servings

Ingredients:
- ¼ cup olive oil
- 1 yellow squash, peeled and chopped
- 1 onion, diced
- 2 garlic cloves, crushed
- 1 lb. (453.592g) Pork mince
- ½ teaspoon cinnamon
- ¼ teaspoon ground cumin
- 1 teaspoon fresh rosemary
- 2 cups tomato passata
- 2 oz. Butter
- ¼ cup flour
- 2 cups almond milk
- ½ cup tasty cheese, grated
- 1 egg
- Salt and black pepper to taste

Directions:
1. Put a wok on moderate heat and add oil to heat.
2. Stir in squash, then sauté for 5 minutes.
3. Add pork, spices, rosemary, garlic, and onion, then stir cook for 8 minutes.
4. Stir in pasta, and tomato paste and cook on a simmer for 5 minutes.
5. Spread this pork mixture in a casserole dish.
6. Prepare the white sauce in a suitable pot.
7. Add oil to heat, then stir in flour and cook for 1 minute.
8. Pour in milk and stir cook until it thickens.
9. Stir in cheese, egg, salt, and black pepper.
10. Spread this white sauce over the pork pasta mixture.
11. Press "power button" of air fry oven and turn the dial to select the "bake" mode.
12. Press the time button and again turn the dial to set the cooking time to 30 minutes.
13. Now push the temp button and rotate the dial to set the temperature at 350 degrees f.
14. Once preheated, place casserole dish in the oven and close its lid.
15. Serve warm.

Nutrition:
Calories 545 Fat 36.4 g Cholesterol 200 mg Sodium 272 mg Carbs 10.7 g Protein 42.5 g

386. Tahini Pork Kebobs

⏱ Prep Time 10 m | ⏱ Cooking Time 18 m | 6 Servings

Ingredients:
- 2 lbs. (907.185g) Pork steaks
- 2 tablespoon tahini
- Zest and juice of 1 lemon
- 1 tablespoon maple syrup
- Handful thyme leaves, chopped

Directions:
1. Mix pork with tahini paste, lemon juice, zest, maple syrup and thyme.
2. Toss well to coat then marinate for 30 minutes.
3. Alternatively, thread the pork on the skewers.
4. Place these pork skewers in the air fry basket.
5. Press "power button" of air fry oven and turn the dial to select the "air fryer" mode.
6. Press the time button and again turn the dial to set the cooking time to 18 minutes.
7. Now push the temp button and rotate the dial to set the temperature at 360 degrees f.
8. Once preheated, place the air fryer basket in the oven and close its lid.
9. Flip the skewers when cooked halfway through then resume cooking.
10. Serve warm.

Nutrition:
Calories 548 Fat 22.9 g Cholesterol 105 mg Sodium 350 mg Carbs 17.5 g Protein 40.1 g

387. Pork Skewers With Garden Salad
⏱ Prep Time 10 m | ⏱ Cooking Time 20 m | 4 Servings

Ingredients:
- 1 ¼ lb. (566.99g) Boneless pork, diced
- 2 teaspoons balsamic vinegar
- 2 tablespoons olive oil
- 1 garlic clove, crushed
- For the salad
- 4 large tomatoes, chopped
- 1 cucumber, chopped
- 1 handful black olives, chopped
- 9 oz. Pack feta cheese, crumbled
- 1 bunch of parsley, chopped

Directions:
1. Whisk balsamic vinegar with garlic and olive oil in a bowl.
2. Toss in pork cubes and mix well to coat. Marinate for 30 minutes.
3. Alternatively, thread the pork on the skewers.
4. Place these pork skewers in the air fry basket.
5. Press "power button" of air fry oven and turn the dial to select the "air fryer" mode.
6. Press the time button and again turn the dial to set the cooking time to 20 minutes.
7. Now push the temp button and rotate the dial to set the temperature at 360 degrees f.
8. Once preheated, place the air fryer basket in the oven and close its lid.
9. Flip the skewers when cooked halfway through then resume cooking.
10. Meanwhile, whisk all the salad ingredients in a salad bowl.
11. Serve the skewers with prepared salad.

Nutrition:

Calories 289 Fat 50.5 g Cholesterol 58 mg Sodium 463 mg Carbs 9.9 g Fiber 1.5 g Protein 29.3 g

388. Wine Soaked Pork Kebobs
⏱ Prep Time 10 m | ⏱ Cooking Time 20 m | 6 Servings

Ingredients:
- 2 ¼ lbs. (1020.583g) Pork shoulder, diced
- 1/3 cup avocado oil
- ½ cup red wine
- 2 teaspoon dried oregano
- Zest and juice 2 limes
- 2 garlic cloves, crushed

Directions:
1. Whisk avocado oil, red wine, oregano, lime juice, zest, and garlic in a suitable bowl.
2. Toss in pork cubes and mix well to coat. Marinate for 30 minutes.
3. Alternatively, thread the pork, onion, and bread on the skewers.
4. Place these pork skewers in the air fry basket.
5. Press "power button" of air fry oven and turn the dial to select the "air fryer" mode.
6. Press the time button and again turn the dial to set the cooking time to 20 minutes.
7. Now push the temp button and rotate the dial to set the temperature at 370 degrees f.
8. Once preheated, place the air fryer basket in the oven and close its lid.
9. Flip the skewers when cooked halfway through then resume cooking.
10. Serve warm.

Nutrition:

Calories 237 Fat 19.8 g Cholesterol 10 mg Sodium 719 mg Carbs 5.1 g Fiber 0.9 g Protein 37.8 g

389. Pork Sausages
⏱ Prep Time 10 m | ⏱ Cooking Time 16 m | 6 Servings

Ingredients:
- 1 lb. (453.592g) Pork mince
- 2 oz. Feta cheese
- 1 large red onion, chopped
- ¼ cup parsley, chopped
- ¼ cup mint, chopped
- 1 tablespoon olive oil
- Juice 1 lemon

Directions:
1. Whisk pork mince with onion, feta, and everything in a bowl.
2. Make 12 sausages out of this mixture then thread them on the skewers.
3. Place these pork skewers in the air fry basket.
4. Press "power button" of air fry oven and turn the dial to select the "bake" mode.
5. Press the time button and again turn the dial to set the cooking time to 16 minutes.
6. Now push the temp button and rotate the dial to set the temperature at 370 degrees f.
7. Once preheated, place the air fryer basket in the oven and close its lid.
8. Flip the skewers when cooked halfway through then resume cooking.
9. Serve warm.

Nutrition: Calories 452 Fat 4 g Cholesterol 65 mg Sodium 220 mg Carbs 23.1 g Fiber 0.3 g Protein 26g

390. Pest Pork Kebobs
⏱ Prep Time 10 m | ⏱ Cooking Time 20 m | 4 Servings

Ingredients:
- 9 ½ oz. Couscous, boiled
- 2 tablespoon pesto paste
- 2/3 lb. (303.9g) Pork steak, diced
- 2 red peppers, cut into chunks
- 2 red onions, cut into chunks
- 1 tablespoon olive oil

Directions:
1. Toss in pork cubes with pesto and oil, then mix well to coat. Marinate for 30 minutes.
2. Alternatively, thread the pork, onion, and peppers on the skewers.
3. Place these pork skewers in the air fry basket.
4. Press "power button" of air fry oven and turn the dial to select the "air fryer" mode.
5. Press the time button and again turn the dial to set the cooking time to 20 minutes.
6. Now push the temp button and rotate the dial to set the temperature at 370 degrees f.
7. Once preheated, place the air fryer basket in the oven and close its lid.
8. Flip the skewers when cooked halfway through then resume cooking.
9. Serve warm with couscous.

Nutrition: Calories 331 Fat 15.8 g Cholesterol 75 mg Sodium 389 mg Cabs 11.7 g Fiber 0.3g Protein 28.2 g

391. Pork Sausage With Yogurt Dip

⏱ Prep Time 10 m | ⏱ Cooking Time 10 m | 8 Servings

Ingredients:

- 2 tablespoon cumin seed
- 2 tablespoon coriander seed
- 2 tablespoon fennel seed
- 1 tablespoon paprika
- 4 garlic cloves, minced
- ½ teaspoon ground cinnamon
- 1 ½ lb. (680.389g) Lean minced pork

- For the yogurt
- 3 zucchinis, grated
- 2 teaspoon cumin seed, toasted
- 9 0z. Greek yogurt
- Small handful chopped the coriander
- A small handful of chopped mint

Directions:

1. Blend all the spices and seeds with garlic and cinnamon in a blender.
2. Add this spice paste to the minced pork then mix well.
3. Make 8 sausages and thread each on the skewers.
4. Place these pork skewers in the air fry basket.
5. Press "power button" of air fry oven and turn the dial to select the "air fryer" mode.
6. Press the time button and again turn the dial to set the cooking time to 10 minutes.
7. Now push the temp button and rotate the dial to set the temperature at 370 degrees f.
8. Once preheated, place the air fryer basket in the oven and close its lid.
9. Flip the skewers when cooked halfway through then resume cooking.
10. Prepare the yogurt ingredients in a bowl.
11. Serve skewers with the yogurt mixture.

Nutrition:

Calories 341 Fat 20.5 g Cholesterol 42 mg Sodium 688 mg Carbs 20.3 g Protein 49 g

392. Pork With Quinoa Salad

⏱ Prep Time 10 m | ⏱ Cooking Time 12 m | 4 Servings

Ingredients:

- 2/3 lbs. (303.9g) Lean pork shoulder, cubed
- 1 teaspoon ground cumin
- ½ teaspoon cayenne pepper
- 1 teaspoon sweet smoked paprika
- 1 tablespoon olive oil
- 24 cherry tomatoes
- Salad:

- ½ cup quinoa, boiled
- ½ cup frozen pea
- 1 large carrot, grated
- Small pack coriander, chopped
- Small pack mint, chopped
- Juice 1 lemon
- 2 tablespoon olive oil

Directions:

1. Toss pork with oil, paprika, pepper, and cumin in a bowl.
2. Alternatively, thread the pork on the skewers.
3. Place these pork skewers in the air fry basket.
4. Press "power button" of air fry oven and turn the dial to select the "air fryer" mode.
5. Press the time button and again turn the dial to set the cooking time to 10 minutes.
6. Now push the temp button and rotate the dial to set the temperature at 370 degrees f.
7. Once preheated, place the air fryer basket in the oven and close its lid.
8. Flip the skewers when cooked halfway through then resume cooking.
9. Meanwhile, sauté carrots and peas with olive oil in a pan for 2 minutes.
10. Stir in mint, lemon juice, coriander, and cooked quinoa.
11. Serve skewers with the couscous salad.

Nutrition:

Calories 331 Fat 20.1 g Cholesterol 110 mg Sodium 941 mg Carbs 20.1 g Fiber 0.9 g Protein 14.6 g

393. Pork Garlic Skewers

⏱ Prep Time 10 m | ⏱ Cooking Time 20 m | 4 Servings

Ingredients:

- 1 lb. (453.592g) Pork, boned and diced
- 1 lemon, juiced and chopped
- 3 tablespoon olive oil
- 20 garlic cloves, chopped

- 1 handful rosemary, chopped
- 3 green peppers, cubed
- 2 red onions, cut into wedges

Directions:

Toss the pork with the rest of the skewer's ingredients in a bowl.
Thread the pork, peppers, garlic, and onion on the skewers, alternately.
Place these pork skewers in the air fry basket.
Press "power button" of air fry oven and turn the dial to select the "air fryer" mode.
Press the time button and again turn the dial to set the cooking time to 20 minutes.

Now push the temp button and rotate the dial to set the temperature at 370 degrees f.
Once preheated, place the air fryer basket in the oven and close its lid.
Flip the skewers when cooked halfway through then resume cooking.
Serve warm.

Nutrition:

Calories 472 Fat 11.1 g Cholesterol 610 mg Sodium 749 mg Carbs 19.9 g Fiber 0.2 g Protein 13.5 g

394. Zesty Pork Skewers

Prep Time 10 m | Cooking Time 20 m | 4 Servings

Ingredients:

- 2 teaspoons ground cumin
- 2 teaspoons ground coriander
- 1 onion, cut into pieces
- 1/4 teaspoon ground cinnamon
- 1/8 teaspoon ground smoked paprika
- 2 teaspoons orange zest
- 1/2 yellow bell pepper, sliced into squares
- 1/2 teaspoon salt
- 1/2 teaspoon black pepper
- 1 tablespoon lemon juice
- 2 teaspoons olive oil
- 1 1/2 lbs. (680.389g) Pork, cubed

Directions:

1. Toss pork with the rest of the skewer's ingredients in a bowl.
2. Thread the pork and veggies on the skewers alternately.
3. Place these pork skewers in the air fry basket.
4. Press "power button" of air fry oven and turn the dial to select the "air fryer" mode.
5. Press the time button and again turn the dial to set the cooking time to 20 minutes.
6. Now push the temp button and rotate the dial to set the temperature at 370 degrees f.
7. Once preheated, place the air fryer basket in the oven and close its lid.
8. Flip the skewers when cooked halfway through then resume cooking.
9. Serve warm.

Nutrition: Calories 327 Fat 3.5 g Cholesterol 162 mg Sodium 142 mg Carbs 13.6 g Fiber 0.4 g Protein 24.5 g

395. Alepo Pork Kebobs

Prep Time 10 m | Cooking Time 16 m | 6 Servings

Ingredients:

- Pork kabobs
- 1 lb. (453.592g) Ground pork
- 1/2 an onion, finely diced
- 3 garlic cloves, finely minced
- 2 teaspoons cumin
- 2 teaspoons coriander
- 2 teaspoons sumac
- 1 teaspoon aleppo chili flakes
- 1 ½ teaspoons salt
- 2 tablespoons chopped mint

Directions:

1. Toss pork with the rest of the kebob ingredients in a bowl.
2. Make 6 sausages out of this mince and thread them on the skewers.
3. Place these pork skewers in the air fry basket.
4. Press "power button" of air fry oven and turn the dial to select the "air fryer" mode.
5. Press the time button and again turn the dial to set the cooking time to 16 minutes.
6. Now push the temp button and rotate the dial to set the temperature at 370 degrees f.
7. Once preheated, place the air fryer basket in the oven and close its lid.
8. Flip the skewers when cooked halfway through then resume cooking.
9. Serve the skewers with yogurt sauce.

Nutrition: Calories 353 Fat 7.5 g Cholesterol 20 mg Sodium 297 mg Carbs 10.4 g Fiber 0.2 g Protein 13.1 g

396. Zucchini Pork Kebobs

Prep Time 10 m | Cooking Time 20 m | 4 Servings

Ingredients:

- 2 garlic cloves
- 1 teaspoon dried oregano
- Olive oil
- 4 pork steaks, diced
- 2 zucchinis, cubed
- 8 fresh bay leaves
- 2 lime, juiced
- A few sprigs parsley, chopped

Directions:

1. Toss pork with the rest of the skewer's ingredients in a bowl.
2. Thread the pork and veggies on the skewers alternately.
3. Place these pork skewers in the air fry basket.
4. Press "power button" of air fry oven and turn the dial to select the "air fryer" mode.
5. Press the time button and again turn the dial to set the cooking time to 20 minutes.
6. Now push the temp button and rotate the dial to set the temperature at 370 degrees f.
7. Once preheated, place the air fryer basket in the oven and close its lid.
8. Flip the skewers when cooked halfway through then resume cooking.
9. Serve warm.

Nutrition: Calories 248 Fat 13 g Cholesterol 387 mg Sodium 353 mg Carbs 12 g Fiber 0.4 g Protein 29 g

397. Lime Glazed Pork Kebobs

Prep Time 10 m | Cooking Time 20 m | 6 Servings

Ingredients:

- 2 lb. (907.185g) Pork, cubed
- 1/2 cup olive oil
- 1 lime juice
- 3 cloves garlic, minced
- 1 onion, sliced
- 1 teaspoon oregano, dried
- 1/4 teaspoon dried thyme,
- 1 teaspoon salt
- 1/4 teaspoon black pepper
- 1 tablespoon parsley, chopped
- 2 red pepper, cut into square
- 1 onion, cut into chunks

Directions:

1. Toss pork with the rest of the kebab ingredients in a bowl.
2. Cover the pork and marinate it for 30 minutes.
3. Thread the pork and veggies on the skewers alternately.
4. Place these pork skewers in the air fry basket.
5. Press "power button" of air fry oven and turn the dial to select the "air fryer" mode.
6. Press the time button and again turn the dial to set the cooking time to 20 minutes.
7. Now push the temp button and rotate the dial to set the temperature at 370 degrees f.
8. Once preheated, place the air fryer basket in the oven and close its lid.
9. Flip the skewers when cooked halfway through then resume cooking.
10. Serve warm.

Nutrition: Calories 457 Fat 19.1 g Cholesterol 262 mg Sodium 557 mg Carbs 18.9 g Fiber 1.7 g Protein 32.5 g

398. Pork Kebab Tacos

Prep Time 10 m | Cooking Time 20 m | 6 Servings

Ingredients:

- Pork kebabs
- 2 lbs. (907.185g) Pork loin chops, diced
- 1 large onion, squares
- Salt, to taste
- For the wrap

- 6 burrito wraps
- 1/4 cup onions, sliced
- 1/2 cup tomatoes, sliced
- 1 1/2 cups romaine lettuce, chopped

Directions:

1. Toss pork and onion with salt in a bowl to season them.
2. Thread the pork and onion on the skewers alternately.
3. Place these pork skewers in the air fry basket.
4. Press "power button" of air fry oven and turn the dial to select the "air fryer" mode.
5. Press the time button and again turn the dial to set the cooking time to 20 minutes.
6. Now push the temp button and rotate the dial to set the temperature at 370 degrees f.
7. Once preheated, place the air fryer basket in the oven and close its lid.
8. Flip the skewers when cooked halfway through then resume cooking.
9. Place the warm burrito wrap on the serving plates.
10. Divide the tortilla ingredients on the tortillas and top them with pork kebabs.
11. Serve warm.

Nutrition:

Calories 392 Fat 16.1 g Cholesterol 231 mg Sodium 466 mg Carbs 3.9 g Fiber 0.9 g Protein 48 g

399. Rainbow Pork Skewers

Prep Time 10 m | Cooking Time 15 m | 4 Servings

Ingredients:

- 1-lb. (453.592g) Boneless pork steaks, diced
- 1 eggplant, diced
- 1 yellow squash, diced
- 1 zucchini, diced
- 1/2 onion

- 4 slices ginger
- 5 cloves garlic
- 1 teaspoon cinnamon, ground
- 1 teaspoon cayenne
- 1 teaspoon salt

Directions:

1. Blend all the spices, ginger, garlic, and onion in a blender.
2. Toss the pork and veggies with prepared spice mixture then thread them over the skewers.
3. Marinate the spiced skewers for 30 minutes.
4. Place these pork skewers in the air fry basket.
5. Press "power button" of air fry oven and turn the dial to select the "air fryer" mode.
6. Press the time button and again turn the dial to set the cooking time to 15 minutes.
7. Now push the temp button and rotate the dial to set the temperature at 350 degrees f.
8. Once preheated, place the air fryer basket in the oven and close its lid.
9. Flip the skewers when cooked halfway through then resume cooking.
10. Serve warm.

Nutrition:

Calories 321 Fat 7.4 g Cholesterol 105 mg Sodium 353 mg Carbs 19.4 g Fiber 2.7 g Protein 37.2 g

400. Tangy Pork Sausages

Prep Time 10 m | Cooking Time 18 m | 4 Servings

Ingredients:

- ¾ lb. (340.194g) Ground pork
- ¼ cup breadcrumbs
- ½ cup egg, beaten
- 1 teaspoon cumin
- 1 teaspoon paprika
- 1 teaspoon garlic powder

- 1 teaspoon onion powder
- ½ teaspoon cinnamon
- ½ teaspoon turmeric
- ½ teaspoon fennel seeds
- ½ teaspoon coriander seed, ground
- ½ teaspoon salt

Directions:

1. Mix pork mince with all the spices and kebab ingredients in a bowl.
2. Make 4 sausages out of this mixture and thread them on the skewers.
3. Refrigerate the pork skewers for 10 minutes to marinate.
4. Place these pork skewers in the air fry basket.
5. Press "power button" of air fry oven and turn the dial to select the "air fryer" mode.
6. Press the time button and again turn the dial to set the cooking time to 8 minutes.
7. Now push the temp button and rotate the dial to set the temperature at 350 degrees f.
8. Once preheated, place the air fryer basket in the oven and close its lid.
9. Flip the skewers when cooked halfway through then resume cooking.
10. Serve warm.

Nutrition:

Calories 248 Fat 15.7 g Cholesterol 75 mg Sodium 94 mg Carbs 31.4 g Fiber 0.4 g Protein 24.9 g

401. Roasted Pork Shoulder
⏱ Prep Time 10 m | ⏱ Cooking Time 1 h 30 m | 12 Servings

Ingredients:
- 6 lb. (2721.55g) Pork shoulder, boneless
- 8 cups buttermilk
- Spice rub:
- 1 cup olive oil
- Juice of 1 lemon
- 1 teaspoon thyme
- 5 teaspoon minced garlic
- Salt to taste
- Black pepper to taste

Directions:
1. Soak the pork shoulder in the buttermilk in a pot and cover to marinate.
2. Refrigerate the pork leg for 8 hours then remove it from the milk.
3. Place the pork shoulder in a baking tray.
4. Whisk spice rub ingredients in a bowl and brush over the pork liberally.
5. Press "power button" of air fry oven and turn the dial to select the "air roast" mode.
6. Press the time button and again turn the dial to set the cooking time to 1 hr. 30 minutes.
7. Now push the temp button and rotate the dial to set the temperature at 370 degrees f.
8. Once preheated, place the pork baking tray in the oven and close its lid.
9. Serve warm.

Nutrition:
Calories 378 Fat 21 g Cholesterol 150 mg Sodium 146 mg Carbs 7.1 g Fiber 0.4 g Protein 23 g

402. Beef And Broccoli
⏱ Prep Time 10 m | ⏱ Cooking Time 14-18 m | 4 Servings

Ingredients:
- 2 tablespoons cornstarch
- ½ cup low-sodium beef broth
- 1 teaspoon low-sodium soy sauce
- 12 ounces sirloin strip steak, cut into 1-inch cubes
- 2½ cups broccoli florets
- 1 onion, chopped
- 1 cup sliced cremini mushrooms (see Tip)
- 1 tablespoon grated fresh ginger
- Brown rice, cooked (optional)

Directions:
1. In a medium bowl, stir together the cornstarch, beef broth, and soy sauce.
2. Add the beef and toss to coat. Let stand for 5 minutes at room temperature.
3. With a slotted spoon, transfer the beef from the broth mixture into a medium metal bowl. Reserve the broth.
4. Add the broccoli, onion, mushrooms, and ginger to the beef. Place the bowl into the air fryer and cook for 12 to 15 minutes, or until the beef reaches at least 145°F on a meat thermometer and the vegetables are tender.
5. Add the reserved broth and cook for 2 to 3 minutes more, or until the sauce boils.
6. Serve immediately over hot cooked brown rice, if desired.

Nutrition:
Calories: 240 Fat: 6g Protein: 19g Carbohydrates: 11g Sodium: 107mg Fiber: 2g Sugar: 3g

403. Beef And Fruit Stir-Fry
⏱ Prep Time 15 m | ⏱ Cooking Time 5-11 m | 4 Servings

Ingredients:
- 12 ounces sirloin tip steak, thinly sliced
- 1 tablespoon freshly squeezed lime juice
- 1 cup canned mandarin orange segments, drained, juice reserved (see Tip)
- 1 cup canned pineapple chunks, drained, juice reserved (see Tip)
- 1 teaspoon low-sodium soy sauce
- 1 tablespoon cornstarch
- 1 teaspoon olive oil
- 2 scallions, white and green parts, sliced
- Brown rice, cooked (optional)

Directions:
1. In a medium bowl, mix the steak with the lime juice. Set aside.
2. In a small bowl, thoroughly mix 3 tablespoons of reserved mandarin orange juice, 3 tablespoons of reserved pineapple juice, the soy sauce, and cornstarch.
3. Drain the beef and transfer it to a medium metal bowl, reserving the juice. Stir the reserved juice into the mandarin-pineapple juice mixture. Set aside.
4. Add the olive oil and scallions to the steak. Place the metal bowl in the air fryer and cook for 3 to 4 minutes, or until the steak is almost cooked, shaking the basket once during cooking.
5. Stir in the mandarin oranges, pineapple, and juice -mixture. Cook for 3 to 7 minutes more, or until the sauce is bubbling and the beef is tender and reaches at least 145°F on a meat thermometer.
6. Stir and serve over hot cooked brown rice, if desired.

Nutrition:
Calories: 212 Fat: 4g Protein: 19g Carbohydrates: 28g Sodium: 105mg Fiber: 2g Sugar: 22g

404. Simple Beef Sirloin Roast

⏱ Prep Time 10 m | ⏱ Cooking Time 50 m | 8 Servings

Ingredients:
- 2½ pounds sirloin roast
- Salt and ground black pepper, as required

Directions:
1. Rub the roast with salt and black pepper generously.
2. Insert the rotisserie rod through the roast.
3. Insert the rotisserie forks, one on each side of the rod to secure the rod to the chicken.
4. Arrange the drip pan in the bottom of Instant Vortex Plus Air Fryer Oven cooking chamber.
5. Select "Roast" and then adjust the temperature to 350 degrees F.
6. Set the timer for 50 minutes and press the "Start".
7. When the display shows "Add Food" press the red lever down and load the left side of the rod into the Vortex.
8. Now, slide the rod's left side into the groove along the metal bar so it doesn't move.
9. Then, close the door and touch "Rotate".
10. When cooking time is complete, press the red lever to release the rod.
11. Remove from the Vortex and place the roast onto a platter for about 10 minutes before slicing.
12. With a sharp knife, cut the roast into desired sized slices and serve.

Nutrition:
Calories 201 Fat 8.8 g Cholesterol 94 mg Sodium 88 mg Carbs 0 g Fiber 0 g Sugar 0 g Protein 28.9 g

405. Seasoned Beef Roast

⏱ Prep Time 10 m | ⏱ Cooking Time 45 m | 10 Servings

Ingredients:
- 3 pounds beef top roast
- 1 tablespoon olive oil
- 2 tablespoons Montreal steak seasoning

Directions:
1. Coat the roast with oil and then rub with the seasoning generously.
2. With kitchen twines, tie the roast to keep it compact.
3. Arrange the roast onto the cooking tray.
4. Arrange the drip pan in the bottom of Instant Vortex Plus Air Fryer Oven cooking chamber.
5. Select "Air Fry" and then adjust the temperature to 360 degrees F.
6. Set the timer for 45 minutes and press the "Start".
7. When the display shows "Add Food" insert the cooking tray in the center position.
8. When the display shows "Turn Food" do nothing.
9. When cooking time is complete, remove the tray from Vortex and place the roast onto a platter for about 10 minutes before slicing.
10. With a sharp knife, cut the roast into desired sized slices and serve.

Nutrition:
Calories 269 Fat 9.9 g Saturated Fat 3.4 g Cholesterol 122 mg Sodium 538 mg

406. Bacon Wrapped Filet Mignon

⏱ Prep Time 10 m | ⏱ Cooking Time 15 m | 2 Servings

Ingredients:
- 2 bacon slices
- 2 (4-ounce) filet mignon
- Salt and ground black pepper, as required
- Olive oil cooking spray

Directions:
1. Wrap 1 bacon slice around each filet mignon and secure with toothpicks.
2. Season the filets with the salt and black pepper lightly.
3. Arrange the filet mignon onto a coking rack and spray with cooking spray.
4. Arrange the drip pan in the bottom of Instant Vortex Plus Air Fryer Oven cooking chamber.
5. Select "Air Fry" and then adjust the temperature to 375 degrees F.
6. Set the timer for 15 minutes and press the "Start".
7. When the display shows "Add Food" insert the cooking rack in the center position.
8. When the display shows "Turn Food" turn the filets.
9. When cooking time is complete, remove the rack from Vortex and serve hot.

Nutrition:
Calories 360 Fat 19.6 g Cholesterol 108 mg Sodium 737 mg Carbs 0.4 g Fiber 0 g Protein 42.6 g

407. Beef Burgers

⏱ Prep Time 15 m | ⏱ Cooking Time 18 m | 4 Servings

Ingredients:
For Burgers:
- 1-pound ground beef
- ½ cup panko breadcrumbs
- ¼ cup onion, chopped finely
- 3 tablespoons Dijon mustard
- 3 teaspoons low-sodium soy sauce
- 2 teaspoons fresh rosemary, chopped finely
- Salt, to taste

For Topping:
- 2 tablespoons Dijon mustard
- 1 tablespoon brown sugar
- 1 teaspoon soy sauce
- 4 Gruyere cheese slices

Directions:
1. In a large bowl, add all the ingredients and mix until well combined.
2. Make 4 equal-sized patties from the mixture.
3. Arrange the patties onto a cooking tray.
4. Arrange the drip pan in the bottom of Instant Vortex Plus Air Fryer Oven cooking chamber.
5. Select "Air Fry" and then adjust the temperature to 370 degrees F.
6. Set the timer for 15 minutes and press the "Start".
7. When the display shows "Add Food" insert the cooking rack in the center position.
8. When the display shows "Turn Food" turn the burgers.
9. Meanwhile, for sauce: in a small bowl, add the mustard, brown sugar and soy sauce and mix well.
10. When cooking time is complete, remove the tray from Vortex and coat the burgers with the sauce.
11. Top each burger with 1 cheese slice.
12. Return the tray to the cooking chamber and select "Broil".
13. Set the timer for 3 minutes and press the "Start".
14. When cooking time is complete, remove the tray from Vortex and serve hot.

Nutrition:
Calories 402 Fat 18 g Cholesterol 133mg Sodium 651 mg Carbs 6.3 g Fiber 0.8 g Protein 44.4 g

408. Beef Jerky

☉ Prep Time 15 m | ☉ Cooking Time 3 h | 4 Servings

Ingredients:

- 1½ pounds beef round, trimmed
- ½ cup Worcestershire sauce
- ½ cup low-sodium soy sauce
- 2 teaspoons honey
- 1 teaspoon liquid smoke
- 2 teaspoons onion powder
- ½ teaspoon red pepper flakes
- Ground black pepper, as required

Directions:

1. In a zip-top bag, place the beef and freeze for 1-2 hours to firm up.
2. Place the meat onto a cutting board and cut against the grain into 1/8-¼-inch strips.
3. In a large bowl, add the remaining ingredients and mix until well combined.
4. Add the steak slices and coat with the mixture generously.
5. Refrigerate to marinate for about 4-6 hours.
6. Remove the beef slices from bowl and with paper towels, pat dry them.
7. Divide the steak strips onto the cooking trays and arrange in an even layer.
8. Select "Dehydrate" and then adjust the temperature to 160 degrees F.
9. Set the timer for 3 hours and press the "Start".
10. When the display shows "Add Food" insert 1 tray in the top position and another in the center position.
11. After 1½ hours, switch the position of cooking trays.
12. Meanwhile, in a small pan, add the remaining ingredients over medium heat and cook for about 10 minutes, stirring occasionally.
13. When cooking time is complete, remove the trays from Vortex.

Nutrition:

Calories 372 Fat 10.7 g Cholesterol 152 mg Sodium 2000 mg Carbs 12 g Fiber 0.2 g Protein 53.8 g

409. Sweet & Spicy Meatballs

☉ Prep Time 20 m | ☉ Cooking Time 30 m | 8 Servings

Ingredients:

For Meatballs:

- 2 pounds lean ground beef
- 2/3 cup quick-cooking oats
- ½ cup Ritz crackers, crushed
- 1 (5-ounce) can evaporated milk
- 2 large eggs, beaten lightly
- 1 teaspoon honey
- 1 tablespoon dried onion, minced
- 1 teaspoon garlic powder
- 1 teaspoon ground cumin
- Salt and ground black pepper, as required

For Sauce:

- 1/3 cup orange marmalade
- 1/3 cup honey
- 1/3 cup brown sugar
- 2 tablespoons cornstarch
- 2 tablespoons soy sauce
- 1-2 tablespoons hot sauce
- 1 tablespoon Worcestershire sauce

Directions:

1. For meatballs: in a large bowl, add all the ingredients and mix until well combined.
2. Make 1½-inch balls from the mixture.
3. Arrange half of the meatballs onto a cooking tray in a single layer.
4. Arrange the drip pan in the bottom of Instant Vortex Plus Air Fryer Oven cooking chamber.
5. Select "Air Fry" and then adjust the temperature to 380 degrees F.
6. Set the timer for 15 minutes and press the "Start".
7. When the display shows "Add Food" insert the cooking tray in the center position.
8. When the display shows "Turn Food" turn the meatballs.
9. When cooking time is complete, remove the tray from Vortex.
10. Repeat with the remaining meatballs.
11. Meanwhile, for sauce: in a small pan, add all the ingredients over medium heat and cook until thickened, stirring continuously.
12. Serve the meatballs with the topping of sauce.

Nutrition:

Calories 411 Fat 11.1 g Cholesterol 153 mg Sodium 448 mg Carbs 38.8 g Fiber 1 g Protein 38.9 g

410. Spiced Pork Shoulder

☉ Prep Time 15 m | ☉ Cooking Time 55 m | 6 Servings

Ingredients:

- 1 teaspoon ground cumin
- 1 teaspoon cayenne pepper
- 1 teaspoon garlic powder
- Salt and ground black pepper, as required
- 2 pounds skin-on pork shoulder

Directions:

1. In a small bowl, mix together the spices, salt and black pepper.
2. Arrange the pork shoulder onto a cutting board, skin-side down.
3. Season the inner side of pork shoulder with salt and black pepper.
4. With kitchen twines, tie the pork shoulder into a long round cylinder shape.
5. Season the outer side of pork shoulder with spice mixture.
6. Insert the rotisserie rod through the pork shoulder.
7. Insert the rotisserie forks, one on each side of the rod to secure the pork shoulder.
8. Arrange the drip pan in the bottom of Instant Vortex Plus Air Fryer Oven cooking chamber.
9. Select "Roast" and then adjust the temperature to 350 degrees F.
10. Set the timer for 55 minutes and press the "Start".
11. When the display shows "Add Food" press the red lever down and load the left side of the rod into the Vortex.
12. Now, slide the rod's left side into the groove along the metal bar so it doesn't move.
13. Then, close the door and touch "Rotate".
14. When cooking time is complete, press the red lever to release the rod.
15. Remove the pork from Vortex and place onto a platter for about 10 minutes before slicing.
16. With a sharp knife, cut the pork shoulder into desired sized slices and serve.

Nutrition:

Calories 445 Fat 32.5 g Cholesterol 136 mg Sodium 131 mg Carbs 0.7 g Fiber 0.2 g Protein 35.4 g

411. Seasoned Pork Tenderloin

⏱ Prep Time 10 m | ⏱ Cooking Time 45 m | 5 Servings

Ingredients:

- 1½ pounds pork tenderloin
- 2-3 tablespoons BBQ pork seasoning

Directions:

1. Rub the pork with seasoning generously.
2. Insert the rotisserie rod through the pork tenderloin.
3. Insert the rotisserie forks, one on each side of the rod to secure the pork tenderloin.
4. Arrange the drip pan in the bottom of Instant Vortex Plus Air Fryer Oven cooking chamber.
5. Select "Roast" and then adjust the temperature to 360 degrees F.
6. Set the timer for 45 minutes and press the "Start".
7. When the display shows "Add Food" press the red lever down and load the left side of the rod into the Vortex.
8. Now, slide the rod's left side into the groove along the metal bar so it doesn't move.
9. Then, close the door and touch "Rotate".
10. When cooking time is complete, press the red lever to release the rod.
11. Remove the pork from Vortex and place onto a platter for about 10 minutes before slicing.
12. With a sharp knife, cut the roast into desired sized slices and serve.

Nutrition:

Calories 195 Fat 4.8 g Cholesterol 99 mg Sodium 116 mg Carbs 0 g Fiber 0 g Protein 35.6 g

412. Garlicky Pork Tenderloin

⏱ Prep Time 15 m | ⏱ Cooking Time 20 m | 5 Servings

Ingredients:

- 1½ pounds pork tenderloin
- Nonstick cooking spray
- 2 small heads roasted garlic
- Salt and ground black pepper, as required

Directions:

1. Lightly, spray all the sides of pork with cooking spray and then, season with salt and black pepper.
2. Now, rub the pork with roasted garlic.
3. Arrange the roast onto the lightly greased cooking tray.
4. Arrange the drip pan in the bottom of Instant Vortex Plus Air Fryer Oven cooking chamber.
5. Select "Air Fry" and then adjust the temperature to 400 degrees F.
6. Set the timer for 20 minutes and press the "Start".
7. When the display shows "Add Food" insert the cooking tray in the center position.
8. When the display shows "Turn Food" turn the pork.
9. When cooking time is complete, remove the tray from Vortex and place the roast onto a platter for about 10 minutes before slicing.
10. With a sharp knife, cut the roast into desired sized slices and serve.

Nutrition:

Calories 202 Fat 4.8 g Cholesterol 99 mg Sodium 109 mg Carbs 1.7 g Fiber 0.1 g Protein 35.9 g

413. Glazed Pork Tenderloin

⏱ Prep Time 15 m | ⏱ Cooking Time 20 m | 3 Servings

Ingredients:

- 1-pound pork tenderloin
- 2 tablespoons Sriracha
- 2 tablespoons honey
- Salt, as required

Directions:

1. Insert the rotisserie rod through the pork tenderloin.
2. Insert the rotisserie forks, one on each side of the rod to secure the pork tenderloin.
3. In a small bowl, add the Sriracha, honey and salt and mix well.
4. Brush the pork tenderloin with honey mixture evenly.
5. Arrange the drip pan in the bottom of Instant Vortex Plus Air Fryer Oven cooking chamber.
6. Select "Air Fry" and then adjust the temperature to 350 degrees F.
7. Set the timer for 20 minutes and press the "Start".
8. When the display shows "Add Food" press the red lever down and load the left side of the rod into the Vortex.
9. Now, slide the rod's left side into the groove along the metal bar so it doesn't move.
10. Then, close the door and touch "Rotate".
11. When cooking time is complete, press the red lever to release the rod.
12. Remove the pork from Vortex and place onto a platter for about 10 minutes before slicing.
13. With a sharp knife, cut the roast into desired sized slices and serve.

Nutrition:

Calories 269 Fat 5.3 g Cholesterol 110 mg Sodium 207 mg Carbs 13.5 g Sugar 11.6 g Protein 39.7 g

414. Honey Mustard Pork Tenderloin

⏱ Prep Time 15 m | ⏱ Cooking Time 25 m | 3 Servings

Ingredients:

- 1-pound pork tenderloin
- 1 tablespoon garlic, minced
- 2 tablespoons soy sauce
- 2 tablespoons honey
- 1 tablespoon Dijon mustard
- 1 tablespoon grain mustard
- 1 teaspoon Sriracha sauce

Directions:

1. In a large bowl, add all the ingredients except pork and mix well.
2. Add the pork tenderloin and coat with the mixture generously.
3. Refrigerate to marinate for 2-3 hours.
4. Remove the pork tenderloin from bowl, reserving the marinade.
5. Place the pork tenderloin onto the lightly greased cooking tray.
6. Arrange the drip pan in the bottom of Instant Vortex Plus Air Fryer Oven cooking chamber.
7. Select "Air Fry" and then adjust the temperature to 380 degrees F.
8. Set the timer for 25 minutes and press the "Start".
9. When the display shows "Add Food" insert the cooking tray in the center position.
10. When the display shows "Turn Food" turn the pork and oat with the reserved marinade.
11. When cooking time is complete, remove the tray from Vortex and place the pork tenderloin onto a platter for about 10 minutes before slicing.
12. With a sharp knife, cut the pork tenderloin into desired sized slices and serve.

Nutrition:

Calories 277 Fat 5.7 g Cholesterol 110 mg Sodium 782 mg Carbs 14.2 g Sugar 11.8 g Protein 40.7 g

415. Seasoned Pork Chops

⏰ Prep Time 10 m | ⏱ Cooking Time 12 m | 4 Servings

Ingredients:

- 4 (6-ounce) boneless pork chops
- 2 tablespoons pork rub
- 1 tablespoon olive oil

Directions:

1. Coat both sides of the pork chops with the oil and then, rub with the pork rub.
2. Place the pork chops onto the lightly greased cooking tray.
3. Arrange the drip pan in the bottom of Instant Vortex Plus Air Fryer Oven cooking chamber.
4. Select "Air Fry" and then adjust the temperature to 400 degrees F.
5. Set the timer for 12 minutes and press the "Start".
6. When the display shows "Add Food" insert the cooking tray in the center position.
7. When the display shows "Turn Food" turn the pork chops.
8. When cooking time is complete, remove the tray from Vortex and serve hot.

Nutrition:

Calories 285 Fat 9.5 g Cholesterol 124 mg Sodium 262 mg Carbs 1.5 g Sugar 0.8 g Protein 44.5 g

416. Perfect Air Fried Pork Chops

⏰ Prep Time 5 m | ⏱ Cooking Time 17 m | 4 Servings

Ingredients:

- 3 cups bread crumbs
- ½ cup grated Parmesan cheese
- 2 tablespoons vegetable oil
- 2 teaspoons salt
- 2 teaspoons sweet paprika
- ½ teaspoon onion powder
- ¼ teaspoon garlic powder
- 6 (½-inch-thick) bone-in pork chops

Directions:

1. Preparing the Ingredients. Spray the Pro Breeze air fryer basket with olive oil. In a large resealable bag, combine the bread crumbs, Parmesan cheese, oil, salt, paprika, onion powder, and garlic powder. Seal the bag and shake it a few times in order for the spices to blend together. Place the pork chops, one by one, in the bag and shake to coat.
2. Air Frying. Place the pork chops in the greased Pro Breeze air fryer basket in a single layer. Be careful not to overcrowd the basket. Spray the chops generously with olive oil to avoid powdery, uncooked breading.
3. Set the temperature of your Pro Breeze AF to 360°F. Set the timer and roast for 10 minutes.
4. Using tongs, flip the chops. Spray them generously with olive oil.
5. Reset the timer and roast for 7 minutes more.
6. Check that the pork has reached an internal temperature of 145°F. Add cooking time if needed.

Nutrition:

Calories: 513 Fat: 23g Carbohydrate: 22g Fiber: 2g Sugar: 3g Protein: 50g Sodium: 1521mg

417. Rustic Pork Ribs

⏰ Prep Time 5 m | ⏱ Cooking Time 15 m | 4 Servings

Ingredients:

- 1 rack of pork ribs
- 3 tablespoons dry red wine
- 1 tablespoon soy sauce
- 1/2 teaspoon dried thyme
- 1/2 teaspoon onion powder
- 1/2 teaspoon garlic powder
- 1/2 teaspoon ground black pepper
- 1 teaspoon smoke salt
- 1 tablespoon cornstarch
- 1/2 teaspoon olive oil

Directions:

1. Preparing the Ingredients. Begin by preheating your Air fryer to 390 degrees F. Place all ingredients in a mixing bowl and let them marinate at least 1 hour.
2. Air Frying. Cook the marinated ribs approximately 25 minutes at 390 degrees F. Serve hot.

Nutrition:

Calories: 119 kcal Protein: 12.26 g Fat: 5.61 g Carbohydrates: 3.64 g

418. Air Fryer Baby Back Ribs

⏰ Prep Time 5 m | ⏱ Cooking Time 25 m | 4 Servings

Ingredients:

- 1 rack baby back ribs
- 1 tablespoon garlic powder
- 1 teaspoon freshly ground black pepper
- 2 tablespoons salt
- 1 cup barbecue sauce (any type)

Directions:

1. Preparing the Ingredients
2. Dry the ribs with a paper towel.
3. Season the ribs with the garlic powder, pepper, and salt.
4. Place the seasoned ribs into the air fryer.
5. Air Frying.
6. Set the temperature of your Pro Breeze AF to 400°F. Set the timer and grill for 10 minutes.
7. Using tongs, flip the ribs.
8. Reset the timer and grill for another 10 minutes.
9. Once the ribs are cooked, use a pastry brush to brush on the barbecue sauce, then set the timer and grill for a final 3 to 5 minutes.

Nutrition:

Calories: 422 Fat: 27g Carbohydrate: 25g Fiber: 1g Sugar: 17g Protein: 18g Sodium: 4273mg

419. Parmesan Crusted Pork Chops
⏱ Prep Time 10 m | ⏱ Cooking Time 15 m | 8 Servings

Ingredients:

- 3 tbsp. grated parmesan cheese
- 1 C. pork rind crumbs
- 2 beaten eggs
- ¼ tsp. chili powder
- ½ tsp. onion powder
- 1 tsp. smoked paprika
- ¼ tsp. pepper
- ½ tsp. salt
- 4-6 thick boneless pork chops

Directions:

1. Preparing the Ingredients. Ensure your air fryer is preheated to 400 degrees.
2. With pepper and salt, season both sides of pork chops.
3. In a food processor, pulse pork rinds into crumbs. Mix crumbs with other seasonings.
4. Beat eggs and add to another bowl.
5. Dip pork chops into eggs then into pork rind crumb mixture.
6. Air Frying. Spray down air fryer with olive oil and add pork chops to the basket. Set temperature to 400°F, and set time to 15 minutes.

Nutrition:
Calories: 422 Fat: 19g Protein:38g Sugar:2g

420. Crispy Dumplings
⏱ Prep Time 10 m | ⏱ Cooking Time 10 m | 8 Servings

Ingredients:

- .5 lb. Ground pork
- 1 tbsp. Olive oil
- .5 tsp each Black pepper and salt
- Half of 1 pkg. Dumpling wrappers

Directions:

1. Set the Air Fryer temperature setting at 390° Fahrenheit.
2. Mix the fixings together.
3. Prepare each dumpling using two teaspoons of the pork mixture.
4. Seal the edges with a portion of water to make the triangle form.
5. Lightly spritz the Air Fryer basket using a cooking oil spray as needed. Add the dumplings to air-fry for eight minutes.
6. Serve when they're ready.

Nutrition:
Calories:110 kcal Protein: 8.14 g Fat: 8.34 g Carbohydrates: 0.27 g

421. Pork Joint
⏱ Prep Time 10 m | ⏱ Cooking Time 20 m | 10 Servings

Ingredients:

- 3 cups Cooked shredded pork tenderloin or chicken
- cups Fat-free shredded mozzarella
- 10 small Flour tortillas
- Lime juice

Directions:

1. Set the Air Fryer at 380° Fahrenheit.
2. Sprinkle the juice over the pork.
3. Microwave five of the tortillas at a time (putting a damp paper towel over them for 10 seconds). Add three ounces of pork and ¼ of a cup of cheese to each tortilla.
4. Tightly roll the tortillas. Line the tortillas onto a greased foil-lined pan.
5. Spray an even coat of cooking oil spray over the tortillas.
6. Air Fry for 7 to 10 minutes or until the tortillas are a golden color, flipping halfway through.

Nutrition:
Calories:334 kcal Protein: 32.03 g Fat: 6.87 g Carbohydrates: 33.92 g

422. Air Fryer Buffalo Cauliflower
🕐 Prep Time 5 m | 🕐 Cooking Time 13 m | 6 Servings

Ingredients

- 2 medium head Cauliflowers which should be carefully chopped to florets that can be eaten in one scoop
- 4-6 tablespoons of red hot spice/sauce.
- ½ teaspoon of salt
- 2 tablespoon of arrowroot starch. You can also use cornstarch
- 3 teaspoons of maple syrup
- 4 spoons of your favorite avocado oil
- 4 tablespoons of nutritional yeast

Directions

1. First of all, make sure to cook with your Air Fryer at 360F.
2. Then add all your ingredients to a large bowl except the cauliflower.
3. Whisk the ingredients in the bowl until it is thorough.
4. Add the cauliflower and toss it to coat evenly.
5. Proceed to add half of your cauliflower to your new Air Fryer.
6. Cook for about 13 minutes and you can shake halfway through the cooking process.
7. If you have leftovers, then you can reheat in your Air Fryer for about 2 minutes.

Nutrition

Calories 118 | Fat 5 g | Protein 31 g | Sugar 5 g

423. Air Fryer Kale Chips
🕐 Prep Time 5 m | 🕐 Cooking Time 5 m | 2 Servings

Ingredients

- 1½ bunch of kale
- 1½ tbsp. oil
- Salt (to taste, preferably a pinch)
- Seasonings (as flavor): ranch or any of your choice

Directions

1. Wash kale under running water and dry.
2. Cut out the leaves and then, into small pieces into a bowl.
3. Pour oil into them and rub it vigorously into the leaves such that every piece is coated with oil.
4. Add salt, shaking the bowl sideways to make sure they are coated well.
5. Arrange kale into the air fryer basket while preventing overlapping and curling of leaves. Don't forget to cook them in batches if they cannot all fit into the basket at once.
6. Preheat the air fryer to 375°F.
7. Set the timer to 3-5 minutes and cook until they are crispy. So that they cook evenly, ensure you shake the basket at least once during cooking.
8. Serve warm while sprinkling the seasoning minimally as flavor to your kale chips.

Nutrition

Calories 345 | Fat 9 g | Protein 27 g | Sugar 7 g

424. Air Fryer Veg Pizza
🕐 Prep Time 10 m | 🕐 Cooking Time 10 m | 4 Servings

Ingredients

- Pizza
- Pizza sauce
- Olives (or other veg toppings of your choice)
- Cheese
- Basil
- Pepper flakes

Directions

1. If you are just fetching the pizza out of the freezer, you might want to warm it. Set the air fryer to 350°F.
2. Once warm, top the pizza with the pizza sauce.
3. Add cheese to the pizza.
4. Add olives to the pizza.
5. Arrange the pizza carefully on the air fryer rack.

(NOTE: you can also set your dough into the air fryer rack before adding the toppings to prevent spills)
6. Preheat the air fryer to 350°F and spray air fryer rack with oil.
7. Set the timer to 5-7 minutes and cook until the cheese is melted.
8. Once cooked, let the cheese set on pizza by waiting for about 2-3 minutes before cutting.
9. Serve warm while topping it with basil and pepper flakes.

Nutrition

Calories 409 | Fat 18 g | Protein 13 g | Sugar 8 g

425. Air Fryer Low Sodium Baked Apple
🕐 Prep Time 15 m | 🕐 Cooking Time 20 m | 2 Servings

Ingredients

- 2 apples
- Oats (as a topping)
- 3 tsp. melted margarine/butter
- ½ tsp. cinnamon
- ½ tsp. nutmeg powder
- 4 tbsp. raisins
- ½ cup of water

Directions

1. Wash and dry apples.
2. Slice the apples in two and use a spoon or knife to cut out some of the flesh.
3. Add the melted margarine, cinnamon, nutmeg powder, chopped raisins, and oats into a small bowl and mix.
4. Preheat the air fryer to 350°F.
5. Place the apples into the drip pan at the bottom of the air fryer.
6. Put the mixture into the center of the apples using a spoon.
7. Pour water into the pan.
8. Set the timer to 15-20 minutes for it to bake till apples are tender and fillings are crisp and browned.
9. Cover the fillings with foil if they seem to be browning quickly.
10. Serve warm and enjoy.

Nutrition

Calories 134 | Fat 7 g | Protein 41 g | Sugar 10 g

426. Air Fried Mozzarella Stalks

⏱ Prep Time 5 m | ⏱ Cooking Time 10 m | 6 Servings

Ingredients

- 15 mozzarella sticks: cut from a block of cheese
- ½ cup general-purpose flour
- 2 Eggs
- 1½ cups breadcrumbs
- Spices: onion powder, garlic powder, smoked paprika (1 tsp. each) and salt (to taste).
- Sauce: any of your choice but for this book, we'll be using marinara

Directions

1. Make your mozzarella sticks by cutting them straight from cheese blocks (you may have them pre-cut though).
2. Arrange cheese sticks on a plate (parchment-lined for ease) and freeze in a freezer for about 40 minutes to prevent melting when placed into the air fryer.
3. You may seize your flour to remove air bubbles and place inside a covered bowl.
4. Break eggs and whisk well in a bowl.
5. Pour and mix spices and breadcrumb into a bowl.
6. Coat the mozzarella sticks evenly by placing them into the covered bowl or container, cover tightly, and shake. Open the bowl, take out the sticks one at a time, place into the whisked egg, and then into the mixture of the spices and crumbs.
7. Place the coated sticks back on the plate and freeze for about 30 minutes more this time around.
8. Get your air fryer out and clean it (you can do that before the whole cooking process though).
9. Grease the air fryer racks lightly.
10. Preheat the air fryer to 390°F.
11. Take out the mozzarella sticks from the freezer and once more, place into the whisked egg, and then into the mixture of the spices and crumbs. Once you are done, transfer them to the air fryer in batches if they cannot all fit into the rack.
12. Set the timer to 7-10 minutes and cook until you have crispy, golden brown mozzarella sticks.
13. Serve with marinara or any sauce of your choice.

Nutrition

Calories 113 | Fat 11 g | Protein 36 g | Sugar 2 g

427. Air Fryer Vegan Fried Ravioli

⏱ Prep Time 5 m | ⏱ Cooking Time 10 m | 2 Servings

Ingredients

- ¼ cup of Panko bread crumbs
- ½ teaspoons of dried basil
- 1 teaspoon of your favorite nutritional yeast flakes
- Pinch of pepper and small salt to taste
- ¼ cup of aquafaba liquid from the can or you can use other beans
- ½ teaspoon of garlic powder
- ½ teaspoon of dried oregano
- ¼ cup of marinara to dip
- 4 ounces of thawed vegan ravioli

Directions

1. Combine the nutritional yeast flakes, dried oregano, salt, pepper, dried basil, garlic powder, and panko bread crumbs on a plate or a clean surface.
2. Put your aquafaba in a separate bowl.
3. Carefully dip the ravioli in the aquafaba, and shake off the excess liquid.
4. After that, dredge it in the bread crumbs mixture while making sure that your ravioli is well covered.
5. Then, move the ravioli into the air fryer basket.
6. Do these steps for all the ravioli you want to cook.
7. Make sure to space the ravioli well in the air fryer basket to ensure that they can turn brown evenly.
8. Then go on to spritz your ravioli with cooking spray in the air fryer basket.
9. Set your air fryer to 390F.
10. Cook for 7 minutes and carefully turn each ravioli on their sides. Try as much as possible not to shake the baskets as you will waste the bread crumbs. After turning, proceed to cook for 2 more minutes.
11. Your ravioli is ready to eat. Make sure to serve with warm marinara as a dipping.
12. Save your leftovers in the refrigerator and reheat when you are ready to eat.

Nutrition

Calories 321 | Fat 2 g | Protein 15 g | Sugar 4 g

428. Air Fryer Buffalo Cauliflower – Onion Dip

⏱ Prep Time 10 m | ⏱ Cooking Time 12 m | 2 Servings

Ingredients

- ¾ head of cauliflower
- ¾ cup of buffalo sauce
- Seasoning and spice: garlic powder (1½ tsp.) and salt (to taste)
- Creamy dipping sauce: French onion dip (or any sauce of your choice)
- Celery
- 3 tbsp. olive oil

Directions

1. Cut the head of cauliflower into tiny florets into a big bowl.
2. Add and mix the cauliflower with the buffalo sauce and the rest of the ingredients apart from the dip sauce and celery sticks.
3. Grease the air fryer rack lightly.
4. Preheat the air fryer to 375°F.
5. Transfer the well-mixed cauliflower to the air fryer in batches if they cannot all fit into the rack.
6. Set the timer to 10-12 minutes and cook until the cauliflower florets are tender and browned a bit.
7. Serve warm with the celery sticks and dipping sauce of your choice. In my case, french onion dip.

Nutrition

Calories 265 | Fat 6 g | Protein 20 g | Sugar 6 g

429. Vegan Air Fryer Eggplant Parmesan Recipe

⏱ Prep Time 15 m | ⏱ Cooking Time 20 m | 4 Servings

Ingredients
- 2 eggplants
- 1 cup whole wheat bread crumbs
- 1 cup flour
- 1 cup almond milk

- 4 tbsp. vegan parmesan
- Spices: onion powder, pepper, garlic powder, and salt (to taste)
- Sauce: marinara
- Toppings: 1 cup mozzarella shreds

Directions
1. Wash and dry eggplants.
2. Cut into slices.
3. Sieve flour to remove air bubbles into a bowl.
4. Mix whole wheat bread crumbs with vegan parmesan, onion powder, pepper, garlic powder, and salt together into a bowl.
5. Take the slices and dip into flour to be coated, then into the almond milk, and lastly into the mixture of vegan parmesan and spices.
6. Preheat air fryer at 375ºF.
7. Place eggplant slices into the air fryer rack.
8. Set the timer to 15-20 minutes, pressing the "Rotate" so that you can turn the slices halfway through.
9. Once golden brown on both sides, top with marinara and the mozzarella shreds and air fry for about 1-2 minutes to melt.
10. Serve warm and enjoy with pasta or any meal of your choice.

Nutrition
Calories 300 | Fat 6 g | Protein 22 g | Sugar 11 g

430. Vegan Cheese Samosa

⏱ Prep Time 20 m | ⏱ Cooking Time 10 m | 3 Servings

Ingredients
For the Samosa:
- ½ tablespoon of pure olive oil
- ¼ cup of water
- 1 package of Samosa pastry sheet
For the Cheese:
- 1 ½ tablespoon of your favorite nutritional yeast
- ½ teaspoon of sea salt

- 1 ½ cup of water
- ¼ cup of raw cashew. It is best if you preboil for 9 minutes
- 2 ½ tablespoon and Tapioca starch (Don't use any other thickener apart from Tapioca, it would yield undesirable results.)
- ½ teaspoon of apple cider vinegar

Directions
1. Use your blender to blend all the cheese ingredients using the "high" option until the mixture is smooth.
2. Transfer the blended mixture into a saucepan then heat on medium temperature. Use a spatula to continuously stir while it cooks.
3. Your mixture will turn into a big mass of cheese at about 4 minutes and you will usually see the process start by the formation of clumps.
4. Cook for additional seconds to make sure it is well done.
5. Put it in the fridge to ensure that it cools before handling. This will take about 20 minutes.
6. After this, place a Samosa pastry sheet on your cutting board and start adding water slightly using a clean pastry brush. This is to make sure that the edges will stick together.
7. Then, add about 1-2 teaspoons of the cheese mixture to the far right corner. Using the bottom right, carefully fold the pastry over the filling to form a triangular shape.
8. Take the top right point of the triangle and proceed to fold horizontally. You should do the previous two steps till you have a triangular-shaped parcel, with the final flap sealed.
9. Repeat this till all your samosa flaps are used.
10. Brush each Samosa with the pastry brush using the pure olive oil. Do this for each side.
11. Place 4-6 parcels of the Samosa in your Air Fryer basket.
12. Cook at 385F for 7-9 minutes until it is crisp and well done.
13. Freeze the leftovers.

Nutrition
Calories 543 | Fat 34 g | Protein 10 g | Sugar 0 g

431. Delicious Air Fryer Potato Chips

⏱ Prep Time 5 m | ⏱ Cooking Time 15 m | 3 Servings

Ingredients
- Grapeseed oil cooking spray or any other cooking spray of your choice.
- Seasonings of choice.

- Pinch of sea salt according to your taste
- 2 medium-sized Russet potato.

Directions
1. Slice your potato after removing the outer cover. Make sure to slice into thin, cylindrical shapes.
2. Use a paper towel to remove as much water from the thin potato slice. Don't do this too hard.
3. Use a teaspoon to add the seasoning of your choice uniformly to the potato slices.
4. Then, spray your Air Fryer Basket with oil spray.
5. Place the sliced potatoes in a single layer inside the basket, you can do this in batches.
6. Go on to spray the top of the potato batches with grape seed oil spray and sprinkle with your sea salt.
7. Cook in your Air Fryer at 450F until the edges of the potatoes become golden brown.
8. Depending on how thin your potato slices are, this should take about 15 minutes to cook in your Air Fryer.
9. Remove the crispy chips from your Fryer and let it cool down before eating.
10. You can store leftovers in the fridge.

Nutrition
Calories 532 | Fat 21 g | Protein 45 g | Sugar 4 g

432. Healthy Green Beans

⏱ Prep Time 5 m | ⏱ Cooking Time 10 m | 6 Servings

Ingredients
- 2 cups green beans, cut in half
- 2 tbsp. olive oil

- 1 tbsp. shawarma spice
- 1/2 tsp salt

Directions
1. Add beans, olive oil, salt, and shawarma into the bowl and toss well.
2. Place beans into the air fryer basket for 10 minutes at 370 F/ 187 C. Shake air fryer basket halfway through.

Nutrition
Calories 243 | Carbohydrates 14g | Protein 12g | Fat 6g

433. Healthy Brussels Sprouts
⏲ Prep Time 8 m | ⏲ Cooking Time 12 m | 3 Servings

Ingredients
- 8 oz. Brussels sprouts
- 1/2 tsp garlic powder
- 1/2 tsp salt
- 1/4 tsp black pepper
- 1 tsp olive oil

Directions
1. Rinse Brussels sprout into the water and dry with a paper towel.
2. Cut Brussels sprouts bottom stem and cut them in half and place them into the bowl.
3. Toss sprouts with garlic powder, salt, pepper, and olive oil and put them into the air fryer basket.
4. Air fry them until they are slightly brown at 360 F/ 182 C for 12 minutes. Shake the air fryer basket halfway through.
5. Transfer Brussels sprouts to the plate and drizzle with fresh lime juice.
6. Serve and enjoy.

Nutrition
Calories 167 | Carbohydrates 7.8g | Protein 32.1g | Fat 15g

434. Mediterranean Vegetables
⏲ Prep Time 5 m | ⏲ Cooking Time 15 m | 2 Servings

Ingredients
- 1/3 cup cherry tomatoes
- 1 parsnip, peel and diced
- 1 carrot, peel and diced
- 1 courgette, sliced
- 1 green pepper, sliced
- 1 tsp mustard
- 1 tsp mixed herbs
- 2 tbsp. honey
- 6 tbsp. olive oil
- 2 tsp garlic paste
- Pepper
- Salt

Directions
1. Add all vegetables into the air fryer basket. Drizzle with 3 tbsp. oil and toss well.
2. Cook into air fryer for 15 minutes at 356 F/ 180 C.
3. Meanwhile, mix remaining ingredients into the air fryer baking dish.
4. Once vegetables are cooked then transfer them into the baking dish and toss well all.
5. Return vegetables into the air fryer basket and cook for 5 minutes more.
6. Serve and enjoy.

Nutrition
Calories 125 | Carbohydrates 8g | Protein 23.1g | Fat 7g

435. Simple Tomatillo Salsa
⏲ Prep Time 5 m | ⏲ Cooking Time 15 m | 5 Servings

Ingredients
- 12 tomatillos wash and remove the husk
- 2 Serrano peppers, cut the stems
- 1 tbsp. olive oil
- 1 cup cilantro, chopped
- 1 tbsp. garlic, minced
- 1 tsp salt

Directions
1. Place the peppers and tomatillos into a heatproof dish and place them into the air fryer basket.
2. Cook in the oven for 15 minutes at 350 F/ 176 C.
3. Once cooking time is over then transfer tomatillos mixture into a blender and blend until pureed.
4. Pour blended mixture into the bowl. Add olive oil, garlic, and salt and stir well.
5. Serve and enjoy.

Nutrition
Calories 365 | Carbohydrates 11.8g | Protein 43.1g | Fat 10g

436. Roasted Zucchini
⏲ Prep Time 13 m | ⏲ Cooking Time 30 m | 3 Servings

Ingredients
- 16 oz. Zucchini, sliced into 1/4inch rounds
- 1 tsp garlic powder
- 1/2 tsp black pepper
- 2 tbsp. olive oil
- 1 tsp kosher salt

Directions
1. Preheat the air fryer at 400 F/ 204 C for 3 minutes.
2. Toss zucchini with olive oil, garlic powder, pepper, and salt.
3. Place seasoned zucchini into the air fryer basket and cook for 30 minutes. Shake sir fryer basket 2-3 times during cooking.
4. Serve and enjoy.

Nutrition
Calories 251 | Carbohydrates 12g | Protein 16g | Fat 2g

437. Tasty Broccoli Bites
⏲ Prep Time 10 m | ⏲ Cooking Time 5 m | 2 Servings

Ingredients
- 3 cups broccoli florets
- 1 tsp onion powder
- 1 tsp garlic powder
- 1 tsp paprika
- 2 tbsp. Nutritional yeast
- 2 tbsp. olive oil
- Pepper
- Salt

Directions
1. Preheat air fryer at 392 F/ 200 C.
2. Add all ingredients into the mixing bowl and toss well to coat.
3. Add broccoli in the air fryer basket and cook for 4-5 minutes.
4. Serve and enjoy.

Nutrition
Calories 265 | Carbohydrates 19g | Protein 22g | Fat 1g

438. Healthy Apple Chips
⏱ Prep Time 2 m | ⏱ Cooking Time 8 m | 4 Servings

Ingredients
- 1 large apple, slice using the slicer
- 1/4 tsp ground nutmeg
- 1/4 tsp ground cinnamon

Directions:
1. Preheat air fryer at 375 F/ 190 C for 3 minutes.
2. Season apple slices with nutmeg and cinnamon.
3. Place apple slice in the air fryer basket and cook for 7-8 minutes.
4. Serve and enjoy.

Nutrition
Calories 312 | Carbohydrates 20g | Protein 40g | Fat 10g

439. Zucchini Chips
⏱ Prep Time 10 m | ⏱ Cooking Time 16 m | 7 Servings

Ingredients
- 1 tbsp. olive oil
- 1 tsp Cajun seasoning
- 1 large zucchini, slice into 1/8" part

Directions
1. Place zucchini slices into the oven basket and drizzle with olive oil.
2. Sprinkle Cajun seasoning on top of zucchini slices.
3. Air-fry them for 187 C/ 370 F for 8 minutes.
4. Turn zucchini chips to the other side and cook for 8 minutes more.
5. Serve and enjoy.

Nutrition
Calories 165 | Carbohydrates 18g | Protein 31g | Fat 2g

440. Roasted Eggplant
⏱ Prep Time 10 m | ⏱ Cooking Time 20 m | 5 Servings

Ingredients
- 2 medium eggplants remove stems and cut into 1-inch pieces
- 1 tbsp. olive oil
- 1 tbsp. lemon juice
- 1 tsp garlic powder
- 1 tsp onion powder
- Pepper
- Salt

Directions
1. Add all ingredients except lemon juice into the bowl and toss well.
2. Place eggplant mixture into the air fryer basket and cook for 15 at 320 F/ 160 C.
3. Toss well and turn temperature to 350 F/ 180 C for 5 minutes.
4. Transfer cooked eggplant into the bowl and drizzle with lemon juice.
5. Serve and enjoy.

Nutrition
Calories 565 | Carbohydrates 26g | Protein 33g | Fat 6g

441. Kale Chips
⏱ Prep Time 5 m | ⏱ Cooking Time 15 m | 7 Servings

Ingredients
- 3 cups kale, wash and cut into bite-size pieces
- 1 tbsp. zaatar seasoning
- 1 tbsp. olive oil
- 1/2 tsp sea salt

Directions
1. Add all necessary ingredients into the bowl and toss well.
2. Place kale mixture into the air fryer basket and cook for 10-15 minutes at 170 C/ 338 F or until kale chips edges brown.
3. Serve and enjoy.

Nutrition
Calories 261 | Carbohydrates 16.5g | Protein 43.1g | Fat 2.3g

442. Roasted Broccoli
⏱ Prep Time 8 m | ⏱ Cooking Time 8 m | 2 Servings

Ingredients
- 3 cups broccoli florets
- 1 tbsp. olive oil
- 1 tbsp. honey
- 2 tbsp. balsamic vinegar

Directions
1. Preheat the air fryer to 374 F/ 190 C for 3 minutes.
2. Add broccoli florets into the air fryer basket and drizzle with olive oil.
3. Cook broccoli in the air fryer for 8 minutes. Shake basket halfway through.
4. Transfer cooked broccoli into the mixing bowl. Add honey and vinegar and toss well to coat.
5. Serve and enjoy.

Nutrition
Calories 276 | Carbohydrates 31g | Protein 14g | Fat 12g

443. Lemon Garlic Broccoli
⏱ Prep Time 8 m | ⏱ Cooking Time 8 m | 12 Servings

Ingredients
- 3 cups broccoli florets
- 1 tbsp. olive oil
- 2 garlic cloves, chopped
- 2 tbsp. lemon juice
- Pepper
- Salt

Directions
1. Preheat the air fryer to 374 F/190 C for 3 minutes.
2. Add broccoli florets into the air fryer basket and drizzle with olive oil.
3. Cook broccoli in the air fryer for 8 minutes. Shake basket halfway through.
4. Transfer cooked broccoli into the mixing bowl. Add garlic, lemon juice, pepper, and salt and toss well.
5. Serve and enjoy.

Nutrition Calories 298 | Carbohydrates 11g | Protein 40g | Fat 10g

444. Roasted Carrots

🕐 Prep Time 10 m | 🕐 Cooking Time 14 m | 4 Servings

Ingredients
- 6 carrots peeled and sliced into thick chips
- 1 tbsp. oregano
- 2 tbsp. olive oil
- 1 tbsp. fresh parsley, chopped
- Pepper
- Salt

Directions
1. Add carrots into the air fryer basket and drizzle with olive oil.
2. Cook carrots in the air fryer for 12 minutes at 360 F/180 C. Shake baskets halfway through.
3. Add oregano, pepper, and salt and shake basket well and cook for 2 minutes more at 400 F/204 C.
4. Garnish with chopped parsley and serve.

Nutrition
Calories 245 | Carbohydrates 28g | Protein 11g | Fat 19g

445. Mushroom and Feta Frittata

🕐 Prep Time 5 m | 🕐 Cooking Time 30 m | 4 Servings

Ingredients:
- cups button mushrooms
- red onion
- tablespoons olive oil
- tablespoons feta cheese, crumbled
- Pinch of salt
- eggs
- Cooking spray

Directions:
1. Add olive oil to pan and sauté mushrooms over medium heat until tender. Remove from heat and pan so that they can cool. Preheat your air fryer to 330 degree F.
2. Add cracked eggs into a bowl, and whisk them, adding a pinch of salt. Coat an 8-inch heat resistant baking dish with cooking spray. Add the eggs into the baking dish, then onion and mushroom mixture, and then add feta cheese.
3. Place the baking dish into air fryer for 30-minutes and serve warm.

Nutrition:
Calories: 246 kcal | Total Fat: 12.3 g | Carbohydrates: 9.2 g | Protein: 10.3 g

446. Cauliflower pizza crust

🕐 Prep Time 26 m | 🕐 Cooking Time 20 m | 4 Servings

Ingredients:
- 1 (12-oz.) Steamer bag cauliflower
- 1 large egg.
- ½ cup shredded sharp cheddar cheese.
- tbsp. Blanched finely ground almond flour
- 1 tsp. Italian blend seasoning

Directions:
1. Cook cauliflower according to package instructions. Remove from bag and place into cheesecloth or paper towel to remove excess water. Place cauliflower into a large bowl.
2. Cut a piece of parchment to fit your air fryer basket. Press cauliflower into 6-inch round circle. Place into the air fryer basket. Adjust the temperature to 360°F and set the timer for 11 minutes. After 7 minutes, flip the pizza crust
3. Add preferred toppings to pizza. Place back into air fryer basket and cook for an additional 4 minutes or until fully cooked and golden. Serve right away.

Nutrition:
Calories: 230 kcal | Protein: 14.9 g | Fiber: 4.7 g | Fat: 14.2 g | Carbohydrates: 10.0 g

447. Olives and artichokes

🕐 Prep Time 20 m | 🕐 Cooking Time 15 m | 4 Servings

Ingredients:
- oz. canned artichoke hearts, drained
- ½ cup tomato sauce
- cups black olives, pitted
- garlic cloves; minced
- 1 tbsp. Olive oil
- 1 tsp. Garlic powder

Directions:
1. In a pan that fits your air fryer, mix the olives with the artichokes and the other ingredients, toss,
2. put the pan in the fryer and cook at 350°f for 15 minutes Divide the mix between plates and serve.

Nutrition:
Calories: 180 kcal | Fat: 4 g | Fiber: 3 g | Carbohydrates: 5 g | Protein: 6 g

448. Lemon asparagus

🕐 Prep Time 17 m | 🕐 Cooking Time 12 m | 4 Servings

Ingredients:
- 1 lb. Asparagus, trimmed
- garlic cloves; minced
- tbsp. Parmesan, grated
- tbsp. Olive oil
- Juice of 1 lemon
- A pinch of salt and black pepper

Directions:
1. Take a bowl and mix the asparagus with the rest of the ingredients and toss.
2. Put the asparagus in your air fryer's basket and cook at 390°F for 12 minutes. Divide between plates and serve!

Nutrition:
Calories: 175 kcal | Fat: 5 g | Fiber: 2 g | Carbohydrates: 4 g | Protein: 8 g

449. Savory cabbage and tomatoes
⏱ Prep Time 20 m | ⏱ Cooking Time 15 m | 4 Servings

Ingredients:

- Spring onions; chopped.
- 1 savoy cabbage, shredded
- 1 tbsp. Parsley; chopped.
- tbsp. Tomato sauce
- Salt and black pepper to taste.

Directions:

1. In a pan that fits your air fryer, mix the cabbage the rest of the ingredients except the parsley, toss, put the pan in the fryer and cook at 360°f for 15 minutes
2. Divide between plates and serve with parsley sprinkled on top.

Nutrition:

Calories: 163 kcal| Fat: 4 g | Fiber: 3 g | Carbohydrates: 6 g| Protein: 7 g

450. Pecan brownies
⏱ Prep Time 30 m | ⏱ Cooking Time 20 m | 6 Servings

Ingredients:

- ¼ cup chopped pecans
- ¼ cup low carb
- Sugar: -free chocolate chips.
- ¼ cup unsalted butter; softened.
- 1 large egg.
- ½ cup blanched finely ground almond flour.
- ½ cup powdered erythritol
- tbsp. Unsweetened cocoa powder
- ½ tsp. Baking powder.

Directions:

1. Take a large bowl, mix almond flour, erythritol, cocoa powder and baking powder. Stir in butter and egg.
2. Adjust the temperature to 300°F and set the timer for 20 minutes. When fully cooked a toothpick inserted in center will come out clean. Allow 20 minutes to fully cool and firm up.

Nutrition:

Calories: 215 kcal| Protein: 4.2 g | Fiber: 2.8 g | Fat: 18.9 g | Carbohydrates: 21.8 g

451. Cheesy endives
⏱ Prep Time 20 m | ⏱ Cooking Time 15 m | 4 Servings

Ingredients:

- endives, trimmed
- ¼ cup goat cheese, crumbled
- 1 tbsp. Lemon juice
- Tbsp. Chives; chopped.
- tbsp. Olive oil
- 1 tsp. Lemon zest, grated
- A pinch of salt and black pepper

Directions:

1. Take a bowl and mix the endives with the other ingredients except the cheese and chives and toss well.
2. Put the endives in your air fryer's basket and cook at 380°F for 15 minutes
3. Divide the corn between plates.
4. Serve with cheese and chives sprinkled on top.

Nutrition:

Calories: 140 kcal |Fat: 4 g | Fiber: 3 g | Carbohydrates: 5 g| Protein: 7 g

452. Cauliflower steak
⏱ Prep Time 12 m | ⏱ Cooking Time 7 m | 4 Servings

Ingredients:

- 1 medium head cauliflower
- ¼ cup blue cheese crumbles
- ¼ cup hot sauce
- ¼ cup full-fat ranch dressing
- Tbsp. Salted butter; melted.

Directions:

1. Remove cauliflower leaves. Slice the head in ½-inch-thick slices.
2. In a small bowl, mix hot sauce and butter. Brush the mixture over the cauliflower.
3. Place each cauliflower steak into the air fryer, working in batches if necessary. Adjust the temperature to 400°F and set the timer for 7 minutes
4. When cooked, edges will begin turning dark and caramelized. To serve, sprinkle steaks with crumbled blue cheese. Drizzle with ranch dressing.

Nutrition:

Calories: 122 kcal |Protein: 4.9 g | Fiber: 3.0 g| Fat: 8.4 g | Carbohydrates: 7.7 g

453. Parmesan Broccoli and Asparagus

⏰ Prep Time 20 m | ⏰ Cooking Time 15 m | 4 Servings

Ingredients:

- ½ lb. asparagus, trimmed
- 1 broccoli head, florets separated
- Juice of 1 lime

- tbsp. parmesan, grated
- tbsp. olive oil
- Salt and black pepper to taste.

Directions:

1. Take a bowl and mix the asparagus with the broccoli and all the other ingredients except the parmesan, toss, transfer to your air fryer's basket and cook at 400°F for 15 minutes

2. Divide between plates, sprinkle the parmesan on top and serve.

Nutrition:

Calories: 172 kcal | Fat: 5 g | Fiber: 2 g | Carbohydrates: 4 g | Protein: 9 g

454. Air Fryer Crunchy Cauliflower

⏰ Prep Time 20 m | ⏰ Cooking Time 15 m | 5 Servings

Ingredients:

- oz. cauliflower
- 1 tbsp. potato starch

- 1 tsp. olive oil
- Salt & pepper to taste

Directions:

1. Set the air fryer toaster oven to 400°F and preheat it for 3 minutes. Slice cauliflower into equal pieces and if you are using potato starch then toss with the florets into bowl.
2. Add some olive oil and mix to coat.
3. Use olive oil cooking spray for spraying the inside of air fryer toaster oven basket then add cauliflower.

4. Cook for eight minutes then shake the basket and cook for another 5 minutes depending on your desired level of crisp. Sprinkle roasted cauliflower with fresh parsley, kosher salt, and your seasonings or sauce of your choice.

Nutrition:

Calories: 36 kcal | Fat: 1 g | Protein: 1 g | Carbs: 5 g | Fiber: 2 g

455. Air Fryer Veg Buffalo Cauliflower

⏰ Prep Time 20 m | ⏰ Cooking Time 15 m | 3 Servings

Ingredients:

- 1 medium head cauliflower
- tsp. avocado oil
- tbsp. red hot sauce
- tbsp. nutritional yeast

- 1 1/2 tsp. maple syrup
- 1/4 tsp. sea salt
- 1 tbsp. cornstarch or arrowroot starch

Directions:

1. Set your air fryer toaster oven to 360°F. Place all the ingredients to bowl except cauliflower. Mix them to combine.
2. Put the cauliflower and mix to coat equally. Put half of your cauliflower to air fryer and cook for 15 minutes but keep shaking them until your get desired consistency.

3. Do the same for the cauliflower which is left except lower Cooking Time to 10 minutes.
4. Keep the cauliflower tightly sealed in refrigerator for 3-4 days. For heating again add back to air fryer for 1-2 minutes until crispness.

Nutrition:

Calories: 248 kcal | Fat: 20g | Protein: 4g | Carbs: 13g | Fiber: 2g

456. Air Fryer Asparagus

⏰ Prep Time 5 m | ⏰ Cooking Time 13 m | 2 Servings

Ingredients:

- Nutritional yeast
- Olive oil nonstick spray

- One bunch of asparagus

Directions:

1. Wash asparagus and then trim off thick, woody ends.
2. Spray asparagus with olive oil spray and sprinkle with yeast.

3. Add the asparagus to air fryer rack/basket in a singular layer. Set temperature to 360°F and set time to 8 minutes. Select START/STOP to begin.

Nutrition:

Calories: 17 kcal | Total Fat: 8 g | Total Carbs: 2 g | Protein: 9 g

457. Almond Flour Battered and Crisped Onion Rings
⏱ Prep Time 5 m | ⏱ Cooking Time 20 m | 3 Servings

Ingredients:

- ½ cup almond flour
- ¾ cup coconut milk
- 1 big white onion, sliced into rings
- 1 egg, beaten
- 1 tablespoon baking powder
- 1 tablespoon smoked paprika
- Salt and pepper to taste

Directions:

1. Preheat the air fryer Oven for 5 minutes.
2. In a mixing bowl, mix the almond flour, baking powder, smoked paprika, salt and pepper.
3. In another bowl, combine the eggs and coconut milk.
4. Soak the onion slices into the egg mixture.
5. Dredge the onion slices in the almond flour mixture.
6. Pour into the Oven rack/basket. Set temperature to 325°F and set time to 15 minutes. Select START/STOP to begin. Shake the fryer basket for even cooking.

Nutrition:

Calories: 217 kcal |Total Fat: 17 g | Total Carbs: 2 g | Fiber: 6 g | Protein: 5 g

458. Divided Balsamic Mustard Greens
⏱ Prep Time 17 m | ⏱ Cooking Time 15 m | 4 Servings

Ingredients:

- mustard greens - 1 bunch, trimmed
- olive oil - 2 tablespoons
- chicken stock - ½ cup
- tomato puree - 2 tablespoons
- garlic cloves - 3, minced
- Salt and black pepper to taste
- balsamic vinegar - 1 tablespoon

Directions:

1. Mix all of the ingredients in a pan that fits right into your air fryer and toss well.
2. Move the pan to the fryer and cook at a temperature of 260 o F for 12 minutes.
3. Divide all of it into different plates, serve your meal, and enjoy!

Nutrition:

Calories 151| Fat 2| Fiber 4 |Carbs 14 |Protein 4

459. Butter Endives Recipe
⏱ Prep Time 15 m | ⏱ Cooking Time 15 m | 4 Servings

Ingredients:

- Endives - 4, trimmed and halved
- Salt and black pepper to taste
- lime juice - 1 tablespoon
- Butter - 1 tablespoon, melted

Directions:

1. Place the endives in your air fryer, then add the salt and pepper to taste, lemon juice, and butter.
2. Cook at a temperature of 360 o F for 10 minutes.
3. Cut into different plates and serve right away.

Nutrition:

Calories 100 |Fat 3 |Fiber 4 |Carbs 8| Protein 4

460. Endives with Bacon Mix
⏱ Prep Time 15 m | ⏱ Cooking Time 15 m | 4 Servings

Ingredients:

- Endives - 4, trimmed and halved
- Salt and black pepper to taste
- olive oil - 1 tablespoon
- bacon - 2 tablespoons, cooked and crumbled
- nutmeg - ½ teaspoon, ground

Directions:

1. Place the endives in your air fryer's basket, then add the salt and pepper to taste as well as oil and nutmeg; ensure to toss gently.
2. Cook at a temperature of 360 o F for 10 minutes.
3. Cut the endives into different plates, then sprinkle the bacon as toppings, and serve.

Nutrition:

Calories 151| fat 6 | fiber 8| carbs 14 | protein 6

461. Sweet Beets Salad

⏲ Prep Time 20 m | ⏲ Cooking Time 15 m | 4 Servings

Ingredients:

- Beets; peeled and quartered-1 ½-pound
- Brown sugar-2 tbsps.
- Scallions; chopped-2
- Cider vinegar-2 tbsps.
- Orange juice-1/2 cup
- Arugula-2 cups
- Mustard-2 tsps.
- Olive oil- a drizzle
- Orange zest; grated-2 tsps.

Directions:

1. Season the beets with orange juice and oil in a bowl.
2. Spread the beets in the air fryer basket and seal the fryer.
3. Cook the beet for 10 minutes at 3500 F on Air fryer mode.
4. Place these cooked beets in a bowl then toss in orange zest, arugula, and scallions.
5. Whisk mustard, vinegar, and sugar in a different bowl.
6. Add this mixture to the beets and mix well.

Nutrition:

Calories 151 |Fat 2| Fiber 4 |Carbs 14| Protein 4

462. Zucchini Parmesan Chips

⏲ Prep Time 5 m | ⏲ Cooking Time 8 m | 10 Servings

Ingredients:

- ½ tsp. paprika
- ½ C. grated parmesan cheese
- ½ C. Italian breadcrumbs
- 1 lightly beaten egg
- thinly sliced zucchinis

Directions:

1. Use a very sharp knife or mandolin slicer to slice zucchini as thinly as you can. Pat off extra moisture.
2. Beat egg with a pinch of pepper and salt and a bit of water.
3. Combine paprika, cheese, and breadcrumbs in a bowl.
4. Dip slices of zucchini into the egg mixture and then into breadcrumb mixture. Press gently to coat.
5. With olive oil cooking spray, mist coated zucchini slices. Place into your air fryer in a single layer.
6. Cook 8 minutes at 350 degrees.
7. Sprinkle with salt and serve with salsa.

Nutrition:

Calories: 211|Fat: 16g| Protein: 8g |Sugar: 0g

463. Avocado Fries

⏲ Prep Time 5 m | ⏲ Cooking Time 5 m | 6 Servings

Ingredients:

- 1 avocado
- ½ tsp. salt
- ½ C. panko breadcrumbs
- Bean liquid (aquafaba) from a 15-ounce can of white or garbanzo beans

Directions:

1. Peel, pit, and slice up avocado.
2. Toss salt and breadcrumbs together in a bowl. Place aquafaba into another bowl.
3. Dredge slices of avocado first in aquafaba and then in panko, making sure you get an even coating.
4. Place coated avocado slices into a single layer in the air fryer.
5. Cook 5 minutes at 390 degrees, shaking at 5 minutes.
6. Serve with your favorite dipping sauce!

Nutrition:

Calories: 102| Fat: 22g |Protein: 9g | Sugar: 1g

464. Jicama Fries

⏲ Prep Time 10 m | ⏲ Cooking Time 20 m | 8 Servings

Ingredients:

- 1 tbsp. dried thyme
- ¾ C. arrowroot flour
- ½ large Jicama
- eggs

Directions:

1. Sliced jicama into fries.
2. Whisk eggs together and pour over fries. Toss to coat.
3. Mix a pinch of salt, thyme, and arrowroot flour together. Toss egg-coated jicama into dry mixture, tossing to coat well.
4. Spray air fryer basket with olive oil and add fries. Cook 20 minutes on CHIPS setting. Toss halfway into the cooking process.

Nutrition:

Calories: 211 |Fat: 19g|Protein: 9g| Sugar: 1g

465. Air Fryer Brussels Sprouts

⏰ Prep Time 5 m | ⏰ Cooking Time 10 m | 5 Servings

Ingredients:

- ¼ tsp. salt
- 1 tbsp. balsamic vinegar
- 1 tbsp. olive oil
- C. Brussels sprouts

Directions:

1 Cut Brussels sprouts in half lengthwise. Toss with salt, vinegar, and olive oil till coated thoroughly.

2 Add coated sprouts to air fryer, cooking 8-10 minutes at 400 degrees. Shake after 5 minutes of cooking.

3 Brussels sprouts are ready to devour when brown and crisp!

Nutrition:

Calories: 118 |Fat: 9g| Protein: 11g | Sugar: 1g

466. Spaghetti Squash Tots

⏰ Prep Time 5 m | ⏰ Cooking Time 15 m | 8-10 Servings

Ingredients:

- ¼ tsp. pepper
- ½ tsp. salt
- 1 thinly sliced scallion
- 1 spaghetti squash

Directions:

1 Wash and cut the squash in half lengthwise. Scrape out the seeds.

2 With a fork, remove spaghetti meat by strands and throw out skins.

3 In a clean towel, toss in squash and wring out as much moisture as possible. Place in a bowl and with a knife slice through meat a few times to cut up smaller.

4 Add pepper, salt, and scallions to squash and mix well.

5 Create "tot" shapes with your hands and place in air fryer. Spray with olive oil.

6 Cook 15 minutes at 350 degrees until golden and crispy!

Nutrition:

Calories: 231 |Fat: 18g |Protein: 5g| Sugar: 0g

467. Cinnamon Butternut Squash Fries

⏰ Prep Time 10 m | ⏰ Cooking Time 10 m | 2 Servings

Ingredients:

- 1 pinch of salt
- 1 tbsp. powdered unprocessed sugar
- ½ tsp. nutmeg
- tsp. cinnamon
- 1 tbsp. coconut oil
- ounces pre-cut butternut squash fries

Directions:

1 In a plastic bag, pour in all ingredients. Coat fries with other components till coated and sugar is dissolved.

2 Spread coated fries into a single layer in the air fryer. Cook 10 minutes at 390 degrees until crispy.

Nutrition:

Calories: 175| Fat: 8g |Protein: 1g| Sugar: 5g

468. Carrot & Zucchini Muffins

⏰ Prep Time 5 m | ⏰ Cooking Time 14 m | 4 Servings

Ingredients:

- tablespoons butter, melted
- ¼ cup carrots, shredded
- ½ cup zucchini, shredded
- 1 ½ cups almond flour
- 1 tablespoon liquid Stevia
- teaspoons baking powder
- Pinch of salt
- eggs
- 1 tablespoon yogurt
- 1 cup milk

Directions:

1 Preheat your air fryer to 350 degree Fahrenheit.

2 Beat the eggs, yogurt, milk, salt, pepper, baking soda, and Stevia.

3 Whisk in the flour gradually.

4 Add zucchini and carrots.

5 Grease muffin tins with butter and pour muffin batter into tins. Cook for 14-minutes and serve.

Nutrition: Calories: 224 |Total Fats: 12.3g | Carbs: 11.2g | Protein: 14.2g

469. Curried Cauliflower Florets

⏰ Prep Time 5 m | ⏰ Cooking Time 10 m | 4 Servings

Ingredients:

- 1/4 cup sultanas or golden raisins
- ¼ teaspoon salt
- 1 tablespoon curry powder
- 1 head cauliflower, broken into small florets
- ¼ cup pine nuts
- ½ cup olive oil

Directions:

1. In a cup of boiling water, soak your sultanas to plump. Preheat your air fryer to 350 degree Fahrenheit.

2. Add oil and pine nuts to air fryer and toast for a minute or so.

3. In a bowl toss the cauliflower and curry powder as well as salt, then add the mix to air fryer mixing well.

4. Cook for 10-minutes. Drain the sultanas, toss with cauliflower, and serve.

Nutrition: Calories: 275 |Total Fat: 11.3g |Carbs: 8.6g |Protein: 9.5g

470. Crispy Rye Bread Snacks with Guacamole and Anchovies

⏱ Prep Time 10 m | ⏱ Cooking Time 10 m | 4 Servings

Ingredients:

- slices of rye bread
- Guacamole
- Anchovies in oil

Directions:

1. Cut each slice of bread into 3 strips of bread.
2. Place in the basket of the air fryer, without piling up, and we go in batches giving it the touch you want to give it. You can select 3500F, 10 minutes.
3. When you have all the crusty rye bread strips, put a layer of guacamole on top, whether homemade or commercial.
4. In each bread, place 2 anchovies on the guacamole.

Nutrition:

Calories: 180| Fat: 11.6g| Carbo 16g |Protein: 6.2g |Sugar: 0g |Cholesterol: 19.6mg

471. Oat and Chia Porridge

⏱ Prep Time 5 m | ⏱ Cooking Time 5 m | 4 Servings

Ingredients:

- tablespoons peanut butter
- teaspoons liquid Stevia
- 1 tablespoon butter, melted
- cups milk
- cups oats
- 1 cup chia seeds

Directions:

1. Preheat your air fryer to 390 degree Fahrenheit.
2. Whisk the peanut butter, butter, milk and Stevia in a bowl.
3. Stir in the oats and chia seeds.
4. Pour the mixture into an oven-proof bowl and place in the air fryer and cook for 5-minutes.

Nutrition:

Calories: 228 |Total Fats: 11.4g |Carbs: 10.2g |Protein: 14.5g

472. Feta & Mushroom Frittata

⏱ Prep Time 15 m | ⏱ Cooking Time 30 m | 4 Servings

Ingredients:

- 1 red onion, thinly sliced
- cups button mushrooms, thinly sliced
- Salt to taste
- tablespoons feta cheese, crumbled
- medium eggs
- Non-stick cooking spray
- tablespoons olive oil

Directions:

1. Sauté the onion and mushrooms in olive oil over medium heat until the vegetables are tender.
2. Remove the vegetables from pan and drain on a paper towel-lined plate.
3. In a mixing bowl, whisk eggs and salt. Coat all sides of baking dish with cooking spray.
4. Preheat your air fryer to 325 degree Fahrenheit. Pour the beaten eggs into prepared baking dish and scatter the sautéed vegetables and crumble feta on top. Bake in the air fryer for 30-minutes. Allow to cool slightly and serve!

Nutrition:

Calories: 226 |Total Fat: 9.3g |Carbs: 8.7g| Protein: 12.6g

473. Butter Glazed Carrots

⏱ Prep Time 20 m | ⏱ Cooking Time 15 m | 4 Servings

Ingredients:

- Baby carrots-2 cups
- Brown sugar-1 tbsps.
- Butter; melted-1/2 tbsps.
- Salt and black pepper- a pinch

Directions:

1. Take a baking dish suitable to fit in your air fryer.
2. Toss carrots with sugar, butter, salt and black peppers in that baking dish.
3. Place this dish in the air fryer basket and seal the fryer.
4. Cook the carrots for 10 minutes at 3500 F on Air fryer mode.
5. Enjoy.

Nutrition:

Calories 151| Fat 2 |Fiber 4| Carbs 14 |Protein 4

474. Air Fryer Asparagus

⏱ Prep Time 5 m | ⏱ Cooking Time 8 m | 2 Servings

Ingredients:

- Nutritional yeast
- Olive oil non-stick spray
- One bunch of asparagus

Directions:

1. Preparing the Ingredients. Wash asparagus and then trim off thick, woody ends.
2. Spray asparagus with olive oil spray and sprinkle with yeast.
3. Air Frying. In your Instant Crisp Air Fryer, lay asparagus in a singular layer. Set the temperature to 360°F, and set time to 8 minutes.

Nutrition:

Calories: 17 |Carbs: 6g| Fat: 4g |Protein: 9g

475. Crispy Ratatouille

🕐 Prep Time 5 m | 🕐 Cooking Time 9 m (Pressure Level: High, Release: Quick | 4 Servings

Ingredients:

- Kosher salt, for salting and seasoning
- 1 small eggplant, peeled and sliced ½ inch thick
- 1 medium zucchini, sliced ½ inch thick
- 2 tablespoons olive oil
- 1 cup chopped onion
- 3 garlic cloves, minced or pressed
- 1 small green bell pepper, cut into ½-inch chunks (about 1 cup)
- 1 small red bell pepper, cut into ½-inch chunks (about 1 cup)
- 1 rib celery, sliced (about 1 cup)
- 1 (14.5-ounce) can diced tomatoes, undrained
- ¼ cup water
- ½ teaspoon dried oregano
- ¼ teaspoon freshly ground black pepper
- 2 tablespoons minced fresh basil
- ¼ cup pitted green or black olives (optional)

Directions:

1. Preparing the Ingredients. Place a rack on a baking sheet. With kosher salt, very liberally salt one side of the eggplant and zucchini slices, and place them, salted-side down, on the rack. Salt the other side. The slices let it sit for 15 to 20 minutes, or until they start to exude water (you'll see it beading up on the surface of the slices and dripping into the sheet pan). Rinse the slices, and blot them dry. Cut the zucchini slices into quarters and the eggplant slices into eighths.
2. Turn the Instant Crisp Air Fryer to "Sauté", heat the olive oil until it shimmers and flows like water. Add the onion and garlic, and sprinkle with a pinch or two of kosher salt. Cook for about 3 minutes, stirring until the onions just begin to brown.
3. Add the eggplant, zucchini, green bell pepper, red bell pepper, celery, and tomatoes with their juice, water, and oregano.
4. High pressure for 4 minutes. Lock the pressure cooking lid on the Instant Crisp Air Fryer and then cook for 4 minutes. To get 4-minutes cook time, press "Pressure" button and use the Time Adjustment button to adjust the cook time to 4 minutes.
5. Pressure Release. Use the quick-release method.
6. Finish the dish. Unlock and remove the lid. Close the Air Fryer Lid, select BROIL, and set the time to 5 minutes. Select START to begin. Cook until top is browned.
7. Stir in the pepper, basil, and olives (if using). For it taste, adjust the seasoning as needed, and serve.
8. While this vegetable dish is usually served on its own, it's great tossed with cooked pasta or served over polenta.

Nutrition:
Calories: 149 Fat: 8g Carbs: 20g Protein: 4g

476. Avocado Fries

🕐 Prep Time 10 m | 🕐 Cooking Time 7 m | 6 Servings

Ingredients:

- 1 avocado
- ½ teaspoon salt
- ½ cup panko breadcrumbs
- Bean liquid (Aquafina) from a 15-ounce can of white or garbanzo beans

Directions:

1. Preparing the Ingredients. Peel, pit, and slice up avocado.
2. Toss salt and breadcrumbs together in a bowl. Place aquafaba into another bowl.
3. Dredge slices of avocado first in aquafaba and then in panko, making sure you get an even coating. Air Frying. Place coated avocado slices into a single layer in the Instant Crisp Air Fryer. Set temperature to 390°F, and set time to 5 minutes.
4. Serve with your favorite keto dipping sauce.

Nutrition:
Calories: 102 Carbs: 15g Fat: 22g Protein: 9g

477. Warm Quinoa and Potato Salad

🕐 Prep Time 5 m | 🕐 Cooking Time 15 m (Pressure Level: High, Release: Quick | 6 Servings

Ingredients:

- ¼ cup white balsamic vinegar
- 1 tablespoon Dijon mustard
- 1 teaspoon sweet paprika
- ½ teaspoon ground black pepper
- ¼ teaspoon celery seeds
- ¼ teaspoon salt
- ¼ cup olive oil
- 1½ pounds tiny white potatoes, halved
- 1 cup blond (white) quinoa
- 1 medium shallot, minced
- 2 medium celery stalks, thinly sliced
- 1 large dill pickle, diced

Directions:

1. Preparing the Ingredients. Whisk the vinegar, mustard, paprika, pepper, celery seeds, and salt in a large serving bowl until smooth; whisk in the olive oil in a thin, steady stream until the dressing is fairly creamy.
2. Place the potatoes and quinoa in the Instant Crisp Air Fryer; add enough cold tap water so that the ingredients are submerged by 3 inches (some of the quinoa may float).
3. High pressure for 10 minutes. Lock the pressure cooking lid on the Instant Crisp Air Fryer and then cook for 10 minutes. To get 10-minutes cook time, press "Pressure" button and use the Time Adjustment button to adjust the cook time to 10 minutes.
4. Pressure Release. Use the quick-release method to bring the pot's pressure back to normal.
5. Finish the dish. Unlock and open the pot. Close the Air Fryer Lid. Select BROIL, and set the time to 5 minutes. Select START to begin. Cook until top is browned. Drain the contents of the pot into a colander lined with paper towels or into a fine-mesh sieve in the sink. Do not rinse.
6. Transfer the potatoes and quinoa to the large bowl with the dressing. Add the shallot, celery, and pickle; toss gently and set aside for a minute or two to warm up the vegetables.

Nutrition:
Calories: 244 Fat: 12g Protein: 12g Carbs: 10.4g

478. Parmesan Breaded Zucchini Chips
Prep Time 15 m | Cooking Time 20 m | 2 Servings

Ingredients:
- For the zucchini chips:
- 2 medium zucchini
- 2 eggs
- 1/3 Cup bread crumbs
- 1/3 Cup grated Parmesan cheese
- Salt
- Pepper
- Cooking oil

- For the lemon aioli:
- ½ cup mayonnaise
- ½ tablespoon olive oil
- Juice of ½ lemon
- 1 teaspoon minced garlic
- Salt
- Pepper

Directions:
1. Preparing the ingredients in making the zucchini chips:
2. Slice the zucchini into thin chips (about 1/8 inch thick) using a knife or mandoline.
3. In a small bowl, beat the eggs. In another small bowl, combine the bread crumbs, Parmesan cheese, and salt and pepper to taste.
4. Spray the Instant Crisp basket with cooking oil.
5. Put the zucchini slices one at a time in the eggs and then the bread crumb mixture. You can also sprinkle the bread crumbs onto the zucchini slices with a spoon.
6. Place the zucchini chips in the Instant Crisp Air Fryer basket, but do not stack.
7. Air Frying. Lock the air fryer lid. Cook in batches. Spray the chips with cooking oil from a distance (otherwise, the breading may fly off). Cook for 10 minutes.
8. Remove the cooked zucchini chips from the Instant Crisp Air Fryer, then repeat step 5 with the remaining zucchini.
9. To make the lemon aioli:
10. While the zucchini is cooking, combine the mayonnaise, olive oil, lemon juice, and garlic in a small bowl, adding salt and pepper to taste. Mix well until fully combined.
11. Cool the zucchini and serve alongside the aioli.

Nutrition: Calories: 192 Carbs: 15g Fat: 13g Protein: 6g

479. Bell Pepper-Corn Wrapped in Tortilla
Prep Time 5 m | Cooking Time 15 m | 4 Servings

Ingredients:
- 1 small red bell pepper, chopped
- 1 small yellow onion, diced
- 1 tablespoon water
- 2 cobs grilled corn kernels

- 4 large tortillas
- 4 pieces commercial vegan nuggets, chopped
- Mixed greens for garnish

Directions:
1. Preparing the Ingredients. Preheat the Instant Crisp Air Fryer to 400°F.
2. In a skillet heated over medium heat, water sauté the vegan nuggets together with the onions, bell peppers, and corn kernels. Set aside.
3. Place filling inside the corn tortillas.
4. Air Frying. Lock the air fryer lid. Fold the tortillas and place inside the Instant Crisp Air Fryer and cook for 15 minutes until the tortilla wraps are crispy.
5. Serve with mix greens on top.

Nutrition: Calories: 548 Carbs: 35g Fat: 20.7g Protein: 46g

480. Spicy Sweet Potato Fries
Prep Time 5 m | Cooking Time 37 m | 4 Servings

Ingredients:
- 2 tablespoons sweet potato fry seasoning mix
- 2 tablespoons olive oil
- 2 sweet potatoes
- Seasoning Mix:
- 2 tablespoons salt

- 1 tablespoons cayenne pepper
- 1 tablespoon dried oregano
- 1 tablespoon fennel
- 2 tablespoons coriander

Directions:
1. Preparing the Ingredients. Slice both ends off sweet potatoes and peel. Slice lengthwise in half and again crosswise to make four pieces from each potato.
2. Slice each potato piece into 2-3 slices, then slice into fries.
3. Grind together all of seasoning mix ingredients and mix in the salt.
4. Ensure the Instant Crisp Air Fryer is preheated to 350 degrees.
5. Toss potato pieces in olive oil, sprinkling with seasoning mix and tossing well to coat thoroughly.
6. Air Frying. Add fries to Instant Crisp Air Fryer basket. Lock the air fryer lid. Set temperature to 350°F, and set time to 27 minutes. Select START to begin.
7. Take out the basket and turn fries. Turn off Instant Crisp Air Fryer and let cook 10-12 minutes till fries are golden.

Nutrition: Calories: 89 Carbs: 25g Fat: 14g Protein: 8gs

481. Air Fried Carrots, Yellow Squash & Zucchini
Prep Time 5 m | Cooking Time 35 m | 4 Servings

Ingredients:
- 1 tbsp. chopped tarragon leaves
- ½ teaspoon white pepper
- 1 teaspoon salt
- 1 pound yellow squash

- 1 pound zucchini
- 6 teaspoon olive oil
- ½ pound carrots

Directions:
1. Preparing the Ingredients. Stem and root the end of squash and zucchini and cut in ¾-inch half-moons. Peel and cut carrots into 1-inch cubes
2. Mixed carrot cubes with 2 teaspoons of olive oil, tossing to combine.
3. Air Frying. Pour into the Instant Crisp Air Fryer basket. Lock the air fryer lid. Set temperature to 400°F, and set time to 5 minutes.
4. As carrots cook, drizzle remaining olive oil over squash and zucchini pieces, then season with pepper and salt. Toss well to coat.
5. Add squash and zucchini when the timer for carrots goes off. Cook 30 minutes, making sure to toss 2-3 times during the cooking process.
6. Once done, take out veggies and toss with tarragon. Serve up warm!

Nutrition: Calories: 122 Fat: 9g Protein: 6g Carbs: 15g

482. Cheesy Cauliflower Fritters

⏲ Prep Time 10 m | ⏲ Cooking Time 7 m | 4 Servings

Ingredients:

- ½ cup chopped parsley
- 1 cup Italian breadcrumbs
- 1/3 cup shredded mozzarella cheese
- 1/3 cup shredded sharp cheddar cheese
- 1 egg
- 2 minced garlic cloves
- 3 chopped scallions
- 1 head of cauliflower

Directions:

1. Preparing the Ingredients. Cut cauliflower up into florets. Wash well and pat dry. Place into a food processor and pulse 20-30 seconds till it looks like rice.
2. Place cauliflower rice in a bowl and mix with pepper, salt, egg, cheeses, breadcrumbs, garlic, and scallions.
3. With hands, form 15 patties of the mixture. Add more breadcrumbs if needed.
4. Air Frying. With olive oil, spritz patties, and place into your Instant Crisp Air Fryer in a single layer. Lock the air fryer lid. Set temperature to 390°F, and set time to 7 minutes, flipping after 7 minutes.

Nutrition:

Calories: 209 Fat: 17g Protein: 6g Carbs: 25g

483. Buttered Carrot-Zucchini with Mayo

⏲ Prep Time 10 m | ⏲ Cooking Time 25 m | 4 Servings

Ingredients:

- 1 tablespoon grated onion
- 2 tablespoons butter, melted
- 1/2-pound carrots, sliced
- 1-1/2 zucchinis, sliced
- 1/4 cup water
- 1/4 cup mayonnaise
- 1/4 teaspoon prepared horseradish
- 1/4 teaspoon salt
- 1/4 teaspoon ground black pepper
- 1/4 cup Italian bread crumbs

Directions:

1. Preparing the Ingredients. Lightly grease baking pan of Instant Crisp Air Fryer with cooking spray. Add carrots. For 8 minutes, cook on 360°F. Put zucchini and continue cooking for another 5 minutes.
2. Meanwhile, in a bowl whisk well pepper, salt, horseradish, onion, mayonnaise, and water. Pour into pan of veggies. Toss well to coat.
3. In a small bowl mix melted butter and bread crumbs. Sprinkle over veggies.
4. Air Frying. Lock the air fryer lid. Cook for 10 minutes at 390°F, until tops are lightly browned.
5. Serve and enjoy.

Nutrition:

Calories: 223 Fat: 17g Protein: 2.7g Carbs: 25

484. Cheddar, Squash, and Zucchini Casserole

⏲ Prep Time 5 m | ⏲ Cooking Time 30 m | 4 Servings

Ingredients:

- 1 egg
- 5 saltine crackers, or as needed, crushed
- 2 tablespoons bread crumbs
- 1/2-pound yellow squash, sliced
- 1/2-pound zucchini, sliced
- 1/2 cup shredded Cheddar cheese
- 1-1/2 teaspoons white sugar
- 1/2 teaspoon salt
- 1/4 onion, diced
- 1/4 cup biscuit baking mix
- 1/4 cup butter

Directions:

1. Preparing the Ingredients. Lightly grease baking pan of Instant Crisp Air Fryer with cooking spray. Add onion, zucchini, and yellow squash. Cover pan with foil and for 15 minutes, cook on 360° F or until tender.
2. Stir in salt, sugar, egg, butter, baking mix, and cheddar cheese. Mix well. Fold in crushed crackers. Top with bread crumbs.
3. Air Frying Lock the air fryer lid. Cook for 15 minutes at 390° F until tops are lightly browned.
4. Serve and enjoy.

Nutrition:

Calories: 285 Fat: 20.5g Protein: 8.6g Carbs: 35g

485. Crispy Roasted Broccoli

⏲ Prep Time 10 m | ⏲ Cooking Time 8 m | 2 Servings

Ingredients:

- ¼ teaspoon Masala
- ½ teaspoon red chili powder
- ½ teaspoon salt
- ¼ teaspoon turmeric powder
- 1 tablespoon chickpea flour
- 2 tablespoons yogurt
- 1 pound broccoli

Directions:

1. Preparing the Ingredients. Cut broccoli up into small. Wash in a bowl of water with 2 teaspoons of salt for at least half an hour to remove impurities.
2. Take out broccoli florets from water and let drain. Wipe down thoroughly.
3. Mix all other ingredients together to create a marinade.
4. Toss broccoli florets in the marinade. Cover and chill 15-30 minutes.
5. Air Frying. Preheat the Instant Crisp Air Fryer to 390 degrees. Place marinated broccoli florets into the fryer, lock the air fryer lid, set temperature to 350°F, and set time to 10 minutes. Florets will be crispy when done.

Nutrition:

Calories: 96 Fat: 1.3g Protein: 7g Carbs: 25g

486. Zucchini Parmesan Chips
⏱ Prep Time 10 m | ⏱ Cooking Time 8 m | 6 Servings

Ingredients:
- ½ teaspoon paprika
- ½ cup grated parmesan cheese
- ½ cup Italian breadcrumbs
- 1 lightly beaten egg
- 2 thinly sliced zucchinis

Directions:
1. Preparing the Ingredients. Use a very sharp knife or mandolin slicer to slice zucchini as thinly as you can. Pat off extra moisture.
2. Beat egg with a pinch of pepper and salt and a bit of water.
3. Combine paprika, cheese, and breadcrumbs in a bowl.
4. Dip slices of zucchini into the egg mixture and then into breadcrumb mixture. Press gently to coat.
5. Air Frying. With olive oil cooking spray, mist coated zucchini slices. Place into your Instant Crisp Air Fryer in a single layer. Lock the air fryer lid. Set temperature to 350°F, and set time to 8 minutes.
6. Sprinkle with salt and serve with salsa.

Nutrition:
Calories: 211 Fat: 16g Protein: 8g Carbs: 15g

487. Jalapeño Cheese Balls
⏱ Prep Time 10 m | ⏱ Cooking Time 8 m | 6 Servings

Ingredients:
- 4 ounces cream cheese
- 1/3 Cup shredded mozzarella cheese
- 1/3 Cup shredded Cheddar cheese
- 2 jalapeños, finely chopped
- ½ cup bread crumbs
- 2 eggs
- ½ cup all-purpose flour
- Salt
- Pepper
- Cooking oil

Directions:
1. Preparing the Ingredients. In a small mixing bowl, mixed the cream cheese, mozzarella, Cheddar, and jalapeños. Mix well.
2. Form the cheese mixture into balls about an inch thick. Using a small ice cream scoop works well.
3. Arrange the cheese balls on a sheet pan and place in the freezer for 15 minutes. This will help the cheese balls maintain their shape while frying.
4. Spray the Instant Crisp Air Fryer basket with cooking oil. Put the bread crumbs in a small bowl. In another small bowl, beat the eggs. In a third small bowl, combine the flour with salt and pepper to taste, and mix well. Remove the cheese balls from the freezer. Put the cheese balls in the flour, then the eggs, and then the bread crumbs.
5. Air Frying. Place the cheese balls in the Instant Crisp Air Fryer. Spray with cooking oil. Lock the air fryer lid. Cook for 8 minutes.
6. Open the Instant Crisp Air Fryer and flip the cheese balls. I recommend flipping them instead of shaking so the balls maintain their form. Cook an additional 4 minutes. Cool before serving.

Nutrition:
Calories: 96 Fat: 6g Protein: 4g Carbs: 15g

488. Crispy Jalapeno Coins
⏱ Prep Time 10 m | ⏱ Cooking Time 5 m | 2 Servings

Ingredients:
- 1 egg
- 2-3 tablespoons coconut flour
- 1 sliced and seeded jalapeno
- Pinch of garlic powder
- Pinch of onion powder
- Pinch of Cajun seasoning (optional)
- Pinch of pepper and salt

Directions:
1. Preparing the Ingredients. Ensure your Instant Crisp Air Fryer is preheated to 400 degrees.
2. Mix together all dry ingredients.
3. Pat jalapeno slices dry. Dip coins into egg wash and then into dry mixture. Toss to thoroughly coat.
4. Add coated jalapeno slices to Instant Crisp Air Fryer in a singular layer. Spray with olive oil.
5. Air Frying. Lock the air fryer lid. Set temperature to 350°F, and set time to 5 minutes. Cook just till crispy.

Nutrition:
Calories: 128 Fat: 8g Protein: 7g Carbs: 15g

489. Steamed Vegetables
⏱ Prep Time 10 m | ⏱ Cooking Time 15 m | 4 Servings

Ingredients
- 3/4 cup water
- 1 head broccoli, chopped
- 1 head cauliflower, chopped
- 2 carrots, chopped
- 1 red pepper, chopped
- 1 yellow pepper, chopped

Directions:
1. Add the 3/4 cup of water to the bottom of the Instant Pot and then place the trivet inside the inner pot. Add veggies, then place the lid on Instant Pot and make sure the valve is set to seal.
2. Press the pressure cook button and set to high, then cook for 0 minutes. Yes, zero minutes is all that's needed to steam! The Instant Pot will take about 5-10 minutes to come to pressure, then notify you it's done by beeping.
3. Press the Cancel button then do a quick release of the pressure on the Instant Pot by flicking the switch at the top with a spoon. Open the lid when the pressure gauge has dropped and the lid opens easily. Season veggies if desired then serve and enjoy!

Nutrition:
Calories: 117 Carbohydrates: 23g Protein: 7g Fat: 1g

490. Mashed Potatoes

Ingredients:

- 5 pounds of potatoes, peeled and halved (see Recipe Notes)
- 4 teaspoons salt, divided
- 2 sticks butter (1 cup)
- 2–4 cloves garlic
- A few sprigs of herbs (sage, thyme, etc.)
- 1 cup cream cheese or sour cream
- 1/4 cup grated Parmesan cheese (optional)
- 1/2 cup broth or milk (optional, for texture)

Directions:

1. Potatoes: Put your potatoes in the Instant Pot and cover with about 6 cups of water – enough to be completely covered. Add 2 teaspoons of salt. Cook on the steam setting for 12 minutes. Release steam right away. Drain the potatoes. They should be fork tender.
2. Garlic Herb Butter: Melt your butter in a large skillet. Add the garlic and herbs and let it just gently cook and infuse the butter with flavor for 10-15 minutes. Pull the herbs and garlic out, and reserve your flavored butter. YUM.
3. Mash and Mix: Using a potato masher or the back of a wooden spoon, mash the potatoes right in the Instant Pot. Add the garlic herb butter, sour cream, Parmesan cheese, and the rest of the salt. Stir to combine. Season with more salt to taste – be generous! Voila. Delicious mashed potatoes are yours!

Nutrition:
Calories: 590 Fat: 40.1g Carbohydrate: 53.4g Protein: 8.2g

491. Mac and Cheese

Ingredients:

- 16 Ounces Uncooked Elbow Macaroni
- 4 Cups Chicken Broth
- 2 Tablespoons Butter
- 1 Teaspoon Hot Pepper Sauce
- 1 Teaspoon Garlic Powder
- 1/2 Teaspoon Pepper
- 1/2 Teaspoon Salt
- 2 Cups Shredded Cheddar Cheese
- 1 Cup Shredded Mozzarella Cheese
- 1/2 Cup Shredded Parmesan Cheese
- 1/2 -1 Cup Milk

Directions:

1. Add the uncooked macaroni, chicken broth, butter, hot sauce, garlic powder, pepper, and salt to the Instant Pot.
2. Place the lid on the pot and set to sealing. Cook on manual function, high pressure for 5 minutes. Then, do a quick release.
3. Add the milk, then the cheese to the pot in 3-4 handfuls, stirring in between each addition until smooth and creamy. Season as necessary to taste.

Nutrition:
Calories: 206 Carbohydrates: 1g Protein: 12g Fat: 16g

492. Portobello Pot Roast

Ingredients:

- 2 tablespoons olive oil, divided (optional - you can sauté in water instead to make the recipe oil free)
- 5 large Portobello mushrooms, sliced into chunky pieces
- 1 large onion, chopped finely
- 3 cloves garlic, chopped finely
- 5 large potatoes, peeled and cut into large chunks (I cut each potato into about 5 pieces).
- 4 large carrots, peeled and cut into 1 inch chunks
- 1½ cups red wine
- ¼ cup soy sauce or Tamari (or gluten-free tamari/soy sauce, or coconut amino).
- 2 cups good quality vegetable or mushroom broth
- 1 teaspoon salt, plus more to taste
- ½ teaspoon black pepper, plus more to taste
- 1 tablespoon sugar
- 4 tablespoons of all-purpose flour, or arrowroot powder, corn starch or gluten free flour. Use the same amount.
- Water, to make a slurry
- 2 springs of fresh thyme
- 1 large sprig fresh rosemary
- 3 to 4 fresh sage leaves

Directions:

1. Set the Instant Pot to sauté and add 1 tablespoon of the olive oil (or use a few tablespoons of water instead if you prefer cooking oil free). Add the mushroom slices and cook until they have a good golden color all over. Then remove to a plate or a bowl and set aside.
2. Add the remaining oil (or more water), and sauté the onions until golden. It's important to get a good color on them because that's what adds lots of flavor. Once golden, turn off the Instant Pot and immediately add the garlic, stirring it in and letting it cook in the residual heat.
3. Add the potatoes, carrots, wine, soy sauce, broth, sugar and seasonings then give it all a good stir. Really scrape into the bottom to get the brown mushroom residue off and into the gravy for extra flavor.
4. Place the fresh herbs on top, place the lid on the Instant Pot and seal it, then set it to Manual (Pressure Cook on newer models), High Pressure for 15 minutes.
5. Once it's done, leave the pressure to release naturally. While waiting, make a slurry with the flour. Add water to it gradually to make a lump free paste then add a little more, stirring constantly until it's pourable like cream.
6. Once the pressure has released turn off the Instant Pot, remove the lid, scoop out the herbs and discard. Turn the Instant Pot to "Sauté" and pour in the slurry, stirring immediately to incorporate.
7. Then add the mushrooms back in and stir gently again. The potatoes will be really soft and might break a little but that's ok. They taste at their best when soft like that in this recipe. Give it a couple of minutes for the gravy to thicken a bit and the mushrooms to warm through then serve.

Nutrition:
Calories: 411 Carbohydrates: 73g Protein: 10.4g Fat: 5g

493. Masoor Dal, Red Lentil Dahl
⏱ Prep Time 15 m | ⏱ Cooking Time 20 m | 6 Servings

Ingredients:

- 1 tablespoon coconut oil (or any vegetable oil. To make the dal oil-free, use 1/4 cup of water to sauté)
- 1 teaspoon mustard seeds
- 1 large onion (finely diced)
- 1 sprig curry leaves (optional, can be replaced with 2 tbsp. chopped cilantro)
- 4 medium tomatoes (finely diced)
- 1-inch piece ginger (grated or crushed into a paste)
- 4 cloves garlic (minced or crushed into a paste)
- 1/2 teaspoon turmeric
- 1 tablespoon ground coriander
- 1/2 to 1 teaspoon red pepper flakes (or if using dry red chili peppers use one or two based on how much heat you can tolerate)
- 1 cup red lentils (masoor dal)
- 1/2 cup coconut milk
- Salt to taste
- Lemon juice for squeezing on top

Directions:

1. Heat the oil in an Instant Pot set to the "Sauté" function set to "Normal". Add the mustard seeds and when they begin to sputter, add the onions, curry leaves, ginger and garlic. (If making this oil-free, add the mustard seeds to the dry Instant Pot liner after it heats up, then, when they sputter, add the onions, ginger and garlic and then add in 1/4 cup water)
2. Sauté, stirring frequently, until the onions soften and just start to brown. Add the tomatoes, turmeric, coriander powder and red pepper flakes and mix well. You can use an Instant Pot glass lid or any glass lid that fits to cover the pot at this time and let the tomatoes cook 3-4 minutes until they are broken down and very pulpy. Stir a couple of times during cooking.
3. Add the dal to the pot and stir to mix, then add in 4 cups of water. Give everything a good stir then click in the Instant Pot lid. Set the Instant Pot at manual pressure for 10 minutes.
4. After cooking, wait either until pressure releases automatically, or, if you're in a rush, wait 10 minutes after the end of cooking, then carefully quick-release according to instructions.
5. Using a ladle, stir in the coconut milk and salt to taste. At this point you can garnish with more cilantro, if you like, or serve as is. Always top the deal with a final squeeze of lemon juice for the perfect finish!

Nutrition:
Calories: 198 Carbohydrates: 26g Protein: 10g Fat: 7g

494. Vegan Air Fryer Eggplant Parmesan Recipe
⏱ Prep Time 20 m | ⏱ Cooking Time 25 m | 2 Servings

Ingredients:

- 1 large Eggplant stems removed and sliced
- 1/2 cup Flour
- 1/2 cup Almond Milk
- 1/2 cup Panko Bread Crumbs
- 2 tablespoons Vegan Grated Parmesan
- Onion Powder to taste
- Garlic Powder to taste
- Salt & Pepper to taste
- To top the eggplant parmesan:
- 1 cup Marinara Sauce plus more for serving
- 1/2 cup Vegan Mozzarella Shreds
- Vegan Grated Parmesan
- For Serving:
- 4 ounces Spaghetti or pasta of your choosing, cooked al dente (about 2 oz. per person)
- Sprinkle Vegan Grated Parmesan
- Parsley for garnish

Directions:

1. Wash, dry and remove stems of eggplant Create slices.
2. Dip the slices into flour, then almond milk and finally, the panko bread crumbs that you have mixed with the vegan parmesan, salt, pepper, and garlic and onion powder.
3. Spray lightly with oil (if desired) and place into the basket of an air fryer at 390 degrees for 15 minutes, flipping halfway through (spray the second side lightly).
4. Alternately, you can do this all in the oven at 400 degrees. Cooking time may vary since air fryer's use a convection type cooking Instructions. Just keep an eye on them.
5. While the eggplant are cooking, go ahead and cook your pasta.
6. Once golden on both sides, spoon on some of the marinara and top with a combination of the two vegan cheeses. Cook just until the cheese begins to melt.
7. Serve with the pasta (and extra sauce), garnishing with fresh parsley and perhaps another sprinkle of the vegan parmesan. Enjoy!

Nutrition:
Calories: 377 Carbs: 36g Fat: 16g Protein: 24g

495. Air Fryer Bow Tie Pasta Chips
⏱ Prep Time 10 m | ⏱ Cooking Time 20 m | 3 Servings

Ingredients:

- 2 cups dry whole wheat bow tie pasta (use brown rice pasta to make it gluten-free)
- 1 tablespoon olive oil (or use aquafaba for oil-free option)
- 1 tablespoon nutritional yeast
- 1 1/2 teaspoon Italian Seasoning Blend
- 1/2 teaspoon salt

Directions:

1. Cook the pasta for 1/2 the time called for on the package. Toss the drained pasta with the olive oil or aquafaba, nutritional yeast, Italian seasoning, and salt.
2. Place about half of the mixture in your air fryer basket if yours is small; larger ones may be able to do cook in one batch.
3. Cook on 390°F for 5 minutes. Shake the basket and cook 3 to 5 minutes more or until crunchy.

Nutrition:
Calories: 113 Carbs: 21g Fat: 1g Protein: 4g

496. Portobello Mushroom Pizzas with Hummus
⏱ Prep Time 15 m | ⏱ Cooking Time 25 m | 6 Servings

Ingredients:
- 4 large Portobello mushrooms
- Balsamic vinegar
- Salt and black pepper
- 4 tablespoons oil-free pasta sauce (such as 365 Organic)
- 1 clove garlic, minced
- 3 ounces zucchini, shredded, chopped, or julienned (about 1/2 medium)
- 2 tablespoons sweet red pepper, diced
- 4 olives kalamata olives, sliced
- 1 teaspoon dried basil
- 1/2 cups hummus (see notes for Kalamata Servings)
- Fresh basil leaves or other herbs, minced

Directions:
1. Wash the Portobello's well. Cut off the stems and remove the gills with a spoon. Pat the insides dry and brush or spray both sides with balsamic vinegar. Sprinkle the inside with salt and pepper.
2. Spread 1 tablespoon of pasta sauce inside each mushroom and sprinkle it with garlic up
3. Air Fryer Instructions
4. Preheat the Air Fryer to 330F. Place as many mushrooms as will fit in a single layer or use a rack to hold two layers. (You may need to do this in batches, depending on the size or your air fryer and Portobello's.) Air Fry for 3 minutes.
5. Remove mushrooms and top each one with equal portions of zucchini, peppers, and olives and sprinkle with dried basil and salt and pepper. Return to the Air Fryer for 3 minutes. Check mushrooms and rearrange if using a rack. Return to the Air Fryer for another 3 minutes or until mushrooms are tender. Place on a plate, drizzle with hummus and sprinkle with basil or other herbs. If you want, you can put the Portobello's back into the air fryer briefly to warm the hummus.

Nutrition:
Calories: 190 Carbs: 24g Fat: 6g Protein: 5g

497. Easy Air Fryer Baked Potatoes
⏱ Prep Time 10 m | ⏱ Cooking Time 50 m | 4 Servings

Ingredients:
- 4 large baking potatoes, cleaned
- 2 tablespoons olive oil
- Coarse kosher salt
- Pepper
- Garlic powder
- Parsley
- 1/2 stick butter (4 tablespoons), divided
- Sour cream, optional

Directions:
1. Rub potatoes with olive oil.
2. Season potatoes with salt, pepper, garlic powder and parsley to taste.
3. Place in air fryer and cook at 400 degrees for 40-50 minutes (depending on size of potatoes).
4. Slice potatoes lengthwise; using both hands, pinch each side of the potatoes, forcing them to open up, forcing the inside of the potato up.
5. Place 1 tablespoon of butter in each of the potatoes and finish with a dollop of sour cream if you'd like.

Nutrition:
Calories: 199 Carbs: 26g Fat: 7g Protein: 7g

498. Air Fryer Toasted Coconut French toast
⏱ Prep Time 10 m | ⏱ Cooking Time 15 m | Servings

Ingredients:
- 2 Slices of Gluten-Free Bread
- 1/2 Cup Lite Culinary Coconut Milk
- 1 teaspoon Baking Powder
- 1/2 Cup Unsweetened Shredded Coconut

Directions:
1. In a wide rimmed bowl, mix together the coconut milk and baking powder.
2. Spread the shredded coconut out on a plate.
3. Take each slice of bread and first soak in the coconut milk mixture and a few seconds before transferring to the shredded coconut plate and fully coating the slice in the coconut.
4. Space both the coated slices of bread in your air fryer, close it, and set the temperature to 350°F and 4 minutes.
5. Once done, remove and top with maple syrup or your favorite French toast toppings!

Nutrition:
Calories: 176 Carbs: 32g Fat: 5g Protein: 4g

499. Air Fryer Kale Chips
⏱ Prep Time 10 m | ⏱ Cooking Time 20 m | 6 Servings

Ingredients:
- 1 bunch kale about 5 cups, 8-10 ounces
- 1 Tablespoon olive oil 15 mL
- ¼ teaspoon salt
- Optional flavorings

Directions:
1. Prep: Wash and dry kale. Cut the leaves away from the spine, then roughly tear the leaves into bite-sized pieces. Massage oil into the leaves, making sure each piece of kale has a thin coat of oil. Sprinkle with salt and toss to coat.
2. Transfer: Lay kale in a single layer in your air fryer basket, uncurling the leaves as much as possible while keeping them from overlapping too much (you may need to cook in batches).
3. Cook: Air fry for 4 to 5 minutes at 375°F (190°C), shaking the pan once to help them cook evenly. Keep a close eye on them after 3 minutes. They're done when crispy!

Nutrition:
Calories: 150 Carbs: 3g Fat: 15g Protein: 2g

500. Air Fryer Mozzarella Sticks

⏱ Prep Time 15 m | ⏲ Cooking Time 15 m | 8 Servings

Ingredients:

- 8 mozzarella sticks
- ¼ cup all-purpose flour
- 1 egg whisked
- 1 cup panko breadcrumbs
- ½ teaspoon each onion powder, garlic powder, smoked paprika, salt

Directions:

1. Freeze Cheese: Unwrap mozzarella sticks (or cut into sticks if starting from a block of cheese). Set on a parchment-lined plate and place in the freezer for 30 minutes.
2. Prep: Meanwhile, set up your breading station. Place flour in a zip lock baggie. Whisk egg in a shallow bowl. Combine panko and seasonings in a separate shallow bowl.
3. Bread Once: Toss mozzarella sticks into the bag with the flour, zip it shut, and shake to evenly coat the cheese. Working one at a time, roll the mozzarella sticks in the egg, then in the panko. Return to the plate and freeze for 30 more minutes.
4. Bread Twice: Lightly grease your air fryer basket or rack, and preheat to 390°F (200°C). Coat the mozzarella sticks in egg then panko one more time, then transfer to the air fryer.
5. Cook: Cook for 6 to 8 minutes, until crispy and golden brown. Serve warm with your favorite dipping sauce, like marinara or ranch.

Nutrition:

Calories: 156 Carbs: 3g Fat: 11g Protein: 13g

501. Crispy Air Fryer Chickpeas

⏱ Prep Time 10 m | ⏲ Cooking Time 15 m | 6 Servings

Ingredients:

- 1 14-oz can chickpeas 425g
- 1 tablespoon olive oil 15 mL
- ½ teaspoon salt or seasoning of choice, see notes

Directions:

1. Prep: Drain and pat chickpeas dry with a paper towel. Toss together with oil and salt (or your chosen seasoning).
2. Cook: Spread in a single layer in your air fryer basket or rack. Cook at 390°F (200°C) for 8 to 10 minutes, or until crispy and lightly browned.

Nutrition:

Calories: 132 Carbs: 25g Fat: 2g Protein: 5g

502. Air Fryer Pizza

⏱ Prep Time 10 m | ⏲ Cooking Time 15 m | 4 Servings

Ingredients:

- Buffalo mozzarella
- Pizza dough 1 12-inch dough will make 2 personal sized pizzas
- Olive oil
- Tomato sauce
- Optional toppings to finish: fresh basil, parmesan cheese, pepper flakes

Directions:

1. Prep: Preheat air fryer to 375°F (190°C). Spray air fryer basket well with oil. Pat mozzarella dry with paper towels (to prevent a soggy pizza).
2. Assemble: Roll out pizza dough to the size of your air fryer baskets carefully transfer it to the air fryer, then brush lightly with a teaspoon or so of olive oil. Spoon on a light layer of tomato sauce and sprinkle with chunks of buffalo mozzarella.
3. Bake: For about 7 minutes until crust is crispy and cheese has melted. Optionally top with basil, grated parmesan, and pepper flakes just before serving
4. .

Nutrition:

Calories: 115 Carbs: 20g Fat: 2g Protein: 0g

503. Air Fryer Brussels sprouts

⏱ Prep Time 10 m | ⏲ Cooking Time 15 m | 3 Servings

Ingredients:

- ½ pound Brussels sprouts 2 to 3 cups
- 1 tablespoon olive oil 15 mL
- Pinch salt and pepper
- Optional: garlic, balsamic reduction, parmesan cheese

Directions:

1. Prep: Remove the tough ends of the Brussels sprouts and remove any damaged outer leaves. Rinse under cold water and pat dry. If your sprouts are on the large side, cut them in half. Toss in oil, salt, and pepper.
2. Cook: Arrange Brussels sprouts in a single layer in your air fryer, working in batches if they don't all fits Cook at 375°F (190°C) for 8 to 12 minutes, shaking the pan halfway through cooking to evenly brown them. They are done when lightly browned and crispy on the edges.
3. Serve: Serve sprouts warm, optionally topped with balsamic reduction and parmesan.

Nutrition:

Calories: 116 Carbs: 10g Fat: 7g Protein: 6g

504. Crispy Air Fried Tofu

⏱ Prep Time 10 m | ⏲ Cooking Time 20 m | 6 Servings

Ingredients:

- 1 16-oz block extra-firm tofu 453 g
- 2 tablespoons soy sauce 30 mL
- 1 Tablespoon toasted sesame oil* 15 mL
- 1 Tablespoon olive oil 15 mL
- 1 clove garlic minced

Directions:

1. Press: Press tofu for at least 15 minutes, using either a tofu press or by setting a heavy pan on top of it, letting the moisture drain. When finished, cut tofu into bite-sized blocks and transfer to a bowl.
2. Flavor: Combine all remaining Ingredients in a small bowl. Drizzle over tofu and let tofu marinate for an additional 15 minutes.
3. Air Fry: Preheat your air fryer to 375 degrees F (190 C). Add tofu blocks to your air fryer basket in a single layer. Cook for 10 to 15 minutes, shaking the pan occasionally to promote even cooking.

Nutrition:

Calories: 212 Carbs: 5g Fat: 16g Protein: 17g

505. Buttermilk Fried Mushrooms
⏰ Prep Time 10 m | ⏰ Cooking Time 20 m | 6 Servings

Ingredients:
- 2 heaping cups oyster mushrooms
- 1 cup buttermilk 240 mL, see notes for vegan substitute
- 1 1/2 cups all-purpose flour 200 g
- 1 teaspoon each salt, pepper, garlic powder, onion powder, smoked paprika, cumin
- 1 Tablespoon oil

Directions:
1. Marinate: Preheat air fryer to 375 degrees F (190 C). Clean mushrooms then toss together with buttermilk in a large bowl. Let marinate for 15 minutes.
2. Breading: In a large bowl combine flour and spices. Spoon mushrooms out of the buttermilk (save the buttermilk). Dip each mushroom in the flour mixture, shake off excess flour, dip once more in the buttermilk, then once more in the flour
3. Cook: Grease the bottom of your air fry pan well, then place mushrooms in a single layer, leaving space between mushrooms. Cook for 5 minutes, then roughly brush all sides with a little oil to promote browning. Continue cooking 5 to 10 more minutes, until golden brown and crispy.

Nutrition:
Calories: 220 Carbs: 10g Fat: 23g Protein: 4g

506. Crispy Baked Avocado Tacos
⏰ Prep Time 15 m | ⏰ Cooking Time 15 m | 4 Servings

Ingredients
- Salsa (can sub your favorite store bought)
- 1 cup finely chopped or crushed pineapple 240 g
- 1 roma tomato finely chopped
- 1/2 red bell pepper finely chopped
- 1/2 of a medium red onion 1/2 cup, finely chopped
- 1 clove garlic minced
- 1/2 jalapeno finely chopped
- Pinch each cumin and salt
- Avocado Tacos
- 1 avocado
- 1/4 cup all-purpose flour 35 g
- 1 large egg whisked
- 1/2 cup panko crumbs 65 g
- Pinch each salt and pepper
- 4 flour tortillas click for recipe
- Adobo Sauce
- 1/4 cup plain yogurt 60 g
- 2 tablespoons mayonnaise 30 g
- 1/4 teaspoon lime juice
- 1 tablespoon adobo sauce from a jar of chipotle peppers

Directions:
1. Salsa: Combine all Salsa Ingredients (finely chop by hand or blitz in the food processor), cover, and set in fridge.
2. Prep Avocado: Cut avocado in half lengthwise and remove pits Place avocado skin side down and cut each half into 4 equal sized pieces, then gently peel the skin off of each.
3. Prep Station: Preheat oven to 450 F (230 C) or air fryer to 375 F (190 C). Arrange your workspace so you have a bowl of flour, a bowl of whisked egg, a bowl of panko with S&P mixed in, and a parchment-lined baking sheet at the end.
4. Coat: Dip each avocado slice first in the flour, then egg, then panko. Place on the prepared baking sheet and either bake or air fry for 10 minutes, flipping halfway through cooking, until lightly browned.
5. Sauce: While avocados are cooking, combine all Sauce Ingredients.
6. Serve: Spoon salsa onto a tortilla, top with 2 pieces of avocado, and drizzle with sauce. Serve immediately and enjoy!

Nutrition:
Calories: 130 Carbs: 20g Fat: 5g Protein: 4g

507. Air Fryer Vegan Tempeh Bacon
⏰ Prep Time 10 m | ⏰ Cooking Time 25 m | 6 Servings

Ingredients:
- 4 ounces Tempeh, sliced thin (organic, non-gmo, preferred brand: Light life Organic Flax
- 1/4 cup low-sodium soy sauce (or tamari if gluten-free)
- 1/2 tablespoon Liquid Smoke
- 1 teaspoon oil
- 1 tablespoon pure maple syrup
- 1/4 teaspoon black pepper
- 1/4 teaspoon garlic powder
- 1/4 teaspoon smoked paprika

Directions:
1. Line the air fryer basket with a round piece of parchment paper, just big enough to cover the bottom.
2. Slice the tempeh thinly.
3. Mix the marinade Ingredients in a shallow bowl; add the tempeh slices and let sit for 10 minutes, flipping over halfway through.
4. Place slices in the parchment lined air fryer basket and drizzle half the remaining marinade over the slices.*
5. Slide the basket into the fryer and set temperature to 350° for 10 minutes.
6. After 5 minutes has elapsed; remove basket, flip slices over and drizzle the remaining marinade. Slide basket back in and the fryer will start up again and continue 'frying' for the remaining 5 minutes.

Nutrition:
Calories: 138 Carbs: 4g Fat: 4g Protein: 20g

508. Air Fryer Tofu Buddha Bowl

🕐 Prep Time 5 m | 🕐 Cooking Time 15 m | 4 Servings

Ingredients:

- 14 oz. extra firm tofu
- 2 tablespoons sesame oil
- 1/4 cup soy sauce
- 3 tablespoons molasses
- 2 tablespoons lime juice
- 1 tablespoon Sirach
- 1 lb. fresh broccoli florets only
- 3 medium carrots peeled and thinly sliced
- 1 red bell pepper thinly sliced
- 8 ounces fresh spinach sautéed with olive oil and garlic
- 2 cups cooked quinoa or brown rice

Directions:

1. Wrap tofu in a several paper towels and set a plate on top to press out excess liquid. Once dry, unwrap tofu and cut into very small cubes (about 100 pieces).
2. Add sesame oil, soy sauce, molasses, lime juice, and Sriracha to a large bowl and whisk until incorporated.
3. Add tofu to the sauce and let marinate for 5--10 minutes, stirring occasionally. While tofu is marinating, prep veggies.
4. Coat air fryer with your choice of oil. Remove tofu from bowl and add to air fryer basket, leaving all marinade in bowl. Cook tofu at 370 degrees F for 15 minutes, shaking basket every 5 minutes.
5. Meanwhile, add broccoli, carrots, and bell pepper to bowl with marinade and mix well every few minutes.
6. Also, while tofu is cooking, cook spinach on the stovetop, just until wilted, making sure not to overcook.
7. Once tofu is done, remove from air fryer and set aside. Then add vegetables to air fryer basket, again leaving marinade in bowl. Cook vegetables for 10 minutes, giving the basket a good shake every few minutes.
8. In a large serving bowl - begin to build your Buddha Bowl. First add cooked quinoa (or rice), then spread the cooked veggies evenly. Next add the cooked spinach, and finally the tofu. Pour over remaining marinade and garnish with sesame seeds. Enjoy!

Nutrition:

Calories: 167 Carbs: 4g Fat: 20g Protein: 8g

509. Roasted Vegetable Salad

🕐 Prep Time 1 h 30 m | 🕐 Cooking Time 25 m | 6 Servings

Ingredients:

- 1 sweet potato, chopped
- 1 red bell pepper, chopped
- 1 onion, chopped
- 4 small potatoes, chopped
- ¼ cup cherry tomatoes, chopped
- Salt and pepper to taste
- ¼ cup parsley, chopped
- 2 tablespoons capers, chopped
- 1 avocado, chopped
- 1 tablespoon lemon juice
- 1 tablespoon olive oil
- 1 can chickpeas mixed with 1 teaspoon mustard powder
- 4 cups lettuce leaves, chopped

Directions:

1. Season all the vegetables (except parsley, capers, lettuce and avocado) with salt and pepper.
2. Toss in oil and cook in the air fryer at 400 degrees for 25 minutes.
3. Transfer to a bowl and refrigerate for 1 hour.
4. Mash avocado and mix with lemon juice and olive oil.
5. Arrange the salad in a bowl by putting the lettuce leaves first and topping with the cooked vegetables and chickpeas.
6. Serve with the avocado dressing.

Nutrition:

Calories 206 Fat 9.2g Carbohydrate 29.6g Protein 3.7g

510. Vegetable & Pasta Salad

🕐 Prep Time 1 h 5 m | 🕐 Cooking Time 1 h 45 m | 4 Servings

Ingredients:

- 3 eggplants, sliced
- 2 tablespoons olive oil, divided
- Salt and pepper to taste
- 3 zucchinis, sliced
- 4 tomatoes, sliced into wedges
- 4 cups macaroni pasta
- Salt to taste
- 8 tablespoons vegan Parmesan cheese, grated
- ½ cup Italian dressing
- Basil leaves, chopped

Directions:

1. Toss eggplant slices in 1 tablespoon olive oil and season with salt and pepper.
2. Cook in the air fryer at 375 degrees F for 40 minutes.
3. Toss the zucchini in the remaining oil and cook in the air fryer for 25 minutes.
4. Cook pasta according to the package **Directions:** Drain and rinse.
5. Toss the pasta with the eggplant and zucchini slices.
6. Drizzle with Italian dressing.
7. Season with salt.
8. Sprinkle cheese and basil on top and serve.

Nutrition:

Calories 336 Fat 11.7g Carbohydrate 52g Protein 9.3g

511. Crispy Tofu & Avocado Salad

🕐 Prep Time 15 m | 🕐 Cooking Time 15 m | 6 Servings

Ingredients:

- Cooking spray
- 2 cups tofu, cubed
- 4 cups mixed greens
- 4 cups Romaine lettuce
- ½ cup onion, sliced
- 1 cup cherry tomatoes, sliced in half
- ½ avocado, sliced into cubes
- ½ cup red wine vinegar
- 1 cup avocado lime dressing

Directions:

1. Spray air fryer basket with oil.
2. Cook the tofu cubes at 375 degrees F for 15 minutes, shaking halfway through.
3. In a bowl, arrange the salad by topping the lettuce and mixed greens with crispy tofu, onion, tomatoes and avocado.
4. Drizzle with red wine vinegar and avocado lime dressing.

Nutrition:

Calories 287 Fat 10.8g Carbohydrate 33.1g Protein 16.8g

512. Radish & Mozzarella Salad

⏱ Prep Time 15 m | ⏱ Cooking Time 30 m | 4 Servings

Ingredients:
- 1 lb. radish, sliced into rounds
- 2 tablespoons olive oil
- Salt and pepper to taste
- ½ lb. vegan mozzarella, sliced into rounds
- 2 tablespoons balsamic glaze

Directions:
1. Toss radish rounds in oil and season with salt and pepper.
2. Cook in the air fryer at 350 degrees F for 30 minutes, shaking once or twice during cooking.
3. Arrange on a serving platter with the vegan mozzarella.
4. Drizzle cheese and radish with balsamic glaze before serving.

Nutrition:
Calories 88 Fat 7.7g Carbohydrate 4g Protein 1.8g

513. Roasted Butternut Squash Salad

⏱ Prep Time 10 m | ⏱ Cooking Time 15 m | 4 Servings

Ingredients:
- 1 butternut squash, sliced into cubes
- 4 tablespoons olive oil, divided
- ¼ teaspoon cayenne pepper
- Salt to taste
- 2 tablespoons fresh lemon juice
- 1 shallot, minced
- 6 oz. arugula
- 1 apple, sliced thinly
- ½ cup almonds, toasted and sliced
- ½ cup vegan Parmesan cheese, grated

Directions:
1. Toss squash cubes in 1 tablespoon olive oil and cayenne pepper.
2. Add to the air fryer and cook at 400 degrees F for 15 minutes, shaking once or twice.
3. In a bowl, mix the salt, remaining olive oil, lemon juice and shallot.
4. Coat arugula with this mixture.
5. Arrange arugula on salad bowls.
6. Top with the squash cubes, apple slices, almonds and Parmesan cheese.

Nutrition:
Calories 295 Fat 20.5g Carbohydrate 28.8g Protein 5.3g

514. Green Salad with Roasted Bell Peppers

⏱ Prep Time 10 m | ⏱ Cooking Time 10 m | 4 Servings

Ingredients:
- 1 red bell pepper
- 1 tablespoon lemon juice
- 2 tablespoons olive oil
- 3 tablespoons vegan yogurt
- Pepper to taste
- 4 cups Romaine lettuce, chopped

Directions:
1. Preheat your air fryer to 400 degrees F.
2. Add the bell pepper inside.
3. Cook for 10 minutes or until slightly charred.
4. Slice the roasted bell peppers.
5. Top the Romaine lettuce with the roasted bell peppers.
6. In a bowl, mix the rest of the ingredients and serve as dressing.

Nutrition:
Calories 205 Fat 14g Carbohydrate 18.3g Protein 3.6g

515. Salad Topped with Garlic Croutons

⏱ Prep Time 10 m | ⏱ Cooking Time 5 m | 4 Servings

Ingredients:
- 4 slices vegan bread, sliced into cubes
- 1 tablespoon olive oil
- Garlic powder to taste
- Salt and pepper to taste
- 1 teaspoon Italian seasoning
- Mixed greens
- 1 cup tomato, chopped
- 1 cup white onion rings

Directions:
1. Coat the bread cubes with olive oil.
2. Season with garlic powder, salt, pepper and Italian seasoning.
3. Cook in the air fryer at 380 degrees F for 5 minutes, shaking a few times.
4. Place the mixed greens in a bowl,
5. Top with the tomato, white onions and croutons.
6. Serve with vegan salad dressing.

Nutrition:
Calories 50 Fat 4.1g Carbohydrate 4g Protein 0.4g

516. Green Bean Salad

⏱ Prep Time 35 m | ⏱ Cooking Time 15 m | 2 Servings

Ingredients:
- 2 cups green beans, trimmed
- ¼ cup water
- ¼ cup vegan mayo
- ¼ cup vegan cheese

Directions:
1. Put the green beans and water in a small heatproof pan.
2. Put the pan in the air fryer basket.
3. Cook in the air fryer at 375 degrees F for 15 minutes.
4. Let cool.
5. Put in the refrigerator for 30 minutes.
6. Mix with mayo and top with cheese.

Nutrition:
Calories 97 Fat 6.1g Carbohydrate 10.1g Protein 2g

517. Salad with Roasted Tomatoes

⏱ Prep Time 5 m | ⏱ Cooking Time 45 m | 4 Servings

Ingredients:

- 2 cups tomatoes, sliced
- Salt to taste
- 4 cups Romaine lettuce leaves
- 2 cups arugula
- 1 cup onion, chopped
- Vegan salad dressing

Directions:

1. Toss tomato slices in olive oil.
2. Season with salt.
3. Cook in the air fryer at 240 degrees F for 45 minutes.
4. Arrange lettuce and arugula on salad bowls.
5. Top with onion and roasted tomatoes.
6. Serve with vegan salad dressing.

Nutrition:

Calories 73 Fat 3.9g Carbohydrate 8.7g Protein 1.6g

518. Prawn Momo's Recipe
⏲ Prep Time 15 m | ⏲ Cooking Time 25 m | 4 Servings

Ingredients
- 1 ½ cup all-purpose flour
- ½ tsp. salt
- 5 tbsp. water

For filling:
- 2 cups minced prawn

- 2 tbsp. oil
- 2 tsp. ginger-garlic paste
- 2 tsp. soya sauce
- 2 tsp. vinegar

Directions
1. Squeeze the dough and cover it with plastic wrap and set aside. Next, cook the ingredients for the filling and try to ensure that the prawn is covered well with the sauce. Roll the dough and cut it into a square.
2. Place the filling in the center. Now, wrap the dough to cover the filling and pinch the edges together. Preheat the Breville smart oven at 200° F for 5 minutes. Place the wontons in the fry basket and close it. Let them cook at the same temperature for another 20 minutes. Recommended sides are chili sauce or ketchup.

Nutrition
Calories 300 | Fat 11 g | Protein 35 g | Sugar 6 g

519. Fish Club Classic Sandwich
⏲ Prep Time 10 m | ⏲ Cooking Time 20 m | 3 Servings

Ingredients
- 2 slices of white bread
- 1 tbsp. softened butter
- 1 tin tuna
- 1 small capsicum

For Barbeque Sauce:
- ¼ tbsp. Worcestershire sauce
- ½ tsp. olive oil
- ½ flake garlic crushed

- ¼ cup chopped onion
- ¼ tsp. mustard powder
- ½ tbsp. sugar
- ¼ tbsp. red chili sauce
- 1 tbsp. tomato ketchup
- ½ cup water.
- Salt and black pepper to taste

Directions
1. Remove the edges of the sliced bread. Now cut the slices horizontally. Cook the ingredients for the sauce and wait till it thickens. Now, add the fish to the sauce and stir till it obtains the flavors. Roast the capsicum and peel the skin off. Cut the capsicum into slices.
2. Mix the ingredients and apply it to the bread slices. Pre-heat the Breville smart oven for 5 minutes at 300 Fahrenheit.
3. Open the basket of the Fryer and place the prepared classic sandwiches in it such that no two classic sandwiches are touching each other. Now keep the fryer at 250 degrees for around 15 minutes. Turn the classic sandwiches in between the cooking process to cook both slices. Serve the classic sandwiches with tomato ketchup or mint sauce.

Nutrition
Calories 232 | Fat 22 g | Protein 25 g | Sugar 5 g

520. Prawn Grandma's Easy to Cook Wontons
⏲ Prep Time 5 m | ⏲ Cooking Time 20 m | 3 Servings

Ingredients
- 1 ½ cup all-purpose flour
- ½ tsp. salt
- 5 tbsp. water
- 2 cups minced prawn

- 2 tbsp. oil
- 2 tsp. ginger-garlic paste
- 2 tsp. soya sauce
- 2 tsp. vinegar

Directions
1. Squeeze out the dough and cover it with plastic wrap and set it aside. Then cook the ingredients for the filling and try to make sure the shrimp are well coated with the sauce. Roll out the dough and place the filling in the center.
2. Now, roll the dough to cover the filling and bring the edges together. Preheat the Breville Smart Oven to 200 ° F for 5 minutes. Place the wontons in the pan and close it. Let them cook at equal temperature for another 20 minutes. Recommended sides are chili sauce or ketchup.

Nutrition
Calories 423 | Fat 20 g | Protein 20 g | Sugar 2 g

521. Prawn Fried Baked Pastry

⏱ Prep Time 15 m | ⏱ Cooking Time 35 m | 4 Servings

Ingredients

- 1 ½ cup all-purpose flour
- 2 tbsp. unsalted butter
- 2 green chilies that are finely chopped or mashed
- Add a lot of water to make the dough stiff and firm
- A pinch of salt to taste
- 1 lb. prawn
- ¼ cup boiled peas
- ½ tsp. cumin
- 1 tsp. coarsely crushed coriander
- 1 dry red chili broken into pieces
- A small amount of salt (to taste)
- ½ tsp. dried mango powder
- 1 tsp. powdered ginger
- ½ tsp. red chili powder
- 1-2 tbsp. coriander

Directions

1. You will first need to make the outer covering. In a large bowl, add the flour, butter, and enough water to knead it into the stiff dough. Transfer this to a container and leave it to rest for five minutes. Place a pan on medium flame and add the oil. Roast the mustard seeds and once roasted, add the coriander seeds and the chopped dry red chilies. Add all the dry ingredients for the filling and mix the ingredients well.
2. Add a little water and continue to mix the ingredients. Make small balls from the dough and wrap them. Cut the wrapped dough in half and spread a little water on the edges to help you fold the halves into a cone.

Add the filling to the cone and close the samosa. Preheat the Breville Smart Oven for about 5 to 6 minutes at 300 Fahrenheit. Place all the samosas in the frying pan and close the basket properly.
3. Keep the Breville Smart Oven at 200 degrees for another 20 to 25 minutes. Around half point, open the basket and turn the samosas for even cooking. After that, fry at 250 degrees for about 10 minutes to give them the desired golden-brown color. Serve hot. Recommended sides are tamarind or mint sauce.

Nutrition

Calories 132 | Fat 1 g | Protein 15 g | Sugar 9 g

522. Fish Spicy Lemon Kebab

⏱ Prep Time 10 m | ⏱ Cooking Time 25 m | 3 Servings

Ingredients

- 1 lb. boneless fish roughly chopped
- 3 onions chopped
- 5 green chilies-roughly chopped
- 1 ½ tbsp. ginger paste
- 1 ½ tsp garlic paste
- 1 ½ tsp salt
- 3 tsp lemon juice
- 2 tsp garam masala
- 4 tbsp. chopped coriander
- 3 tbsp. cream
- 2 tbsp. coriander powder
- 4 tbsp. fresh mint chopped
- 3 tbsp. chopped capsicum
- 3 eggs
- 2 ½ tbsp. white sesame seeds

Directions

1. Take all the ingredients mentioned under the first heading and mix them in a bowl. Grind them thoroughly to make a smooth paste. Take the eggs in a different bowl and beat them. Add a pinch of salt and leave them aside. Take a flat plate and in it, mix the sesame seeds and breadcrumbs. Mold the mixture of fish into small balls and flatten them into round and flat kebabs. Dip these kebabs in the egg and salt mixture

and then in the mixture of breadcrumbs and sesame seeds. Leave these kebabs in the fridge for an hour or so to set.
2. Preheat the Breville smart oven at 160 degrees Fahrenheit for around 5 minutes. Place the kebabs in the basket and let them cook for another 25 minutes at the same temperature. Turn the kebabs over in between the cooking process to get a uniform cook. Serve the kebabs with mint sauce.

Nutrition

Calories 432 | Fat 3 g | Protein 22 g | Sugar 1 g

523. Fish Oregano Fingers

⏱ Prep Time 10 m | ⏱ Cooking Time 25 m | 5 Servings

Ingredients

- ½ lb. firm white fish fillet cut into Oregano Fingers
- 1 tbsp. lemon juice
- 2 cups of dry breadcrumbs
- 1 cup oil for frying
- 1 ½ tbsp. ginger-garlic paste
- 3 tbsp. lemon juice
- 2 tsp salt
- 1 ½ tsp pepper powder
- 1 tsp red chili
- 3 eggs
- 5 tbsp. corn flour
- 2 tsp tomato ketchup

Directions

1. Rub a little lemon juice on the oregano fingers and set aside. Wash the fish after an hour and pat dry. Make the marinade and transfer the oregano fingers into the marinade. Allow them to dry on a plate for fifteen minutes. Now cover the oregano fingers with the crumbs and set aside to dry for fifteen minutes.

2. Preheat the Breville smart oven at 160 degrees Fahrenheit for 5 minutes or so. Keep the fish in the fry basket now and close it properly.
3. Let the oregano fingers cook at the same temperature for another 25 minutes. In between the cooking process, toss the fish once in a while to avoid burning the food. Serve either with tomato ketchup or chili sauce. Mint sauce also works well with the fish.

Nutrition

Calories 234 | Fat 3 g | Protein 35 g | Sugar 0 g

524. Tuna Sandwich
Prep Time 5 m | Cooking Time 15 m | 4 Servings

Ingredients
- 2 slices of white bread
- 1 tbsp. softened butter
- 1 tin tuna
- 1 small capsicum
- For Barbeque Sauce:
- ¼ tbsp. Worcestershire sauce
- ½ tsp. olive oil
- ¼ tsp. mustard powder

- ½ flake garlic crushed
- ¼ cup chopped onion
- ½ tbsp. sugar
- 1 tbsp. tomato ketchup
- ½ cup water.
- ¼ tbsp. red chili sauce
- Salt and black pepper to taste

Directions
1. Remove the edges of the slices of bread. Now cut the slices horizontally. Cook the ingredients for the sauce and wait till it thickens. Now, add the lamb to the sauce and stir till it obtains the flavors. Roast the capsicum and peel the skin off. Cut the capsicum into slices. Mix the ingredients and apply it to the bread slices.

2. Pre-heat the Breville smart oven for 5 minutes at 300 Fahrenheit. Open the basket of the Fryer and place the prepared classic sandwiches in it such that no two classic sandwiches are touching each other. Now keep the fryer at 250 degrees for around 15 minutes. Turn the classic sandwiches in between the cooking process to cook both slices. Serve the classic sandwiches with tomato ketchup or mint sauce.

Nutrition
Calories 460 | Fat 1 g | Protein 11 g | Sugar 5 g

525. Shrimp Momo's Recipe
Prep Time 10 m | Cooking Time 20 m | 7 Servings

Ingredients
- 1 ½ cup all-purpose flour
- ½ tsp. salt
- 5 tbsp. water
For filling:
- 2 cups minced shrimp

- 2 tbsp. oil
- 2 tsp. ginger-garlic paste
- 2 tsp. soya sauce
- 2 tsp. vinegar

Directions
1. Squeeze out the dough and cover it with plastic wrap and set it aside. Then cook the ingredients for the filling and try to make sure the shrimp are well coated with the sauce. Roll up the dough and cut it into squares. Place the filling in the center.

2. Now, roll the dough to cover the filling and bring the edges together. Preheat the Breville Smart Oven to 200 ° F for 5 minutes. Place the wontons in the pan and close it. Let them cook at an equal temperature for another 20 minutes. Recommended sides are chili sauce or ketchup.

Nutrition
Calories 103 | Fat 0 g | Protein 34 g | Sugar 11 g

526. Salmon Tandoor
Prep Time 10 m | Cooking Time 20 m | 5 Servings

Ingredients
- 2 lb. boneless salmon filets
1st Marinade:
- 3 tbsp. vinegar or lemon juice
- 2 or 3 tsp. paprika
- 1 tsp. black pepper
- 1 tsp. salt
- 3 tsp. ginger-garlic paste
2nd Marinade:
- 1 cup yogurt

- 4 tsp. tandoori masala
- 2 tbsp. dry fenugreek leaves
- 1 tsp. black salt
- 1 tsp. chat masala
- 1 tsp. garam masala powder
- 1 tsp. red chili powder
- 1 tsp. salt
- 3 drops of red color

Directions
1. Make the first marinade and soak the fileted salmon in it for four hours. While this is happening, make the second marinade and soak the salmon in it overnight to let the flavors blend. Preheat the Breville smart oven at 160 degrees Fahrenheit for 5 minutes.

2. Put the oregano fingers in the pan and close it. Let them cook at an equal temperature for another 15 minutes or so. Toss the oregano fingers well so that they are well cooked. Serve with mint sauce.

Nutrition
Calories 187 | Fat 2 g | Protein 30 g | Sugar 0 g

527. Salmon Fries
Prep Time 5 m | Cooking Time 15 m | 3 Servings

Ingredients
- 1 lb. boneless salmon filets
- 2 cup dry breadcrumbs
- 2 tsp. oregano
- 2 tsp. red chili flakes
- 1 ½ tbsp. ginger-garlic paste
- 4 tbsp. lemon juice

- 2 tsp. salt
- 1 tsp. pepper powder
- 1 tsp. red chili powder
- 6 tbsp. corn flour
- 4 eggs

Directions
1. Mix every ingredient for the marinade and put the salmon fillets and leave to rest overnight. Mix the toast, oregano, and red chili flakes well and place the marinated oregano fingers in this mixture. Cover with cling film and leave until served.

2. Preheat the Breville smart oven to 160 degrees Fahrenheit for 5 minutes.
3. Put the oregano fingers in the pan and close it. Let them cook at an equal temperature for another 15 minutes or so. Toss the oregano fingers well so that they are well cooked.

Nutrition
Calories 300 | Fat 3 g | Protein 16 g | Sugar 2 g

528. Carp Best Homemade Croquette

⏱ Prep Time 15 m | ⏱ Cooking Time 25 m | 3 Servings

Ingredients

- 1 lb. Carp filets
- 3 onions chopped
- 5 green chilies-roughly chopped
- 1 ½ tbsp. ginger paste
- 1 ½ tsp garlic paste
- 1 ½ tsp salt
- 3 tsp lemon juice
- 2 tsp garam masala

- 4 tbsp. chopped coriander
- 3 tbsp. cream
- 2 tbsp. coriander powder
- 4 tbsp. fresh mint chopped
- 3 tbsp. chopped capsicum
- 3 eggs
- 2 ½ tbsp. white sesame seeds

Directions

1. Take all the ingredients mentioned under the first heading and mix them in a bowl. Grind them thoroughly to make a smooth paste. Take the eggs in a different bowl and beat them. Add a pinch of salt and leave them aside. Mold the fish mixture into small balls and flatten them into round and flat Best Homemade Croquettes. Dip these croquettes in the egg and salt mixture and then in the mixture of breadcrumbs and sesame seeds.

2. Leave these croquettes in the fridge for an hour or so to set. Preheat the Breville smart oven at 160 degrees Fahrenheit for around 5 minutes. Place the croquettes in the basket and let them cook for another 25 minutes at the same temperature. Turn the croquettes over in between the cooking process to get a uniform cook. Serve the croquettes with mint sauce.

Nutrition

Calories 209 | Fat 4 g | Protein 49 g | Sugar 1g

529. Cheese Carp Fries

⏱ Prep Time 15 m | ⏱ Cooking Time 25 m | 4 Servings

Ingredients

- 1 lb. carp oregano fingers
- Ingredients for the marinade:
- 1 tbsp. olive oil
- 1 tsp. mixed herbs
- ½ tsp. red chili flakes

- A pinch of salt to taste
- 1 tbsp. lemon juice
- For the garnish:
- 1 cup melted cheddar cheese

Directions

1. Take all the ingredients mentioned in the heading "For the marinade" and mix well. Cook the oregano fingers and dip them in the marinade.
2. Preheat the Breville smart oven for about 5 minutes at 300 Fahrenheit. Take the basket out of the fryer and place the tent in it. Close the basket. Now keep the fryer at 220 Fahrenheit for 20 to 25 minutes.

3. Between the process, toss the potatoes two or three times so they are cooked through. Towards the rare end of the cooking process (the last 2 minutes or so), sprinkle the melted cheddar cheese over the potatoes and serve hot.

Nutrition

Calories 502 | Fat 22 g | Protein 40 g | Sugar: 14 g

530. Lobster Grandma's Easy to Cook Wontons

⏱ Prep Time 10 m | ⏱ Cooking Time 20 m | 4 Servings

Ingredients

- 1 ½ cup all-purpose flour
- ½ tsp. salt
- 5 tbsp. water
- For filling:
- 2 cups minced lobster

- 2 tbsp. oil
- 2 tsp. ginger-garlic paste
- 2 tsp. soya sauce
- 2 tsp. vinegar

Directions

1. Squeeze out the dough and cover it with plastic wrap and set it aside. Then cook the ingredients for the filling and try to make sure the lobster is well coated with the sauce.
2. Roll out the dough and place the filling in the center. Now, roll the dough to cover the filling and bring the edges together.

3. Preheat the Breville Smart Oven to 200 ° F for 5 minutes. Place the wontons in the pan and close it. Let them cook at an equal temperature for another 20 minutes. Recommended sides are chili sauce or ketchup.

Nutrition

Calories 600 | Fat 13 g | Protein 21 g | Sugar 9 g

531. Crab Cakes

⏱ Prep Time 5 m | ⏱ Cooking Time 10 m | 4 Servings

Ingredients

- 8 ounces jumbo lump crabmeat
- 1 tablespoon Old Bay seasoning
- ⅓ cup bread crumbs
- ¼ cup diced red bell pepper
- ¼ cup diced green bell pepper

- 1 egg
- ¼ cup mayonnaise
- Juice of ½ lemon
- 1 teaspoon flour
- Cooking oil

Directions

1. In a bowl, combine the crab meat, Old Bay seasoning, bread crumbs, red bell pepper, green bell pepper, egg, mayo, and lemon juice. Mix gently to combine.
2. Form the mixture into 4 patties. Sprinkle ¼ teaspoon of flour on top of each patty.

3. Place the crab cakes in the air fryer. Spray them with cooking oil. Cook for 10 minutes.
4. Serve.
5. Ingredient tip: You can make your own crab seasoning using ¼ teaspoon of each of the following: celery salt, black pepper, red pepper flakes, and paprika.

Nutrition

Calories 176 | Fat 8g | Saturated Fat 1g | Cholesterol 101mg | Sodium 826mg | Carbohydrates 12g | Fiber 1g | Protein 15g

532. Oyster Club Sandwich

🕐 Prep Time 10 m | 🕐 Cooking Time 15 m | 4 Servings

Ingredients

- 2 slices of white bread
- 1 tbsp. softened butter
- ½ lb. shelled oyster
- 1 small capsicum

For Barbeque Sauce:

- ¼ tbsp. Worcestershire sauce
- ½ tsp. olive oil
- ½ flake garlic crushed

- ¼ cup chopped onion
- ¼ tsp. mustard powder
- 1 tbsp. tomato ketchup
- ½ tbsp. sugar
- ¼ tbsp. red chili sauce
- ½ cup water.
- Salt and black pepper to taste

Directions

1. Remove the edges of the slices of bread. Now cut the slices horizontally. Cook the ingredients for the sauce and wait till it thickens. Now, add the oyster to the sauce and stir till it obtains the flavors.
2. Roast the capsicum and peel the skin off. Cut the capsicum into slices. Mix all ingredients together and apply it to the bread slices. Pre-heat the Breville smart oven for 5 minutes at 300 Fahrenheit. Open the basket of the Fryer and place the prepared classic sandwiches in it such that no two classic sandwiches are touching each other. Now keep the fryer at 250 degrees for around 15 minutes.
3. Turn the classic sandwiches in between the cooking process to cook both slices. Serve the Classic Sandwiches with tomato ketchup or mint sauce.

Nutrition

Calories 407 | Fat 10 g | Protein 31 g | Sugar 11 g

533. Seafood Pizza

🕐 Prep Time 10 m | 🕐 Cooking Time 22 m | 4 Servings

Ingredients

- One pizza base
- Grated pizza cheese (mozzarella cheese preferably) for topping
- Some pizza topping sauce
- Use cooking oil for brushing and topping purposes

Ingredients for topping:

- 2 onions chopped
- 2 cups mixed seafood

- 2 capsicums chopped
- 2 tomatoes that have been deseeded and chopped
- 1 tbsp. (optional) mushrooms/corns
- 2 tsp. pizza seasoning
- Some cottage cheese that has been cut into small cubes (optional)

Directions

1. Put the pizza base in a pre-heated Breville smart oven for around 5 minutes. (Preheated to 340 Fahrenheit). Take out the base. Pour some pizza sauce on top of the base at the center. Using a spoon, spread the sauce over the base making sure that you leave some gap around the circumference. Grate some mozzarella cheese and sprinkle it over the sauce layer. Take all the vegetables and the seafood and mix them in a bowl. Add some oil and seasoning.
2. Also, add some salt and pepper according to taste. Mix them properly. Put this topping over the layer of cheese on the pizza. Now sprinkle some more grated cheese and pizza seasoning on top of this layer. Preheat the Breville smart oven at 250 Fahrenheit for around 5 minutes.
3. Open the fry basket and place the pizza inside. Close the basket and keep the fryer at 170 degrees for another 10 minutes. If you feel that it is undercooked, you may put it at the same temperature for another 2 minutes or so.

Nutrition

Calories 116 | Fat 23 g | Protein 29 g | Sugar 1 g

534. Cilantro-Lime Fried Shrimp

🕐 Prep Time 10 m | 🕐 Cooking Time 10 m | 4 Servings

Ingredients

- ½ cup chopped fresh cilantro
- Juice of 1 lime
- 1 pound of raw shrimp, deveined and peeled with tails on or off
- 1 egg
- ½ cup all-purpose flour

- ¾ cup bread crumbs
- Salt
- Pepper
- Cooking oil
- ½ cup cocktail sauce (optional)

Directions

1. Place the shrimp in a plastic bag. Add the cilantro and lime juice. Seal the bag. Shake to combine. Marinate in the refrigerator for 30 minutes.
2. In a small bowl, beat the egg. In another small bowl, place the flour. Place the crumbs of bread in a third small bowl, and season with salt and pepper to taste.
3. Spray cooking oil to the air fryer basket.
4. Remove the shrimp from the plastic bag. Wet each in the flour, then the egg, and then the bread crumbs.
5. Place the shrimp in the air fryer. It is okay to stack them. Spray the shrimp with cooking oil. Cook for 4 minutes.
6. Open the air fryer and flip the shrimp. I recommend flipping individually instead of shaking to keep the breading intact. Cook for another 4 minutes, or until crisp.
7. Cool before serving. Serve with cocktail sauce if desired.
8. Substitution tip: You can reduce the number of calories and fat in this recipe by substituting an egg white for the whole egg.
9. Preparation tip: If using frozen shrimp, place the shrimp in a large bowl of cold water to thaw. Let the shrimp soak for 15 minutes.

Nutrition

Calories 254 | Fat 4g | Saturated Fat 1g | Cholesterol 221mg | Sodium 334mg | Carbohydrates 27g | Fiber 1g | Protein 29g

535. Salmon Croquettes

⏱ Prep Time 5 m | ⏱ Cooking Time 15 m | 6 Servings

Ingredients

- 1 (14.75-ounce) can Alaskan pink salmon, drained and bones removed
- 1 egg, beaten
- ½ cup bread crumbs
- 2 scallions, diced
- 1 teaspoon garlic powder
- Salt
- Pepper
- Cooking oil

Directions

1. In a large bowl, combine the salmon, beaten egg, bread crumbs, and scallions. Season with the garlic powder and salt and pepper to taste.
2. Form the mixture into 6 patties.
3. Place the croquettes in the air fryer. It is okay to stack them. Spray the croquettes with cooking oil. Cook for 7 minutes.
4. Open the air fryer and flip the patties. Cook for an additional 3 to 4 minutes, or until golden brown.

Nutrition

Calories 142 | Fat 6g | Saturated Fat 1g | Cholesterol 58mg | Sodium 135mg | Carbohydrates 7g | Fiber 1g | Protein 16g

536. Beer-Battered Fish and Chips

⏱ Prep Time 5 m | ⏱ Cooking Time 30 m | 4 Servings

Ingredients

- 2 eggs
- 1 cup malty beer, such as Pabst Blue Ribbon
- 1 cup all-purpose flour
- ½ cup cornstarch
- 1 teaspoon garlic powder
- Salt
- Pepper
- Cooking oil
- 4 (4-ounce) cod fillets

Directions

1. Beat the eggs with the beer. In another medium bowl, combine the flour and cornstarch, and season with the garlic powder and salt and pepper to taste.
2. Spray cooking oil to the air fryer basket.
3. Dip each cod fillet in the flour and cornstarch mixture and then in the egg and beer mixture. Dip the cod in the flour and cornstarch a second time.
4. Place the cod in the air fryer. Do not stack. Cook in batches. Spray with cooking oil. Cook for 8 minutes.
5. Open the air fryer and flip the cod. Cook for an additional 7 minutes.
6. Remove the cooked cod from the air fryer, then repeat steps 4 and 5 for the remaining fillets.
7. Serve with Classic French Fries or prepare air-fried frozen fries. Frozen fries will need to be cooked for 18 to 20 minutes at 400°F.
8. Cool before serving.

Nutrition

Calories 325 | Fat 4g | Saturated Fat 1g | Cholesterol 137mg | Sodium 144mg | Carbohydrates 41g | Fiber 1g | Protein 26g

537. Firecracker Shrimp

⏱ Prep Time 10 m | ⏱ Cooking Time 10 m | 4 Servings

Ingredients

For the shrimp:
- 1-pound raw shrimp, peeled and deveined
- Salt
- Pepper
- 1 egg
- ½ cup all-purpose flour
- ¾ cup panko bread crumbs
- Cooking oil

For the firecracker sauce:
- ⅓ cup sour cream
- 2 tablespoons Sriracha
- ¼ cup sweet chili sauce

Directions

To make the shrimp:
1. Add the shrimp with pepper and salt to taste.
2. In a small bowl, beat the egg.
3. In another small bowl, place the flour. In another small bowl, add the panko bread crumbs.
4. Spray cooking oil to the air fryer basket.
5. Dip the shrimp in the flour, then the egg, and then the bread crumbs.
6. Place the shrimp in the fryer basket. It is okay to stack them. Spray the shrimp with cooking oil. Cook for 4 minutes.
7. Open the air fryer and flip the shrimp. I recommend flipping individually instead of shaking to keep the breading intact.
8. Cook for another 4 minutes or until crisp.

To make the firecracker sauce:
9. While the shrimp is cooking, make the firecracker sauce: In a small bowl, combine the sour cream, Sriracha, and sweet chili sauce. Mix well.
10. Serve with the shrimp.

Substitution tip: In place of sour cream, use nonfat plain Greek yogurt. This saves calories and fat while providing 5.5 grams of additional protein.

Nutrition

Calories 266 | Fat 6g | Saturated Fat 3g | Cholesterol 229mg | Sodium 393mg | Carbohydrates 23g | Fiber 1g | Protein 27g

538. oconut Shrimp

⏲ Prep Time 10 m | ⏲ Cooking Time 10 m | 4 Servings

Ingredients

- 1-pound raw shrimp, peeled and deveined
- 1 egg
- ¼ cup all-purpose flour
- ⅓ cup shredded unsweetened coconut

- ¼ cup panko bread crumbs
- Salt
- Pepper
- Cooking oil

Directions

1. Dry the shrimp with paper towels.
2. In a small bowl, beat the egg. In another small bowl, place the flour. In a third small bowl, combine the coconut and panko bread crumbs, and season with salt and pepper to taste. Mix well.
3. Spray cooking oil to the air fryer basket.
4. Dip the shrimp in the flour, then the egg, and then the coconut and bread crumb mixture.
5. Place the shrimp in the air fryer. It is okay to stack them. Cook for 4 minutes.
6. Open the air fryer and flip the shrimp. I recommend flipping individually instead of shaking, which keeps the breading intact. Cook for another 4 minutes or until crisp.
7. Cool before serving.

Nutrition

Calories 182 | Fat 6g | Saturated Fat 3g | Cholesterol 246mg | Sodium 780mg | Carbohydrates 8g | Fiber 1g | Protein 24g

539. Spicy Shrimp Kebab

⏲ Prep Time 25 m | ⏲ Cooking Time 20 m | 4 Servings

Ingredients

- 1 ½ pounds jumbo shrimp, cleaned, shelled, and deveined
- 1-pound cherry tomatoes
- 2 tablespoons butter, melted
- 1 tablespoons sriracha sauce
- Sea salt and ground black pepper

- 1/2 teaspoon dried oregano
- 1/2 teaspoon dried basil
- 1 teaspoon dried parsley flakes
- 1/2 teaspoon marjoram
- 1/2 teaspoon mustard seeds

Directions

1. Toss all elements in a mixing bowl until the shrimp and tomatoes are covered on all sides.
2. Let the wooden skewers be soaked in water for 15 minutes.
3. Thread the jumbo shrimp and cherry tomatoes onto skewers. Cook in the preheated air fryer at a temperature of 400 degrees F for 5 minutes, working with batches.

Nutrition

Calories 247 | Fat 8.4g | Carbohydrates 6g | Protein 36.4g | Sugar 3.5g | Fiber 1.8g

540. Lemon-Pepper Tilapia with Garlic Aioli

⏲ Prep Time 5 m | ⏲ Cooking Time 15 m | 4 Servings

Ingredients

For the tilapia:

- 4 tilapia fillets
- 1 tablespoon extra-virgin olive oil
- 1 teaspoon paprika
- 1 teaspoon garlic powder
- 1 teaspoon dried basil
- Lemon-pepper seasoning (such as McCormick Perfect Pinch Lemon & Pepper Seasoning)

For the garlic aioli:

- 2 garlic cloves, minced
- 1 tablespoon mayonnaise
- 1 teaspoon extra-virgin olive oil
- Juice of ½ lemon
- Salt
- Pepper

Directions

1. To make the tilapia:
2. Coat the fish with the olive oil. Season with the paprika, garlic powder, dried basil, and lemon-pepper seasoning.
3. Place the fish in the air fryer. It is okay to stack the fish. Cook for 8 minutes.
4. Open the fryer and flip the fish. Cook for an additional 7 minutes.
5. To make the garlic aioli:
6. In a bowl, put together the garlic, mayonnaise, olive oil, lemon juice, and salt and pepper to taste. Whisk well to combine.
7. Serve alongside the fish.

Nutrition

Calories 155 | Total fat: 7g | Saturated fat: 1g | Cholesterol: 56mg | Sodium: 107mg | Carbohydrates: 2g | Fiber: 0g | Protein: 21g

541. Blackened Shrimp

⏲ Prep Time 5 m | ⏲ Cooking Time 10 m | 4 Servings

Ingredients

- 1-pound raw shrimp, peeled and deveined
- 1 teaspoon paprika
- ½ teaspoon dried oregano
- ½ teaspoon cayenne pepper

- Juice of ½ lemon
- Salt
- Pepper
- Cooking oil

Directions

1. Put the shrimp in a sealable plastic bag then add the paprika, oregano, cayenne pepper, lemon juice, and salt and pepper to taste. Seal the bag. Shake well to combine.
2. Spray a grill pan or the air fryer basket with cooking oil.
3. Place the shrimp in the air fryer. It is okay to stack the shrimp. Cook for 4 minutes.
4. Open the air fryer then after that, shake the basket. Heat for an additional of 3 to 4 minutes, or til the shrimp has blackened.
5. Cool before serving.

Nutrition

Calories 101 | Total fat: 2g | Saturated fat: 2g | Cholesterol: 168mg | Sodium: 759mg | Carbohydrates: 0g | Fiber: 0g | Protein: 21g

542. Fried Catfish Nuggets

⏰ Prep Time 5 m | ⏰ Cooking Time 40 m | 4 Servings

Ingredients

- 1-pound catfish fillets, cut into 1-inch chunks
- ½ cup seasoned fish fry breading mix (such as Louisiana Fish Fry)
- Cooking oil

Directions

1. Rinse and thoroughly dry the catfish. Pour the seasoned fish fry breading mix into a sealable plastic bag and add the catfish. (You may need to use two bags depending on the size of your nuggets.) Seal the bag and shake to coat the fish with breading evenly.
2. Spray cooking oil to the air fryer basket.
3. Transfer the catfish nuggets to the air fryer. Do not overcrowd the basket. You may need to cook the nuggets in two batches. Spray the nuggets with cooking oil. Cook for 10 minutes.
4. Open the air fryer then after that, shake the basket. Cook for an additional of 8 to 10 minutes, or till the fish is crisp.
5. If necessary, remove the cooked catfish nuggets from the air fryer, then repeat steps 3 and 4 for the remaining fish.
6. Cool before serving.

Ingredient tip: You may be able to purchase catfish nuggets at the fish counter of your grocery store. It's worth asking!

Cooking tip: Open the air fryer and check in on the fish a few times throughout the cooking process. When the fish has turned golden brown on both sides, it has finished cooking.

Nutrition

Calories 183 | Total fat: 9g | Saturated fat: 2g | Cholesterol: 56mg | Sodium: 199mg | Carbohydrates: 5g | Fiber: 0g | Protein: 19g

543. Crumbed Fish Fillets with Tarragon

⏰ Prep Time 25 m | ⏰ Cooking Time 20 m | 4 Servings

Ingredients

- 2 eggs, beaten
- 1 2 teaspoon tarragon
- 4 fish fillets, halved
- 2 tablespoons dry white wine
- 1/3 cup parmesan cheese, grated
- 1 teaspoon seasoned salt
- 1/3 teaspoon mixed peppercorns
- 1/2 teaspoon fennel seed

Directions

1. Add the parmesan cheese, salt, peppercorns, fennel seeds, and tarragon to your food processor; blitz for about 20 seconds.
2. Drizzle fish fillets with dry white wine. Dump the egg into a shallow dish.
3. Now, coat the fish fillets with the beaten egg on all sides; then, coat them with the seasoned cracker mix.
4. Air-fry at 345 degrees F for about 17 minutes.

Nutrition

305 calories | 17.7g fat | 6.3g Carbohydrates | 27.2g protein | 0.3g sugar | 0.1g fiber

544. Cornmeal Shrimp Po'boy

⏰ Prep Time 10 m | ⏰ Cooking Time 10 m | 4 Servings

Ingredients

For the shrimp:
- 1-pound shrimp, peeled and deveined
- 1 egg
- ½ cup flour
- ¾ cup cornmeal
- Salt
- Pepper
- Cooking oil

For the remoulade:
- ½ cup mayonnaise
- 1 teaspoon mustard (I use Dijon)
- 1 teaspoon Worcestershire
- 1 teaspoon minced garlic
- Juice of ½ lemon
- 1 teaspoon Sriracha
- ½ teaspoon Creole seasoning

For the po'boys:
- 4 rolls
- 2 cups shredded lettuce
- 8 slices tomato

Directions

1. To make the shrimp:
2. Dry the shrimp with paper towels.
3. In a small bowl, beat the egg. In another small bowl, place the flour. Place the cornmeal in a third small bowl, and season with salt and pepper to taste.
4. Spray cooking oil to the air fryer basket.
5. Dip the shrimp in the flour, then the egg, and then the cornmeal.
6. Place the shrimp in the air fryer. Cook for 4 minutes. Open the basket and flip the shrimp. Cook for another 4 minutes, or till crisp.
7. To make the remoulade:
8. While the shrimp is cooking, in a small bowl, combine the mayonnaise, mustard, Worcestershire, garlic, lemon juice, Sriracha, and Creole seasoning. Mix well.
9. To make the po'boys:
10. Split the rolls and spread them with the remoulade.
11. Let the shrimp cool slightly before assembling the po'boys.
12. Fill each roll with a quarter of the shrimp, ½ cup of shredded lettuce, and 2 slices of tomato. Serve.

Nutrition

Calories 483 | Total fat: 15g | Saturated fat: 2g | Cholesterol: 229mg | Sodium: 690mg | Carbohydrates: 58g | Fiber: 6g | Protein: 32g

545. Smoked and Creamed White Fish
🕐 Prep Time 20 m | 🕐 Cooking Time 15 m | 4 Servings

Ingredients

- 1/2 tablespoon yogurt
- 1/3 cup spring garlic, finely chopped
- Fresh chopped chives, for garnish
- 3 eggs, beaten
- 1/2 teaspoon dried dill weed
- 1 teaspoon dried rosemary
- 1/3 cup scallions, chopped

- 1/3 cup smoked white fish, chopped
- 1 ½ tablespoon crème Fraiche
- 1 teaspoon kosher salt
- 1 teaspoon dried marjoram
- 1/3 teaspoon ground black pepper, or more to taste
- Cooking spray

Directions

1. Firstly, spritz four oven-safe ramekins with cooking spray. Then, divide smoked whitefish, spring garlic, and scallions among greased ramekins.
2. Crack an egg into each ramekin; add the crème, yogurt, and all seasonings.

3. Now, air-fry approximately 13 minutes at 355 degrees f. Taste for doneness and eat warm garnished with fresh chives.

Nutrition

249 Calories | 22.1g Fat | 7.6g Carbohydrates | 5.3g Protein | 3.1g Sugars | 0.7g Fiber

546. Parmesan and Paprika Baked Tilapia
🕐 Prep Time 20 m | 🕐 Cooking Time 15 m | 6 Servings

Ingredients

- 1 cup parmesan cheese, grated
- 1 teaspoon paprika
- 1 teaspoon dried dill weed
- 2 pounds tilapia fillets

- 1/3 cup mayonnaise
- 1/2 tablespoon lime juice
- Salt and ground black pepper, to taste

Directions

1. Mix the mayonnaise, parmesan, paprika, salt, black pepper, and dill weed until everything is thoroughly combined.
2. Then, drizzle tilapia fillets with the lime juice.

3. Cover each fish fillet with parmesan mayo mixture; roll them in parmesan paprika mixture. Bake to your fryer at 335 for about 10 minutes. Serve and eat warm.

Nutrition

294 calories | 16.1g fat | 2.7g Carbohydrates | 35.9g protein | 0.1g sugars | 0.2g fiber

547. Tangy Cod Fillets
🕐 Prep Time 20 m | 🕐 Cooking Time 15 m | 2 Servings

Ingredients

1 ½ tablespoons sesame oil
1/2 heaping teaspoon dried parsley flakes
1/3 teaspoon fresh lemon zest, finely grated
2 medium-sized cod fillets

1 teaspoon sea salt flakes
A pinch of salt and pepper
1/3 teaspoon ground black pepper, or more to savor
1/2 tablespoon fresh lemon juice

Directions

1. Set the air fryer to cook at 375 degrees f. Season each cod fillet with sea salt flakes, black pepper, and dried parsley flakes. Now, drizzle them with sesame oil.
2. Place the seasoned cod fillets in a single layer at the bottom of the cooking basket; air-fry approximately 10 minutes.

3. While the fillets are cooking, prepare the sauce by mixing the other ingredients. Serve cod fillets on four individual plates garnished with the creamy citrus sauce.

Nutrition

291 calories | 11.1g fat | 2.7g Carbohydrates | 41.6g protein | 1.2g sugars | 0.5g fiber

548. Fish and Cauliflower Cakes
🕐 Prep Time 2 h 20 m | 🕐 Cooking Time 13 m | 4 Servings

Ingredients

- 1/2-pound cauliflower florets
- 1/2 teaspoon English mustard
- 2 tablespoons butter, room temperature
- 1/2 tablespoon cilantro, minced

- 2 tablespoons sour cream
- 2 ½ cups cooked white fish
- Salt and freshly cracked black pepper, to savor

Directions

1. Boil the cauliflower until tender. Then, purée the cauliflower in your blender. Transfer to a mixing dish.
2. Now, stir in the fish, cilantro, salt, and black pepper.

3. Add the sour cream, English mustard, and butter; mix until everything's well incorporated. Using your hands, shape into patties.
4. Place inside the refrigerator for around two hours. Cook in your fryer for 13 minutes at 395 degrees F. Serve with some extra English mustard.

Nutrition

285 calories | 15.1g fat | 4.3g Carbohydrates | 31.1g protein | 1.6g sugars | 1.3g fiber

549. Prawn Momo's Recipe
⏱ Prep Time 15 m | ⏱ Cooking Time 25 m | 4 Servings

Ingredients:

- 1 ½ cup all-purpose flour
- ½ tsp. salt
- 5 tbsp. water
- For filling:
- 2 cups minced prawn
- 2 tbsp. oil
- 2 tsp. ginger-garlic paste
- 2 tsp. soya sauce
- 2 tsp. vinegar

Directions:

1. Squeeze the dough and cover it with plastic wrap and set aside. Next, cook the ingredients for the filling and try to ensure that the prawn is covered well with the sauce. Roll the dough and cut it into a square.

2. Place the filling in the center. Now, wrap the dough to cover the filling and pinch the edges together. Pre heat the smart oven at 200° F for 5 minutes. Place the wontons in the fry basket and close it. Let them cook at the same temperature for another 20 minutes. Recommended sides are chili sauce or ketchup.

Nutrition:

Calories: 300 | Fat: 11g| Protein: 35g| Sugar: 6

550. Fish club Classic Sandwich
⏱ Prep Time 10 m | ⏱ Cooking Time 20 m | 3 Servings

Ingredients:

- 2 slices of white bread
- 1 tbsp. softened butter
- 1 tin tuna
- 1 small capsicum
- For Barbeque Sauce:
- ¼ tbsp. Worcestershire sauce
- ½ tsp. olive oil
- ½ flake garlic crushed
- ¼ cup chopped onion
- ¼ tsp. mustard powder
- ½ tbsp. sugar
- ¼ tbsp. red chili sauce
- 1 tbsp. tomato ketchup
- ½ cup water.
- Salt and black pepper to taste

Directions:

1. Remove the edges of the slice bread. Now cut the slices horizontally. Cook the ingredients for the sauce and wait till it thickens. Now, add the fish to the sauce and stir till it obtains the flavors. Roast the capsicum and peel the skin off. Cut the capsicum into slices.

2. Mix the ingredients and apply it to the bread slices. Pre-heat the smart oven for 5 minutes at 300 Fahrenheit.

3. Open the basket of the Fryer and place the prepared Classic Sandwiches in it such that no two Classic Sandwiches are touching each other. Now keep the fryer at 250 degrees for around 15 minutes. Turn the Classic Sandwiches in between the cooking process to cook both slices. Serve the Classic Sandwiches with tomato ketchup or mint sauce.

Nutrition:

Calories: 232 | Fat: 22g| Protein: 25g| Sugar: 5

551. Prawn Fried Baked Pastry
⏱ Prep Time 15 m | ⏱ Cooking Time 35 m | 4 Servings

Ingredients:

- 1 ½ cup all-purpose flour
- 2 tbsp. unsalted butter
- 2 green chilies that are finely chopped or mashed
- Add a lot of water to make the dough stiff and firm
- A pinch of salt to taste
- 1 lb. prawn
- ¼ cup boiled peas
- ½ tsp. cumin
- 1 tsp. coarsely crushed coriander
- 1 dry red chili broken into pieces
- A small amount of salt (to taste)
- ½ tsp. dried mango powder
- 1 tsp. powdered ginger
- ½ tsp. red chili power.
- 1-2 tbsp. coriander.

Directions:

1. You will first need to make the outer covering. In a large bowl, add the flour, butter and enough water to knead it into dough that is stiff. Transfer this to a container and leave it to rest for five minutes. Place a pan on medium flame and add the oil. Roast the mustard seeds and once roasted, add the coriander seeds and the chopped dry red chilies. Add all the dry ingredients for the filling and mix the ingredients well.

2. Add a little water and continue to mix the ingredients. Make small balls from the dough and wrap them. Cut the wrapped dough in half and spread a little water on the edges to help you fold the

halves into a cone. Add the filling to the cone and close the samosa. Preheat the Smart Oven for about 5 to 6 minutes at 300 Fahrenheit. Place all the samosas in the frying pan and close the basket properly.

3. Keep the Smart Oven at 200 degrees for another 20 to 25 minutes. Around half point, open the basket and turn the samosas for even cooking. After that, fry at 250 degrees for about 10 minutes to give them the desired golden-brown color. Serve hot. Recommended sides are tamarind or mint sauce.

Nutrition:

Calories: 132 | Fat: 1g | Protein: 15g | Sugar: 9

552. Fish Spicy Lemon Kebab

⏱ Prep Time 10 m | ⏱ Cooking Time 25 m | 3 Servings

Ingredients:

- 1 lb. boneless fish roughly chopped
- 3 onions chopped
- 5 green chilies-roughly chopped
- 1 ½ tbsp. ginger paste
- 1 ½ tsp garlic paste
- 1 ½ tsp salt
- 3 tsp lemon juice
- 2 tsp garam masala
- 4 tbsp. chopped coriander
- 3 tbsp. cream
- 2 tbsp. coriander powder
- 4 tbsp. fresh mint chopped
- 3 tbsp. chopped capsicum
- 3 eggs
- 2 ½ tbsp. white sesame seeds

Directions:

1. Take all the ingredients mentioned under the first heading and mix them in a bowl. Grind them thoroughly to make a smooth paste. Take the eggs in a different bowl and beat them. Add a pinch of salt and leave them aside. Take a flat plate and in it mix the sesame seeds and breadcrumbs. Mold the mixture of fish into small balls and flatten them into round and flat kebabs. Dip these kebabs in the egg and salt mixture and then in the mixture of breadcrumbs and sesame seeds. Leave these kebabs in the fridge for an hour or so to set.

2. Pre heat the smart oven at 160 degrees Fahrenheit for around 5 minutes. Place the kebabs in the basket and let them cook for another 25 minutes at the same temperature. Turn the kebabs over in between the cooking process to get a uniform cook. Serve the kebabs with mint sauce.

Nutrition:

Calories: 432| Fat: 3g |Protein: 22g |Sugar: 1

553. Fish Oregano Fingers

⏱ Prep Time 10 m | ⏱ Cooking Time 25 m | 4 Servings

Ingredients:

- ½ lb. firm white fish fillet cut into Oregano Fingers
- 1 tbsp. lemon juice
- 2 cups of dry breadcrumbs
- 1 cup oil for frying
- 1 ½ tbsp. ginger-garlic paste
- 3 tbsp. lemon juice
- 2 tsp salt
- 1 ½ tsp pepper powder
- 1 tsp red chili
- 3 eggs
- 5 tbsp. corn flour
- 2 tsp tomato ketchup

Directions:

1. Rub a little lemon juice on the Oregano Fingers and set aside. Wash the fish after an hour and pat dry. Make the marinade and transfer the Oregano Fingers into the marinade. Allow them to dry on a plate for fifteen minutes. Now cover the Oregano Fingers with the crumbs and set aside to dry for fifteen minutes.

2. Pre heat the smart oven at 160 degrees Fahrenheit for 5 minutes or so. Keep the fish in the fry basket now and close it properly.

3. Let the Oregano Fingers cook at the same temperature for another 25 minutes. In between the cooking process, toss the fish once in a while to avoid burning the food. Serve either with tomato ketchup or chili sauce. Mint sauce also works well with the fish.

Nutrition:

Calories: 234 |Fat: 3g| Protein: 35g| Sugar: 0

554. Prawn Grandma's Easy to Cook Wontons

⏱ Prep Time 5 m | ⏱ Cooking Time 20 m | 3 Servings

Ingredients:

- 1 ½ cup all-purpose flour
- ½ tsp. salt
- 5 tbsp. water
- 2 cups minced prawn
- 2 tbsp. oil
- 2 tsp. ginger-garlic paste
- 2 tsp. soya sauce
- 2 tsp. vinegar

Directions:

1. Squeeze out the dough and cover it with plastic wrap and set it aside. Then cook the ingredients for the filling and try to make sure the shrimp are well coated with the sauce. Roll out the dough and place the filling in the center.

2. Now, roll the dough to cover the filling and bring the edges together. Preheat the Smart Oven to 200 ° F for 5 minutes. Place the wontons in the pan and close it. Let them cook at equal temperature for another 20 minutes. Recommended sides are chili sauce or ketchup.

Nutrition:

Calories: 423| Fat: 20g |Protein: 20g |Sugar: 2

555. Tuna Sandwich

☉ Prep Time 5 m | ☉ Cooking Time 15 m | 4 Servings

Ingredients:

- 2 slices of white bread
- 1 tbsp. softened butter
- 1 tin tuna
- 1 small capsicum
- For Barbeque Sauce:
- ¼ tbsp. Worcestershire sauce
- ½ tsp. olive oil
- ¼ tsp. mustard powder

- ½ flake garlic crushed
- ¼ cup chopped onion
- ½ tbsp. sugar
- 1 tbsp. tomato ketchup
- ½ cup water.
- ¼ tbsp. red chili sauce
- Salt and black pepper to taste

Directions:

1. Remove the edges of the slices bread. Now cut the slices horizontally. Cook the ingredients for the sauce and wait till it thickens. Now, add the lamb to the sauce and stir till it obtains the flavors. Roast the capsicum and peel the skin off. Cut the capsicum into slices. Mix the ingredients and apply it to the bread slices.

2. Pre-heat the smart oven for 5 minutes at 300 Fahrenheit. Open the basket of the Fryer and place the prepared Classic Sandwiches in it such that no two Classic Sandwiches are touching each other. Now keep the fryer at 250 degrees for around 15 minutes. Turn the Classic Sandwiches in between the cooking process to cook both slices. Serve the Classic Sandwiches with tomato ketchup or mint sauce.

Nutrition:

Calories: 460 |Fat: 1g| Protein: 11g |Sugar: 5

556. Salmon Tandoor

☉ Prep Time 10 m | ☉ Cooking Time 20 m | 5 Servings

Ingredients:

- 2 lb. boneless salmon filets
- 1st Marinade:
- 3 tbsp. vinegar or lemon juice
- 2 or 3 tsp. paprika
- 1 tsp. black pepper
- 1 tsp. salt
- 3 tsp. ginger-garlic paste
- 2nd Marinade:
- 1 cup yogurt

- 4 tsp. tandoori masala
- 2 tbsp. dry fenugreek leaves
- 1 tsp. black salt
- 1 tsp. chat masala
- 1 tsp. garam masala powder
- 1 tsp. red chili powder
- 1 tsp. salt
- 3 drops of red color

Directions:

1. Make the first marinade and soak the fileted salmon in it for four hours. While this is happening, make the second marinade and soak the salmon in it overnight to let the flavors blend. Pre heat the smart oven at 160 degrees Fahrenheit for 5 minutes.

2. Put the oregano fingers in the pan and close it. Let them cook at the equal temperature for another 15 minutes or so. Toss the oregano fingers well so that they are well cooked. Serve with mint sauce.

Nutrition:

Calories: 187 |Fat: 2g |Protein: 30g|Sugar: 0

557. Shrimp Momo's Recipe

☉ Prep Time 10 m | ☉ Cooking Time 20 m | 7 Servings

Ingredients:

- 1 ½ cup all-purpose flour
- ½ tsp. salt
- 5 tbsp. water
- For filling:
- 2 cups minced shrimp

- 2 tbsp. oil
- 2 tsp. ginger-garlic paste
- 2 tsp. soya sauce
- 2 tsp. vinegar

Directions:

1. Squeeze out the dough and cover it with plastic wrap and set it aside. Then cook the ingredients for the filling and try to make sure the shrimp are well coated with the sauce. Roll up the dough and cut it into squares. Place the filling in the center.

2. Now, roll the dough to cover the filling and bring the edges together. Preheat the Smart Oven to 200 ° F for 5 minutes. Place the wontons in the pan and close it. Let them cook at the equal temperature for another 20 minutes. Recommended sides are chili sauce or ketchup.

Nutrition:

Calories: 103 |Fat: 0g| Protein: 34g| Sugar: 11

558. Carp Best Homemade Croquette
⏱ Prep Time 15 m | ⏱ Cooking Time 25 m | 3 Servings

Ingredients:

- 1 lb. Carp filets
- 3 onions chopped
- 5 green chilies-roughly chopped
- 1 ½ tbsp. ginger paste
- 1 ½ tsp garlic paste
- 1 ½ tsp salt
- 3 tsp lemon juice
- 2 tsp garam masala
- 4 tbsp. chopped coriander
- 3 tbsp. cream
- 2 tbsp. coriander powder
- 4 tbsp. fresh mint chopped
- 3 tbsp. chopped capsicum
- 3 eggs
- 2 ½ tbsp. white sesame seeds

Directions:

1. Take all the ingredients mentioned under the first heading and mix them in a bowl. Grind them thoroughly to make a smooth paste. Take the eggs in a different bowl and beat them. Add a pinch of salt and leave them aside. Mold the fish mixture into small balls and flatten them into round and flat Best Homemade Croquettes. Dip these Best Homemade Croquettes in the egg and salt mixture and then in the mixture of breadcrumbs and sesame seeds.

2. Leave these Best Homemade Croquettes in the fridge for an hour or so to set. Pre heat the smart oven at 160 degrees Fahrenheit for around 5 minutes. Place the Best Homemade Croquettes in the basket and let them cook for another 25 minutes at the same temperature. Turn the Best Homemade Croquettes over in between the cooking process to get a uniform cook. Serve the Best Homemade Croquettes with mint sauce.

Nutrition:
Calories: 209 | Fat: 4g | Protein: 49g | Sugar: 1

559. Salmon fries
⏱ Prep Time 5 m | ⏱ Cooking Time 15 m | 3 Servings

Ingredients:

- 1 lb. boneless salmon filets
- 2 cup dry breadcrumbs
- 2 tsp. oregano
- 2 tsp. red chili flakes
- 1 ½ tbsp. ginger-garlic paste
- 4 tbsp. lemon juice
- 2 tsp. salt
- 1 tsp. pepper powder
- 1 tsp. red chili powder
- tbsp. corn flour
- 4 eggs

Directions:

1. Mix each and every ingredients for the marinade and put the salmon fillets and leave to rest overnight. Mix the toast, oregano, and red chili flakes well and place the marinated oregano fingers in this mixture. Cover with cling film and leave until served.

2. Preheat the smart oven to 160 degrees Fahrenheit for 5 minutes.

3. Put the oregano fingers in the pan and close it. Let them cook at the equal temperature for another 15 minutes or so. Toss the oregano fingers well so that they are well cooked.

Nutrition:
Calories: 300 | Fat: 3g | Protein: 16g | Sugar: 2

560. Oyster Club Sandwich
⏱ Prep Time 10 m | ⏱ Cooking Time 15 m | 4 Servings

Ingredients:

- 2 slices of white bread
- 1 tbsp. softened butter
- ½ lb. shelled oyster
- 1 small capsicum
- For Barbeque Sauce:
- ¼ tbsp. Worcestershire sauce
- ½ tsp. olive oil
- ½ flake garlic crushed
- ¼ cup chopped onion
- ¼ tsp. mustard powder
- 1 tbsp. tomato ketchup
- ½ tbsp. sugar
- ¼ tbsp. red chili sauce
- ½ cup water.
- Salt and black pepper to taste

Directions:

1. Remove the edges of the slice bread. Now cut the slices horizontally. Cook the ingredients for the sauce and wait till it thickens. Now, add the oyster to the sauce and stir till it obtains the flavors.

2. Roast the capsicum and peel the skin off. Cut the capsicum into slices. Mix all ingredients together and apply it to the bread slices. Pre-heat the smart oven for 5 minutes at 300 Fahrenheit. Open the basket of the Fryer and place the prepared Classic Sandwiches in it such that no two Classic Sandwiches are touching each other. Now keep the fryer at 250 degrees for around 15 minutes.

3. Turn the Classic Sandwiches in between the cooking process to cook both slices. Serve the Classic Sandwiches with tomato ketchup or mint sauce.

Nutrition:
Calories: 407 | Fat: 10g | Protein: 31g | Sugar: 11

561. Cheese Carp Fries

⏱ Prep Time 15 m | ⏱ Cooking Time 25 m | 4 Servings

Ingredients:

- 1 lb. carp Oregano Fingers
- Ingredients for the marinade:
- 1 tbsp. olive oil
- 1 tsp. mixed herbs
- ½ tsp. red chili flakes

- A pinch of salt to taste
- 1 tbsp. lemon juice
- For the garnish:
- 1 cup melted cheddar cheese

Directions:

1. Take all the ingredients mentioned in the heading "For the marinade" and mix well. Cook the oregano fingers and dip them in the marinade.
2. Preheat the smart oven for about 5 minutes at 300 Fahrenheit. Take the basket out of the fryer and place the tent in it. Close the basket. Now keep the fryer at 220 Fahrenheit for 20 to 25 minutes.
3. Between the processes, toss the potatoes two or three times so they are cooked through. Towards the rare end of the cooking process (the last 2 minutes or so), sprinkle the melted cheddar cheese over the potatoes and serve hot.

Nutrition:

Calories: 502 | Fat: 22g | Protein: 40g | Sugar: 14g

562. Seafood Pizza

⏱ Prep Time 10 m | ⏱ Cooking Time 22 m | 4 Servings

Ingredients:

- One pizza base
- Grated pizza cheese (mozzarella cheese preferably) for topping
- Some pizza topping sauce
- Use cooking oil for brushing and topping purposes
- Ingredients for topping:
- 2 onions chopped

- 2 cups mixed seafood
- 2 capsicums chopped
- 2 tomatoes that have been deseeded and chopped
- 1 tbsp. (optional) mushrooms/corns
- 2 tsp. pizza seasoning
- Some cottage cheese that has been cut into small cubes (optional)

Directions:

1. Put the pizza base in a pre-heated smart oven for around 5 minutes. (Pre heated to 340 Fahrenheit). Take out the base. Pour some pizza sauce on top of the base at the center. Using a spoon spread the sauce over the base making sure that you leave some gap around the circumference. Grate some mozzarella cheese and sprinkle it over the sauce layer. Take all the vegetables and the seafood and mix them in a bowl. Add some oil and seasoning.
2. Also add some salt and pepper according to taste. Mix them properly. Put this topping over the layer of cheese on the pizza. Now sprinkle some more grated cheese and pizza seasoning on top of this layer. Pre heat the smart oven at 250 Fahrenheit for around 5 minutes.
3. Open the fry basket and place the pizza inside. Close the basket and keep the fryer at 170 degrees for another 10 minutes. If you feel that it is undercooked you may put it at the same temperature for another 2 minutes or so.

Nutrition:

Calories: 116 | Fat: 23g | Protein: 29g | Sugar: 1

563. Lobster Grandma's Easy to Cook Wontons

⏱ Prep Time 10 m | ⏱ Cooking Time 20 m | 4 Servings

Ingredients:

- 1 ½ cup all-purpose flour
- ½ tsp. salt
- tbsp. water
- For filling:
- 2 cups minced lobster
- 2 tbsp. oil
- 2 tsp. ginger-garlic paste
- 2 tsp. soya sauce
- 2 tsp. vinegar

Directions:

1. Squeeze out the dough and cover it with plastic wrap and set it aside. Then cook the ingredients for the filling and try to make sure the lobster is well coated with the sauce.
2. Roll out the dough and place the filling in the center. Now, roll the dough to cover the filling and bring the edges together.
3. Preheat the Smart Oven to 200 ° F for 5 minutes. Place the wontons in the pan and close it. Let them cook at the equal temperature for another 20 minutes. Recommended sides are chili sauce or ketchup.

Nutrition:

Calories: 600 | Fat: 13g Protein: 21g Sugar 9g

564. Cilantro-Lime Fried Shrimp
Prep Time 10 m | Cooking Time 10 m | 4 Servings

Ingredients:

- ½ cup chopped fresh cilantro
- Juice of 1 lime
- 1 pound of raw shrimp, deveined and peeled with tails on or off
- 1 egg
- ½ cup all-purpose flour
- ¾ cup bread crumbs
- Salt
- Pepper
- Cooking oil
- ½ cup cocktail sauce (optional)

Directions:

1. Place the shrimp in a plastic bag. Add the cilantro and lime juice. Seal the bag. Shake to combine. Marinate in the refrigerator for 30 minutes.
2. In a small bowl, beat the egg. In another small bowl, place the flour. Place the crumbs of bread in a third small bowl, and season with salt and pepper to taste.
3. Spray cooking oil to the air fryer basket.
4. Remove the shrimp from the plastic bag. Wet each in the flour, then the egg, and then the bread crumbs.
5. Place the shrimp in the air fryer. It is okay to stack them. Spray the shrimp with cooking oil. Cook for 4 minutes.
6. Open the air fryer and flip the shrimp. I recommend flipping individually instead of shaking to keep the breading intact. Cook for another 4 minutes, or until crisp.
7. Cool before serving. Serve with cocktail sauce if desired.
8. Substitution tip: You can reduce the number of calories and fat in this recipe by substituting an egg white for the whole egg.
9. Preparation tip: If using frozen shrimp, place the shrimp in a large bowl of cold water to thaw. Let the shrimp to soak for 15 minutes.

Nutrition:

Calories: 254 | Fat: 4g | Cholesterol: 221mg | Sodium: 334mg | Carbo 27g | Fiber: 1g | Protein: 29g

565. Salmon Croquettes
Prep Time 5 m | Cooking Time 15 m | 6 Servings

Ingredients:

- 1 (14.75-ounce) can Alaskan pink salmon, drained and bones removed
- 1 egg, beaten
- ½ cup bread crumbs
- 2 scallions, diced
- 1 teaspoon garlic powder
- Salt
- Pepper
- Cooking oil

Directions:

1. In a large bowl, combine the salmon, beaten egg, bread crumbs, and scallions. Season with the garlic powder and salt and pepper to taste.
2. Form the mixture into 6 patties.
3. Place the croquettes in the air fryer. It is okay to stack them. Spray the croquettes with cooking oil. Cook for 7 minutes.
4. Open the air fryer and flip the patties. Cook for an additional 3 to 4 minutes, or until golden brown.
5. Serve.

Nutrition:

Calories: 142 | Fat: 6g | Cholesterol: 58mg | Sodium: 135mg | Carbo 7g | Fiber: 1g | Protein: 16g

566. Beer-Battered Fish and Chips
Prep Time 5 m | Cooking Time 30 m | 4 Servings

Ingredients:

- 2 eggs
- 1 cup malty beer, such as Pabst Blue Ribbon
- 1 cup all-purpose flour
- ½ cup cornstarch
- 1 teaspoon garlic powder
- Salt
- Pepper
- Cooking oil
- (4-ounce) cod fillets

Directions:

1. Beat the eggs with the beer. In another medium bowl, combine the flour and cornstarch, and season with the garlic powder and salt and pepper to taste.
2. Spray cooking oil to the air fryer basket.
3. Dip each cod fillet in the flour and cornstarch mixture and then in the egg and beer mixture. Dip the cod in the flour and cornstarch a second time.
4. Place the cod in the air fryer. Do not stack. Cook in batches. Spray with cooking oil. Cook for 8 minutes.
5. Open the air fryer and flip the cod. Cook for an additional 7 minutes.
6. Remove the cooked cod from the air fryer, then repeat steps 4 and 5 for the remaining fillets.
7. Serve with Classic French Fries or prepare air-fried frozen fries. Frozen fries will need to be cooked for 18 to 20 minutes at 400°F.

Nutrition:

Calories: 325 | Fat: 4g | Cholesterol: 137mg | Sodium: 144mg | Carbo 41g | Fiber: 1g | Protein: 26g

567. Firecracker Shrimp

⏱ Prep Time 10 m | ⏱ Cooking Time 10 m | 4 Servings

Ingredients:

For the shrimp:

- 1-pound raw shrimp, peeled and deveined
- Salt
- Pepper
- 1 egg
- ½ cup all-purpose flour

- ¾ cup panko bread crumbs
- Cooking oil

For the firecracker sauce:

1. 1/3 cup sour cream
2. tablespoons Sriracha
3. ¼ cup sweet chili sauce

Directions:

1. To make the shrimp
2. Add the shrimp with pepper and salt to taste.
3. In a small bowl, beat the egg.
4. In another small bowl, place the flour. In another small bowl, add the panko bread crumbs.
5. Spray cooking oil to the air fryer basket.
6. Dip the shrimp in the flour, then the egg, and then the bread crumbs.
7. Place the shrimp in the fryer basket. It is okay to stack them. Spray the shrimp with cooking oil. Cook for 4 minutes.
8. Open the air fryer and flip the shrimp. I recommend flipping individually instead of shaking to keep the breading intact.
9. Cook for another 4 minutes or until crisp.
10. To make the firecracker sauce
11. While the shrimp is cooking, make the firecracker sauce: In a small bowl, combine the sour cream, Sriracha, and sweet chili sauce. Mix well.
12. Serve with the shrimp.
13. Substitution tip: In place of sour cream, use nonfat plain Greek yogurt. This saves calories and fat while providing 5.5 grams additional protein.

Nutrition:

Calories: 266 | Fat: 6g | Cholesterol: 229mg | Sodium: 393mg | Carbo 23g | Fiber: 1g | Protein: 27g

568. Crab Cakes

⏱ Prep Time 5 m | ⏱ Cooking Time 10 m | 4 Servings

Ingredients:

- ounces jumbo lump crabmeat
- 1 tablespoon Old Bay Seasoning
- 1/3 cup bread crumbs
- ¼ cup diced red bell pepper
- ¼ cup diced green bell pepper

- 1 egg
- ¼ cup mayonnaise
- Juice of ½ lemon
- 1 teaspoon flour
- Cooking oil

Directions:

1. In a bowl, combine the crab meat, Old Bay Seasoning, bread crumbs, red bell pepper, green bell pepper, egg, mayo, and lemon juice. Mix gently to combine.
2. Form the mixture into 4 patties. Sprinkle ¼ teaspoon of flour on top of each patty.
3. Place the crab cakes in the air fryer. Spray them with cooking oil. Cook for 10 minutes.
4. Serve.
5. Ingredient tip: You can make your own crab seasoning using ¼ teaspoon of each of the following: celery salt, black pepper, red pepper flakes, and paprika.

Nutrition:

Calories: 176 | Fat: 8g | Cholesterol: 101mg | Sodium: 826mg | Carbo 12g | Fiber: 1g | Protein: 15g

569. Coconut Shrimp

⏱ Prep Time 10 m | ⏱ Cooking Time 10 m | 4 Servings

Ingredients:

- 1-pound raw shrimp, peeled and deveined
- 1 egg
- ¼ cup all-purpose flour
- 1/3 cup shredded unsweetened coconut

- ¼ cup panko bread crumbs
- Salt
- Pepper
- Cooking oil

Directions:

1. Dry the shrimp with paper towels.
2. In a small bowl, beat the egg. In another small bowl, place the flour. In a third small bowl, combine the coconut and panko bread crumbs, and season with salt and pepper to taste. Mix well.
3. Spray cooking oil to the air fryer basket.
4. Dip the shrimp in the flour, then the egg, and then the coconut and bread crumb mixture.
5. Place the shrimp in the air fryer. It is okay to stack them. Cook for 4 minutes.
6. Open the air fryer and flip the shrimp. I recommend flipping individually instead of shaking, which keeps the breading intact. Cook for another 4 minutes or until crisp.

Nutrition:

Calories: 182 | Fat: 6g | Cholesterol: 246mg | Sodium: 780mg | Carbo 8g | Fiber: 1g | Protein: 24g

570. Lemon-Pepper Tilapia with Garlic Aioli
Prep Time 5 m | Cooking Time 15 m | 4 Servings

Ingredients:

- For the tilapia
- tilapia fillets
- 1 tablespoon extra-virgin olive oil
- 1 teaspoon paprika
- 1 teaspoon garlic powder
- 1 teaspoon dried basil
- Lemon-pepper seasoning (such as McCormick Perfect Pinch Lemon & Pepper Seasoning)

- For the garlic aioli
- 2 garlic cloves, minced
- 1 tablespoon mayonnaise
- 1 teaspoon extra-virgin olive oil
- Juice of ½ lemon
- Salt
- Pepper

Directions:

1. To make the tilapia
2. Coat the fish with the olive oil. Season with the paprika, garlic powder, dried basil, and lemon-pepper seasoning.
3. Place the fish in the air fryer. It is okay to stack the fish. Cook for 8 minutes.
4. Open the fryer and flip the fish. Cook for an additional 7 minutes.
5. To make the garlic aioli
6. In a bowl, put together the garlic, mayonnaise, olive oil, lemon juice, and salt and pepper to taste. Whisk well to combine.
7. Serve alongside the fish.
8. Variation tip: This recipe can be made gluten-free by using gluten-free mayonnaise; be sure to check the label.
9. Ingredient tip: You can make your own lemon-pepper seasoning using the juice of ½ lemon and pepper to taste.
10. Preparation tip: If using frozen tilapia, the best way to thaw it is in a covered bowl in the refrigerator, overnight. You can keep the fish in a sealed plastic bag as well and submerge the bag in cold water for 15 minutes or till thawed.

Nutrition:

Calories: 155 | Fat: 7g | Cholesterol: 56mg | Sodium: 107mg | Carbo 2g | Fiber: 0g | Protein: 21g

571. Blackened Shrimp
Prep Time 5 m | Cooking Time 10 m | 4 Servings

Ingredients:

- 1-pound raw shrimp, peeled and deveined
- 1 teaspoon paprika
- ½ teaspoon dried oregano
- ½ teaspoon cayenne pepper

- Juice of ½ lemon
- Salt
- Pepper
- Cooking oil

Directions:

1. Put the shrimp in a sealable plastic bag then add the paprika, oregano, cayenne pepper, lemon juice, and salt and pepper to taste. Seal the bag. Shake well to combine.
2. Spray a grill pan or the air fryer basket with cooking oil.
3. Place the shrimp in the air fryer. It is okay to stack the shrimp. Cook for 4 minutes.
4. Open the air fryer then after that, shake the basket. Heat for an additional 3 to 4 minutes, or til the shrimp has blackened.
5. Cool before serving.
6. Variation tip: This shrimp is delicious over a green salad with avocado. Dress it with a simple cilantro-lime vinaigrette made from chopped fresh cilantro, lime juice, and olive oil.

Nutrition:

Calories: 101 | Fat: 2g | Cholesterol: 168mg | Sodium: 759mg | Carbo 0g | Fiber: 0g | Protein: 21g

572. Spicy Shrimp Kebab
Prep Time 25 m | Cooking Time 20 m | 4 Servings

Ingredients:

- 1 ½ pounds jumbo shrimp, cleaned, shelled and deveined
- 1-pound cherry tomatoes
- 2 tablespoons butter, melted
- 1 tablespoons Sirach sauce
- Sea salt and ground black pepper

- 1 2 teaspoon dried oregano
- 1 2 teaspoon dried basil
- 1 teaspoon dried parsley flakes
- 1 2 teaspoon marjoram
- 1 2 teaspoon mustard seeds

Directions:

1. Toss all elements in a mixing bowl until the shrimp and tomatoes are covered on all sides.
2. Let the wooden skewers be soaked in water for 15 minutes.
3. Thread the jumbo shrimp and cherry tomatoes onto skewers. Cook in the preheated air fryer at a temperature of 400 degrees f for 5 minutes, working with batches.

Nutrition:

247 Calories | 8.4g Fat | 6g Carbo | 36.4gProtein | 3.5g Sugars | 1.8g Fiber

573. Fried Catfish Nuggets

⏱ Prep Time 5 m | ⏱ Cooking Time 40 m | 4 Servings

Ingredients:

- 1-pound catfish fillets, cut into 1-inch chunks
- ½ cup seasoned fish fry breading mix (such as Louisiana Fish Fry)
- Cooking oil

Directions:

1. Rinse and thoroughly dry the catfish. Pour the seasoned fish fry breading mix into a sealable plastic bag and add the catfish. (You may need to use two bags depending on the size of your nuggets.) Seal the bag and shake to coat the fish with breading evenly.
2. Spray cooking oil to the air fryer basket.
3. Transfer the catfish nuggets to the air fryer. Do not overcrowd the basket. You may need to cook the nuggets in two batches. Spray the nuggets with cooking oil. Cook for 10 minutes.
4. Open the air fryer then after that, shake the basket. Cook for an additional of 8 to 10 minutes, or till the fish is crisp.
5. If necessary, remove the cooked catfish nuggets from the air fryer, then repeat steps 3 and 4 for the remaining fish.
6. Cool before serving.
7. Ingredient tip: You may be able to purchase catfish nuggets at the fish counter of your grocery store. It's worth asking!
8. Cooking tip: Open the air fryer and check in on the fish a few times throughout the cooking process. When the fish has turned golden brown on both sides, it has finished cooking.

Nutrition:

Calories: 183 | Fat: 9g | Cholesterol: 56mg | Sodium: 199mg | Carbo 5g | Fiber: 0g | Protein: 19g

574. Cornmeal Shrimp Po'boy

⏱ Prep Time 10 m | ⏱ Cooking Time 10 m | 4 Servings

Ingredients:

- For the shrimp
- 1-pound shrimp, peeled and deveined
- 1 egg
- ½ cup flour
- ¾ cup cornmeal
- Salt
- Pepper
- Cooking oil
- For the remoulade
- ½ cup mayonnaise
- 1 teaspoon mustard (I use Dijon)
- 1 teaspoon Worcestershire
- 1 teaspoon minced garlic
- Juice of ½ lemon
- 1 teaspoon Sriracha
- ½ teaspoon Creole seasoning
- For the po'boys
- rolls
- 2 cups shredded lettuce
- slices tomato

Directions:

1. To make the shrimp
2. Dry the shrimp with paper towels.
3. In a small bowl, beat the egg. In another small bowl, place the flour. Place the cornmeal in a third small bowl, and season with salt and pepper to taste.
4. Spray cooking oil to the air fryer basket.
5. Dip the shrimp in the flour, then the egg, and then the cornmeal.
6. Place the shrimp in the air fryer. Cook for 4 minutes. Open the basket and flip the shrimp. Cook for another 4 minutes, or till crisp.
7. To make the remoulade
8. While the shrimp is cooking, in a small bowl, combine the mayonnaise, mustard, Worcestershire, garlic, lemon juice, Sriracha, and Creole seasoning. Mix well.
9. To make the po'boys
10. Split the rolls and spread them with the remoulade.
11. Let the shrimp cool slightly before assembling the po'boys.
12. Fill each roll with a quarter of the shrimp, ½ cup of shredded lettuce, and 2 slices of tomato. Serve.

Nutrition:

Calories: 483 | Fat: 15g | Cholesterol: 229mg | Sodium: 690mg | Carbo 58g | Fiber: 6g | Protein: 32g

575. Crumbed Fish Fillets with Tarragon

⏱ Prep Time 25 m | ⏱ Cooking Time 20 m | 4 Servings

Ingredients:

- 2 eggs, beaten
- 1 2 teaspoon tarragon
- fish fillets, halved
- 2 tablespoons dry white wine
- 1 3 cup parmesan cheese, grated
- 1 teaspoon seasoned salt
- 1 3 teaspoon mixed peppercorns
- 1 2 teaspoon fennel seed

Directions:

1. Add the parmesan cheese, salt, peppercorns, fennel seeds, and tarragon to your food processor; blitz for about 20 seconds.
2. Drizzle fish fillets with dry white wine. Dump the egg into a shallow dish.
3. Now, coat the fish fillets with the beaten egg on all sides; then, coat them with the seasoned cracker mix.
4. Air-fry at 345 degrees f for about 17 minutes.

Nutrition:

305 calories | 17.7g fat | 6.3g Carbo | 27.2g protein | 0.3g sugars | 0.1g fiber

576. Smoked and Creamed White Fish
🕑 Prep Time 20 m | 🕑 Cooking Time 15 m | 4 Servings

Ingredients:

- 1 2 tablespoon yogurt
- 1 3 cup spring garlic, finely chopped
- Fresh chopped chives, for garnish
- eggs, beaten
- 1 2 teaspoon dried dill weed
- 1 teaspoon dried rosemary
- 1 3 cup scallions, chopped

- 1 3 cup smoked white fish, chopped
- 1 ½ tablespoons crème fraiche
- 1 teaspoon kosher salt
- 1 teaspoon dried marjoram
- 1 3 teaspoon ground black pepper, or more to taste
- Cooking spray

Directions:

1. Firstly, spritz four oven safe ramekins with cooking spray. Then, divide smoked whitefish, spring garlic, and scallions among greased ramekins.
2. Crack an egg into each ramekin; add the crème, yogurt and all seasonings.
3. Now, air-fry approximately 13 minutes at 355 degrees f. Taste for doneness and eat warm garnished with fresh chives.

Nutrition:

249 Calories | 22.1g Fat | 7.6g Carbo | 5.3g Protein | 3.1g Sugars | 0.7g Fiber

577. Parmesan and Paprika Baked Tilapia
🕑 Prep Time 20 m | 🕑 Cooking Time 15 m | 6 Servings

Ingredients:

- 1 cup parmesan cheese, grated
- 1 teaspoon paprika
- 1 teaspoon dried dill weed
- 2 pounds tilapia fillets

- 1 3 cup mayonnaise
- 1 2 tablespoon lime juice
- Salt and ground black pepper, to taste

Directions:

1. Mix the mayonnaise, parmesan, paprika, salt, black pepper, and dill weed until everything is thoroughly combined.
2. Then, drizzle tilapia fillets with the lime juice.
3. Cover each fish fillet with parmesan mayo mixture; roll them in parmesan paprika mixture. Bake to your fryer at 335 for about 10 minutes. Serve and eat warm.

Nutrition:

294 calories | 16.1g fat | 2.7g Carbo | 35.9g protein | 0.1g sugars | 0.2g fiber

578. Tangy Cod Fillets
🕑 Prep Time 20 m | 🕑 Cooking Time 15 m | 2 Servings

Ingredients:

- 1 ½ tablespoons sesame oil
- 1 2 heaping teaspoon dried parsley flakes
- 1 3 teaspoon fresh lemon zest, finely grated
- 2 medium-sized cod fillets

- 1 teaspoon sea salt flakes
- A pinch of salt and pepper
- 1 3 teaspoon ground black pepper, or more to savor
- 1 2 tablespoon fresh lemon juice

Directions:

1. Set the air fryer to cook at 375 degrees f. Season each cod fillet with sea salt flakes, black pepper and dried parsley flakes. Now, drizzle them with sesame oil.
2. Place the seasoned cod fillets in a single layer at the bottom of the cooking basket; air-fry approximately 10 minutes.
3. While the fillets are cooking, prepare the sauce by mixing the other ingredients. Serve cod fillets on four individual plates garnished with the creamy citrus sauce.

Nutrition:

291 calories | 11.1g fat | 2.7g Carbo | 41.6g protein | 1.2g sugars | 0.5g fiber

579. Fish and Cauliflower Cakes
🕑 Prep Time 2 h 20 m | 🕑 Cooking Time 13 m | 4 Servings

Ingredients:

- 1 2-pound cauliflower florets
- 1 2 teaspoon English mustard
- 2 tablespoons butter, room temperature
- 1 2 tablespoon cilantro, minced

- 2 tablespoons sour cream
- 2 ½ cups cooked white fish
- Salt and freshly cracked black pepper, to savor

Directions:

1. Boil the cauliflower until tender. Then, purée the cauliflower in your blender. Transfer to a mixing dish.
2. Now, stir in the fish, cilantro, salt, and black pepper.
3. Add the sour cream, English mustard, and butter; mix until everything's well incorporated. Using your hands, shape into patties.
4. Place inside the refrigerator for around two hours. Cook in your fryer for 13 minutes at 395 degrees f. Serve with some extra English mustard.

Nutrition:

285 calories | 15.1g fat | 4.3g Carbohydrates | 31.1g protein | 1.6g sugars

580. Crisp-fried Salmon

⏰ Prep Time 5 m | ⏰ Cooking Time 10 m | 2 Servings

Ingredients:

- ½ teaspoon thyme leaves
- 1 teaspoon brown sugar
- 2 tablespoons Whole grain mustard
- Salt and ground black pepper to taste
- 2 (6 oz.) salmon fillets
- 2 teaspoons extra-virgin olive oil
- 1 clove of garlic, minced

Directions:

1. Rub salmon with salt and pepper.
2. Using a small bowl, add the mustard, garlic, sugar, thyme and oil. Whisk to blend. Scatter the mixture on top of the salmon.
3. Arrange salmon in the air fryer basket and the set air fryer to 400 degrees F. Cook for 10 minutes until the salmon turns brown and crispy.
4. Serve and enjoy.

Nutrition: Calories 317 Carbohydrates: 10.33 g Fat: 14.38 g Protein: 36.66 g

581. Air Fryer Tuna Patties

⏰ Prep Time 15 m | ⏰ Cooking Time 10 m | 6 Servings

Ingredients:

- ½ teaspoon dried herbs: oregano, dill, basil, thyme or any combo
- 2-3 large eggs
- 15 ounces canned tuna, drained
- Zest of 1 medium lemon
- Freshly cracked black pepper to taste
- ½ cup bread crumbs
- 1 tablespoon lemon juice
- 3 tablespoons grated Parmesan cheese
- 3 tablespoons onion, minced
- 1 stalk of celery, finely chopped
- ½ teaspoon garlic powder
- Optional tartar sauce, ranch, lemon slices, mayonnaise for serving
- ¼ teaspoon kosher salt
- 2 lemon slices for garnish

Directions:

1. Combine eggs, Parmesan cheese, bread crumbs, lemon zest, lemon juice, garlic powder, onions, celery, and dried herbs in a bowl. Season with salt and pepper to taste. Gently fold in the tuna and stir thoroughly to combine.
2. Form the mixture into 3" x 3" patties. This recipe makes about 10 patties. If the patties turn out too soft, chill in the fridge for about an hour to harden.
3. Line each layer of the air fryer basket with parchment paper and spray with olive oil before arranging patties inside in a single layer to avoid overcrowding.
4. Lay the second layer of the air fryer basket with patties on top of the first layer. Also, spray with olive oil.
5. Place the 2-layered air fryer basket inside the instant pot unit and cover with the air fryer lid.
6. Air-fry for about 10 minutes at 360 degrees F, flipping halfway. Spray with olive oil after flipping.
7. Garnish with lemon slices and serve with your favorite sauce.

Nutrition: Calories 68 Fat 2.29 g Carbohydrates 2.33 g Protein 9.63 g

582. Air Fryer Garlic-lemon Shrimp

⏰ Prep Time 10 m | ⏰ Cooking Time 15 m | 3 Servings

Ingredients:

- 1 lb. raw shrimp, peeled and deveined
- ¼ teaspoon garlic powder
- 2 lemon wedges, juiced
- 1 tablespoon vegetable oil or spray for coating
- Salt and black pepper to taste
- A pinch of parsley, minced
- Optional: a dash of chili flakes

Directions:

1. Add shrimp in a bowl. Pour oil and toss to combine.
2. Add garlic powder and season with salt and pepper. Toss to coat evenly.
3. Place shrimp in a single-layered instant pot air fryer basket.
4. Attach to the instant pot duo crisp air fryer lid and securely cover the pot.
5. Set to air frying mode and cook at 400 degrees F for 10-14 minutes, flipping halfway for even cooking.
6. Once the timer is off or when the shrimp is cooked, transfer to a plate and squeeze lemon juice over it.
7. Sprinkle with parsley or chili flakes or both.
8. Serve while hot.

Nutrition: Calories 243 Fat 4.34 g Carbohydrates 4.11 g Protein - 46.93 g

583. Air-fried Shrimps with Lemon

⏰ Prep Time 10 m | ⏰ Cooking Time 15 m | 3 Servings

Ingredients:

- ¼ teaspoon garlic powder
- 1 pound raw shrimps, peeled and deveined
- A dash of vegetable oil or cooking spray, for coating
- A pinch of parsley or chili flakes, optional
- Black pepper and salt to taste
- 2 lemon wedges, juiced

Directions:

1. In a bowl, combine shrimps with oil and add salt, pepper and garlic. Toss thoroughly to mix well.
2. Place shrimps in the air fryer basket and insert the basket inside the instant pot. Attach the air fryer lid and set to air-fry at 400 degrees F for 10-14 minutes. Gently shake the air fryer basket to flip halfway through cooking.
3. Once done, transfer the shrimp dish to a bowl and drizzle lemon juice over it.
4. Sprinkle parsley or chili flakes on top and serve hot.

Nutrition: Calories 117 Fat 1.66 g Carbohydrates 2.07 g Protein 23.46 g

584. Air Fried White Fish with Garlic & Lemon

⏲ Prep Time 5 m | ⏲ Cooking Time 10 m | 2 Servings

Ingredients:

- Freshly cracked black pepper to taste
- ½ teaspoon lemon powder
- 12 ounces tilapia fillets or white fish
- 1 tablespoon freshly chopped parsley
- ½ teaspoon garlic powder
- 4 lemon wedges
- ½ teaspoon onion powder, optional
- Salt to taste

Directions:

1. Cleanse and pat dry fish fillets and make sure to coat it with the olive oil and season with onion powder, garlic powder and lemon powder. Season with salt and pepper. Make sure fillets are evenly coated.
2. Line air fryer basket with parchment paper and lightly grease with cooking spray.
3. Arrange fish on top, adding few lemon wedges. Insert the air fryer basket to the instant pot duo crisp and attach the air fryer lid. Secure lock and air-fry at 360 degrees F for about 6-12 minutes or until fish can be flaked. Expect thicker fillets to take longer time to cook so adjust cooking time.
4. Sprinkle chopped parsley on the cooked dish and serve immediately with roasted lemon wedges.

Nutrition: Calories 308 Fat 16.47 g Carbohydrates 6.88 g Protein 33.08 g

585. Air-fried Crumbed Fish

⏲ Prep Time 10 m | ⏲ Cooking Time 12 m | 4 Servings

Ingredients:

- ¼ cup vegetable oil
- 1 egg, beaten
- 4 flounder fillets
- 1 cup dry bread crumbs
- 1 lemon, sliced

Directions:

1. In a mixing bowl, mix oil and bread crumbs. Stir to combine.
2. Dredge fillets into the egg, shaking off excess liquid.
3. Dip fillets into the bread crumbs to coat evenly on all sides.
4. Lay coated fillets on the air fryer basket and place inside the instant pot. Attach the air fryer lid and cook at 350 degrees F for about 12 minutes. Flip halfway through cooking.
5. Garnish with lemon slices and serve.

Nutrition:
Calories 357 Carbohydrates 22.5g Fat 17.7g Protein 26.9g

586. Air Fryer Coconut Shrimp

⏲ Prep Time 30 m | ⏲ Cooking Time 10 m | 4 Servings

Ingredients:

- 2 large eggs
- ½ teaspoon ground black pepper
- 3 cups panko bread crumbs
- ½ cup all-purpose flour
- ¼ cup honey
- 3 cups flaked coconut, unsweetened
- 12 ounces medium-sized raw shrimps, peeled and deveined
- 1 Serrano chili, thinly sliced
- ½ teaspoon kosher salt, divided
- 2 teaspoons fresh cilantro, chopped
- ¼ cup lime juice

Directions:

1. Combine pepper and flour in a shallow dish. Stir to combine.
2. In another shallow dish, add the lightly beaten eggs.
3. Add coconut and bread crumbs in another shallow dish.
4. Dredge shrimps in the shallow dish with flour. Shake lightly to remove excess flour.
5. One by one, dip shrimp to the dish with the egg mixture. Allow excess liquid to drip off. Transfer to the third dish with coconut-bread crumbs mixture. Coat shrimps evenly on all sides and lay them inside the 2-layered air fryer basket of the instant pot duo crisp lined with parchment paper. Coat shrimps with cooking spray, avoiding overcrowding.
6. Place the air fryer inside the instant pot and cover with air fryer lid. Lock in place and air fry at 200 degrees F for about 3 minutes, flip and cook for another 3 minutes. Season with salt to taste.
7. In a small bowl, combine honey, Serrano chili and lime juice. Whisk together for the dip.
8. Serve crisp shrimps sprinkled with cilantro and the sauce for dipping.

Nutrition:
Calories 247 Fat 9.1 g Carbohydrates 27.6 g Protein 13.8 g

587. Air Fryer Fish Sticks
⏱ Prep Time 10 m | ⏱ Cooking Time 10 m | 4 Servings

Ingredients
- ½ cup all-purpose flour
- 1 lb. white fish fillet, tilapia or cod
- 1 large egg
- ½ cup Parmesan cheese, grated
- ½ cup panko bread crumbs
- 1 teaspoon paprika
- 1 tablespoon parsley flakes
- 1 teaspoon black pepper
- Cooking spray

Directions:
1. Cleanse fish and pat dry with paper towels. Cut into 1"x3" sticks.
2. Prepare 3 shallow dishes. Put flour in the first dish. Beat egg in the second dish and mix Parmesan cheese, panko bread crumbs and seasonings in the third dish.
3. Coat fish sticks evenly with flour and then dip to the dish with beaten eggs. Shake off excess liquid. Dip in the seasoned bread crumbs to coat and shake off excess bread crumbs.
4. Line air fryer basket with parchment paper and spray cooking oil.
5. Arrange fish sticks on the air fryer basket and spray cooking oil on top before putting inside the instant pot. Cover with the air fryer lid and air fry at 400 degrees F for 5 minutes. Flip fish sticks after the timer ended and cook for an additional 5 minutes.
6. Serve in a platter.

Nutrition:
Calories 208 Carbohydrates 16.5.g Fat 4.1g Protein 26.3g

588. Lobster Tails with Lemon-garlic Butter
⏱ Prep Time 10 m | ⏱ Cooking Time 10 m | 2 Servings

Ingredients:
- 4 tablespoons Butter
- 2 (4 oz.) lobster tails
- 1 teaspoon lemon zest
- 1 teaspoon fresh parsley, chopped
- 1 clove of garlic, minced and grated
- 2 lemon wedges
- Salt and ground black pepper to taste

Directions:
1. Use kitchen shears to cut the lobster tails lengthwise through the center hard shell and flesh but not through the other side of the shell.
2. Spread tails apart and place them in the air fryer basket with the lobster's meat facing upward.
3. Add butter, lemon zest and garlic to the instant pot duo and attach the pressure cooker lid. Set to sauté function for 30 seconds. Once the butter has melted and garlic is tender, transfer 2 tablespoons of butter mixture to the small bowl and brush onto the lobster. Season lobster with salt and pepper.
4. Place the air fryer into the instant pot. Detach the pressure cooker lid and attach the air fryer lid and air fry at 380 degrees F for 5-7 minutes.
5. Once done, remove the lobster tails from the air fryer and transfer to a platter. Spoon some melted butter from the inner pot over the dish and top with lemon wedges and parsley.

Nutrition:
Calories 318 Fat 25.8g Carbohydrates 3.3g Protein 18.1 g

589. Air Fried Shrimps
⏱ Prep Time 5 m | ⏱ Cooking Time 8 m | 4 Servings

Ingredients:
- 1 lb. large shrimps, peeled and deveined
- 1 tablespoon butter
- ½ teaspoon garlic granules
- 1 teaspoon lemon juice
- 1/8 cup Parmesan cheese, freshly grated
- 1/8 teaspoon salt

Directions:
1. Remove shrimps' tails.
2. Mix in garlic granules, lemon, and salt to a bowl with the melted butter.
3. Add the shrimps and toss to coat evenly on all sides.
4. Line the air fryer basket with parchment paper and place shrimps inside. Sprinkle Parmesan cheese over shrimps.
5. Place the air fryer basket inside the instant pot duo crisp and attach the air fryer lid.
6. Set to air fry at 400 degrees F for 8 minutes. Cook until shrimps become bright red and the meat is opaque.

Nutrition:
Calories 122 Carbohydrates 0.5g Fat 4.6g Protein 19.6g

590. Coconut Shrimp
🕐 Prep Time 10 m | 🕐 Cooking Time 15 m | 3 Servings

Ingredients:
- ½ cup flour
- 1 teaspoon kosher salt
- 3/4 cup plain breadcrumbs
- 1/2 cup shredded unsweetened coconut chopped
- ½ teaspoon white pepper
- 2 egg whites lightly beaten
- 1 pound Shrimp peeled and deveined
- Sweet chili sauce or duck sauce
- 2 teaspoon lime zest
- 1 teaspoon salt

Directions:
1. Combine flour, salt, and white pepper in a dish. Add egg whites to a second dish. Combine breadcrumbs, coconut, lime zest, and salt in a third shallow dish.
2. Dredge the shrimp first in a flour mixture, then in the egg mixture, place the shrimp in the mixture of breadcrumb and press the crumbs firmly on all sides.
3. Divide the coated shrimp onto the cooking trays, leaving space between each piece.
4. Place the drip pan in the Instant Pot Duo Crisp Air Fryer basket. Using the display panel, select the option Air Fry, then adjust the temperature to 400°F and the time to 12 minutes.
5. Press start to begin preheating by closing the lid of Instant Pot Duo Crisp Air Fryer basket.
6. Turn the food over after 5 minutes and switch the cooking trays so that the one that was in the top-most position is now in the bottom-most position, and vice-versa.
7. When the program is complete, remove the shrimp and serve with your choice of dipping sauce.

Nutrition:
Calories 406 Fat 9.2g Carbs 48.4g Protein 32.4g

591. Baked Shrimp Scampi
🕐 Prep Time 10 m | 🕐 Cooking Time 10 m | 4 Servings

Ingredients:
- 1 pound large shrimp
- 8 tablespoons butter
- 1 tablespoon minced garlic (use 2 for extra garlic flavor)
- 5 teaspoons white wine or cooking sherry
- 1/2 teaspoon salt
- 1/4 teaspoon cayenne pepper
- 1/4 teaspoon paprika
- 1/2 teaspoon onion powder
- 3/4 cup bread crumbs

Directions:
1. Using a mixing bowl, mix the bread crumbs with dry seasonings.
2. On the stovetop (or in the Instant Pot on sauté), melt the butter with the garlic and the white wine.
3. Remove from heat and add the shrimp and the bread crumb mix.
4. Transfer the mix to a casserole dish.
5. Choose the Bake operation and add food to the Instant Pot Duo Crisp Air Fryer. Close the lid and Bake at 350°F for 10 minutes or until they are browned. Serve and enjoy.

Nutrition:
Calories 422 Fat 26g Carbs 18g Protein 29 g

592. Air Fryer Marinated Salmon
🕐 Prep Time 5 m | 🕐 Cooking Time 12 m | 4 Servings

Ingredients:
- 4 salmon fillets or 1 1lb fillet cut into 4 pieces
- 1 tablespoon brown sugar
- ½ tablespoon Minced Garlic
- 6 tablespoons Soy Sauce
- ¼ cup Dijon Mustard
- 1 Green onions finely chopped

Directions:
1. Take a bowl and whisk together soy sauce, Dijon mustard, brown sugar, and minced garlic. Pour this mixture over salmon fillets, making sure that all the fillets are covered. Refrigerate and marinate for 20-30 minutes.
2. Remove salmon fillets from marinade and place them in greased or lined on the tray in the Instant Pot Duo Crisp Air Fryer basket, close the lid.
3. Select the Air Fry option and Air Fry for around 12 minutes at 400°F.
4. Remove from Instant Pot Duo Crisp Air Fryer and top with chopped green onions.

Nutrition:
Calories 267 Fat 11g Carbs 5g Protein 37g

593. Crusted Salmon Mix
🕐 Prep Time 10 m | 🕐 Cooking Time 15 m | 4 Servings

Ingredients:
- 1 cup of Pistachios (chopped)
- 4 salmon fillets
- 1/4 cup of lemon juice
- 2 tablespoon of honey
- 1 teaspoon of Dill (chopped)
- Salt and black pepper to taste
- 1 tablespoon of mustard

Directions:
1. Mix pistachios with mustard, honey, lemon juice, salt, black pepper and dill in a clean bowl.
2. Whisk properly and spread over the salmon.
3. Put inside your air fryer and cook at a temperature of 350 degrees F for 10 minutes.
4. Divide into different plates and serve with a side salad.

Nutrition:
Calories: 260 Fat: 5g Carbs: 5g Protein: 30g

594. Coconut Shrimp with Dip

⏱ Prep Time 10 m | ⏲ Cooking Time 9 m | 4 Servings

Ingredients:

- 1 pound deveined and peeled shrimp with tail on
- 2 eggs beaten
- ¼ cup Panko Breadcrumbs
- 1 teaspoon salt
- ¼ teaspoon black pepper
- ½ cup All-Purpose Flour
- ½ cup unsweetened shredded coconut
- Oil for spraying

Directions:

1. Clean and dry the shrimp. Set it aside.
2. Take 3 bowls. Put flour in the first bowl. Beat eggs in the second bowl. Mix coconut, breadcrumbs, salt, and black pepper in the third bowl.
3. Select the Air Fry option and adjust the temperature to 390°F. Push start and preheating will start.
4. Dip each shrimp in flour followed by the egg and then coconut mixture, ensuring shrimp is covered on all sides during each dip.
5. Once the preheating is done, place shrimp in a single layer on greased tray in the basket of the Instant Pot Duo Crisp Air Fryer.
6. Spray the shrimp with oil lightly, and then close the Air Fryer basket lid. Cook for around 4 minutes.
7. After 4 minutes, open the Air Fryer basket lid and flip the shrimp over. Respray the shrimp with oil, close the Air Fryer basket lid, and cook for five more minutes.
8. Remove shrimp from the basket and serve with Thai Sweet Chili Sauce.

Nutrition:

Calories 279 Fat 11g Carbs 17g Protein 28g

595. Air Fryer Fish

⏱ Prep Time 10 m | ⏲ Cooking Time 17 m | 4 Servings

Ingredients:

- 4-6 Whiting Fish fillets cut in half
- Oil to mist
- Fish Seasoning
- ¾ cup very fine cornmeal
- ¼ cup flour
- 2 teaspoon old bay
- 1 ½ teaspoon salt
- 1 teaspoon paprika
- ½ teaspoon garlic powder
- ½ teaspoon black pepper

Directions:

1. Put the ingredients for fish seasoning in a Zip lock bag and shake it well. Set aside.
2. Wash with running water and pat dry the fish fillets with paper towels. Make sure that they still are damp.
3. Place the fish fillets in a zip lock bag and shake until they are completely covered with seasoning.
4. Place the fillets on a baking rack to let any excess flour to fall off.
5. Grease the bottom of the Instant Pot Duo Crisp Air Fryer basket tray and place the fillets on the tray. Close the lid, select the Air Fry option and cook filets on 400°F for 10 minutes.
6. Open the Air Fryer lid and spray the fish with oil on the side facing up before flipping it over, ensure that the fish is fully coated. Flip and cook another side of the fish for 7 minutes. Remove the fish and serve.

Nutrition:

Calories 193 Fat 1g Carbs 27g Protein 19g

596. Shrimp and Cauliflower Mix

⏱ Prep Time 15 m | ⏲ Cooking Time 20 m | 2 Servings

Ingredients:

- 1 tablespoon of butter
- Cooking spray
- 1 riced cauliflower head
- 1 pound of shrimp (peeled and deveined)
- 1/4 cup of heavy cream
- 8 ounces of mushrooms (roughly chopped)
- A pinch of red pepper flakes
- Salt and black pepper to taste
- 2 garlic cloves (minced)
- 4 bacon (slices, cooked and crumbled)
- 1/2 cup of beef stock
- 1 tablespoon of parsley (finely chopped)
- 1 tablespoon of chives (chopped)

Directions:

1. Season shrimp with salt and pepper, spray with cooking oil, place in your air fryer and cook at 360 degrees F for 7 minutes.
2. Meanwhile, heat up a pan with butter over medium heat, add mushrooms, stir and cook for 3-4 minutes.
3. Add garlic, cauliflower rice, pepper flakes, stock, cream, chives, and parsley.
4. Sprinkle salt and pepper to taste.
5. Stir gently, and cook for some minutes before turning off the heat.
6. Divide the shrimp on different plates.
7. Then add cauliflower mix on the side.
8. Sprinkle bacon as topping.
9. Serve immediately.

Nutrition:

Calories: 74 Carbs: 7g Fat: 3g Protein: 0g

597. Stuffed Calamari Mix
Prep Time 10 m | Cooking Time 30 m | 4 Servings

Ingredients:

- 4 big calamari (tentacles separated and chopped and tubes reserved)
- 2 tablespoon of Parsley (chopped)
- 5 ounces of Kale (chopped)
- 2 garlic cloves (minced)
- 1 red bell pepper (chopped)
- 1 tablespoon of olive oil
- 2 ounces of canned tomato puree
- 1 yellow onion (chopped)
- Salt and black pepper to taste

Directions:

1. Heat up a pan containing oil over medium heat, and add onion and garlic.
2. Stir gently and cook for about 2 minutes.
3. Add bell pepper, tomato puree, calamari tentacles, kale, salt and pepper, stir gently.
4. Cook for about 10 minutes and remove the heat.
5. Stir gently and cook for 3 minutes.
6. Stuffed calamari tubes in the mix.
7. Hold firmly with toothpicks, then put in your air fryer.
8. Cook at a temperature of 360 degrees F for 20 minutes.
9. Divide the calamari on different plates
10. Sprinkle parsley all over and serve.

Nutrition:
Calories: 110 Fat: 5g Carbs: 15g Protein: 18g

598. Salmon and Avocado Sauce Mix using Air Fryer
Prep Time 10 m | Cooking Time 15 m | 4 Servings

Ingredients:

- 1 Avocado (pitted, peeled and chopped)
- 4 salmon fillets (boneless)
- 1/4 cup of Cilantro (chopped)
- 1/3 cup of coconut milk
- 1 tablespoon of lime juice
- 1 tablespoon of lime zest (grated)
- 1 teaspoon of onion powder
- 1 teaspoon of garlic powder
- Salt and black pepper to taste

Directions:

1. Season with salt, pepper and lime zest the salmon fillets then rub well.
2. Place inside the air fryer, cook at a temperature of 350 degrees F for 9 minutes, flipping once.
3. Then divide into different plates
4. Mix the avocado with cilantro, garlic powder, onion powder, lime juice, salt, pepper and coconut milk in a different bowl.
5. Blend properly, and drizzle over salmon
6. Serve immediately.

Nutrition:
Calories: 240 Fat: 5g Carbs: 11g Protein: 14g

599. Salmon and Orange Marmalade with Side Salad
Prep Time 10 m | Cooking Time 25 m | 4 Servings

Ingredients:

- 1 pound of wild salmon (skinless, boneless and cubed)
- 2 lemons (sliced)
- 1/4 cup of balsamic vinegar
- 1/4 cup of orange juice
- 1/3 cup of orange marmalade
- A pinch of salt
- Black pepper

Directions:

1. Heat up a pot containing vinegar over medium-high heat.
2. Then add marmalade as well as orange juice.
3. Stir gently, and bring to a simmer.
4. Cook for about a minute and remove the heat.
5. Thread salmon cubes and lemon slices on skewers, season with salt and black pepper to taste.
6. Brush them with half of the orange marmalade mix.
7. Place neatly in your air fryer's basket; then cook at 360 degrees F for about 3 minutes on each side.
8. Brush skewers with the remaining vinegar mix.
9. Divide into different plates
10. Serve immediately with a side salad and enjoy.

Nutrition:
Calories 240 Fat 9g Carbs 14g Protein 10g

600. Hot and Creamy Salmon
Prep Time 10 m | Cooking Time 15 m | 4 Servings

Ingredients:

- 4 salmon fillets (boneless)
- 1 tablespoon of olive oil
- Salt and black pepper to taste
- 1/3 cup of cheddar cheese (grated)
- 1 and 1/2 teaspoon of mustard
- 1/2 cup of coconut cream

Directions:

1. Season with salt and pepper the salmon, drizzle the oil and rub well.
2. Mix coconut cream with cheddar, mustard, salt and pepper in a bowl and stir well.
3. Transfer salmon to a pan that fits your air fryer, add coconut cream mix, introduce in your air fryer and cook at a temperature of 320 degrees F for about 10 minutes.
4. Divide into different plates
5. Serve immediately. Enjoy!

Nutrition:
Calories: 240 Fat: 3g Carbs: 12g Protein: 20g

601. Salmon with Lemon Dill Sauce

⏱ Prep Time 15 m | ⏱ Cooking Time 3 m | 4 Servings

Ingredients:

- Pressure cooker salmon
- 1 cup water
- 4 5- to 6- ounce skin-on center-cut salmon fillets 3/4 to 1 inch thick
- 1 lemon thinly sliced
- Salt and pepper
- Lemon dill sauce
- 3/4 cup dry white wine
- 3 Tablespoons chopped shallot
- 2 Tablespoons lemon juice
- 1/2 cup unsalted butter cut into 6 pieces
- 1 1/2 Tablespoons chopped fresh dill
- Salt and pepper to taste

Directions:

1. Pour water into the pressure cooker and place Silicone Pressure Cooker Rack on top.
2. Place salmon, skin side down on rack, in a single layer.
3. Sprinkle it with salt and pepper and cover with lemon slices.
4. Put the lid on the pot, and lock into place. Set valve to sealing.
5. Cook on "" (high pressure) for 3 minutes (5 minutes for frozen). It will take about 10 minutes for the pressure to build, then the countdown timer will begin.
6. Once the timer goes off, press the "Cancel" button, and quickly release the pressure.
7. While the salmon cooks, make the lemon dill sauce.
8. Boil wine, shallot and lemon juice in a medium saucepan over high heat until reduced to 1/4 cup, about 6 minutes. Reduce heat to low; add butter, 1 piece at a time, whisking until melted before adding more. Remove pan from heat. Stir in dill. Season to taste with salt and pepper.
9. Serve salmon fillets with lemon-dill sauce spooned on top.

Nutrition:

Calories: 255 Fat: 23g Carbohydrates: 5g Protein: 15g

602. Shrimp Boil

⏱ Prep Time 15 m | ⏱ Cooking Time 20 m | 4-6 Servings

Ingredients:

- 1 1/2 pounds baby red potatoes
- 1 (12.8-ounce) package smoked Andouille sausage, thinly sliced
- 1/2 medium sweet onion, chopped
- 4 teaspoons Old Bay seasoning, divided
- 1 tablespoon hot sauce
- 3 ears corn, halved
- 1 (16-ounce) pilsner or lager beer
- 1 1/2 pounds medium shrimp, shell-on
- 1/4 cup unsalted butter
- 3 cloves garlic, minced
- 2 tablespoons chopped fresh parsley leaves
- 1 lemon, cut into wedges

Directions:

1. Place potatoes, sausage, onion, 3 teaspoons Old Bay seasoning and hot sauce into a 6-qt Instant Pot. Stir until well combined. Top with corn and beer.
2. Select "Manual" setting; adjust pressure to high, and set time for 5 minutes. When finished cooking, quick-release pressure according to the manufacturer's directions.
3. Add shrimp. Select "Manual" setting; adjust pressure to high, and set time for 1 minute. When finished cooking, quick-release pressure according to the manufacturer's directions.
4. Melt butter in a small skillet over medium low heat. Stir in garlic and remaining 1 teaspoon Old Bay seasoning until fragrant, about 1-2 minutes.
5. Serve shrimp mixture immediately, drizzled with butter mixture, garnished with parsley and lemon, if desired.

Nutrition:

Calories: 385.3 Fat: 12.9g Carbohydrates: 38.8g Protein: 30.5g

603. Salmon with Chili-Lime Sauce
🕐 Prep Time 15 m | 🕐 Cooking Time 3 m | 2 Servings

Ingredients:
- Salmon
- 2 (5- to 7-ounce) fresh or frozen salmon fillets, 1 inch thick in the thickest part (can be skin on or off)
- 1 cup water
- 1/4 teaspoon table salt
- 1/4 teaspoon ground black pepper
- Optional nonstick oil spray
- Chili Lime Sauce
- 2 cloves garlic, minced (I use a garlic press)
- 1 tablespoon sriracha sauce
- 1 tablespoon freshly squeezed lime juice
- 1 tablespoon finely chopped fresh cilantro leaves (can be substituted with parsley)
- 2 teaspoons hot water
- 1/2 teaspoon smoked paprika
- 1/2 teaspoon ground cumin

Directions:
1. Stir all sauce ingredients together with a spoon in a small bowl until well-mixed. Set aside at room temperature to let the flavors develop while you prepare the salmon.
2. Pour water into the pressure cooker pot (I use a 6-quart Instant Pot). Place a steam rack inside the pot; I use the trivet that came with my Instant Pot, with its handles resting on the sides of the pot. If you are using skin-off salmon, spray the trivet with a nonstick oil spray to help release the salmon after cooking; this is usually not necessary for skin-on salmon which releases easily.
3. Place salmon fillets side-by-side on top of the trivet; if skin-on, place them skin side facing down. Evenly season the tops of fillets with salt and pepper.
4. Secure and seal the lid; make sure the knob is not set to venting. Select the "Steam" mode at "High Pressure". For Fresh Salmon: Set the cooking time to 3 minutes. For Frozen Salmon: Set the cooking time to 8 minutes.
5. After pressure cooking (as soon as the timer beeps), immediately do a quick pressure release to stop the cooking process to avoid overcooking the fish.
6. Uncover, and use a spatula and/or tongs to carefully transfer the salmon to serving plates. Cooked salmon is soft and flaky, and may fall apart or stick to the trivet if you're not careful.
7. Give the chili lime sauce a quick stir, and spoon it over salmon fillets. Serve immediately while warm, since the salmon will cool quickly.

Nutrition:
Calories: 310 Fat: 18g Carb: 3g Protein 28g

604. Tuna Noodle Casserole
🕐 Prep Time 15 m | 🕐 Cooking Time 20 m | 8 Servings

Ingredients
- 1/4 cup unsalted butter
- 8 ounces fresh mushrooms, sliced
- 1 medium onion, chopped
- 1 medium bell pepper, diced
- 1 teaspoon salt, divided
- 1 teaspoon pepper, divided
- 2 cloves garlic, minced
- 1/4 cup all-purpose flour
- 2 cups reduced-sodium chicken broth
- 2 cups half and half
- 8 ounces (4 cups) uncooked egg noodles
- 3 (5 ounces each) cans light tuna in water, drained
- 2 tablespoons lemon juice
- 2 cups shredded Colby-Jack cheese
- 2 cups frozen peas, thawed
- 2 cups crushed potato chips

Directions:
1. Select the "Sauté" setting on a 6-quart Instant Pot or electric pressure cooker. Add the butter. When the butter melts, add the mushrooms, onion, and sweet pepper. Cook, stirring, until the vegetables are tender, about 6-8 minutes. Season with 1/2 teaspoon of salt and 1/2 teaspoon of pepper. Add the garlic and cook for an additional minute.
2. Stir in the flour and cook for another minute. Gradually whisk in the chicken broth. Bring the mixture to a boil, stirring constantly, until it thickens slightly, about 1-2 minutes. Stir in the cream and the noodles.
3. Place the top on the Instant Pot and lock the lid. Make sure the vent is closed. Select the "Manual", adjust the pressure to high and set the time to 3 minutes.
4. When the time is finished, do a quick-release to release any remaining pressure.
5. Combine the tuna, lemon juice and the remaining 1/2 teaspoon salt and 1/2 teaspoon pepper in a small bowl.
6. Select the "Sauté" setting on the Instant Pot and stir in the tuna mixture, the cheese, and the peas. Cook for a few minutes, just until heated through.
7. Serve the tuna casserole topped with the crushed potato chips.

Nutrition:
Calories: 497 Fat: 28g Carbohydrates: 34g Protein: 30g

605. Seafood Gumbo

🕐 Prep Time 15 m | 🕐 Cooking Time 25 m | 8 Servings

Ingredients

- 24 ounces sea bass filets patted dry and cut into 2" chunks
- 3 tablespoons ghee or avocado oil
- 3 tablespoons Cajun seasoning or creole seasoning
- 2 yellow onions diced
- 2 bell peppers diced
- 4 celery ribs diced
- 28 ounces diced tomatoes
- 1/4 cup tomato paste
- 3 bay leaves
- 1 1/2 cups bone broth
- 2 pounds medium to large raw shrimp deveined
- Sea salt to taste
- Black pepper to taste

Directions:

1. Season the barramundi with some salt and pepper, and make sure they are as evenly coated as possible. Sprinkle half of the Cajun seasoning onto the fish and give it a stir- make sure it is coated well and set aside.
2. Put the ghee in the Instant Pot and push "Sauté". Wait until it reads "Hot" and add the barramundi chunks. Sauté for about 4 minutes, until it looks cooked on both sides. Use a slotted spoon to transfer the fish to a large plate.
3. Add the onions, pepper, celery and the rest of the Cajun seasoning to the pot and saute for 2 minutes until fragrant. Push "Cancel/Keep Warm". Add the cooked fish, diced tomatoes, tomato paste, bay leaves and bone broth to the pot and give it a nice stir. Put the lid back on the pot and set it to "Sealing." Push "Manual" and set the time for just 5 minutes! The Instant Pot will slowly build up to a high pressure point and once it reaches that point, the gumbo will cook for 5 minutes.
4. Once the 5 minutes have ended, push the "Keep warm/Cancel" button. Cautiously change the "Sealing" valve over to "Venting," which will manually release all of the pressure. Once the pressure has been released (this will take a couple of minutes), remove the lid and change the setting to "Sauté" again. Add the shrimp and cook for about 3-4 minutes, or until the shrimp have become opaque. Add some more sea salt and black pepper, to taste. Serve hot and top off with some cauliflower rice and chives.

Nutrition:

Calories: 343 Carbohydrates: 9g Protein: 49g Fat: 12g

606. Low Country Boil

🕐 Prep Time 15 m | 🕐 Cooking Time 10 m | 4 Servings

Ingredients

- 1/2 pounds (226.8 g) smoked sausages, cut into four pieces
- 4 ears corn
- 2 red potatoes cut in half
- 1 tablespoon (1 tablespoon) Louisiana Shrimp and Crab Boil
- Water to cover the above
- To add to pot later
- 1/2 pounds (226.8 g) raw shrimp
- For sauce
- 6 tablespoons (6 tablespoon) Butter
- 1 tablespoon (1 tablespoon) Garlic, minced
- 1/8 teaspoon (0.13 teaspoon) Cajun Seasoning
- 1/4 teaspoons (0.25 teaspoons) Old Bay seasoning
- 3-5 shakes (3 shakes) Louisiana Hot Sauce, such as Louisiana Hot sauce or Tabasco
- 1/8 teaspoon (0.13 teaspoons) lemon pepper
- 1/2 (0.5) Lemon, juiced

Directions:

1. Place the sausage, corn, and potatoes in the pot and cover with water.
2. Add in the Louisiana Shrimp and Crab Boil Mix.
3. Set your Instant Pot to high pressure for 4 minutes.
4. Meanwhile in a pan over medium-high heat, melt the better.
5. Add minced garlic and sauté well while stirring, allowing the butter to boil and take on the garlic flavor.
6. Add all other spices and mix well, and taste it. Be sparing with these spices otherwise, your sauce will get quite salty. Most of the flavor will come from the butter and garlic, anyway, and you can add the plain hot sauce for heat if you need. Leave this sauce to warm in the pan. By this time your Instant Pot should be done.
7. Once your Instant Pot is done, perform a Quick Pressure Release, and open the lid carefully. Check to ensure the potatoes are cooked. Mine were very tender, but not mushy.
8. Throw in your shrimp and stir. As soon as the shrimp turn pink, take them out, and then take out the corn, potatoes, and sausage.
9. Put everything a bit into the sauce, stirring well to coat everything with the spiced butter goodness, starting with the shrimp so they have to cook just a little more.
10. Serve immediately and be prepared for everyone to want to dip their food into the sauce left in the serving pot.
11. Adjust this as you need to feed children or adults who can't tolerate spice, by simply relying on butter, garlic, lemon juice, and lemon pepper to add flavor to the butter.

Nutrition:

Calories: 459 Carbohydrates: 18g Protein: 22g Fat: 33g

607. Shrimp and Grits

Prep Time 15 m | Cooking Time 45 m | 4 Servings

Ingredients:

- Shrimp Ingredients
- 1 pound shrimp peeled and deveined
- 2 teaspoon Old Bay seasoning or more to taste
- 3 strips smoked bacon diced
- 1/3 cup onion chopped
- 1/2 cup bell peppers red and/or green, chopped
- 1 tablespoon garlic minced
- 2 tablespoons dry white wine
- 1 1/2 cups canned diced tomatoes
- 2 tablespoons lemon juice or to taste
- 1/4 cup chicken broth
- 1/4 teaspoon Tabasco sauce or hot sauce, more to taste
- 1/2 teaspoon salt or to taste
- 1/4 teaspoon black pepper
- 1/4 cup heavy cream
- 1/4 cup scallions sliced thin (green parts only)
- Grits Ingredients
- 1/2 cup grits
- 1 cup milk
- 1 cup water
- Salt and pepper to taste
- 1 tablespoon butter optional

Directions:

1. Pat shrimp dry and sprinkle with Old Bay seasoning. Set aside.
2. On "Sauté" mode, cook bacon until crisp, about 3 minutes. Using a slotted spoon, remove to a plate and set aside.
3. Sauté onions and bell peppers in the rendered bacon fat till onion is translucent, about 2 to 3 minutes.
4. Add garlic and sauté briefly. Turn Instant Pot off.
5. Deglaze with white wine, and stir well to remove any browned bits, allowing the wine to mostly evaporate.
6. Stir in tomatoes, lemon juice, broth, hot sauce, salt and pepper. Place trivet in the Instant Pot.
7. In a medium bowl that will fit in the Instant Pot, stir together grits, milk, water, salt and pepper. Place bowl on trivet.
8. Close Instant Pot Lid, and make sure the steam release handle is in the "Sealing" position.
9. Cook on "Manual" (or "Pressure Cook") mode for 10 minutes. Allow the pressure to release naturally.
10. Open the Instant Pot, remove the grits and set aside. Remove the trivet. Carefully stir in shrimp.
11. Close the Instant Pot immediately and allow the shrimp to finish cooking in the residual heat. Instant Pot will be in "Keep Warm" mode.
12. While shrimp is cooking, fluff grits with a fork, adding in a tablespoon of butter.
13. After 10 minutes, open the Instant Pot. Gently stir the shrimp. Turn on 'Sauté' mode and stir in cream. Heat through (don't boil) and turn off Instant Pot.
14. Garnish with scallions and bacon. Serve grits topped with shrimp and sauce.

Nutrition:

Calories: 292 Carbohydrates: 18g Protein: 30g Fat: 9g

608. Crust less Crab Quiche

Prep Time 15 m | Cooking Time 50 m | 4 Servings

Ingredients

- 4 Eggs
- 1/2 -1 teaspoon Salt
- 1 teaspoon (1 teaspoon) Ground Black Pepper
- 1 teaspoon (1 teaspoon) Smoked Paprika
- 1 teaspoon (1 teaspoon) Herbs de Provence
- 1 cup (108 g) shredded parmesan or Swiss cheese
- 1 cup (100 g) Green Onions, green and white parts
- 8 ounces (226.8 g) imitation crab meat, about 2 cups OR
- 8 ounces real crab meat, or a mix of crab and chopped raw shrimp

Directions:

1. In a large bowl, beat together eggs and half-and-half with a whisk. (I don't know if this will work with non-dairy milk since it needs to set).
2. Add salt, pepper, sweet smoked paprika, Herbs de Provence, and shredded cheese, and stir with a fork to mix.
3. Stir in chopped green onions.
4. Add in EITHER the imitation crab meat OR the real crab meat OR some combination of crab meat and chopped raw shrimp. You only want 2 cups of seafood however you do this
5. Lay out a sheet of aluminum foil that is cut bigger than the pan you intend to use. Place the spring form pan on this sheet and crimp the sheet about the bottom
6. You are doing this as most spring form pans can leak a little with liquids. The aluminum foil reduces the mess a little.
7. Pour in the egg mixture into your spring form pan. Cover loosely with foil or a silicone lid.
8. Into the inner pot of your Instant Pot or pressure cooker, place 2 cups of water. Place a steamer rack in the pot.
9. Place the covered spring form pan on the trivet. Cook at high pressure for 40 minutes. Let the pot sit undisturbed for 10 minutes and then release all remaining pressure.
10. Very carefully take out the hot silicone pan. Using a knife, loosen the edges of the quiche from the pan. Remove the outer ring, and serve your delicious crab quiche either hot or at room temperature.

Nutrition:

Calories: 395 Carbohydrates: 19g Protein: 22g Fat: 25g

609. Lemon Pepper Salmon

⏰ Prep Time 15 m | ⏰ Cooking Time 10 m | 3-4 Servings

Ingredients:

- ¾ cup water
- A few sprigs of parsley dill, tarragon, basil or a combo
- 1 pound salmon filet skin on
- 3 teaspoons ghee or other healthy fat divided
- ¼ teaspoon salt or to taste
- ½ teaspoon pepper or to taste
- 1/2 lemon thinly sliced
- 1 zucchini julienned
- 1 red bell pepper julienned
- 1 carrot julienned

Directions:

1. Put water and herbs in the Instant Pot and then put in the steamer rack making sure the handles are extended up.
2. Place salmon, skin down on rack.
3. Drizzle salmon with ghee/fat, season with salt and pepper, and cover with lemon slices.
4. Close the Instant Pot and make sure the vent is turned to "Sealing". Plug it in, press "Steam" and press the + or – buttons to set it to 3 minutes.
5. While salmon cooks, julienne your veggies.
6. When the Instant Pot beeps that it's done, quick release the pressure, being careful to stay out of the way of the steam that will shoot up. Press the "Warm/Cancel" button. Remove the lid, and using hot pads, carefully remove the rack with salmon and set on a plate.
7. Remove herbs and discard. Add veggies and put the lid back on. Press "Saute" and let the veggies cook for just 1 or 2 minutes.
8. Serve veggies with salmon and add remaining teaspoon of fat to the pot and pour a little of the sauce over them if desired.

Nutrition:

Calories: 296 Fat: 15g Carbohydrates 8g Protein: 31g

610. Shrimp with Tomatoes and Feta

⏰ Prep Time 15 m | ⏰ Cooking Time 12 m | 6 Servings

Ingredients:

- Cook Together
- 2 tablespoons (2 tablespoons) Butter
- 1 tablespoon (1 tablespoon) Garlic
- 1/2 teaspoon (0.5 teaspoon) Red Pepper Flakes, adjust to taste
- cups (32 g) onions, chopped
- 1 14.5-oz (1 14.5-oz) Canned Tomatoes
- 1 teaspoon (1 teaspoon) Dried Oregano
- 1 teaspoons (1 teaspoons) Salt
- 1 pound (453.59 g) frozen shrimp, 21-25 count, shelled
- Add after cooking
- 1 cup (150 g) crumbled feta cheese
- 1/2 cup (67.5 g) sliced black olives
- 1/4 cup (15 g) Chopped Parsley

Directions:

1. For the Instant Pot. Turn your Instant Pot or Pressure cooker to "Saute" and once it is hot, add the butter. Let it melt a little and then add garlic and red pepper flakes.
2. Add in onions, tomatoes, oregano and salt. Pour in the frozen shrimp.
3. Set your Instant pot to "Low" pressure 1 minute. Once the pot is done cooking, release all pressure immediately.
4. Mix in the shrimp with the rest of the lovely tomato broth. Allow it to cool slightly. Right before serving, sprinkle the feta cheese, olives, and parsley.
5. This dish makes a soupy broth, so it's great for dipping buttered French bread into, or eating over rice, or riced cauliflower.

Nutrition:

Calories: 211 Carbohydrates: 6g Protein: 19g Fat: 11g

611. Scallops And Spring Veggies

⏰ Prep Time 10 m | ⏰ Cooking Time 8 m | 4 Servings

Ingredients

- ½ pound (226.8g) asparagus, ends trimmed, cut into 2-inch pieces
- 1 cup sugar snap peas
- 1 pound (453.592g) sea scallops
- 1 tablespoon lemon juice
- 2 teaspoons olive oil
- ½ teaspoon dried thyme
- Pinch salt
- Freshly ground black pepper

Directions:

1. Place the asparagus and sugar snap peas in the air fryer basket.
2. Cook for 2 to 3 minutes or until the vegetables are just starting to get tender.
3. Meanwhile, check the scallops for a small muscle attached to the side, and pull it off and discard.
4. In a medium bowl, toss the scallops with the lemon juice, olive oil, thyme, salt, and pepper. Place into the air fryer oven basket on top of the vegetables.
5. Steam for 5 to 7 minutes, tossing the basket once during cooking time, until the scallops are just firm when tested with your finger and are opaque in the center, and the vegetables are tender. Serve immediately.

Nutrition:

calories: 162; carbs:10g; fat: 4g; protein:22g; fiber:3g

612. Air Fryer Salmon Patties

⏰ Prep Time 8 m | ⏰ Cooking Time 7 m | 4 Servings

Ingredients

- 1 tbsp. Olive oil
- 1 tbsp. Ghee
- ¼ tsp. Salt
- 1/8 tsp. Pepper
- 1 egg
- 1 c. Almond flour
- 1 can wild alaskan pink salmon

Directions:

1. Drain can of salmon into a bowl and keep liquid. Discard skin and bones.
2. Add salt, pepper, and egg to salmon, mixing well with hands to incorporate. Make patties.
3. Dredge in flour and remaining egg. If it seems dry, spoon reserved salmon liquid from the can onto patties.

Nutrition:
calories: 437; carbs:55; fat: 12g; protein:24g; sugar:2g

613. Salmon Noodles

Prep Time 5 m | Cooking Time 16 m | 4 Servings

Ingredients
- 1 salmon fillet
- 1 tbsp teriyaki marinade
- 3 ½ ozs soba noodles, cooked and drained
- 10 ozs firm tofu
- 7 ozs mixed salad
- 1 cup broccoli
- Olive oil
- Salt and pepper to taste

Directions:
1. Season the salmon with salt and pepper to taste, then coat with the teriyaki marinate. Set aside for 15 minutes
2. Preheat the air fryer oven at 350 degrees, then cook the salmon for 8 minutes.
3. Whilst the air fryer is cooking the salmon, start slicing the tofu into small cubes.
4. Next, slice the broccoli into smaller chunks. Drizzle with olive oil.
5. Once the salmon is cooked, put the broccoli and tofu into the air fryer oven tray for 8 minutes.
6. Plate the salmon and broccoli tofu mixture over the soba noodles. Add the mixed salad to the side and serve.

614. Beer-battered fish and chips

Prep Time 5 m | Cooking Time 30 m | 4 Servings

Ingredients
- 2 eggs
- 1 cup malty beer, such as pabst blue ribbon
- 1 cup all-purpose flour
- ½ cup cornstarch
- 1 teaspoon garlic powder
- Salt
- Pepper
- Cooking oil
- (4-ounce) cod fillets

Directions:
1. In a medium bowl, beat the eggs with the beer. In another medium bowl, combine the flour and cornstarch, and season with the garlic powder and salt and pepper to taste.
2. Spray the air fryer basket with cooking oil.
3. Dip each cod fillet in the flour and cornstarch mixture and then in the egg and beer mixture. Dip the cod in the flour and cornstarch a second time.
4. Place the cod in the air fryer oven. Do not stack. Cook in batches. Spray with cooking oil. Cook for 8 minutes.
5. Open the air fryer oven and flip the cod. Cook for an additional 7 minutes.
6. Remove the cooked cod from the air fryer, then repeat steps 4 and 5 for the remaining fillets.
7. Serve with prepared air fried frozen fries. Frozen fries will need to be cooked for 18 to 20 minutes at 400°f.
8. Cool before serving.

Nutrition:
calories: 325; carbs:41; fat: 4g; protein:26g; fiber:1g

615. Tuna Stuffed Potatoes

☺ Prep Time 5 m | ☺ Cooking Time 30 m | 4 Servings

Ingredients

- 4 starchy potatoes
- ½ tablespoon olive oil
- 1 (6-ounce) can tuna, drained
- 2 tablespoons plain greek yogurt

- 1 teaspoon red chili powder
- Salt and freshly ground black pepper, to taste
- 1 scallion, chopped and divided
- 1 tablespoon capers

Directions:

- In a large bowl of water, soak the potatoes for about 30 minutes. Drain well and pat dry with paper towel.
- Preheat the air fryer to 355 degrees f. Place the potatoes in a fryer basket.
- Cook for about 30 minutes.
- Meanwhile in a bowl, add tuna, yogurt, red chili powder, salt, black pepper and half of scallion and with a potato masher, mash the mixture completely.

- Remove the potatoes from the air fryer oven and place onto a smooth surface.
- Carefully, cut each potato from top side lengthwise.
- With your fingers, press the open side of potato halves slightly. Stuff the potato open portion with tuna mixture evenly.
- Sprinkle with the capers and remaining scallion. Serve immediately.

Nutrition:
Calories: 795, Protein: 109.77g, Fat: g, Carbs: g

616. Fried Calamari

☺ Prep Time 8 m | ☺ Cooking Time 7 m | 6-8 Servings

Ingredients

- ½ tsp. Salt
- ½ tsp. Old bay seasoning
- 1/3 c. Plain cornmeal
- ½ c. Semolina flour

- ½ c. Almond flour
- 5-6 c. Olive oil
- 1 ½ pounds (680.389g) baby squid

Directions:

1   Rinse squid in cold water and slice tentacles, keeping just ¼-inch of the hood in one piece.
2   Combine 1-2 pinches of pepper, salt, old bay seasoning, cornmeal, and both flours together. Dredge squid pieces into flour mixture and place into the air fryer basket.
3   Spray liberally with olive oil. Cook 15 minutes at 345 degrees till coating turns a golden brown.

Nutrition:
Calories: 211; carbs:55; fat: 6g; protein:21g; sugar:1g

617. Soy And Ginger Shrimp

☺ Prep Time 8 m | ☺ Cooking Time 10 m | 4 Servings

Ingredients

- 2 tablespoons olive oil
- 2 tablespoons scallions, finely chopped
- 2 cloves garlic, chopped
- 1 teaspoon fresh ginger, grated
- 1 tablespoon dry white wine

- 1 tablespoon balsamic vinegar
- 1/4 cup soy sauce
- 1 tablespoon sugar
- 1 pound (453.592g) shrimp
- Salt and ground black pepper, to taste

Directions:

- To make the marinade, warm the oil in a saucepan; cook all ingredients, except the shrimp, salt, and black pepper. Now, let it cool.
- Marinate the shrimp, covered, at least an hour, in the refrigerator.

- After that, pour into the oven rack/basket. Place the rack on the middle-shelf of the air fryer oven. Set temperature to 350°f, and set time to 10 minutes. Bake the shrimp at 350 degrees f for 8 to 10 minutes (depending on the size), turning once or twice. Season prepared shrimp with salt and black pepper and serve.

Nutrition:
Calories: 233, Protein: 24.55g, Fat: 10.28g, Carbs: 10.86g

618. Crispy Cheesy Fish Fingers

☺ Prep Time 10 m | ☺ Cooking Time 20 m | 4 Servings

Ingredients

- Large cod fish filet, approximately 6-8 ounces, fresh or frozen and thawed, cut into 1 ½-inch strips
- 2 raw eggs
- ½ cup of breadcrumbs (we like panko, but any brand or home recipe will do)

- 2 tablespoons of shredded or powdered parmesan cheese
- 1 tablespoons of shredded cheddar cheese
- Pinch of salt and pepper

Directions:

1   Cover the basket of the air fryer oven with a lining of tin foil, leaving the edges uncovered to allow air to circulate through the basket.
2   Preheat the air fryer oven to 350 degrees.
3   In a large mixing bowl, beat the eggs until fluffy and until the yolks and whites are fully combined.
4   Dunk all the fish strips in the beaten eggs, fully submerging.
5   In a separate mixing bowl, combine the bread crumbs with the parmesan, cheddar, and salt and pepper, until evenly mixed.
6   One by one, coat the egg-covered fish strips in the mixed dry ingredients so that they're fully covered, and place on the foil-lined air fryer basket.
7   Set the air fryer oven timer to 20 minutes.
8   Halfway through the cooking time, shake the handle of the air fryer so that the breaded fish jostles inside and fry coverage is even.
9   After 20 minutes, when the fryer shuts off, the fish strips will be perfectly cooked and their breaded crust golden-brown and delicious! Using tongs, remove from the air fryer and set on a serving dish to cool.

Nutrition:
Calories: 124, Protein: 6.86g, Fat: 5.93g, Carbs: 12.26g

619. Panko-Crusted Tilapia
⏱ Prep Time 5 m | ⏱ Cooking Time 10 m | 3 Servings

Ingredients

- 2 tsp. Italian seasoning
- 2 tsp. Lemon pepper
- 1/3 c. Panko breadcrumbs
- 1/3 c. Egg whites
- 1/3 c. Almond flour
- tilapia fillets
- Olive oil

Directions:

1 Place panko, egg whites, and flour into separate bowls. Mix lemon pepper and italian seasoning in with breadcrumbs.
2 Pat tilapia fillets dry. Dredge in flour, then egg, then breadcrumb mixture.
3 Add to the air fryer basket and spray lightly with olive oil.
4 Cook 10-11 minutes at 400 degrees, making sure to flip halfway through cooking.

Nutrition:
Calories: 256; fat: 9g; protein:39g; sugar:5g

620. Potato Crusted Salmon
⏱ Prep Time 10 m | ⏱ Cooking Time 15 m | 4 Servings

Ingredients

- 1 pound (453.592g) salmon, swordfish or arctic char fillets, 3/4 inch thick
- 1 egg white
- 2 tablespoons water
- 1/3 cup dry instant mashed potatoes
- 2 teaspoons cornstarch
- 1 teaspoon paprika
- 1 teaspoon lemon pepper seasoning

Directions:

1 Remove and skin from the fish and cut it into 4 serving pieces mix together the egg white and water. Mix together all of the dry ingredients. Dip the filets into the egg white mixture then press into the potato mix to coat evenly.
2 Pour into the oven rack/basket. Place the rack on the middle-shelf of the air fryer oven. Set temperature to 360°f, and set time to 15 minutes, flip the filets halfway through.

Nutrition:
Calories:176; fat: 7g; protein:23g; :5g

621. Salmon Croquettes
⏱ Prep Time 5 m | ⏱ Cooking Time 10 m | 6-8 Servings

Ingredients

- Panko breadcrumbs
- Almond flour
- egg whites
- 2 tbsp. Chopped chives
- 2 tbsp. Minced garlic cloves
- ½ c. Chopped onion
- 2/3 c. Grated carrots
- 1 pound (453.592g) chopped salmon fillet

Directions:

1 Mix together all ingredients minus breadcrumbs, flour, and egg whites.
2 Shape mixture into balls. Then coat them in flour, then egg, and then breadcrumbs. Drizzle with olive oil.
3 Pour the coated salmon balls into the oven rack/basket. Place the rack on the middle-shelf of the air fryer oven. Set temperature to 350°f, and set time to 6 minutes. Shake and cook an additional 4 minutes until golden in color.

Nutrition:
Calories: 503 carbs:61g fat: 9g; protein:5g; sugar:4g

622. Snapper Scampi
⏱ Prep Time 5 m | ⏱ Cooking Time 10 m | 4 Servings

Ingredients

- (6-ounce) skinless snapper or arctic char fillets
- 1 tablespoon olive oil
- tablespoons lemon juice, divided
- ½ teaspoon dried basil
- Pinch salt
- Freshly ground black pepper
- 2 tablespoons butter
- Cloves garlic, minced

Directions:

1 Rub the fish fillets with olive oil and 1 tablespoon of the lemon juice. Sprinkle with the basil, salt, and pepper, and place in the air fryer oven basket.
2 Grill the fish for 7 to 8 minutes or until the fish just flakes when tested with a fork. Remove the fish from the basket and put on a serving plate. Cover to keep warm. In a 6-by-6-by-2-inch pan, combine the butter, remaining 2 tablespoons lemon juice, and garlic. Cook in the air fryer oven for 1 to 2 minutes or until the garlic is sizzling. Pour this mixture over the fish and serve.

Nutrition:
Calories: 265; carbs:1g; fat: 11g; protein:39g; fiber:0g

623. Thai Fish Cakes With Mango Relish

⏱ Prep Time 5 m | ⏱ Cooking Time 10 m | 4 Servings

Ingredients

- 1 lb (453.592g) white fish fillets
- tbsps ground coconut
- 1 ripened mango
- ½ tsps chili paste
- Tbsps fresh parsley
- 1 green onion
- 1 lime
- 1 tsp salt
- 1 egg

Directions:

1. To make the relish, peel and dice the mango into cubes. Combine with a half teaspoon of chili paste, a tablespoon of parsley, and the zest and juice of half a lime.
2. In a food processor, pulse the fish until it forms a smooth texture. Place into a bowl and add the salt, egg, chopped green onion, parsley, two tablespoons of the coconut, and the remainder of the chili paste and lime zest and juice. Combine well
3. Portion the mixture into 10 equal balls and flatten them into small patties. Pour the reserved tablespoon of coconut onto a dish and roll the patties over to coat.
4. Preheat the air fryer oven to 390 degrees
5. Place the fish cakes into the air fryer oven and cook for 8 minutes. They should be crisp and lightly browned when ready
6. Serve hot with mango relish

Nutrition:

Calories: 169, Protein: 22.41g, Fat: 5.36g, Carbs: 6.91g

624. Air Fryer Fish Tacos

⏱ Prep Time 5 m | ⏱ Cooking Time 15 m | 4 Servings

Ingredients

- 1 pound (453.592g) cod
- 1 tbsp. Cumin
- ½ tbsp. Chili powder
- 1 ½ c. Almond flour
- 1 ½ c. Coconut flour
- ounces mexican beer
- eggs

Directions:

1. Whisk beer and eggs together.
2. Whisk flours, pepper, salt, cumin, and chili powder together.
3. Slice cod into large pieces and coat in egg mixture then flour mixture.
4. Spray bottom of your air fryer oven basket with olive oil and add coated codpieces. Cook 15 minutes at 375 degrees.
5. Serve on lettuce leaves topped with homemade salsa.

Nutrition:

Calories: 178; carbs:61g; fat:10g; protein:19g; sugar:1g

625. Firecracker shrimp

⏱ Prep Time 10 m | ⏱ Cooking Time 8 m | 4 Servings

Ingredients

- For the shrimp
- 1 pound (453.592g) raw shrimp, peeled and deveined
- Salt
- Pepper
- 1 egg
- ½ cup all-purpose flour
- ¾ cup panko bread crumbs
- Cooking oil
- For the firecracker sauce
- ⅓ cup sour cream
- tablespoons sriracha
- ¼ cup sweet chili sauce

Directions:

1. Season the shrimp with salt and pepper to taste. In a small bowl, beat the egg. In another small bowl, place the flour. In a third small bowl, add the panko bread crumbs.
2. Spray the air fryer oven basket with cooking oil. Dip the shrimp in the flour, then the egg, and then the bread crumbs. Place the shrimp in the air fryer basket. It is okay to stack them. Spray the shrimp with cooking oil.
3. Cook for 4 minutes. Open the air fryer oven and flip the shrimp. I recommend flipping individually instead of shaking to keep the breading intact. Cook for an additional 4 minutes or until crisp.
4. While the shrimp is cooking, make the firecracker sauce: in a small bowl, combine the sour cream, sriracha, and sweet chili sauce. Mix well. Serve with the shrimp.

Nutrition:

Calories: 266; carbs:23g; fat:6g; protein:27g; fiber:1g

626. Sesame Seeds Coated Fish

⏱ Prep Time 10 m | ⏱ Cooking Time 8 m | 5 Servings

Ingredients

- tablespoons plain flour
- eggs
- ½ cup sesame seeds, toasted
- ½ cup breadcrumbs
- 1/8 teaspoon dried rosemary, crushed
- Pinch of salt
- Pinch of black pepper
- tablespoons olive oil
- frozen fish fillets (white fish of your choice)

Directions:

1. In a shallow dish, place flour. In a second shallow dish, beat the eggs. In a third shallow dish, add remaining ingredients except fish fillets and mix till a crumbly mixture forms.
2. Coat the fillets with flour and shake off the excess flour.
3. Next, dip the fillets in egg.
4. Then coat the fillets with sesame seeds mixture generously.
5. Preheat the air fryer oven to 390 degrees f.
6. Line an air fryer basket with a piece of foil. Arrange the fillets into prepared basket.
7. Cook for about 14 minutes, flipping once after 10 minutes.

Nutrition:

Calories: 393, Protein: 13.41g, Fat: 30.44g, Carbs: 18.09g

627. Bacon Wrapped Scallops
🕐 Prep Time 5 m | 🕐 Cooking Time 5 m | 4 Servings

Ingredients
- 1 tsp. Paprika
- 1 tsp. Lemon pepper
- slices of center-cut bacon
- 20 raw sea scallops

Directions:
1. Rinse and drain scallops, placing on paper towels to soak up excess moisture.
2. Cut slices of bacon into 4 pieces.
3. Wrap each scallop with a piece of bacon, using toothpicks to secure. Sprinkle wrapped scallops with paprika and lemon pepper.
4. Spray air fryer basket with olive oil and add scallops.
5. Cook 5-6 minutes at 400 degrees, making sure to flip halfway through.

Nutrition:
Calories: 389; carbs:63g; fat:17g; protein:21g; sugar:1g

628. Crispy Paprika Fish Fillets
🕐 Prep Time 5 m | 🕐 Cooking Time 15 m | 4 Servings

Ingredients
- 1/2 cup seasoned breadcrumbs
- 1 tablespoon balsamic vinegar
- 1/2 teaspoon seasoned salt
- 1 teaspoon paprika
- 1/2 teaspoon ground black pepper
- 1 teaspoon celery seed
- fish fillets, halved
- 1 egg, beaten

Directions:
1. Add the breadcrumbs, vinegar, salt, paprika, ground black pepper, and celery seeds to your food processor. Process for about 30 seconds.
2. Coat the fish fillets with the beaten egg; then, coat them with the breadcrumbs mixture.
3. Pour the fish fillets into the oven rack/basket. Place the rack on the middle-shelf of the air fryer oven. Set temperature to 350°f, and set time to 15 minutes.

Nutrition:
Calories: 187, Protein: 13.59g, Fat: 7.93g, Carbs: 11.61g

629. Parmesan Shrimp
🕐 Prep Time 5 m | 🕐 Cooking Time 10 m | 4 Servings

Ingredients
- tbsp. Olive oil
- 1 tsp. Onion powder
- 1 tsp. Basil
- ½ tsp. Oregano
- 1 tsp. Pepper
- 2/3 c. Grated parmesan cheese
- minced garlic cloves
- Pounds of jumbo cooked shrimp (peeled/deveined)

Directions:
1. Mix all seasonings together and gently toss shrimp with mixture.
2. Spray olive oil into the air fryer basket and add seasoned shrimp.
3. Cook 8-10 minutes at 350 degrees.
4. Squeeze lemon juice over shrimp right before devouring!

Nutrition:
Calories: 351; fat:11g; protein:19g; sugar:1g

630. Flaky Fish Quesadilla
🕐 Prep Time 10 m | 🕐 Cooking Time 12 m | 4 Servings

Ingredients
- Two 6-inch corn or flour tortilla shells
- 1 medium-sized tilapia fillet, approximately 4 ounces
- ½ medium-sized lemon, sliced
- ½ an avocado, peeled, pitted and sliced
- 1 clove of garlic, peeled and finely minced
- Pinch of salt and pepper
- ½ teaspoon of lemon juice
- ¼ cup of shredded cheddar cheese
- ¼ cup of shredded mozzarella cheese

Directions:
1. Preheat the air fryer oven to 350 degrees.
2. In the air fryer oven, grill the tilapia with a little salt and lemon slices in foil on high heat for 20 minutes.
3. Remove fish in foil from the oven, and break the fish meat apart into bite-sized pieces with a fork – it should be flaky and chunky when cooked.
4. While the fish is cooling, combine the avocado, garlic, salt, pepper, and lemon juice in a small mixing bowl; mash lightly, but don't whip - keep the avocado slightly chunky.
5. Spread the guacamole on one of the tortillas, then cover with the fish flakes, and then with the cheese. Top with the second tortilla.
6. Place directly on hot surface of the air frying basket.
7. Set the air fryer oven timer for 6 minutes.
8. After 6 minutes, when the air fryer shuts off, flip the tortillas onto the other side with a spatula; the cheese should be melted enough that it won't fall apart.
9. Reset air fryer oven to 350 degrees for another 6 minutes.
10. After 6 minutes, when the air fryer shuts off, the tortillas should be browned and crisp, and the fish, guacamole and cheese will be hot and delicious inside. Remove with spatula and let sit on a serving plate to cool for a few minutes before slicing.

Nutrition:
Calories: 85, Protein: 8.81g, Fat: 4.23g, Carbs: 4.21g

631. Quick Fried Catfish

Prep Time 5 m | Cooking Time 15 m | 4 Servings

Ingredients

- 3/4 cups original bisquick™ mix
- 1/2 cup yellow cornmeal
- 1 tablespoon seafood seasoning
- catfish fillets (4 to 6 ounces each)
- 1/2 cup ranch dressing
- Lemon wedges

Directions:

1. In a shallow bowl mix together the bisquick mix, cornmeal, and seafood seasoning. Pat the filets dry, then brush them with ranch dressing.
2. Press the filets into the bisquick mix on both sides until the filet is evenly coated.
3. Cook in your air fryer oven at 360 degrees for 15 minutes, flip the filets halfway through.
4. Serve with a lemon garnish.

Nutrition:
Calories: 372; fat:16g; protein:28g; fiber:1.7g

632. Honey Glazed Salmon

Prep Time 5 m | Cooking Time 8 m | 2 Servings

Ingredients

- 1 tsp. Water
- tsp. Rice wine vinegar
- tbsp. Low-sodium soy sauce
- tbsp. Raw honey
- salmon fillets

Directions:

1. Combine water, vinegar, honey, and soy sauce together. Pour half of this mixture into a bowl.
2. Place salmon in one bowl of marinade and let chill 2 hours.
3. Ensure your air fryer oven is preheated to 356 degrees and add salmon.
4. Cook 8 minutes, flipping halfway through. Baste salmon with some of the remaining marinade mixture and cook another 5 minutes.
5. To make a sauce to serve salmon with, pour remaining marinade mixture into a saucepan, heating till simmering. Let simmer 2 minutes. Serve drizzled over salmon!

Nutrition:
Calories: 348; fat:12g; protein:20g; sugar:3g

633. Fish And Chips

Prep Time 10 m | Cooking Time 20 m | 4 Servings

Ingredients

- (4-ounce) fish fillets
- Pinch salt
- Freshly ground black pepper
- ½ teaspoon dried thyme
- 1 egg white
- ¾ cup crushed potato chips
- tablespoons olive oil, divided
- russet potatoes, peeled and cut into strips

Directions:

1. Pat the fish fillets dry and sprinkle with salt, pepper, and thyme. Set aside.
2. In a shallow bowl, beat the egg white until foamy. In another bowl, combine the potato chips and 1 tablespoon of olive oil and mix until combined.
3. Dip the fish fillets into the egg white, then into the crushed potato chip mixture to coat.
4. Toss the fresh potato strips with the remaining 1 tablespoon olive oil.
5. Use your separator to divide the air fryer basket in half, then fry the chips and fish. The chips will take about 20 minutes; the fish will take about 10 to 12 minutes to cook.

Nutrition:
Calories: 374; fat:16g; protein:30g; fiber:4g

634. Fish Sandwiches

Prep Time 10 m | Cooking Time 20 m | 4 Servings

Ingredients

- white fish fillets
- 1/4 cup yellow cornmeal
- 2 tsp greek seasoning
- Salt and pepper to taste
- 2 ½ cups plain flour
- 2tsps baking powder
- cups beer
- hamburger buns
- Mayonnaise
- Lettuce leaves
- 1 tomato, sliced
- 2 egg

Directions:

1. Cut the fish fillets into burger patty sized strips. Season with salt and pepper to desired taste.
2. In a medium bowl, mix together the beer, egg, baking powder, plain flour, cornmeal, greek seasoning and additional salt and pepper
3. Heat the air fryer oven to 340 degrees
4. Place each seasoned fish strip into the batter, ensuring that it is well coated
5. Place battered fish into the air fryer tray and cook in batches for 6 minutes or until crispy
6. Compile the sandwich by topping each bun with mayonnaise, then a lettuce leaf, tomato slices, and finally the cooked fish strip.

Nutrition:
Calories: 632, Protein: 25.85g, Fat: 23.15g, Carbs: 76.98g

635. Crab Cakes

🕐 Prep Time 5 m | 🕐 Cooking Time 10 m | 4 Servings

Ingredients

- ounces jumbo lump crabmeat
- tablespoon old bay seasoning
- ⅓ cup bread crumbs
- ¼ cup diced red bell pepper
- ¼ cup diced green bell pepper
- 1 egg
- ¼ cup mayonnaise
- Juice of ½ lemon
- 1 teaspoon flour
- Cooking oil

Directions:

1. In a large bowl, combine the crabmeat, old bay seasoning, bread crumbs, red bell pepper, green bell pepper, egg, mayo, and lemon juice. Mix gently to combine.
2. Form the mixture into 4 patties. Sprinkle ¼ teaspoon of flour on top of each patty.
3. Place the crab cakes in the air fryer oven. Spray them with cooking oil. Cook for 10 minutes.
4. Serve.

Nutrition:
Calories: 142, Protein: 4.18g, Fat: 11.24g, Carbs: 7.11g

636. Crispy Air Fried Sushi Roll

🕐 Prep Time 10 m | 🕐 Cooking Time 5 m | 12 Servings

Ingredients

- Kale salad:
  - tbsp. Sesame seeds
- ¾ tsp. Soy sauce
- ¼ tsp. Ginger
- 1/8 tsp. Garlic powder
- ¾ tsp. Toasted sesame oil
- ½ tsp. Rice vinegar
- 1 ½ c. Chopped kale
- Sushi rolls:
- ½ of a sliced avocado
  - sheets of sushi nori
- 1 batch cauliflower rice
- Sriracha mayo:
- Sriracha sauce
- ¼ c. Vegan mayo
- Coating:
- ½ c. Panko breadcrumbs

Directions:

1. Combine all of kale salad ingredients together, tossing well. Set to the side.
2. Lay out a sheet of nori and spread a handful of rice on. Then place 2-3 tbsp. Of kale salad over rice, followed by avocado. Roll up sushi.
3. To make mayo, whisk mayo ingredients together until smooth.
4. Add breadcrumbs to a bowl.
5. Coat sushi rolls in crumbs till coated and add to the air fryer oven.
6. Cook rolls 10 minutes at 390 degrees, shaking gently at 5 minutes.
7. Slice each roll into 6-8 pieces and enjoy!

Nutrition:
Calories: 267; fat:13g; protein:6g; sugar:3g

637. Rosemary Buttery Prawns

🕐 Prep Time 10 m | 🕐 Cooking Time 10 m | 4 Servings

Ingredients

- large prawns
- rosemary sprig, chopped
- ½ tbsp melted butter
- Salt and black pepper to taste

Directions

1. Combine butter, rosemary, salt and pepper, in a bowl. Add the prawns to the bowl and mix to coat them well. Cover the bowl and refrigerate for 1 hour. Preheat air fryer on air fry to 350 f, and cook for 10 minutes.

Nutrition:
Calories: 55, Protein: 0.63g, Fat: 4.8g, Carbs: 3.23g

638. Parmesan Fish With Pine Nuts

🕐 Prep Time 15 m | 🕐 Cooking Time 8 m | 6 Servings

Ingredients

- bunch of basil
- garlic cloves, minced
- 1 tbsp olive oil
- 1 tbsp parmesan cheese, grated
- Black pepper and salt to taste
- tbsp pine nuts
- white fish fillet
- tbsp olive oil

Directions

1. Season the fillets with salt and pepper. Preheat air fryer on air fry function to 350 f, and cook the fillets inside for 8 minutes. In a bowl, add basil, oil, pine nuts, garlic and parmesan cheese; mix with hand. Serve with the fish.

Nutrition:
Calories: 214, Protein: 27.11g, Fat: 10.72g, Carbs: 1.16g

639. Honey and Wine Chicken Breasts
⏱ Prep Time 5 m | ⏱ Cooking Time 15 m | 4 Servings

Ingredients
- 2 chicken breasts, rinsed and halved
- 1 tablespoon melted butter
- A pinch of salt and 1/2 tsp freshly ground pepper to taste
- 3/4 teaspoon sea salt, or to taste
- 1 teaspoon paprika
- 1 teaspoon dried rosemary
- 2 tablespoons dry white wine
- 1 tablespoon honey

Directions
1. Firstly, pat the chicken breasts dry. Lightly coat them with the melted butter.
2. Then, add the remaining ingredients.
3. Transfer them to the air fryer rack/basket; bake about 15 minutes at 330 degrees F. Serve warm and enjoy

Nutrition
Calories 189 | Fat: 14g | Protein:11g | Sugar:1 g

640. Crispy Honey Garlic Chicken Wings
⏱ Prep Time 10 m | ⏱ Cooking Time 25 m | 8 Servings

Ingredients
- 1/8 C. water
- ½ tsp. salt
- 4 tbsp. minced garlic
- ¼ C. vegan butter
- ¼ C. raw honey
- ¾ C. almond flour
- 16 chicken wings

Directions
1. Rinse off and dry chicken wings well.
2. Spray air fryer rack/basket with olive oil.
3. Coat chicken wings with almond flour and add coated wings to the Air fryer oven.
4. Set temperature to 380°F, and set time to 25 minutes. Cook shaking every 5 minutes.
5. When the timer goes off, cook 5-10 minutes at 400 degrees till the skin becomes crispy and dry.
6. As chicken cooks, melt butter in a saucepan and add garlic. Sauté garlic 5 minutes. Add salt and honey, simmer 20 minutes. Make sure to stir every so often, so the sauce does not burn. Add a bit of water after 15 minutes to ensure the sauce does not harden.
7. Take out chicken wings from the air fryer and coat in sauce. Enjoy!

Nutrition
Calories: 435 | Fat: 19g | Protein:31g | Sugar 6 g

641. Lemon-Pepper Chicken Wings
⏱ Prep Time 10 m | ⏱ Cooking Time 20 m | 4 Servings

Ingredients
- 8 whole chicken wings
- Juice of ½ lemon
- ½ teaspoon garlic powder
- 1 teaspoon onion powder
- Salt
- Pepper
- ¼ cup low-fat buttermilk
- ½ cup all-purpose flour
- Cooking oil

Directions
1. Place the wings in a sealed plastic bag. Drizzle the wings with the lemon juice. Season the wings with the garlic powder, onion powder, and salt and pepper to taste.
2. Seal the bag. Shake thoroughly to combine the seasonings and coat the wings.
3. Pour the buttermilk and the flour into separate bowls large enough to dip the wings.
4. Spray the oven rack/basket with cooking oil.
5. One at a time, dip the wings in the buttermilk and then the flour.
6. Place the wings in the oven rack/basket. It is okay to stack them on top of each other. Spray the wings with cooking oil, being sure to spray the bottom layer. Place the tray rack on the middle shelf of the Air fryer oven. Set temperature to 360°F and cook for 5 minutes.
7. Remove the basket and shake it to ensure all of the pieces will cook fully.
8. Return the basket to the Air fryer oven and continue to cook the chicken. Repeat shaking every 5 minutes until a total of 20 minutes has passed.
9. Cool before serving.

Nutrition
Calories: 347 | Fat: 12g | Protein:46g | Fiber:1g

642. Cheesy Chicken in Leek-Tomato Sauce
⏱ Prep Time 10 m | ⏱ Cooking Time 20 m | 4 Servings

Ingredients
- Large-sized chicken breasts, cut in half lengthwise
- Salt and ground black pepper, to taste
- Ounces cheddar cheese, cut into sticks
- 1 tablespoon sesame oil
- 1 cup leeks, chopped
- 2 cloves garlic, minced
- 2/3 cup roasted vegetable stock
- 2/3 cup tomato puree
- 1 teaspoon dried rosemary
- 1 teaspoon dried thyme

Directions
1. Firstly, season chicken breasts with the salt and black pepper; place a piece of cheddar cheese in the middle. Then, tie it using a kitchen string; drizzle with sesame oil and reserve.
2. Add the leeks and garlic to the oven-safe bowl.
3. Cook in the Air fryer oven at 390 degrees F for 5 minutes or until tender.
4. Add the reserved chicken. Throw in the other ingredients and cook for 12 to 13 minutes more or until the chicken is done. Enjoy!

643. Mexican Chicken Burgers

⏱ Prep Time 10 m | ⏱ Cooking Time 10 m | 6 Servings

Ingredients

- 1 jalapeno pepper
- 1 tsp. cayenne pepper
- 1 tbsp. mustard powder
- 1 tbsp. oregano
- 1 tbsp. thyme
- 3 tbsp. smoked paprika
- 1 beaten egg
- 1 small head of cauliflower
- Chicken breasts

Directions

1. Ensure your Air fryer oven is preheated to 350 degrees.
2. Add seasonings to a blender. Slice cauliflower into florets and add to blender.
3. Pulse till mixture resembles that of breadcrumbs.
4. Take out ¾ of the cauliflower mixture and add to a bowl. Set to the side. In another bowl, beat your egg and set it to the side.
5. Remove skin and bones from chicken breasts and add to blender with remaining cauliflower mixture. Season with pepper and salt.
6. Take out the mixture and form into burger shapes. Roll each patty in cauliflower crumbs, then the egg, and back into crumbs again.
7. Place coated patties into the Air fryer oven. Set temperature to 350°F, and set time to 10 minutes.
8. Flip over at a 10-minute mark. They are done when crispy!

Nutrition

Calories: 234 | Fat: 18g | Protein: 24g | Sugar: 1g

644. Fried Chicken Livers

⏱ Prep Time 5 m | ⏱ Cooking Time 10 m | 4 Servings

Ingredients

- 1 pound chicken livers
- 1 cup flour
- 1/2 cup cornmeal
- 2 teaspoons your favorite seasoning blend
- eggs
- 2 tablespoons milk

Directions

1. Clean and rinse the livers, pat dry.
2. Beat eggs in a shallow bowl and mix in milk.
3. In another bowl combine flour, cornmeal, and seasoning, mixing until even.
4. Dip the livers in the egg mix, then toss them in the flour mix.
5. Air-fry at 375 degrees for 10 minutes using your Air fryer oven. Toss at least once halfway through.

Nutrition

Calories 409 | Fat 11g | Protein 36g | Fiber 2g

645. Minty Chicken-Fried Pork Chops

⏱ Prep Time 10 m | ⏱ Cooking Time 30 m | 6 Servings

Ingredients

- Medium-sized pork chops, approximately 3.5 ounces each
- 1 cup of breadcrumbs (Panko brand works well)
- 2 medium-sized eggs
- Pinch of salt and pepper
- ½ tablespoon of mint, either dried and ground; or fresh, rinsed and finely chopped

Directions

1. Cover the basket of the Air fryer oven with a lining of tin foil, leaving the edges uncovered to allow air to circulate through the basket. Preheat the Air fryer oven to 350 degrees.
2. In a bowl, beat the eggs until fluffy and until the yolks and whites are completely combined and set aside.
3. In a separate bowl, combine the crumbs, mint, salt, and pepper and set aside. One at a time, dip each raw pork chop into the dry ingredient bowl, coat all sides, then dip it into the wet ingredient bowl, then dip it back into the dry ingredients. This double layer will ensure cooler air.

    Place the breaded pork chops on the oven rack, in a single flat layer. Place the air fryer rack on the middle shelf of the fryer.

4. Set the Air Fryer timer to 15 minutes. After 15 minutes the Air Fryer oven will turn off and the pork should cook in the middle and the bread layer should start to brown. Using tweezers, flip each piece of meat over to secure a full pair of pants. Return the fryer to 320 degrees for 15 minutes.
5. After 15 minutes, when the fryer is off, remove the fried pork chops with tongs and place them in a source. Eat as fresh as you can, and enjoy it!

Nutrition

Calories 213 | Fat 9g | Protein 12g | Fiber 3g

646. Crispy Southern Fried Chicken

⏱ Prep Time 10 m | ⏱ Cooking Time 25 m | 4 Servings

Ingredients

- 1 tsp. cayenne pepper
- 2 tbsp. mustard powder
- 2 tbsp. oregano
- 2 tbsp. thyme
- 3 tbsp. coconut milk
- 1 beaten egg
- ¼ C. cauliflower
- ¼ C. gluten-free oats
- 8 chicken drumsticks

Directions

1. Ensure the Air fryer oven is preheated to 350 degrees.
2. Lay out the chicken and season with pepper and salt on all sides.
3. Add all other ingredients to a blender, blending till a smooth-like breadcrumb mixture is created. Place in a bowl and add a beaten egg to another bowl.
4. Dip chicken into breadcrumbs, then into the egg, and breadcrumbs once more.
5. Place coated drumsticks into the Air fryer oven. Set temperature to 350°F, and set time to 20 minutes, and cook 20 minutes. Bump up the temperature to 390 degrees and cook another 5 minutes till crispy.

Nutrition

Calories 504 | Fat 18g | Protein 35g | Sugar 5g

647. Tex-Mex Turkey Burgers
Prep Time 10 m | Cooking Time 15 m | 4 Servings

Ingredients
- ⅓ cup finely crushed corn tortilla chips
- 1 egg, beaten
- ¼ cup salsa
- ⅓ cup shredded pepper Jack cheese
- Pinch salt
- Freshly ground black pepper
- 1 pound ground turkey
- 1 tablespoon olive oil
- 1 teaspoon paprika

Directions
1. In a small bowl, combine the tortilla chips, egg, salsa, cheese, salt, and pepper, and mix well.
2. Add the turkey and mix gently but thoroughly with clean hands.
3. Form the meat mixture into patties about ½ inch thick. Make an indentation in the center of each patty with your thumb, so the burgers don't puff up while cooking.
4. Brush the patties on each side with the olive oil and sprinkle with paprika.
5. Put in the oven rack/basket. Place the tray rack on the middle shelf of the Air fryer oven. Grill for 14 to 16 minutes or until the meat registers at least 165°F.

Nutrition
Calories 354 | Fat 21g | Protein 36g | Fiber 2g

648. Air Fryer Turkey Breast
Prep Time 5 m | Cooking Time 60 m | 6 Servings

Ingredients
- Pepper and salt
- 1 oven-ready turkey breast
- Turkey seasonings of choice

Directions
1. Preheat the Air fryer oven to 350 degrees.
2. Season turkey with pepper, salt, and other desired seasonings.
3. Place turkey in the oven rack/basket. Place the tray Rack on the middle-shelf of the Air fryer oven.
4. Set temperature to 350°F, and set time to 60 minutes. Cook 60 minutes. The meat should be at 165 degrees when done.
5. Allow resting 10-15 minutes before slicing. Enjoy!

Nutrition
Calories 212 | Fat 12g | Protein 24g | Sugar 0g

649. Mustard Chicken Tenders
Prep Time 5 m | Cooking Time 20 m | 4 Servings

Ingredients
- ½ C. coconut flour
- 1 tbsp. spicy brown mustard
- Beaten eggs
- 1 pound of chicken tenders

Directions
1. Season tenders with pepper and salt.
2. Place a thin layer of mustard onto tenders and then dredge in flour and dip in egg.
3. Add to the Air fryer oven, set the temperature to 390°F, and set time to 20 minutes.

Nutrition
Calories 403 | Fat 20g | Protein 22g | Sugar 4g

650. Chicken Nuggets
Prep Time 10 m | Cooking Time 20 m | 4 Servings

Ingredients
- 1 pound boneless, skinless chicken breasts
- Chicken seasoning or rub
- Salt
- Pepper
- Eggs
- Tablespoons bread crumbs
- Tablespoons panko bread crumbs
- Cooking oil

Directions
1. Cut the chicken breasts into 1-inch pieces.
2. In a large bowl, add together the chicken pieces with the chicken seasoning, salt, and pepper.
3. In a small bowl, beat the eggs. In another bowl, combine breadcrumbs and countertop.
4. Dip the chicken pieces in the eggs and then the breadcrumbs.
5. Place the pepitas in the deep fryer. Don't overdo the basket. Cook in batches. Drizzle the seeds with cooking oil.
6. Cook for 4 minutes. Open the air fryer oven and shake the basket. Set temperature to 360°F. Cook for an additional 4 minutes. Remove the cooked nuggets from the air fryer oven, then repeat steps 5 and 6 for the remaining chicken nuggets. Cool before serving.

Nutrition
Calories 206 | Fat 5g | Protein 31g | Fiber 1g

651. Air Fryer Chicken Parmesan
Prep Time 5 m | Cooking Time 9 m | 4 Servings

Ingredients
- ½ C. keto marinara
- tbsp. mozzarella cheese
- 1 tbsp. melted ghee
- tbsp. grated parmesan cheese
- tbsp. gluten-free seasoned breadcrumbs
- 8-ounce chicken breasts

Directions
1. Ensure air fryer is preheated to 360 degrees. Spray the basket with olive oil.
2. Mix parmesan cheese and breadcrumbs together. Melt ghee.
3. Brush melted ghee onto the chicken and dip into breadcrumb mixture.
4. Place coated chicken in the air fryer and top with olive oil.
5. Set temperature to 360°F, and set time to 6 minutes. Cook 2 breasts for 6 minutes and top each breast with a tablespoon of sauce and 1½ tablespoons of mozzarella cheese. Cook another 3 minutes to melt the cheese.
6. Keep cooked pieces warm as you repeat the process with remaining breasts.

Nutrition
Calories 251 | Fat 10g | Protein 31g | Sugar 0g

652. Cheesy Chicken Fritters

☉ Prep Time 5 m | ☉ Cooking Time 20 m | 17 Servings

Ingredients

Chicken Fritters:

- ½ tsp. salt
- 1/8 tsp. pepper
- 1 ½ tbsp. fresh dill
- 1 1/3 C. shredded mozzarella cheese
- 1/3 C. coconut flour
- 1/3 C. vegan mayo
- 2 eggs
- 1 ½ pounds chicken breasts

Garlic Dip:

- 1/8 tsp. pepper
- ¼ tsp. salt
- ½ tbsp. lemon juice
- 1 pressed garlic cloves
- 1/3 C. vegan mayo

Directions

1. Slice chicken breasts into 1/3" pieces and place in a bowl. Add all remaining fritter ingredients to the bowl and stir well. Cover and chill 2 hours or overnight.
2. Ensure your air fryer is preheated to 350 degrees. Spray basket with a bit of olive oil.
3. Add marinated chicken to the air fryer oven. Set temperature to 350°F, and set time to 20 minutes and cook 20 minutes, making sure to turn halfway through the cooking process.
4. To make the dipping sauce, combine all the dip ingredients until smooth.

Nutrition

Calories 467 | Fat 27g | Protein 21g | Sugar 3g

653. Ricotta and Parsley Stuffed Turkey Breasts

☉ Prep Time 5 m | ☉ Cooking Time 25 m | 4 Servings

Ingredients

- 1 turkey breast, quartered
- 1 cup Ricotta cheese
- 1/4 cup fresh Italian parsley, chopped
- 1 teaspoon garlic powder
- 1/2 teaspoon cumin powder
- 1 egg, beaten
- 1 teaspoon paprika
- Salt and ground black pepper, to taste
- Crushed tortilla chips
- 1 ½ tablespoons extra-virgin olive oil

Directions

1. Firstly, flatten out each piece of turkey breast with a rolling pin. Prepare three mixing bowls.
2. In a shallow bowl, combine Ricotta cheese with the parsley, garlic powder, and cumin powder.
3. Place the Ricotta/parsley mixture in the middle of each piece. Repeat with the remaining pieces of the turkey breast and roll them up.
4. In another shallow bowl, whisk the egg together with paprika. In the third shallow bowl, combine the salt, pepper, and crushed tortilla chips.
5. Dip each roll in the whisked egg, then, roll them over the tortilla chips mixture.
6. Transfer prepared rolls to the oven rack/basket. Drizzle olive oil over all the rolls. Place the tray Rack on the middle-shelf of the Air fryer oven.
7. Cook for 25 minutes at 350 degrees F, working in batches. Serve warm, garnished with some extra parsley, if desired.

Nutrition

Calories 509 | Fat 23g | Protein 26g | Fiber 5g

654. Deviled chicken

☉ Prep Time 10 m | ☉ Cooking Time 40 m | 8 Servings

Ingredients

- tablespoons butter
- cloves garlic, chopped
- 1 cup Dijon mustard
- 1/2 teaspoon cayenne pepper
- 1 1/2 cups panko breadcrumbs
- 3/4 cup parmesan, freshly grated
- 1/4 cup chives, chopped
- teaspoons paprika
- small bone-in chicken thighs, skin removed

Directions:

1. Toss the chicken thighs with crumbs, cheese, chives, butter, and spices in a bowl and mix well to coat.
2. Transfer the chicken along with its spice mix to a baking pan.
3. Press "power button" of air fry oven and turn the dial to select the "air fry" mode.
4. Press the time button and again turn the dial to set the cooking time to 40 minutes.
5. Now push the temp button and rotate the dial to set the temperature at 350 degrees f.
6. Once preheated, place the baking pan inside and close its lid.
7. Serve warm.

Nutrition:

Calories 380 | Fat 20 g | Cholesterol 151 mg | Sodium 686 mg | Carbs 33 g | Fiber 1 g | Protein 21 g

655. Marinated chicken parmesan

🕑 Prep Time 10 m | 🕑 Cooking Time 20 m | 4 Servings

Ingredients

- cups breadcrumbs
- 1 teaspoon dried oregano
- 1/2 teaspoon garlic powder
- teaspoons paprika
- 1/2 teaspoon salt
- 1/2 teaspoon black pepper
- egg whites

- 1/2 cup skim milk
- 1/2 cup flour
- oz. Chicken breast halves
- Cooking spray
- 1 jar marinara sauce
- 3/4 cup mozzarella cheese, shredded
- tablespoons parmesan, shredded

Directions:

1. Whisk the flour with all the spices in a bowl and beat the eggs in another.
2. Coat the pounded chicken with flour then dip in the egg whites.
3. Dredge the chicken breast through the crumbs well.
4. Spread marinara sauce in a baking dish and place the crusted chicken on it.
5. Drizzle cheese on top of the chicken.
6. Press "power button" of air fry oven and turn the dial to select the "bake" mode.
7. Press the time button and again turn the dial to set the cooking time to 20 minutes.
8. Now push the temp button and rotate the dial to set the temperature at 400 degrees f.
9. Once preheated, place the baking pan inside and close its lid.
10. Serve warm.

Nutrition:
Calories 361 | Fat 16.3 g Cholesterol 114 mg | Sodium 515 mg | Carbs 19.3g | Fiber 0.1g | Protein 33.3 g

656. Rosemary lemon chicken

🕑 Prep Time 10 m | 🕑 Cooking Time 45 m | 8 Servings

Ingredients

- 4-lb. (1814.37g) Chicken, cut into pieces
- Salt and black pepper, to taste
- Flour for dredging
- tablespoons olive oil
- 1 large onion, sliced
- Peel of ½ lemon

- large garlic cloves, minced
- 1 1/2 teaspoons rosemary leaves
- 1 tablespoon honey
- 1/4 cup lemon juice
- 1 cup chicken broth

Directions:

1. Dredges the chicken through the flour then place in the baking pan.
2. Whisk broth with the rest of the ingredients in a bowl.
3. Pour this mixture over the dredged chicken in the pan.
4. Press "power button" of air fry oven and turn the dial to select the "bake" mode.
5. Press the time button and again turn the dial to set the cooking time to 45 minutes.
6. Now push the temp button and rotate the dial to set the temperature at 400 degrees f.
7. Once preheated, place the baking pan inside and close its lid.
8. Baste the chicken with its sauce every 15 minutes.
9. Serve warm.

Nutrition:
Calories 405 | Fat 22.7 g | Cholesterol 4 mg | Sodium 227 mg | Carbs 26.1 g | Fiber 1.4 g | Protein 45.2 g

657. Spanish chicken bake

🕑 Prep Time 10 m | 🕑 Cooking Time 25 m | 4 Servings

Ingredients

- ½ onion, quartered
- ½ red onion, quartered
- ½ lb. (226.8g) Potatoes, quartered
- garlic cloves
- tomatoes, quartered
- 1/8 cup chorizo

- ¼ teaspoon paprika powder
- chicken thighs, boneless
- ¼ teaspoon dried oregano
- ½ green bell pepper, julienned
- Salt
- Black pepper

Directions:

1. Toss chicken, veggies, and all the ingredients in a baking tray.
2. Press "power button" of air fry oven and turn the dial to select the "bake" mode.
3. Press the time button and again turn the dial to set the cooking time to 25 minutes.
4. Now push the temp button and rotate the dial to set the temperature at 425 degrees f.
5. Once preheated, place the baking pan inside and close its lid.

Nutrition:
Calories 301 | Fat 8.9 g | Cholesterol 57 mg | Sodium 340 mg | Carbs 24.7 g | Fiber 1.2 g | Protein 15.3 g

658. Garlic chicken potatoes
Prep Time 10 m | Cooking Time 30 m | 4 Servings

Ingredients

- lbs. (907.185g) Red potatoes, quartered
- tablespoons olive oil
- 1/2 teaspoon cumin seeds
- Salt and black pepper, to taste
- garlic cloves, chopped
- tablespoons brown sugar
- 1 lemon (1/2 juiced and 1/2 cut into wedges)
- Pinch of red pepper flakes
- skinless, boneless chicken breasts
- tablespoons cilantro, chopped

Directions:

1. Place the chicken, lemon, garlic, and potatoes in a baking pan.
2. Toss the spices, herbs, oil, and sugar in a bowl.
3. Add this mixture to the chicken and veggies then toss well to coat.
4. Press "power button" of air fry oven and turn the dial to select the "bake" mode.
5. Press the time button and again turn the dial to set the cooking time to 30 minutes.
6. Now push the temp button and rotate the dial to set the temperature at 400 degrees f.
7. Once preheated, place the baking pan inside and close its lid.
8. Serve warm.

Nutrition:

Calories 545 | Fat 36.4 g | Cholesterol 200 mg | Sodium 272mg | Carbs 40.7g | Fiber 0.2g | Protein 42.5 g

659. Chicken potato bake
Prep Time 10 m | Cooking Time 25 m | 4 Servings

Ingredients

- potatoes, diced
- 1 tablespoon garlic, minced
- 1.5 tablespoons olive oil
- 1/8 teaspoon salt
- 1/8 teaspoon pepper
- 1.5 lbs. (680.389g) Boneless skinless chicken
- 3/4 cup mozzarella cheese, shredded
- Parsley chopped

Directions:

1. Toss chicken and potatoes with all the spices and oil in a baking pan.
2. Drizzle the cheese on top of the chicken and potato.
3. Press "power button" of air fry oven and turn the dial to select the "bake" mode.
4. Press the time button and again turn the dial to set the cooking time to 25 minutes.
5. Now push the temp button and rotate the dial to set the temperature at 375 degrees f.
6. Once preheated, place the baking pan inside and close its lid.
7. Serve warm.

Nutrition:

Calories 695 | Fat 17.5 g | Cholesterol 283mg | Sodium 355mg | Carbs 26.4g | Fiber 1.8g | Protein 117.4g

660. Chicken pasta bake
Prep Time 10 m | Cooking Time 22 m | 4 Servings

Ingredients

- 9oz penne, boiled
- 1 onion, roughly chopped
- chicken breasts, cut into strips
- tablespoon olive oil
- 1 tablespoon paprika
- Salt and black pepper
- Sauce
- 1¾oz butter
- 1¾oz plain flour
- 1 pint 6 fly oz. hot milk
- 1 teaspoon dijon mustard
- 3½oz parmesan cheese, grated
- large tomatoes, deseeded and cubed

Directions:

1. Butter a casserole dish and toss chicken with pasta, onion, oil, paprika, salt, and black pepper in it.
2. Prepare the sauce in a suitable pan. Add butter and melt over moderate heat.
3. Stir in flour and whisk well for 2 minutes, then pour in hot milk.
4. Mix until smooth, then add tomatoes, mustard, and cheese.
5. Toss well and pour this sauce over the chicken mix in the casserole dish.
6. Press "power button" of air fry oven and turn the dial to select the "bake" mode.
7. Press the time button and again turn the dial to set the cooking time to 20 minutes.
8. Now push the temp button and rotate the dial to set the temperature at 375 degrees f.
9. Once preheated, place the casserole dish inside and close its lid.
10. Serve warm.

Nutrition:

Calories 548 | Fat 22.9 g | Cholesterol 105 mg | Sodium 350mg | Carbs 17.5g | Fiber 6.3g | Protein 40.1 g

661. Creamy chicken casserole

Prep Time 10 m | Cooking Time 45 m | 6 Servings

Ingredients

- Chicken and mushroom casserole:
- 1/2 lbs. (1133.98g) Chicken breasts, cut into strips
- 1 1/2 teaspoon salt
- 1/4 teaspoon black pepper
- 1 cup all-purpose flour
- tablespoon olive oil
- 1-lb. (453.592g) White mushrooms, sliced
- 1 medium onion, diced
- garlic cloves, minced
- Sauce:
- tablespoon unsalted butter
- tablespoon all-purpose flour
- 1 1/2 cups chicken broth
- 1 tablespoon lemon juice
- 1 cup half and half cream

Directions:

1. Butter a casserole dish and toss in chicken with mushrooms and all the casserole ingredients.
2. Prepare the sauce in a suitable pan. Add butter and melt over moderate heat.
3. Stir in flour and whisk well for 2 minutes, then pour in milk, lemon juice, and cream.
4. Mix well and pour milk this sauce over the chicken mix in the casserole dish.
5. Press "power button" of air fry oven and turn the dial to select the "bake" mode.
6. Press the time button and again turn the dial to set the cooking time to 45 minutes.
7. Now push the temp button and rotate the dial to set the temperature at 350 degrees f.
8. Once preheated, place the casserole dish inside and close its lid.
9. Serve warm.

Nutrition:

Calories 409 | Fat 50.5 g | Cholesterol 58 mg | Sodium 463 mg | Carbs 9.9 g | Fiber 1.5 g | Protein 29.3 g

662. Italian chicken bake

Prep Time 10 m | Cooking Time 25 m | 6 Servings

Ingredients:

- ¾ lbs. (340.194g) Chicken breasts
- tablespoons pesto sauce
- ½ (14 oz.) can tomatoes, diced
- 1 cup mozzarella cheese, shredded
- tablespoon fresh basil, chopped

Directions:

1. Place the flattened chicken breasts in a baking pan and top them with pesto.
2. Add tomatoes, cheese, and basil on top of each chicken piece.
3. Press "power button" of air fry oven and turn the dial to select the "bake" mode.
4. Press the time button and again turn the dial to set the cooking time to 25 minutes.
5. Now push the button and rotate the dial to set the temperature at 355 degrees f.
6. Once preheated, place the baking dish inside and close its lid.
7. Serve warm.

Nutrition:

Calories 537 | Fat 19.8 g | Cholesterol 10 mg | Sodium 719 mg | Carbs 25.1 g | Fiber 0.9g | Protein 37.8 g

663. Pesto chicken bake

Prep Time 10 m | Cooking Time 35 m | 3 Servings

Ingredients

- chicken breasts
- 1 (6 oz.) Jar basil pesto
- medium fresh tomatoes, sliced
- mozzarella cheese slices

Directions:

1. Spread the tomato slices in a casserole dish and top them with chicken.
2. Add pesto and cheese on top of the chicken and spread evenly.
3. Press "power button" of air fry oven and turn the dial to select the "air fry" mode.
4. Press the time button and again turn the dial to set the cooking time to 30 minutes.
5. Now push the temp button and rotate the dial to set the temperature at 350 degrees f.
6. Once preheated, place the casserole dish inside and close its lid.
7. After it is baked, switch the oven to broil mode and broil for 5 minutes.
8. Serve warm.

Nutrition:

Calories 452 | Fat 4 g | Cholesterol 65 mg | Sodium 220 mg | Carbs 23.1 g | Fiber 0.3 g | Protein 26g

664. Baked duck
Prep Time 10 m | Cooking Time 20 m | 6 Servings

Ingredients

- 1 ½ sprig of fresh rosemary
- ½ nutmeg
- Black pepper
- Juice from 1 orange
- 1 whole duck
- cloves garlic, chopped
- 1 ½ red onions, chopped
- A few stalks celery
- 1 ½ carrot
- cm piece fresh ginger
- 1 ½ bay leaves
- lbs. (907.185g) Piper potatoes
- cups chicken stock

Directions:

1. Place duck in a large cooking pot and add broth along with all the ingredients.
2. Cook this duck for 2 hours on a simmer then transfer to the baking tray.
3. Press "power button" of air fry oven and turn the dial to select the "air fry" mode.
4. Press the time button and again turn the dial to set the cooking time to 20 minutes.
5. Now push the temp button and rotate the dial to set the temperature at 350 degrees f.
6. Once preheated, place the baking tray inside and close its lid.
7. Serve warm.

Nutrition:

Calories 308 | Fat 20.5 g | Cholesterol 42 mg | Sodium 688 mg | Carbs 40.3 g | Fiber 4.3 g | Protein 49 g

665. Roasted goose
Prep Time 10 m | Cooking Time 40 m | 12 Servings

Ingredients

- lbs. (3628.74g) Goose
- Juice of a lemon
- Salt and pepper
- 1/2 yellow onion, peeled and chopped
- 1 head garlic, peeled and chopped
- 1/2 cup wine
- 1 teaspoon dried thyme

Directions:

1. Place the goose in a baking tray and whisk the rest of the ingredients in a bowl.
2. Pour this thick sauce over the goose and brush it liberally.
3. Press "power button" of air fry oven and turn the dial to select the "air roast" mode.
4. Press the time button and again turn the dial to set the cooking time to 40 minutes.
5. Now push the temp button and rotate to set the temperature at 355 degrees f.
6. Once preheated, place the casserole dish inside and close its lid.
7. Serve warm.

Nutrition:

Calories 231 | Fat 20.1 g | Cholesterol 110 mg | Sodium 941mg | Carbs 20.1g | Fiber 0.9g | Protein 14.6 g

666. Christmas roast goose
Prep Time 10 m | Cooking Time 60 m | 12 Servings

Ingredients

- goose
- lemons, sliced
- 1 ½ lime, sliced
- ½ teaspoon Chinese five-spice powder
- ½ handful parsley, chopped
- ½ handful sprigs, chopped
- ½ handful thyme, chopped
- ½ handful sage, chopped
- 1 ½ tablespoon clear honey
- ½ tablespoon thyme leaves

Directions:

1. Place the goose in a baking dish and brush it with honey.
2. Set the lemon and lime slices on top of the goose.
3. Add all the herbs and spice powder over the lemon slices.
4. Press "power button" of air fry oven and turn the dial to select the "air roast" mode.
5. Press the time button and again turn the dial to set the cooking time to 60 minutes.
6. Now push the temp button and rotate the dial to set the temperature at 375 degrees f.
7. Once preheated, place the baking dish inside and close its lid.
8. Serve warm.

Nutrition:

Calories 472 | Fat 11.1 g | Cholesterol 610mg | Sodium 749mg | Carbs 19.9g | Fiber 0.2g | Protein 13.5 g

667. Chicken kebabs
⏱ Prep Time 10 m | ⏱ Cooking Time 20 m | 2 Servings

Ingredients

- oz. skinless chicken breasts, cubed
- tablespoons soy sauce
- ½ zucchini sliced
- 1 tablespoon chicken seasoning
- 1 teaspoon bbq seasoning
- Salt and pepper to taste
- ½ green pepper sliced
- ½ red pepper sliced
- ½ yellow pepper sliced
- ¼ red onion sliced
- cherry tomatoes
- Cooking spray

Directions:

1. Toss chicken and veggies with all the spices and seasoning in a bowl.
2. Alternatively, thread them on skewers and place these skewers in the air fryer basket.
3. Press "power button" of air fry oven and turn the dial to select the "air fry" mode.
4. Press the time button and again turn the dial to set the cooking time to 20 minutes.
5. Now push the temp button and rotate the dial to set the temperature at 350 degrees f.
6. Once preheated, place the baking dish inside and close its lid.
7. Flip the skewers when cooked halfway through then resume cooking.
8. Serve warm.

Nutrition:

Calories 327 | Fat 3.5 g | Cholesterol 162 mg | Sodium 142mg | Carbs 33.6g | Fiber 0.4g | Protein 24.5 g

668. Asian chicken kebabs
⏱ Prep Time 10 m | ⏱ Cooking Time 12 m | 6 Servings

Ingredients

- lbs. (907.185g) Chicken breasts, cubed
- 1/2 cup soy sauce
- cloves garlic, crushed
- 1 teaspoon fresh ginger, grated
- 1/2 cup golden sweetener
- 1 red pepper, chopped
- 1/2 red onion, chopped
- mushrooms, halved
- cups zucchini, chopped

Directions:

1. Toss chicken and veggies with all the spices and seasoning in a bowl.
2. Alternatively, thread them on skewers and place these skewers in the air fryer basket.
3. Press "power button" of air fry oven and turn the dial to select the "air fry" mode.
4. Press the time button and again turn the dial to set the cooking time to 12 minutes.
5. Now push the temp button and rotate the dial to set the temperature at 380 degrees f.
6. Once preheated, place the baking dish inside and close its lid.
7. Flip the skewers when cooked halfway through then resume cooking.
8. Serve warm.

Nutrition:

Calories 353 | Fat 7.5 g | Cholesterol 20 mg | Sodium 297 mg | Carbs 10.4 g | Fiber 0.2 g | Protein 13.1 g

669. Kebab tavuk sheesh
⏱ Prep Time 10 m | ⏱ Cooking Time 10 m | 2 Servings

Ingredients

- 1/4 cup plain yogurt
- 1 tablespoon garlic, minced
- 1 tablespoon tomato paste
- 1 tablespoon olive oil
- 1 tablespoon lemon juice
- 1 teaspoon salt
- 1 teaspoon ground cumin
- 1 teaspoon smoked paprika
- 1/2 teaspoon ground cinnamon
- 1/2 teaspoon ground black pepper
- 1/2 teaspoon cayenne
- 1 lb. (453.592g) Boneless skinless chicken thighs, quartered

Directions:

1. Mix chicken with yogurt and all the seasonings in a bowl.
2. Marinate the yogurt chicken for 30 minutes in the refrigerator.
3. Thread chicken pieces on the skewers and place these skewers in the air fryer basket.
4. Press "power button" of air fry oven and turn the dial to select the "air fry" mode.
5. Press the time button and again turn the dial to set the cooking time to 10 minutes.
6. Now push the temp button and rotate the dial to set the temperature at 370 degrees f.
7. Once preheated, place the baking dish inside and close its lid.
8. Flip the skewers when cooked halfway through then resume cooking.

Nutrition:

Calories 248 | Fat 13 g | Cholesterol 387 mg | Sodium 353 mg | Carbs 1 g | Fiber 0.4 g | Protein 29 g

670. Chicken mushroom kebab

⏱ Prep Time 10 m | ⏱ Cooking Time 15 m | 4 Servings

Ingredients

- 1/3 cup honey
- 1/3 cup soy sauce
- Salt, to taste
- mushrooms chop in half
- bell peppers, cubed
- chicken breasts diced

Directions:

1. Toss chicken, mushrooms and veggies with all the honey, and seasoning in a bowl.
2. Alternatively, thread them on skewers and place these skewers in the air fryer basket.
3. Press "power button" of air fry oven and turn the dial to select the "air fry" mode.
4. Press the time button and again turn the dial to set the cooking time to 15 minutes.
5. Now push the temp button and rotate the dial to set the temperature at 350 degrees f.
6. Once preheated, place the baking dish inside and close its lid.
7. Flip the skewers when cooked halfway through then resume cooking.
8. Serve warm.

Nutrition:

Calories 457 | Fat 19.1g | Cholesterol 262 mg | Sodium 557 mg | Carbs 18.9g | Fiber 1.7g | Protein 32.5 g

671. Chicken fajita skewers

⏱ Prep Time 10 m | ⏱ Cooking Time 8 m | 2 Servings

Ingredients

- 1 lb. (453.592g) Chicken breasts, diced
- 1 tablespoon lemon juice
- 1 teaspoon chili powder
- 1 teaspoon cumin
- 1 orange bell pepper, cut into squares
- 1 red bell pepper, cut into squares
- tablespoon olive oil
- 1 teaspoon garlic powder
- 1 large red onion, cut into squares
- 1 teaspoon salt
- 1 teaspoon ground black pepper
- 1 teaspoon oregano
- 1 teaspoon parsley flakes
- 1 teaspoon paprika

Directions:

1. Toss chicken and veggies with all the spices and seasoning in a bowl.
2. Alternatively, thread them on skewers and place these skewers in the air fryer basket.
3. Press "power button" of air fry oven and turn the dial to select the "air fry" mode.
4. Press the time button and again turn the dial to set the cooking time to 8 minutes.
5. Now push the temp button and rotate the dial to set the temperature at 360 degrees f.
6. Once preheated, place the baking dish inside and close its lid.
7. Flip the skewers when cooked halfway through then resume cooking.
8. Serve warm.

Nutrition:

Calories 392 | Fat 16.1 g | Cholesterol 231 mg | Sodium 466 mg | Carbs 13.9g | Fiber 0.9g | Protein 48 g

672. Zucchini chicken kebabs

⏱ Prep Time 10 m | ⏱ Cooking Time 16 m | 4 Servings

Ingredients

- 1 large zucchini, cut into squares
- chicken breasts boneless, skinless, cubed
- 1 onion yellow, cut into squares
- 1.5 cup grape tomatoes
- 1 clove garlic minced
- 1 lemon juiced
- 1/4 c olive oil
- 1 tablespoon olive oil
- tablespoon red wine vinegar
- 1 teaspoon oregano

Directions:

1. Toss chicken and veggies with all the spices and seasoning in a bowl.
2. Alternatively, thread them on skewers and place these skewers in the air fryer basket.
3. Press "power button" of air fry oven and turn the dial to select the "air fry" mode.
4. Press the time button and again turn the dial to set the cooking time to 16 minutes.
5. Now push the temp button and rotate the dial to set the temperature at 380 degrees f.
6. Once preheated, place the baking dish inside and close its lid.
7. Flip the skewers when cooked halfway through then resume cooking.
8. Serve warm.

Nutrition:

Calories 321 | Fat 7.4 g | Cholesterol 105 mg | Sodium 353 mg | Carbs 19.4 g | Fiber 2.7g | Protein 37.2 g

673. Chicken soy skewers

⏰ Prep Time 10 m | ⏱ Cooking Time 7 m | 4 Servings

Ingredients

- 1-lb. (453.592g) Boneless chicken tenders, diced
- 1/2 cup soy sauce
- 1/2 cup pineapple juice
- 1/4 cup sesame seed oil
- garlic cloves, chopped
- scallions, chopped
- 1 tablespoon grated ginger
- teaspoons toasted sesame seeds
- Black pepper

Directions:

1. Toss chicken with all the sauces and seasonings in a baking pan.
2. Press "power button" of air fry oven and turn the dial to select the "air fry" mode.
3. Press the time button and again turn the dial to set the cooking time to 7 minutes.
4. Now push the temp button and rotate the dial to set the temperature at 390 degrees f.
5. Once preheated, place the baking dish inside and close its lid.
6. Serve warm.

Nutrition:

Calories 248 | Fat 15.7 g | Cholesterol 75 mg | Sodium 94 mg | Carbs 31.4 g | Fiber 0.4 g | Protein 24.9 g

674. Chicken Popcorn

⏰ Prep Time 10 m | ⏱ Cooking Time 10 m | 6 Servings

Ingredients:

- 4 eggs
- 1 1/2 lb. chicken breasts, cut into small chunks
- 1 tsp paprika
- 1/2 tsp garlic powder
- 1 tsp onion powder
- 2 1/2 cups pork rind, crushed
- 1/4 cup coconut flour
- Pepper
- Salt

Directions::

1. In a small bowl, mix together coconut flour, pepper, and salt.
2. In another bowl, whisk eggs until combined.
3. Take one more bowl and mix together pork panko, paprika, garlic powder, and onion powder.
4. Add chicken pieces in a large mixing bowl. Sprinkle coconut flour mixture over chicken and toss well.
5. Dip chicken pieces in the egg mixture and coat with pork panko mixture and place on a plate.
6. Spray air fryer basket with cooking spray.
7. Preheat the air fryer to 400 F.
8. Add half prepared chicken in air fryer basket and cook for 10-12 minutes. Shake basket halfway through.
9. Cook remaining half using the same method.
10. Serve and enjoy.

Nutrition:

Calories 265 Fat 11 g Carbohydrates 3 g Sugar 0.5 g Protein 35 g Cholesterol 195 mg

675. Delicious Whole Chicken

⏰ Prep Time 10 m | ⏱ Cooking Time 50 m | 4 Servings

Ingredients:

- 3 lbs. whole chicken, remove giblets and pat dry chicken
- 1 tsp Italian seasoning
- 1/2 tsp garlic powder
- 1/2 tsp onion powder
- 1/4 tsp paprika
- 1/4 tsp pepper
- 1 1/2 tsp salt

Directions::

1. In a small bowl, mix together Italian seasoning, garlic powder, onion powder, paprika, pepper, and salt.
2. Rub spice mixture from inside and outside of the chicken.
3. Place chicken breast side down in air fryer basket.
4. Roast chicken for 30 minutes at 360 F.
5. Turn chicken and roast for 20 minutes more or internal temperature of chicken reaches at 165 F.
6. Serve and enjoy.

Nutrition:

Calories 356 Fat 25 g Carbohydrates 1 g Sugar 1 g Protein 30 g Cholesterol 120 mg

676. Quick & Easy Meatballs

⏰ Prep Time 10 m | ⏱ Cooking Time 10 m | 4 Servings

Ingredients:

- 1 lb. ground chicken
- 1 egg, lightly beaten
- 1/2 cup mozzarella cheese, shredded
- 1 1/2 tbsp taco seasoning
- 3 garlic cloves, minced
- 3 tbsp fresh parsley, chopped
- 1 small onion, minced
- Pepper
- Salt

Directions::

1. Add all ingredients into the large mixing bowl and mix until well combined.
2. Make small balls from mixture and place in the air fryer basket.
3. Cook meatballs for 10 minutes at 400 F.
4. Serve and enjoy.

Nutrition:

Calories 253 Fat 10 g Carbohydrates 2 g Sugar 0.9 g Protein 35 g Cholesterol 144 mg

677. Lemon Pepper Chicken Wings

⏰ Prep Time 10 m | ⏰ Cooking Time 16 m | 4 Servings

Ingredients:
- 1 lb. chicken wings
- 1 tsp lemon pepper
- 1 tbsp olive oil
- 1 tsp salt

Directions::
1. Add chicken wings into the large mixing bowl.
2. Add remaining ingredients over chicken and toss well to coat.
3. Place chicken wings in the air fryer basket.
4. Cook chicken wings for 8 minutes at 400 F.
5. Turn chicken wings to another side and cook for 8 minutes more.
6. Serve and enjoy.

Nutrition:
Calories 247 Fat 11 g Carbohydrates 0.3 g Sugar 0 g Protein 32 g Cholesterol 101 mg

678. BBQ Chicken Wings

⏰ Prep Time 10 m | ⏰ Cooking Time 20 m | 4 Servings

Ingredients:
- 1 1/2 lbs. chicken wings
- 2 tbsp unsweetened BBQ sauce
- 1 tsp paprika
- 1 tbsp olive oil
- 1 tsp garlic powder
- Pepper
- Salt

Directions::
1. In a large bowl, toss chicken wings with garlic powder, oil, paprika, pepper, and salt.
2. Preheat the air fryer to 360 F.
3. Add chicken wings in air fryer basket and cook for 12 minutes.
4. Turn chicken wings to another side and cook for 5 minutes more.
5. Remove chicken wings from air fryer and toss with BBQ sauce.
6. Return chicken wings in air fryer basket and cook for 2 minutes more.
7. Serve and enjoy.

Nutrition:
Calories 372 Fat 16.2 g Carbohydrates 4.3 g Sugar 3.7 g Protein 49.4 g Cholesterol 151 mg

679. Flavorful Fried Chicken

⏰ Prep Time 10 m | ⏰ Cooking Time 40 m | 10 Servings

Ingredients:
- 5 lbs. chicken, about 10 pieces
- 1 tbsp coconut oil
- 2 1/2 tsp white pepper
- 1 tsp ground ginger
- 1 1/2 tsp garlic salt
- 1 tbsp paprika
- 1 tsp dried mustard
- 1 tsp pepper
- 1 tsp celery salt
- 1/3 tsp oregano
- 1/2 tsp basil
- 1/2 tsp thyme
- 2 cups pork rinds, crushed
- 1 tbsp vinegar
- 1 cup unsweetened almond milk
- 1/2 tsp salt

Directions::
1. Add chicken in a large mixing bowl.
2. Add milk and vinegar over chicken and place in the refrigerator for 2 hours.
3. I a shallow dish, mix together pork rinds, white pepper, ginger, garlic salt, paprika, mustard, pepper, celery salt, oregano, basil, thyme, and salt.
4. Coat air fryer basket with coconut oil.
5. Coat each chicken piece with pork rind mixture and place on a plate.
6. Place half coated chicken in the air fryer basket.
7. Cook chicken at 360 F for 10 minutes then turn chicken to another side and cook for 10 minutes more or until internal temperature reaches at 165 F.
8. Cook remaining chicken using the same method.
9. Serve and enjoy.

Nutrition:
Calories 539 Fat 37 g Carbohydrates 1 g Sugar 0 g Protein 45 g Cholesterol 175 mg

680. Yummy Chicken Nuggets

⏰ Prep Time 10 m | ⏰ Cooking Time 12 m | 4 Servings

Ingredients:
- 1 lb. chicken breast, skinless, boneless and cut into chunks
- 6 tbsp sesame seeds, toasted
- 4 egg whites
- 1/2 tsp ground ginger
- 1/4 cup coconut flour
- 1 tsp sesame oil
- Pinch of salt

Directions::
1. Preheat the air fryer to 400 F.
2. Toss chicken with oil and salt in a bowl until well coated.
3. Add coconut flour and ginger in a zip-lock bag and shake to mix. Add chicken to the bag and shake well to coat.
4. In a large bowl, add egg whites. Add chicken in egg whites and toss until well coated.
5. Add sesame seeds in a large zip-lock bag.
6. Shake excess egg off from chicken and add chicken in sesame seed bag. Shake bag until chicken well coated with sesame seeds.
7. Spray air fryer basket with cooking spray.
8. Place chicken in air fryer basket and cook for 6 minutes.
9. Turn chicken to another side and cook for 6 minutes more.
10. Serve and enjoy.

Nutrition:
Calories 265 Fat 11.5 g Carbohydrates 8.6 g Sugar 0.3 g Protein 31.1 g Cholesterol 73 mg

681. Italian Seasoned Chicken Tenders

⏱ Prep Time 10 m | ⏱ Cooking Time 10 m | 2 Servings

Ingredients:

- 2 eggs, lightly beaten
- 1 1/2 lbs. chicken tenders
- 1/2 tsp onion powder
- 1/2 tsp garlic powder
- 1 tsp paprika
- 1 tsp Italian seasoning
- 2 tbsp ground flax seed
- 1 cup almond flour
- 1/2 tsp pepper
- 1 tsp sea salt

Directions::

1. Preheat the air fryer to 400 F.
2. Season chicken with pepper and salt.
3. In a medium bowl, whisk eggs to combine.
4. In a shallow dish, mix together almond flour, all seasonings, and flaxseed.
5. Dip chicken into the egg then coats with almond flour mixture and place on a plate.
6. Spray air fryer basket with cooking spray.
7. Place half chicken tenders in air fryer basket and cook for 10 minutes. Turn halfway through.
8. Cook remaining chicken tenders using same steps.
9. Serve and enjoy.

Nutrition:
Calories 315 Fat 21 g Carbohydrates 12 g Sugar 0.6 g Protein 17 g Cholesterol 184 mg

682. Classic Chicken Wings

⏱ Prep Time 10 m | ⏱ Cooking Time 40 m | 4 Servings

Ingredients:

- 2 lbs. chicken wings
- For sauce:
- 1/4 tsp Tabasco
- 1/4 tsp Worcestershire sauce
- 6 tbsp butter, melted
- 12 oz hot sauce

Directions::

1. Spray air fryer basket with cooking spray.
2. Add chicken wings in air fryer basket and cook for 25 minutes at 380 F. Shake basket after every 5 minutes.
3. After 25 minutes turn temperature to 400 F and cook for 10-15 minutes more.
4. Meanwhile, in a large bowl, mix together all sauce ingredients.
5. Add cooked chicken wings in a sauce bowl and toss well to coat.
6. Serve and enjoy.

Nutrition:
Calories 593 Fat 34.4 g Carbohydrates 1.6 g Sugar 1.1 g Protein 66.2 g Cholesterol 248 mg

683. Simple Spice Chicken Wings

⏱ Prep Time 10 m | ⏱ Cooking Time 30 m | 3 Servings

Ingredients:

- 1 1/2 lbs. chicken wings
- 1 tbsp baking powder, gluten-free
- 1/2 tsp onion powder
- 1/2 tsp garlic powder
- 1/2 tsp smoked paprika
- 1 tbsp olive oil
- 1/2 tsp pepper
- 1/4 tsp sea salt

Directions::

1. Add chicken wings and oil in a large mixing bowl and toss well.
2. Mix together remaining ingredients and sprinkle over chicken wings and toss to coat.
3. Spray air fryer basket with cooking spray.
4. Add chicken wings in air fryer basket and cook at 400 F for 15 minutes. Toss well.
5. Turn chicken wings to another side and cook for 15 minutes more.
6. Serve and enjoy.

Nutrition:
Calories 280 Fat 19 g   Carbohydrates 2 g Sugar 0 g Protein 22 g Cholesterol 94 mg

684. Easy & Crispy Chicken Wings

⏱ Prep Time 5 m | ⏱ Cooking Time 20 m | 8 Servings

Ingredients:

- 1 1/2 lbs. chicken wings
- 2 tbsp olive oil
- Pepper
- Salt

Directions::

1. Toss chicken wings with oil and place in the air fryer basket.
2. Cook chicken wings at 370 F for 15 minutes.
3. Shake basket and cook at 400 F for 5 minutes more.
4. Season chicken wings with pepper and salt.
5. Serve and enjoy.

Nutrition:
Calories 192 Fat 9.8 g Carbohydrates 0 g Sugar 0 g Protein 24.6 g Cholesterol 76 mg

685. Herb Seasoned Turkey Breast

⏱ Prep Time 10 m | ⏱ Cooking Time 35 m | 4 Servings

Ingredients:

- 2 lbs. turkey breast
- 1 tsp fresh sage, chopped
- 1 tsp fresh rosemary, chopped
- 1 tsp fresh thyme, chopped
- Pepper
- Salt

Directions::

1. Spray air fryer basket with cooking spray.
2. In a small bowl, mix together sage, rosemary, and thyme.
3. Season turkey breast with pepper and salt and rub with herb mixture.
4. Place turkey breast in air fryer basket and cook at 390 F for 30-35 minutes.
5. Slice and serve.

Nutrition: Calories 238 Fat 3.9 g Carbohydrates 10 g Sugar 8 g Protein 38.8 g Cholesterol 98 mg

686. Tasty Rotisserie Chicken
⏱ Prep Time 10 m | ⏱ Cooking Time 20 m | 6 Servings

Ingredients:

- 3 lbs. chicken, cut into eight pieces
- 1/4 tsp cayenne
- 1 tsp paprika
- 2 tsp onion powder
- 1 1/2 tsp garlic powder
- 1 1/2 tsp dried oregano
- 1/2 tbsp dried thyme
- Pepper
- Salt

Directions::

1. Season chicken with pepper and salt.
2. In a bowl, mix together spices and herbs and rub spice mixture over chicken pieces.
3. Spray air fryer basket with cooking spray.
4. Place chicken in air fryer basket and cook at 350 F for 10 minutes.
5. Turn chicken to another side and cook for 10 minutes more or until the internal temperature of chicken reaches at 165 F.
6. Serve and enjoy.

Nutrition:
Calories 350 Fat 7 g Carbohydrates 1.8 g Sugar 0.5 g Protein 66 g Cholesterol 175 mg

687. Spicy Asian Chicken Thighs
⏱ Prep Time 10 m | ⏱ Cooking Time 20 m | 4 Servings

Ingredients:

- 4 chicken thighs, skin-on, and bone-in
- 2 tsp ginger, grated
- 1 lime juice
- 2 tbsp chili garlic sauce
- 1/4 cup olive oil
- 1/3 cup soy sauce

Directions::

1. In a large bowl, whisk together ginger, lime juice, chili garlic sauce, oil, and soy sauce.
2. Add chicken in bowl and coat well with marinade and place in the refrigerator for 30 minutes.
3. Place marinated chicken in air fryer basket and cook at 400 F for 15-20 minutes or until the internal temperature of chicken reaches at 165 F. Turn chicken halfway through.
4. Serve and enjoy.

Nutrition:
Calories 403 Fat 23.5 g Carbohydrates 3.2 g Sugar 0.6 g Protein 43.7 g Cholesterol 130 mg

688. Chicken with Broccoli
⏱ Prep Time 10 m | ⏱ Cooking Time 20 m | 4 Servings

Ingredients:

- 1 lb. chicken breast, skinless, boneless, and cut into chunks
- 2 cups broccoli florets
- 2 tsp hot sauce
- 2 tsp vinegar
- 1 tsp sesame oil
- 1 tbsp soy sauce
- 1 tbsp ginger, minced
- 1/2 tsp garlic powder
- 1 tbsp olive oil
- 1/2 onion, sliced
- Pepper
- Salt

Directions::

1. Add all ingredients into the large mixing bowl and toss well.
2. Spray air fryer basket with cooking spray.
3. Transfer chicken and broccoli mixture into the air fryer basket.
4. Cook at 380 F for 15-20 minutes. Shake halfway through.
5. Serve and enjoy.

Nutrition:
Calories 199 Fat 7.7 g Carbohydrates 5.9 g Sugar 1.6 g Protein 25.9 g Cholesterol 73 mg

689. Zaatar Chicken
⏱ Prep Time 10 m | ⏱ Cooking Time 35 m | 4 Servings

Ingredients:

- 4 chicken thighs
- 2 sprigs thyme
- 1 onion, cut into chunks
- 2 1/2 tbsp zaatar
- 1/2 tsp cinnamon
- 2 garlic cloves, smashed
- 1 lemon juice
- 1 lemon zest
- 1/4 cup olive oil
- 1/4 tsp pepper
- 1 tsp salt

Directions::

1. Add oil, lemon juice, lemon zest, cinnamon, garlic, pepper, 2 tbsp zaatar, and salt in a large zip-lock bag and shake well.
2. Add chicken, thyme, and onion to bag and shake well to coat. Place in refrigerator for overnight.
3. Preheat the air fryer to 380 F.
4. Add marinated chicken in air fryer basket and cook at 380 F for 15 minutes.
5. Turn chicken to another side and sprinkle with remaining zaatar spice and cook at 380 F for 15-18 minutes more.
6. Serve and enjoy.

Nutrition:
Calories 415 Fat 24.1 g Carbohydrates 5.2 g Sugar 1.5 g Protein 43 g Cholesterol 130 mg

690. Teriyaki Chicken

⏰ Prep Time 10 m | ⏰ Cooking Time 20 m | 6 Servings

Ingredients:

- 6 chicken drumsticks
- 1 cup keto teriyaki sauce
- 1 tbsp sesame seeds, toasted
- 2 tbsp green onion, sliced

Directions::

1. Add chicken and teriyaki sauce into the large zip-lock bag. Shake well and place in the refrigerator for 1 hour.
2. Preheat the air fryer to 360 F.
3. Add marinated chicken drumsticks into the air fryer basket and cook for 20 minutes. Shake basket twice.
4. Garnish with green onion and sesame seeds.
5. Serve and enjoy.

Nutrition:

Calories 165 Fat 7 g Carbohydrates 7 g Sugar 6 g Protein 16 g Cholesterol 65 mg

691. Crispy & Juicy Whole Chicken

⏰ Prep Time 10 m | ⏰ Cooking Time 60 m | 8 Servings

Ingredients:

- 5 lbs. chicken, wash and remove giblets
- 1/2 tsp onion powder
- 1/2 tsp pepper
- 1 tsp paprika
- 1 tsp dried oregano
- 1 tsp dried basil
- 1 1/2 tsp salt

Directions::

1. Preheat the air fryer to 360 F.
2. Mix together all spices and rub over chicken.
3. Place chicken into the air fryer basket. Make sure the chicken breast side down.
4. Cook chicken for 30 minutes then turn to another side and cook for 30 minutes more.
5. Slice and serve.

Nutrition:

Calories 430 Fat 8.6 g Carbohydrates 0.5 g Sugar 0.1 g Protein 82.3 g Cholesterol 218 mg

692. Juicy Turkey Breast Tenderloin

⏰ Prep Time 10 m | ⏰ Cooking Time 25 m | 3 Servings

Ingredients:

- 1 turkey breast tenderloin
- 1/2 tsp sage
- 1/2 tsp smoked paprika
- 1/2 tsp pepper
- 1/2 tsp thyme
- 1/2 tsp salt

Directions::

1. Preheat the air fryer to 350 F.
2. Spray air fryer basket with cooking spray.
3. Rub turkey breast tenderloin with paprika, pepper, thyme, sage, and salt and place in the air fryer basket.
4. Cook for 25 minutes. Turn halfway through.
5. Slice and serve.

Nutrition:

Calories 61 Fat 1 g Carbohydrates 1 g Sugar 1 g Protein 12 g Cholesterol 25 mg

693. Flavorful Cornish Hen

⏰ Prep Time 10 m | ⏰ Cooking Time 25 m | 3 Servings

Ingredients:

- 1 Cornish hen, wash and pat dry
- 1 tbsp olive oil
- 1 tsp smoked paprika
- 1/2 tsp garlic powder
- Pepper
- Salt

Directions::

1. Coat Cornish hen with olive oil and rub with paprika, garlic powder, pepper, and salt.
2. Place Cornish hen in the air fryer basket.
3. Cook at 390 F for 25 minutes. Turn halfway through.
4. Slice and serve.

Nutrition:

Calories 301 Fat 5 g Carbohydrates 2 g Sugar 0.5 g Protein 25 g Cholesterol 150 mg

694. Chicken Vegetable Fry

⏰ Prep Time 10 m | ⏰ Cooking Time 15 m | 2 Servings

Ingredients:

- 6 oz chicken breast, boneless and cut into cubes
- 1/4 tsp dried thyme
- 1/2 tsp garlic powder
- 1 tsp dried oregano
- 1/4 onion, sliced
- 1/2 bell pepper, chopped
- 1/2 zucchini, chopped
- 1 tbsp olive oil

695. Flavorful Chicken Drumsticks

⏱ Prep Time 10 m | ⏱ Cooking Time 30 m | 4 Servings

- **Ingredients:**
- 8 chicken drumsticks
- ¼ tsp cayenne pepper
- 1 tbsp onion powder
- 1 tbsp garlic powder
- 1 ½ tbsp honey
- 1 ½ tbsp fresh lemon juice

- 1 tbsp Worcestershire sauce
- ¼ cup soy sauce, low sodium
- 1 tbsp sesame oil
- 2 tbsp olive oil
- ½ tsp kosher salt

Directions::
1. Add all ingredients except chicken in a large mixing bowl and mix well.
2. Add chicken drumsticks to the bowl and mix until well coated.
3. Place chicken drumsticks on the instant vortex air fryer rack air fry at 400 F for 15 minutes.
4. Turn chicken drumsticks to another side and cook for 15 minutes more.
5. Serve and enjoy.

Nutrition:
Calories 296 Fat 15.8 g Carbohydrates 11.6 g Sugar 8.7 g Protein 26.9 g Cholesterol 81 mg

696. Gluten-Free Air Fried Chicken

⏱ Prep Time 10 m | ⏱ Cooking Time 25 m | 6 Servings

Ingredients:
- 6 chicken drumsticks, rinse and pat dry with a paper towel
- 1 tsp ginger
- 1 tsp onion powder
- 1 tsp garlic powder
- 1 tsp paprika
- 1 cup buttermilk

- ¼ cup brown sugar
- ½ cup breadcrumbs
- 1 cup all-purpose flour
- ½ tsp pepper
- 1 tsp salt

Directions::
1. Preheat the instant vortex air fryer using bake mode at 390 F.
2. Add breadcrumbs, spices, and flour into the zip-lock bag and mix well.
3. In a bowl, mix together chicken and buttermilk and let sit for 2 minutes.
4. Now put a single piece of chicken into the zip-lock bag and shake it until chicken is evenly coated with breadcrumb mixture. Do this same with remaining chicken pieces.
5. Spray coated chicken with cooking spray.
6. Place chicken into the bottom tray of instant vortex air fryer and bake for 25 minutes.
7. Serve and enjoy.

Nutrition:
Calories 234 Fat 3.8 g Carbohydrates 31.5 g Sugar 8.7 g Protein 17.6 g Cholesterol 42 mg

697. Parmesan Garlic Chicken Wings

⏱ Prep Time 10 m | ⏱ Cooking Time 21 m | 4 Servings

Ingredients:
- 1 lb. chicken wings
- 1 tsp parsley
- 2 tbsp garlic, minced
- ¾ cup parmesan cheese, grated

- 1 tbsp butter, melted
- ¼ tsp pepper
- 1 tsp salt

Directions::
1. Arrange chicken wings on instant vortex air fryer tray and air fry at 400 F for 7 minutes.
2. Turn chicken wings to the other side and air fry for 7 minutes more.
3. Turn chicken wings again and air fry for another 7 minutes.
4. In a mixing bowl, mix together cheese, butter, parsley, garlic, pepper, and salt.
5. Once chicken wings are done then transfer in mixing bowl and toss well with cheese mixture until well coated.
6. Serve and enjoy.

Nutrition:
Calories 398 Fat 20.3 g Carbohydrates 1.5 g Sugar 0 g Protein 45.2 g Cholesterol 139 mg

698. Healthy Chicken Popcorn

⏱ Prep Time 10 m | ⏱ Cooking Time 10 m | 4 Servings

Ingredients:
- 1 lb. chicken breast, skinless, boneless, and cut into 1-inch pieces
- 1 egg, lightly beaten
- ½ tbsp Tabasco sauce
- 1 cup buttermilk

- 1 tsp baking powder
- 1 cup all-purpose flour
- ½ tsp pepper
- 1 tsp salt

Directions::
1. Season chicken pieces with pepper and salt.
2. In a medium bowl, mix together all-purpose flour and baking powder.
3. In another mixing bowl, mix together egg, buttermilk, and Tabasco sauce.
4. Coat chicken with flour mixture then dip chicken into the egg mixture then again coat with flour mixture.
5. Place coated chicken pieces on instant vortex air fryer tray. Spray coated chicken pieces with cooking spray.
6. Air fry chicken popcorn at 400 F for minutes. Turn chicken popcorn to another side and air fry for 5 minutes more.
7. Serve and enjoy.

Nutrition:
Calories 285 Fat 4.8 g Carbohydrates 27.6 g Sugar 3.1 g Protein 30.7 g Cholesterol 116 mg

699. Cuban Chicken Wings

⏱ Prep Time 10 m | ⏱ Cooking Time 35 m | 4 Servings

Ingredients:
- 12 chicken wings
- 2 tbsp water
- 1 tbsp sazon seasoning
- 1 tbsp adobo seasoning
- 1 tsp salt

Directions::
1. Place chicken wings in a large mixing bowl.
2. Add remaining ingredients over chicken and toss until chicken is well coated.
3. Add chicken into the rotisserie basket and place basket into the instant vortex air fryer.
4. Air fry chicken at 375 F for 35 minutes.
5. Serve and enjoy.

Nutrition:
Calories 476 Fat 32.1 g Carbohydrates 16.1 g Sugar 0 g Protein 29.2 g Cholesterol 116 mg

700. Red Thai Turkey Drumsticks in Coconut Milk

⏱ Prep Time 25 m | ⏱ Cooking Time 23 m | 2 Servings

Ingredients:
- 1 tablespoon red curry paste
- 1/2 teaspoon cayenne pepper
- 1 ½ tablespoons minced ginger
- 2 turkey drumsticks
- 1/4 cup coconut milk
- 1 teaspoon kosher salt, or more to taste
- 1/3 teaspoon ground pepper, to more to taste

Directions:
1. First, place turkey drumsticks with all ingredients in your refrigerator; let it marinate overnight.
2. Cook turkey drumsticks at 380 degrees f for 23 minutes; make sure to flip them over at half-time. Serve with the salad on the side.

Nutrition:
Calories 298 Fat 20.3 g Carbohydrates 1.5 g Sugar 0 g Protein 45.2 g Cholesterol 139 mg

701. Fried Turkey with Lemon and Herbs

⏱ Prep Time 45 m | ⏱ Cooking Time 28 m | 6 Servings

Ingredients:
- 1 ½ tablespoons yellow mustard
- 1 ½ tablespoons herb seasoning blend
- 1/3 cup tamari sauce
- 1 ½ tablespoons olive oil
- 1/2 lemon, juiced
- 3 turkey drumsticks
- 1/3 cup pear or apple cider vinegar
- 2 sprigs rosemary, chopped

Directions:
1. Dump all ingredients into a mixing dish. Let it marinate overnight.
2. Set your air fryer to cook at 355 degrees f.
3. Season turkey drumsticks with salt and black pepper and roast them at 355 degrees f for 28 minutes. Cook one drumstick at a time.
4. Pause the machine after 14 minutes and flip turkey drumstick.

Nutrition:
Calories 323 Fat 20.3 g Carbohydrates 1.5 g Sugar 0 g Protein 45.2 g Cholesterol 139 mg

702. Chicken Sausage with Nestled Eggs

⏱ Prep Time 20 m | ⏱ Cooking Time 17 m | 6 Servings

Ingredients:
- 6 eggs
- 2 bell peppers, seeded and sliced
- 1 teaspoon dried oregano
- 1 teaspoon hot paprika
- 1 teaspoon freshly cracked black pepper
- 6 chicken sausages
- 1 teaspoon sea salt
- 1 1/2 shallots, cut into wedges
- 1 teaspoon dried basil

Directions:
1. Take four ramekins and divide chicken sausages, shallot, and bell pepper among those ramekins. Cook at 315 degrees f for about 12 minutes.
2. Now, crack an egg into each ramekin. Sprinkle the eggs with hot paprika, basil, oregano, salt, and cracked black pepper. Cook for 5 more minutes at 405 degrees f.

Nutrition:
Calories 221 Fat 20.3 g Carbohydrates 1.5 g Sugar 0 g Protein 45.2 g Cholesterol 139 mg

703. Tangy and Buttery Chicken

⏱ Prep Time 20 m | ⏱ Cooking Time 13 m | 4 Servings

Ingredients:
- ½ tablespoon Worcestershire sauce
- 1 teaspoon finely grated orange zest
- 2 tablespoons melted butter
- ½ teaspoon smoked paprika
- 4 chicken drumsticks, rinsed and halved
- 1 teaspoon sea salt flakes
- 1 tablespoon cider vinegar
- 1/2 teaspoon mixed peppercorns, freshly cracked

Directions:
1. Firstly, pat the chicken drumsticks dry. Coat them with the melted butter on all sides. Toss the chicken drumsticks with the other ingredients.
2. Transfer them to the air fryer cooking basket and roast for about 13 minutes at 345 degrees f.

Nutrition:
Calories 264 Fat 20.3 g Carbohydrates 1.5 g Sugar 0 g Protein 45.2 g Cholesterol 139 mg

704. Easy Turkey Kabobs
Prep Time 15 m | Cooking Time 10 m | 8 Servings

Ingredients:
- 1 cup parmesan cheese, grated
- 1 ½ cups of water
- 14 ounces ground turkey
- 2 small eggs, beaten
- 1 teaspoon ground ginger
- 2 ½ tablespoons vegetable oil
- 1 cup chopped fresh parsley
- 2 tablespoons almond meal
- 3/4 teaspoon salt
- 1 heaping teaspoon fresh rosemary, finely chopped
- 1/2 teaspoon ground allspice

Directions:
1. Mix all the above ingredients in a bowl. Knead the mixture with your hands.
2. Then, take small portions and gently roll them into balls.
3. Now, preheat your air fryer to 380 degrees f. Air fry for 8 to 10 minutes in the air fryer basket. Serve on a serving platter with skewers and eat with your favorite dipping sauce.

Nutrition:
Calories 360 Fat 20.3 g Carbohydrates 1.5 g Sugar 0 g Protein 45.2 g Cholesterol 139 mg

705. Turkey Breasts with Greek Mustard Sauce
Prep Time 1 h 13 m | Cooking Time 18 m | 4 Servings

Ingredients:
- 1/2 teaspoon cumin powder
- 2 pounds turkey breasts, quartered
- 2 cloves garlic, smashed
- ½ teaspoon hot paprika
- 2 tablespoons melted butter
- 1 teaspoon fine sea salt
- Freshly cracked mixed peppercorns, to savor
- Fresh juice of 1 lemon
- For the mustard sauce:
- 1 ½ tablespoons mayonnaise
- 1 ½ cups Greek yogurt
- 1/2 tablespoon yellow mustard

Directions:
1. Grab a medium-sized mixing dish and combine the garlic and melted butter; rub this mixture evenly over the surface of the turkey.
2. Add the cumin powder, followed by paprika, salt, peppercorns, and lemon juice. Place in your refrigerator at least 55 minutes.
3. Set your air fryer to cook at 375 degrees f. Roast the turkey for 18 minutes, turning halfway through; roast in batches.
4. In the meantime, make the mustard sauce by mixing all ingredients for the sauce. Serve warm roasted turkey with the mustard sauce.

Nutrition:
Calories 471 Fat 20.3 g Carbohydrates 1.5 g Sugar 0 g Protein 45.2 g Cholesterol 139 mg

706. Country-Style Nutty Turkey Breast
Prep Time 30 m | Cooking Time 25 m | 2 Servings

Ingredients:
- 1 ½ tablespoons coconut amines
- 1/2 tablespoon xanthan gum
- 2 bay leaves
- 1/3 cup dry sherry
- 1 ½ tablespoons chopped walnuts
- 1 teaspoon shallot powder
- 1-pound turkey breasts, sliced
- 1 teaspoon garlic powder
- 2 teaspoons olive oil
- 1/2 teaspoon onion salt
- 1/2 teaspoon red pepper flakes, crushed
- 1 teaspoon ground black pepper

Directions:
1. Begin by preheating your air fryer to 395 degrees f. Place all ingredients, minus chopped walnuts, in a mixing bowl and let them marinate at least 1 hour.
2. After that, cook the marinated turkey breast approximately 23 minutes or until heated through.
3. Pause the machine, scatter chopped walnuts over the top and air-fry an additional 5 minutes.

Nutrition:
Calories 365 Fat 20.3 g Carbohydrates 1.5 g Sugar 0 g Protein 45.2 g Cholesterol 139 mg

707. Eggs and Sausage with Keto Rolls
Prep Time 40 m | Cooking Time 14 m | 6 Servings

Ingredients:
- 1 teaspoon dried dill weed
- 1 teaspoon mustard seeds
- 6 turkey sausages
- 3 bell peppers, seeded and thinly sliced
- 6 medium-sized eggs
- 1/2 teaspoon fennel seeds
- 1 teaspoon sea salt
- 1/3 teaspoon freshly cracked pink peppercorns
- Keto rolls:
- 1/2 cup ricotta cheese, crumbled
- 1 cup part skim mozzarella cheese, shredded
- 1 egg
- 1/2 cup coconut flour
- 1/2 cup almond flour
- 1 teaspoon baking soda
- 2 tablespoons plain whey protein isolate

Directions:
1. Set your air fryer to cook at 325 degrees f. Cook the sausages and bell peppers in the air fryer cooking basket for 8 minutes.
2. Crack the eggs into the ramekins; sprinkle them with salt, dill weed, mustard seeds, fennel seeds, and cracked peppercorns. Cook an additional 12 minutes at 395 degrees f.
3. To make the keto rolls, microwave the cheese for 1 minute 30 seconds, stirring twice. Add the cheese to the bowl of a food processor and blend well. Fold in the egg and mix again.
4. Add in the flour, baking soda, and plain whey protein isolate; blend again. Scrape the batter onto the center of a lightly greased cling film.
5. Form the dough into a disk and transfer to your freezer to cool; cut into 6 pieces and transfer to a parchment-lined baking pan (make sure to grease your hands.
6. Bake in the preheated oven at 400 degrees f for about 14 minutes.
7. Serve eggs and sausages on keto rolls.

Nutrition:
Calories 398 Fat 20.3 g Carbohydrates 1.5 g Sugar 0 g Protein 45.2 g Cholesterol 139 mg

708. Bacon-Wrapped Turkey with Cheese
⏱ Prep Time 20 m | ⏱ Cooking Time 13 m | 12 Servings

Ingredients:
- 1 ½ small-sized turkey breast, chop into 12 pieces
- 12 thin slices asiago cheese
- Paprika, to taste
- Fine sea salt and ground black pepper, to savor
- 12 rashers bacon

Directions:
1. Lay out the bacon rashers; place 1 slice of asiago cheese on each bacon piece.
2. Top with turkey, season with paprika, salt, and pepper, and roll them up; secure with a cocktail stick.
3. Air-fry at 365 degrees f for 13 minutes.

Nutrition:
Calories 534 Fat 20.3 g Carbohydrates 1.5 g Sugar 0 g Protein 45.2 g Cholesterol 139 mg

709. Italian-Style Spicy Chicken Breasts
⏱ Prep Time 20 m | ⏱ Cooking Time 11 m | 4 Servings

Ingredients:
- 2 ounces asiago cheese, cut into sticks
- 1/3 cup tomato paste
- 1/2 teaspoon garlic paste
- 2 chicken breasts, cut in half lengthwise
- 1/2 cup green onions, chopped
- 1 tablespoon chili sauce
- 1/2 cup roasted vegetable stock
- 1 tablespoon sesame oil
- 1 teaspoon salt
- 2 teaspoons unsweetened cocoa
- 1/2 teaspoon sweet paprika, or more to taste

Directions:
1. Sprinkle chicken breasts with the salt and sweet paprika; drizzle with chili sauce. Now, place a stick of asiago cheese in the middle of each chicken breast.
2. Then, tie the whole thing using a kitchen string; give a drizzle of sesame oil.
3. Transfer the stuffed chicken to the cooking basket. Add the other ingredients and toss to coat the chicken.
4. Afterward, cook for about 11 minutes at 395 degrees f. Serve the chicken on two serving plates, garnish with fresh or pickled salad and serve immediately.

Nutrition:
Calories 398 Fat 20.3 g Carbohydrates 1.5 g Sugar 0 g Protein 45.2 g Cholesterol 139 mg

710. Classic Chicken Nuggets
⏱ Prep Time 20 m | ⏱ Cooking Time 10 m | 4 Servings

Ingredients:
- 1 ½ pounds chicken tenderloins, cut into small pieces
- 1/2 teaspoon garlic salt
- 1/2 teaspoon cayenne pepper
- 1/4 teaspoon black pepper, freshly cracked
- 4 tablespoons olive oil
- 2 scoops low-carb unflavored protein powder
- 4 tablespoons parmesan cheese, freshly grated

Directions:
1. Start by preheating your air fryer to 390 degrees f.
2. Season each piece of the chicken with garlic salt, cayenne pepper, and black pepper.
3. In a mixing bowl, thoroughly combine the olive oil with protein powder and parmesan cheese. Dip each piece of chicken in the parmesan mixture.
4. Cook for 8 minutes, working in batches.
5. Later, if you want to warm the chicken nuggets, add them to the basket and cook for 1 minute more.

Nutrition:
Calories 327 Fat 20.3 g Carbohydrates 1.5 g Sugar 0 g Protein 45.2 g Cholesterol 139 mg

711. Thai Chicken with Bacon
⏱ Prep Time 50 m | ⏱ Cooking Time 20 m | 2 Servings

Ingredients:
- 4 rashers smoked bacon
- 2 chicken filets
- 1/2 teaspoon coarse sea salt
- 1/4 teaspoon black pepper, preferably freshly ground
- 1 teaspoon garlic, minced
- 1 (2-inch piece ginger, peeled and minced
- 1 teaspoon black mustard seeds
- 1 teaspoon mild curry powder
- 1/2 cup coconut milk
- 1/2 cup parmesan cheese, grated

Directions:
1. Start by preheating your air fryer to 400 degrees f. Add the smoked bacon and cook in the preheated air fryer for 5 to 7 minutes. Reserve.
2. In a mixing bowl, place the chicken fillets, salt, black pepper, garlic, ginger, mustard seeds, curry powder, and milk. Let it marinate in your refrigerator about 30 minutes.
3. In another bowl, place the grated parmesan cheese.
4. Dredge the chicken fillets through the parmesan mixture and transfer them to the cooking basket. Reduce the temperature to 380 degrees f and cook the chicken for 6 minutes.
5. Turn them over and cook for a further 6 minutes. Repeat the process until you have run out of ingredients.
6. Serve with reserved bacon. Enjoy!

Nutrition:
Calories 612 Fat 20.3 g Carbohydrates 1.5 g Sugar 0 g Protein 45.2 g Cholesterol 139 mg

712. Thanksgiving Turkey with Mustard Gravy

⏱ Prep Time 50 m | ⏱ Cooking Time 45 m | 6 Servings

Ingredients:

- 2 teaspoons butter, softened
- 1 teaspoon dried sage
- 2 sprigs rosemary, chopped
- 1 teaspoon salt
- 1/4 teaspoon freshly ground black pepper, or more to taste
- 1 whole turkey breast
- 2 tablespoons turkey broth
- 2 tablespoons whole-grain mustard
- 1 tablespoon butter

Directions:

1. Start by preheating your air fryer to 360 degrees f.
2. To make the rub, combine 2 tablespoons of butter, sage, rosemary, salt, and pepper; mix well to combine and spread it evenly over the surface of the turkey breast.
3. Roast for 20 minutes in an air fryer cooking basket. Flip the turkey breast over and cook for a further 15 to 16 minutes. Now, flip it back over and roast for 12 minutes more.
4. While the turkey is roasting, whisk the other ingredients in a saucepan. After that, spread the gravy all over the turkey breast.
5. Let the turkey rest for a few minutes before carving.

Nutrition:

Calories 376 Fat 20.3 g Carbohydrates 1.5 g Sugar 0 g Protein 45.2 g Cholesterol 139 mg

713. Pretzel Crusted Chicken With Spicy Mustard Sauce

⏱ Prep Time 15 m | ⏱ Cooking Time 20 m | 6 Servings

Ingredients:

- 2 eggs
- 1 ½ pound chicken breasts, boneless, skinless, cut into bite-sized chunks
- 1/2 cup crushed pretzels
- 1 teaspoon shallot powder
- 1 teaspoon paprika
- Sea salt and ground black pepper, to taste
- 1/2 cup vegetable broth
- 1 tablespoon cornstarch
- 3 tablespoons Worcestershire sauce
- 3 tablespoons tomato paste
- 1 tablespoon apple cider vinegar
- 2 tablespoons olive oil
- 2 garlic cloves, chopped
- 1 jalapeno pepper, minced
- 1 teaspoon yellow mustard

Directions:

1. Start by preheating your Air Fryer to 390 degrees F.
2. In a mixing dish, whisk the eggs until frothy; toss the chicken chunks into the whisked eggs and coat well.
3. In another dish, combine the crushed pretzels with shallot powder, paprika, salt and pepper. Then, lay the chicken chunks in the pretzel mixture; turn it over until well coated.
4. Place the chicken pieces in the air fryer basket. Cook the chicken for 12 minutes, shaking the basket halfway through.
5. Meanwhile, whisk the vegetable broth with cornstarch, Worcestershire sauce, tomato paste, and apple cider vinegar.
6. Preheat a cast-iron skillet over medium flame. Heat the olive oil and sauté the garlic with jalapeno pepper for 30 to 40 seconds, stirring frequently.
7. Add the cornstarch mixture and let it simmer until the sauce has thickened a little. Now, add the air-fried chicken and mustard; let it simmer for 2 minutes more or until heated through.
8. Serve immediately and enjoy!

Nutrition:

357 Calories 17.6g Fat 20.3g Carbs 28.1g Protein 2.8g Sugars

714. Chinese-Style Sticky Turkey Thighs

⏱ Prep Time 20 m | ⏱ Cooking Time 35 m | 6 Servings

Ingredients:

- 1 tablespoon sesame oil
- 2 pounds turkey thighs
- 1 teaspoon Chinese Five-spice powder
- 1 teaspoon pink Himalayan salt
- 1/4 teaspoon Sichuan pepper
- 6 tablespoons honey
- 1 tablespoon Chinese rice vinegar
- 2 tablespoons soy sauce
- 1 tablespoon sweet chili sauce
- 1 tablespoon mustard

Directions:

1. Preheat your Air Fryer to 360 degrees F.
2. Brush the sesame oil all over the turkey thighs. Season them with spices.
3. Cook for 23 minutes, turning over once or twice. Make sure to work in batches to ensure even cooking
4. In the meantime, combine the remaining ingredients in a wok (or similar type pan) that is preheated over medium-high heat. Cook and stir until the sauce reduces by about a third.
5. Add the fried turkey thighs to the wok; gently stir to coat with the sauce.
6. Let the turkey rest for 10 minutes before slicing and serving. Enjoy!

Nutrition:

279 Calories 10.1g Fat 19g Carbs 27.7g Protein 17.9g Sugars

715. Easy Hot Chicken Drumsticks

⏱ Prep Time 40 m | ⏱ Cooking Time 30 m | 6 Servings

Ingredients:

- 6 chicken drumsticks
- Sauce:
- 6 ounces hot sauce
- 3 tablespoons olive oil
- 3 tablespoons tamari sauce
- 1 teaspoon dried thyme
- 1/2 teaspoon dried oregano

Directions:

1. Spritz the sides and bottom of the cooking basket with a nonstick cooking spray.
2. Cook the chicken drumsticks at 380 degrees F for 35 minutes, flipping them over halfway through.
3. Meanwhile, heat the hot sauce, olive oil, tamari sauce, thyme, and oregano in a pan over medium-low heat; reserve.
4. Drizzle the sauce over the prepared chicken drumsticks; toss to coat well and serve. Bon appétit!

Nutrition:

280 Calories 18.7g Fat 2.6g Carbs 24.1g Protein 1.4g Sugars

716. Crunchy Munchy Chicken Tenders With Peanuts

⏱ Prep Time 25 m | ⏱ Cooking Time 20 m | 4 Servings

Ingredients:

- 1 ½ pounds chicken tenderloins
- 2 tablespoons peanut oil
- 1/2 cup tortilla chips, crushed
- Sea salt and ground black pepper, to taste
- 1/2 teaspoon garlic powder
- 1 teaspoon red pepper flakes
- 2 tablespoons peanuts, roasted and roughly chopped

Directions:

1. Start by preheating your Air Fryer to 360 degrees F.
2. Brush the chicken tenderloins with peanut oil on all sides.
3. In a mixing bowl, thoroughly combine the crushed chips, salt, black pepper, garlic powder, and red pepper flakes. Dredge the chicken in the breading, shaking off any residual coating.
4. Lay the chicken tenderloins into the cooking basket. Cook for 12 to 13 minutes or until it is no longer pink in the center. Work in batches; an instant-read thermometer should read at least 165 degrees F.
5. Serve garnished with roasted peanuts. Bon appétit!

Nutrition:

343 Calories 16.4g Fat 10.6g Carbs 36.8g Protein 1g Sugar

717. Tarragon Turkey Tenderloins With Baby Potatoes

⏱ Prep Time 50 m | ⏱ Cooking Time 50 m | 6 Servings

Ingredients:

- 2 pounds turkey tenderloins
- 2 teaspoons olive oil
- Salt and ground black pepper, to taste
- 1 teaspoon smoked paprika
- 2 tablespoons dry white wine
- 1 tablespoon fresh tarragon leaves, chopped
- 1-pound baby potatoes, rubbed

Directions:

1. Brush the turkey tenderloins with olive oil. Season with salt, black pepper, and paprika.
2. Afterwards, add the white wine and tarragon.
3. Cook the turkey tenderloins at 350 degrees F for 30 minutes, flipping them over halfway through. Let them rest for 5 to 9 minutes before slicing and serving.
4. After that, spritz the sides and bottom of the cooking basket with the remaining 1 teaspoon of olive oil.
5. Then, preheat your Air Fryer to 400 degrees F; cook the baby potatoes for 15 minutes. Serve with the turkey and enjoy!

Nutrition:

317 Calories 7.4g Fat 14.2g Carbs 45.7g Protein 1.1g Sugars

718. Mediterranean Chicken Breasts With Roasted Tomatoes

⏱ Prep Time 1 h | ⏱ Cooking Time 30 m | 8 Servings

Ingredients:

- 2 teaspoons olive oil, melted
- 3 pounds chicken breasts, bone-in
- 1/2 teaspoon black pepper, freshly ground
- 1/2 teaspoon salt
- 1 teaspoon cayenne pepper
- 2 tablespoons fresh parsley, minced
- 1 teaspoon fresh basil, minced
- 1 teaspoon fresh rosemary, minced
- 4 medium-sized Roma tomatoes, halved

Directions:

1. Start by preheating your Air Fryer to 370 degrees F. Brush the cooking basket with 1 teaspoon of olive oil.
2. Sprinkle the chicken breasts with all seasonings listed above.
3. Cook for 25 minutes or until chicken breasts are slightly browned. Work in batches.
4. Arrange the tomatoes in the cooking basket and brush them with the remaining teaspoon of olive oil. Season with sea salt.
5. Cook the tomatoes at 350 degrees F for 10 minutes, shaking halfway through the cooking time. Serve with chicken breasts. Bon appétit!

Nutrition:

315 Calories 17.1g Fat 2.7g Carbs 36g Protein 1.7g Sugars

719. Thai Red Duck With Candy Onion

⏱ Prep Time 25 m | ⏱ Cooking Time 25 m | 4 Servings

Ingredients:

- 1 ½ pounds duck breasts, skin removed
- 1 teaspoon kosher salt
- 1/2 teaspoon cayenne pepper
- 1/3 teaspoon black pepper
- 1/2 teaspoon smoked paprika
- 1 tablespoon Thai red curry paste
- 1 cup candy onions, halved
- 1/4 small pack coriander, chopped

Directions:

1. Place the duck breasts between 2 sheets of foil; then, use a rolling pin to bash the duck until they are 1-inch thick.
2. Preheat your Air Fryer to 395 degrees F.
3. Rub the duck breasts with salt, cayenne pepper, black pepper, paprika, and red curry paste. Place the duck breast in the cooking basket.
4. Cook for 11 to 12 minutes. Top with candy onions and cook for another 10 to 11 minutes.
5. Serve garnished with coriander and enjoy!

Nutrition:

362 Calories 18.7g Fat 4g Carbs 42.3g Protein 1.3g Sugars

720. Rustic Chicken Legs With Turnip Chips

⏱ Prep Time 30 m | ⏱ Cooking Time 20 m | 3 Servings

Ingredients:

- 1-pound chicken legs
- 1 teaspoon Himalayan salt
- 1 teaspoon paprika
- 1/2 teaspoon ground black pepper
- 1 teaspoon butter, melted
- 1 turnip, trimmed and sliced

Directions:

1. Spritz the sides and bottom of the cooking basket with a nonstick cooking spray.
2. Season the chicken legs with salt, paprika, and ground black pepper.
3. Cook at 370 degrees F for 10 minutes. Increase the temperature to 380 degrees F.
4. Drizzle turnip slices with melted butter and transfer them to the cooking basket with the chicken. Cook the turnips and chicken for 15 minutes more, flipping them halfway through the cooking time.
5. As for the chicken, an instant-read thermometer should read at least 165 degrees F.
6. Serve and enjoy!

Nutrition:

207 Calories 7.8g Fat 3.4g Carbs 29.5g Protein 1.6g Sugars

721. Old-Fashioned Chicken Drumettes
Prep Time 30 m | Cooking Time 22 m | 3 Servings

Ingredients:
- 1/3 cup all-purpose flour
- 1/2 teaspoon ground white pepper
- 1 teaspoon seasoning salt
- 1 teaspoon garlic paste
- 1 teaspoon rosemary
- 1 whole egg + 1 egg white
- 6 chicken drumettes
- 1 heaping tablespoon fresh chives, chopped

Directions:
1. Start by preheating your Air Fryer to 390 degrees.
2. Mix the flour with white pepper, salt, garlic paste, and rosemary in a small-sized bowl.
3. In another bowl, beat the eggs until frothy.
4. Dip the chicken into the flour mixture, then into the beaten eggs; coat with the flour mixture one more time.
5. Cook the chicken drumettes for 22 minutes. Serve warm, garnished with chives.

Nutrition:
347 Calories 9.1g Fat 11.3g Carbs 41g Protein 0.1g Sugars

722. Easy Ritzy Chicken Nuggets
Prep Time 20 m | Cooking Time 8 m | 4 Servings

Ingredients:
- 1 ½ pounds chicken tenderloins, cut into small pieces
- 1/2 teaspoon garlic salt
- 1/2 teaspoon cayenne pepper
- 1/4 teaspoon black pepper, freshly cracked
- 4 tablespoons olive oil
- 1/3 cup saltines (e.g. Ritz crackers), crushed
- 4 tablespoons Parmesan cheese, freshly grated

Directions:
1. Start by preheating your Air Fryer to 390 degrees F.
2. Season each piece of the chicken with garlic salt, cayenne pepper, and black pepper.
3. In a mixing bowl, thoroughly combine the olive oil with crushed saltines. Dip each piece of chicken in the cracker mixture.
4. Finally, roll the chicken pieces over the Parmesan cheese. Cook for 8 minutes, working in batches.
5. Later, if you want to warm the chicken nuggets, add them to the basket and cook for 1 minute more. Serve with French fries, if desired.

Nutrition:
355 Calories 20.1g Fat 5.3g Carbs 36.6g Protein 0.2g Sugars

723. Asian Chicken Filets With Cheese
Prep Time 50 m | Cooking Time 20 m | 2 Servings

Ingredients:
- 4 rashers smoked bacon
- 2 chicken filets
- 1/2 teaspoon coarse sea salt
- 1/4 teaspoon black pepper, preferably freshly ground
- 1 teaspoon garlic, minced
- 1 (2-inch) piece ginger, peeled and minced
- 1 teaspoon black mustard seeds
- 1 teaspoon mild curry powder
- 1/2 cup coconut milk
- 1/3 cup tortilla chips, crushed
- 1/2 cup Pecorino Romano cheese, freshly grated

Directions:
1. Start by preheating your Air Fryer to 400 degrees F. Add the smoked bacon and cook in the preheated Air Fryer for 5 to 7 minutes. Reserve.
2. In a mixing bowl, place the chicken fillets, salt, black pepper, garlic, ginger, mustard seeds, curry powder, and milk. Let it marinate in your refrigerator about 30 minutes.
3. In another bowl, mix the crushed chips and grated Pecorino Romano cheese.
4. Dredge the chicken fillets through the chips mixture and transfer them to the cooking basket. Reduce the temperature to 380 degrees F and cook the chicken for 6 minutes.
5. Turn them over and cook for a further 6 minutes. Repeat the process until you have run out of ingredients.
6. Serve with reserved bacon. Enjoy!

Nutrition:
376 Calories 19.6g Fat 12.1g Carbs 36.2g Protein 3.4g Sugars

724. Paprika Chicken Legs With Brussels Sprouts
Prep Time 30 m | Cooking Time 20 m | 2 Servings

Ingredients:
- 2 chicken legs
- 1/2 teaspoon paprika
- 1/2 teaspoon kosher salt
- 1/2 teaspoon black pepper
- 1-pound Brussels sprouts
- 1 teaspoon dill, fresh or dried

Directions:
1. Start by preheating your Air Fryer to 370 degrees F.
2. Now, season your chicken with paprika, salt, and pepper. Transfer the chicken legs to the cooking basket. Cook for 10 minutes.
3. Flip the chicken legs and cook an additional 10 minutes. Reserve.
4. Add the Brussels sprouts to the cooking basket; sprinkle with dill. Cook at 380 degrees F for 15 minutes, shaking the basket halfway through.
5. Serve with the reserved chicken legs. Bon appétit!

Nutrition:
355 Calories 20.1g Fat 5.3g Carbs 36.6g Protein 0.2g Sugars

725. Chinese Duck

🕐 Prep Time 30 m | 🕐 Cooking Time 20 m | 6 Servings

Ingredients:

- 2 pounds duck breast, boneless
- 2 green onions, chopped
- 1 tablespoon light soy sauce
- 1 teaspoon Chinese 5-spice powder
- 1 teaspoon Szechuan peppercorns
- 3 tablespoons Shaoxing rice wine
- 1 teaspoon coarse salt
- 1/2 teaspoon ground black pepper

Glaze:

- 1/4 cup molasses
- 3 tablespoons orange juice
- 1 tablespoon soy sauce

Directions:

1. In a ceramic bowl, place the duck breasts, green onions, light soy sauce, Chinese 5-spice powder, Szechuan peppercorns, and Shaoxing rice wine. Let it marinate for 1 hour in your refrigerator.
2. Preheat your Air Fryer to 400 degrees F for 5 minutes.
3. Now, discard the marinade and season the duck breasts with salt and pepper. Cook the duck breasts for 12 to 15 minutes or until they are golden brown. Repeat with the other ingredients.
4. In the meantime, add the reserved marinade to the saucepan that is preheated over medium-high heat. Add the molasses, orange juice, and 1 tablespoon of soy sauce.
5. Bring to a simmer and then, whisk constantly until it gets syrupy. Brush the surface of duck breasts with glaze so they are completely covered.
6. Place duck breasts back in the Air Fryer basket; cook an additional 5 minutes. Enjoy!

Nutrition:

403 Calories 25.3g Fat 16.4g Carbs 27.5g Protein 13.2g Sugars

726. Turkey Bacon With Scrambled Eggs

🕐 Prep Time 25 m | 🕐 Cooking Time 20 m | 4 Servings

Ingredients:

- 1/2-pound turkey bacon
- 4 eggs
- 1/3 cup milk
- 2 tablespoons yogurt
- 1/2 teaspoon sea salt
- 1 bell pepper, finely chopped
- 2 green onions, finely chopped
- 1/2 cup Colby cheese, shredded

Directions:

1. Place the turkey bacon in the cooking basket.
2. Cook at 360 degrees F for 9 to 11 minutes. Work in batches. Reserve the fried bacon.
3. In a mixing bowl, thoroughly whisk the eggs with milk and yogurt. Add salt, bell pepper, and green onions.
4. Brush the sides and bottom of the baking pan with the reserved 1 teaspoon of bacon grease.
5. Pour the egg mixture into the baking pan. Cook at 355 degrees F about 5 minutes. Top with shredded Colby cheese and cook for 5 to 6 minutes more.
6. Serve the scrambled eggs with the reserved bacon and enjoy!

Nutrition:

456 Calories 38.3g Fat 6.3g Carbs 1.4g Protein 4.5g Sugars

727. Italian Chicken And Cheese Frittata

🕐 Prep Time 25 m | 🕐 Cooking Time 20 m | 4 Servings

Ingredients:

- 1 (1-pound) fillet chicken breast
- Sea salt and ground black pepper, to taste
- 1 tablespoon olive oil
- 4 eggs
- 1/2 teaspoon cayenne pepper
- 1/2 cup Mascarpone cream
- 1/4 cup Asiago cheese, freshly grated

Directions:

1. Flatten the chicken breast with a meat mallet. Season with salt and pepper.
2. Heat the olive oil in a frying pan over medium flame. Cook the chicken for 10 to 12 minutes; slice into small strips, and reserve.
3. Then, in a mixing bowl, thoroughly combine the eggs, and cayenne pepper; season with salt to taste. Add the cheese and stir to combine.
4. Add the reserved chicken. Then, pour the mixture into a lightly greased pan; put the pan into the cooking basket.
5. Cook in the preheated Air Fryer at 355 degrees F for 10 minutes, flipping over halfway through.

Nutrition:

329 Calories 25.3g Fat 3.4g Carbs 21.1g Protein 2.3g Sugars

728. Parmigiana Chicken

🕐 Prep Time 3 m | 🕐 Cooking Time 12 m | 4 Servings

Ingredients:

- 2 eggs
- ½ cup Parmesan cheese, grated
- 1 cup seasoned bread crumbs
- 1-pound (454 g) chicken breast halves
- 2 sprigs rosemary, chopped
- From the cupboard:
- Salt and ground black pepper, to taste

Directions:

1. Preheat the air fryer to 380°F (193°C). Spritz the air fryer basket with cooking spray.
2. Beat the egg in a first bowl and sprinkle with salt and black pepper. Combine the Parmesan and bread crumbs in the second bowl.
3. Dredge the chicken in the first bowl to coat well, then in the second the bowl. Shake the excess off.
4. Cook the chicken in the preheated air fryer for 12 minutes or until the internal temperature reaches at least 165°F (74°C). Flip the chicken halfway through the cooking time.
5. Transfer the chicken to a plate and serve with rosemary on top.

Nutrition:

Calories: 430 Fat: 25.0g Carbs: 21.5g Protein: 48.0g

729. Easy Paprika Chicken

⏱ Prep Time 7 m | ⏱ Cooking Time 18 m | 4 Servings

Ingredients:

- 4 chicken breasts
- 1 tablespoon paprika
- ¼ teaspoon garlic powder
- 2 tablespoons fresh thyme, chopped

- From the cupboard:
- Salt and ground black pepper, to taste
- 2 tablespoons butter, melted

Directions:

1. Preheat the air fryer to 360°F (182°C). Spritz the air fryer basket with cooking spray.
2. On a clean work surface, rub the chicken breasts with paprika, garlic powder, salt, and black pepper, then brush with butter.
3. Cook the chicken in the preheated air fryer for 18 minutes or until the internal temperature reaches at least 165°F (74°C). Flip the chicken with tongs halfway through the cooking time.
4. Serve the cooked chicken on a plate immediately with thyme on top.

Nutrition:
Calories: 368 Fat: 14.1g Carbs: 2.3g Protein: 57.9g

730. Spinach And Cheese Stuffed Chicken Breasts

⏱ Prep Time 3 m | ⏱ Cooking Time 12 m | 4 Servings

Ingredients:

- 1 cup spinach, chopped
- 4 tablespoons cottage cheese
- 2 chicken breasts
- 2 tablespoons Italian seasoning

- Juice of ½ lime
- Special Equipment:
- 2 or 4 toothpicks, soaked for at least 30 minutes

Directions:

1. Preheat the air fryer to 390°F (199°C). Spritz the air fryer basket with cooking spray.
2. Combine the chopped spinach and cheese in a large bowl. Set aside.
3. Butterfly the chicken breasts and flatten with a rolling pin. Sprinkle with Italian seasoning, then wrap the spinach and cheese mixture in the butterflied chicken breasts. Secure with toothpicks.
4. Place the chicken in the air fryer basket and spritz with cooking spray.
5. Cook for 12 minutes or until the internal temperature reaches at least 165°F (74°C). Flip the chicken halfway through the cooking time.
6. Remove the chicken from the air fryer basket. Discard the toothpicks and serve drizzled with lemon juice.

Nutrition:
Calories: 248 Fat: 11.0g Carbs: 4.1g Protein: 31.0g

731. Texas Thighs

⏱ Prep Time 10 m | ⏱ Cooking Time 20 m | 8 Servings

Ingredients:

- 8 chicken thighs
- 2 teaspoons Texas BBQ Jerky seasoning
- 2 tablespoons cilantro, chopped

- From the Cupboard:
- 1 tablespoon olive oil
- Salt and ground black pepper, to taste

Directions:

1. Preheat air fryer to 380°F (193°C). Spritz the air fryer basket with cooking spray.
2. Arrange the chicken thighs in the air fryer basket, then brush with olive oil on all sides. Sprinkle with BBQ seasoning, salt, and black pepper.
3. Cook for 20 minutes or until the internal temperature of the thighs reaches at least 165°F (74°C). Flip the thighs three times during the cooking time.
4. Remove the chicken thighs from the air fryer basket and serve with cilantro on top.

Nutrition:
Calories: 444 Fat: 33.8g Carbs: 1.0g Protein: 31.9g

732. Chicken Wings With Sweet Chili Sauce

⏱ Prep Time 6 m | ⏱ Cooking Time 14 m | 4 Servings

Ingredients:

- 1-pound (454 g) chicken wings
- 1 teaspoon garlic powder
- 1 tablespoon tamarind powder

- ¼ cup sweet chili sauce
- From the Cupboard:
- Salt and ground black pepper, to taste

Directions:

1. Preheat the air fryer to 390°F (199°C). Spritz the air fryer with cooking spray.
2. On a clean work surface, rub the chicken wings with garlic powder, tamarind powder, salt, and black pepper.
3. Place the wings in the basket and cook for 6 minutes, then spread the chili sauce on top and cook for an additional 8 minutes or until the internal temperature of the wings reaches at least 165°F (74°C).
4. Remove the wings from the air fryer. Allow to cool for a few minutes and serve.

Nutrition:
Calories: 165 Fat: 4.1g Carbs: 4.5g Protein: 25.5g

733. Crunchy Golden Nuggets

⏱ Prep Time 5 m | ⏱ Cooking Time 10 m | 4 Servings

Ingredients:

- 2 chicken breasts, cut into nuggets
- 4 tablespoons sour cream
- ½ cup bread crumbs
- ½ tablespoon garlic powder

From the Cupboard:

- ½ teaspoon cayenne pepper
- Salt and ground black pepper, to taste

Directions:

1. Preheat the air fryer to 360°F (182°C). Spritz the air fryer basket with cooking spray.
2. Put the sour cream in a large bowl. Combine the bread crumbs, cayenne pepper, garlic powder, salt, and black pepper on a large plate.
3. Dredge the chicken nuggets in the bowl of sour cream, shake the excess off, then roll the nuggets through the bread crumbs mixture to coat well.
4. Place the nuggets in the air fryer basket and cook for 10 minutes or until the chicken nuggets are golden brown and crispy. Flip the nuggets halfway through the cooking time.
5. Remove the nuggets from the basket and serve warm.

Nutrition:
Calories: 324 Fat: 15.5g Carbs: 11.7g Protein: 32.7g

734. Roasted Whole Chicken

⏱ Prep Time 10 m | ⏱ Cooking Time 40 m | 4 Servings

Ingredients:

- 1 (3-pound / 1.4-kg) chicken, rinsed and patted dry
- 1 garlic bulb
- 1 sprig fresh tarragon
- 1 lemon, cut into wedges

- From the Cupboard:
- 2 tablespoons butter, melted
- Salt and ground black pepper, to taste

Directions:

1. Preheat the air fryer to 380°F (193°C). Spritz the air fryer basket with cooking spray.
2. On a clean work surface, brush the chicken with butter and rub with salt and black pepper. Stuff the chicken with garlic, tarragon, and lemon wedges.
3. Arrange the chicken in the air fryer basket and roast for 40 minutes or until an instant-read thermometer inserted in the thickest part of the chicken registers at least 165°F (74°C).
4. Remove the chicken from the basket and put on a large platter. Carve the chicken and slice to serve.

Nutrition:
Calories: 440 Fat: 15.0g Carbs: 2.6g Protein: 69.7g

735. Cheesy Chicken Thighs With Marinara Sauce

⏱ Prep Time 10 m | ⏱ Cooking Time 10 m | 4 Servings

Ingredients:

- 2 tablespoons grated Parmesan cheese
- ½ cup Italian bread crumbs
- 4 chicken thighs
- ½ cup shredded Monterrey Jack cheese

- ½ cup marinara sauce
From the Cupboard:
- 1 tablespoon butter, melted

Directions:

1. Preheat the air fryer to 380°F (193°C). Spritz the air fryer basket with cooking spray.
2. Combine the Parmesan and bread crumbs in a bowl.
3. On a clean work surface, brush the chicken thighs with butter, then dredge the thighs in the Parmesan mixture to coat.
4. Place the chicken thighs in the preheated air fryer and cook for 5 minutes, then spread the Monterrey Jack cheese over and pour the marinara sauce on the thighs, and then cook for 4 more minutes until the thighs are golden brown and the cheese melts.
5. Transfer the thighs onto a plate and serve warm.

Nutrition:
Calories: 617 Fat: 42.1g Carbs: 17.7g Protein: 39.6g

736. Chicken In Bacon Wrap

⏱ Prep Time 5 m | ⏱ Cooking Time 15 m | 4 Servings

Ingredients:

- 2 chicken breasts
- 8 ounces (227 g) onion and chive cream cheese
- 6 slices turkey bacon
- 1 tablespoon fresh parsley, chopped
- Juice from ½ lemon

- From the Cupboard:
- 1 tablespoon butter
- Salt, to taste
- Special Equipment:
- 2 or 4 toothpicks, soaked for at least 30 minutes

Directions:

1. Preheat the air fryer to 390°F (199°C). Spritz the air fryer basket with cooking spray.
2. On a clean work surface, brush the chicken breasts with cream cheese and butter on both sides. Sprinkle with salt.
3. Wrap each chicken breast with 3 slices of bacon and secure with 1 or 2 toothpicks.
4. Arrange the bacon-wrapped chicken in the preheated air fryer and cook for 14 minutes or until the bacon is well browned and a meat thermometer inserted in the chicken reads at least 165°F (74°C). Flip them halfway through the cooking time.
5. Remove them from the air fryer basket and serve with parsley and lemon juice on top.

Nutrition:
Calories: 437 Fat: 28.6g Carbs: 5.2g Protein: 39.8g

737. Chicken Thighs With Honey-Dijon Sauce
⏱ Prep Time 5 m | ⏱ Cooking Time 35 m | 4 Servings

Ingredients:
- 8 bone-in and skinless chicken thighs
- Chicken seasoning or rub, to taste
- ½ cup honey
- ¼ cup Dijon mustard
- 2 garlic cloves, minced
- From the Cupboard:
- Salt and ground black pepper, to taste

Directions:
1. Preheat the air fryer to 400°F (205°C). Spritz the air fryer basket with cooking spray.
2. On a clean work surface, rub the chicken thighs with chicken seasoning, salt, and black pepper.
3. Cook the chicken thighs in the preheated air fryer for 15 minutes or until the internal temperature of the chicken thighs reaches at least 165°F (74°C). Flip the thighs halfway through the cooking time. You may need to work in batches to avoid overcrowding.
4. Meanwhile, combine the honey, Dijon mustard, and garlic in a saucepan, and cook over medium-high heat for 3 to 4 minutes until the sauce reduced by one third. Keep stirring during the cooking.
5. Remove the chicken thighs from the air fryer basket and put on a dish. Baste the thighs with the cooked sauce and serve warm.

Nutrition: Calories: 382 Fat: 18.0g Carbs: 36.0g Protein: 21.0g

738. Lemon And Honey Glazed Game Hen
⏱ Prep Time 10 m | ⏱ Cooking Time 20 m | 2 Servings

Ingredients:
- 1 (2-pound / 907-g) Cornish game hen, split in half
- ¼ teaspoon dried thyme
- Juice and zest of 1 lemon
- ¼ cup honey
- 1½ teaspoons chopped fresh thyme leaves
- From the Cupboard:
- 1 tablespoon olive oil
- Salt and ground black pepper, to taste
- ½ teaspoon soy sauce

Directions:
1. Preheat the air fryer to 390°F (199°C). Spritz the air fryer basket with cooking spray.
2. On a clean work surface, brush the game hen halves with olive oil, then sprinkle with dried thyme, salt, and black pepper to season.
3. Cook the hen in the preheated air fryer for 15 minutes or until the hen is lightly browned. Flip the hen halfway through.
4. Meanwhile, mix the lemon juice and zest, honey, thyme leaves, soy sauce, and black pepper in a bowl.
5. Baste the game hen with the honey glaze, then cook for an additional 4 minutes or until the hen is well glazed and a meat thermometer inserted in the hen reads at least 165°F (74°C).
6. Remove the game hen from the air fryer basket. Allow to cool for a few minutes and slice to serve.

Nutrition: Calories: 724 Fat: 22.0g Carbs: 37.5g Protein: 91.3g

739. Cheesy Spinach Stuffed Chicken Breasts
⏱ Prep Time 20 m | ⏱ Cooking Time 25 m | 4 Servings

Ingredients:
- 1 (10-ounce / 284-g) package frozen spinach, thawed and drained well
- 1 cup feta cheese, crumbled
- 4 boneless chicken breasts
- From the Cupboard:
- Salt and ground black pepper, to taste
- Special Equipment:
- 4 or 8 toothpicks, soaked for at least 30 minutes

Directions:
1. Preheat the air fryer to 380°F (193°C). Spritz the air fryer basket with cooking spray.
2. Make the filling: Chop the spinach and put in a large bowl, then add the feta cheese and ½ teaspoon of ground black pepper. Stir to mix well.
3. On a clean work surface, using a knife, cut a 1-inch incision into the thicker side of each chicken breast horizontally. Make a 3-inch long pocket from the incision and keep the sides and bottom intact.
4. Stuff the chicken pockets with the filling and secure with 1 or 2 toothpicks.
5. Arrange the stuffed chicken breasts in the preheated air fryer. Sprinkle with salt and black pepper and spritz with cooking spray. You may need to work in batches to avoid overcrowding.
6. Cook for 12 minutes or until the internal temperature of the chicken reads at least 165°F (74°C). Flip the chicken halfway through the cooking time.
7. Remove the chicken from the air fryer basket. Discard the toothpicks and allow to cool for 10 minutes before slicing to serve.

Nutrition: Calories: 648 Fat: 38.7g Carbs: 4.5g Protein: 68.2g

740. Turkey And Pepper Sandwich
⏱ Prep Time 5 m | ⏱ Cooking Time 5 m | 1 Servings

Ingredients:
- 2 slices whole grain bread
- 2 teaspoons Dijon mustard
- 2 ounces (57 g) cooked turkey breast, thinly sliced
- 2 slices low-fat Swiss cheese
- 3 strips roasted red bell pepper
- From the Cupboard:
- Salt and ground black pepper, to taste

Directions:
1. Preheat the air fryer to 330°F (166°C). Spritz the air fryer basket with cooking spray.
2. Assemble the sandwich: On a dish, place a slice of bread, then top the bread with 1 teaspoon of Dijon mustard, use a knife to smear the mustard evenly.
3. Layer the turkey slices, Swiss cheese slices, and red pepper strips on the bread according to your favorite order. Top them with remaining teaspoon of Dijon mustard and remaining bread slice.
4. Place the sandwich in the preheated air fryer and spritz with cooking spray. Sprinkle with salt and black pepper.
5. Cook for 5 minutes until the cheese melts and the bread is lightly browned. Flip the sandwich halfway through the cooking time.

Nutrition: Calories: 328 Fat: 5.0g Carbs: 38.0g Protein: 29.0g

741. Spicy Turkey Breast

⏱ Prep Time 5 m | ⏱ Cooking Time 40 m | 4 Servings

Ingredients:

- 2-pound (907 g) turkey breast
- 2 teaspoons taco seasonings
- 1 teaspoon ground cumin
- 1 teaspoon red pepper flakes

From the Cupboard:

- Salt and ground black pepper, to taste

Directions:

1. Preheat the air fryer to 350°F (180°C). Spritz the air fryer basket with cooking spray.
2. On a clean work surface, rub the turkey breast with taco seasoning, ground cumin, red pepper flakes, salt, and black pepper.
3. Arrange the turkey in the preheated air fryer and cook for 40 minutes or until the internal temperature of the turkey reads at least 165°F (74°C). Flip the turkey breast halfway through the cooking time.
4. Remove the turkey from the basket. Allow to cool for 15 minutes before slicing to serve.

Nutrition:

Calories: 235 Fat: 5.6g Carbs: 6.6g Protein: 37.3g

742. Chicken, Mushroom, And Pepper Kabobs

⏱ Prep Time 1 h 5 m | ⏱ Cooking Time 15-20 m | 4 Servings

Ingredients:

- ⅓ cup raw honey
- 2 tablespoons sesame seeds
- 2 boneless chicken breasts, cut into cubes
- 6 white mushrooms, cut in halves
- 3 green or red bell peppers, diced

From the Cupboard:

- ⅓ cup soy sauce
- Salt and ground black pepper, to taste
- Special Equipment:
- 4 wooden skewers, soaked for at least 30 minutes

Directions:

1. Combine the honey, soy sauce, sesame seeds, salt, and black pepper in a large bowl. Stir to mix well.
2. Dunk the chicken cubes in this bowl, then wrap the bowl in plastic and refrigerate to marinate for at least an hour.
3. Preheat the air fryer to 390°F (199°C). Spritz the air fryer basket with cooking spray.
4. Remove the chicken cubes from the marinade, then run the skewers through the chicken cubes, mushrooms, and bell peppers alternatively.
5. Baste the chicken, mushrooms, and bell peppers with the marinade, then arrange them in the preheated air fryer.
6. Spritz them with cooking spray and cook for 15 to 20 minutes or until the mushrooms and bell peppers are tender and the chicken cubes are well browned. Flip them halfway through the cooking time.
7. Transfer the skewers to a large plate and serve hot.

Nutrition:

Calories: 380 Fat: 16.0g Carbs: 26.1g Protein: 34.0g

743. Chicken & Zucchini

⏱ Prep Time 30 m | ⏱ Cooking Time 20 m | 6 Servings

Ingredients:

- 1/4 cup olive oil
- 1 tablespoon lemon juice
- 2 tablespoons red wine vinegar
- 1 teaspoon oregano
- 1 tablespoon garlic, chopped
- 2 chicken breast fillet, sliced into cubes
- 1 zucchini, sliced
- 1 red onion, sliced
- 1 cup cherry tomatoes, sliced
- Salt and pepper to taste

Directions:

1. In a bowl, mix the olive oil, lemon juice, vinegar, oregano and garlic.
2. Pour half of mixture into another bowl.
3. Toss chicken in half of the mixture.
4. Cover and marinate for 15 minutes.
5. Toss the veggies in the remaining mixture.
6. Season both chicken and veggies with salt and pepper.
7. Add chicken to the air fryer basket.
8. Spread veggies on top.
9. Select air fry function. Seal and cook at 380 degrees f for 15 to 20 minutes.

Nutrition:

Calories: 282 kcal Protein: 21.87 g Fat: 19.04 g Carbohydrates: 5.31 g

744. Chicken Quesadilla

⏱ Prep Time 20 m | ⏱ Cooking Time 30 m | 8 Servings

Ingredients:

- 4 tortillas
- Cooking spray
- 1/2 cup sour cream
- 1/2 cup salsa
- Hot sauce
- 12 oz. chicken breast fillet, chopped and grilled
- 3 jalapeño peppers, diced
- 2 cups cheddar cheese, shredded
- Chopped scallions

Directions:

1. Add grill grate to the Ninja Foodi Grill.
2. Close the hood.
3. Choose grill setting.
4. Preheat for 5 minutes.
5. While waiting, spray tortillas with oil.
6. In a bowl, mix sour cream, salsa and hot sauce. Set aside.
7. Add tortilla to the grate.
8. Grill for 1 minute.
9. Repeat with the other tortillas.
10. Spread the toasted tortilla with the salsa mixture, chicken, jalapeño peppers, cheese and scallions.
11. Place a tortilla on top. Press.
12. Repeat these steps with the remaining 2 tortillas.
13. Take the grill out of the pot.
14. Choose roast setting.
15. Cook the Quesadillas at 350F for 25 minutes.

Nutrition: Calories:184 kcal Protein: 12.66 g Fat: 7.66 g Carbohydrates: 15.87 g

745. Buffalo Chicken Wings
⏱ Prep Time 15 m | ⏱ Cooking Time 30 m | 4 Servings

Ingredients:
- 2 lb. chicken wings
- 2 tablespoons oil
- 1/2 cup Buffalo sauce

Directions:
1. Coat the chicken wings with oil.
2. Add these to an air fryer basket.
3. Choose air fry function.
4. Cook at 390 degrees F for 15 minutes.
5. Shake and then cook for another 15 minutes.
6. Dip in Buffalo sauce before serving.

Nutrition:
Calories: 376 kcal Protein: 51.93 g Fat: 16.4 g Carbohydrates: 2.18 g

746. Mustard Chicken
⏱ Prep Time 20 m | ⏱ Cooking Time 50 m | 4 Servings

Ingredients:
- 1/4 cup Dijon mustard
- 1/4 cup cooking oil
- Salt and pepper to taste
- 2 tablespoons honey
- 1 tablespoon dry oregano
- 2 teaspoons dry Italian seasoning
- 1 tablespoon lemon juice
- 6 chicken pieces

Directions:
1. Combine all the ingredients except chicken in a bowl.
2. Mix well.
3. Toss the chicken in the mixture.
4. Add roasting rack to your Ninja Foodi Grill.
5. Choose roast function.
6. Set it to 350 degrees F.
7. Cook for 30 minutes.
Flip and cook for another 15 to 20 minutes.

Nutrition:
Calories: 1781 kcal Protein: 293.44 g Fat: 54.33 g Carbohydrates: 11.71 g

747. Honey & Rosemary Chicken
⏱ Prep Time 15 m | ⏱ Cooking Time 35 m | 6 Servings

Ingredients:
- 1 teaspoon paprika
- Salt to taste
- 1/2 teaspoon baking powder
- 2 lb. chicken wings
- 1/4 cup honey
- 1 tablespoon lemon juice
- 1 tablespoon garlic, minced
- 1 tablespoon rosemary, chopped

Directions:
1. Choose air fry setting in your Ninja Foodi Grill.
2. Set it to 390 degrees F.
3. Set the time to 30 minutes.
4. Press start to preheat.
5. While waiting, mix the paprika, salt and baking powder in a bowl.
6. Add the wings to the crisper basket.
7. Close and cook for 15 minutes.
8. Flip and cook for another 15 minutes.
9. In a bowl, mix the remaining ingredients.
10. Coat the wings with the sauce and cook for another 5 minutes.

Nutrition:
Calories:251 kcal Protein: 34.49 g Fat: 6.44 g Carbohydrates: 12.56 g

748. Grilled Chicken With Veggies
⏱ Prep Time 20 m | ⏱ Cooking Time 25 m | 2 Servings

Ingredients:
- 2 chicken thighs and legs
- 2 tablespoons oil, divided
- Salt and pepper to taste
- 1 onion, diced
- 1/4 cup mushrooms, sliced
- 1 cup potatoes, diced
- 1 tablespoon lemon juice
- 1 tablespoon honey
- 4 sprigs fresh thyme, chopped
- 2 cloves garlic, crushed and minced

Directions:
1. Add the grill grate to your Ninja Foodi Grill.
2. Put the veggie tray on top of the grill grate.
3. Close the hood.
4. Choose grill function and set it to high.
5. Press start to preheat.
6. Brush the chicken with half of oil.
7. Season with salt and pepper.
8. Toss the onion, mushrooms and potatoes in the remaining oil.
9. Sprinkle with salt and pepper.
10. Add chicken to the grill grate.
11. Add the potato mixture to the veggie tray.
12. Close the hood and cook for 10 to 15 minutes.
13. Flip chicken and toss potatoes.
14. Cook for another 10 minutes.

Nutrition:
715 kcal Protein: 37.93 g Fat: 48.89 g Carbohydrates: 31.05 g

749. Grilled Garlic Chicken
⏱ Prep Time 10 m | ⏱ Cooking Time 20 m | 8 Servings

Ingredients:
- 3 lb. chicken thigh fillets
- Garlic salt to taste

Directions:
1. Add grill plate to the Ninja Foodi Grill.
2. Preheat to medium heat.
3. Sprinkle chicken with garlic salt on both sides.
4. Cook for 8 to 10 minutes.
5. Flip and cook for another 7 minutes.

Nutrition:
Calories: 386 kcal Protein: 28.9 g Fat: 29.01 g Carbohydrates: 0.43 g

750. Grilled Balsamic Chicken Breast
⏱ Prep Time 45 m | ⏱ Cooking Time 45 m | 4 Servings

Ingredients:
- 1/4 cup olive oil
- 2 tablespoons balsamic vinegar
- 3 teaspoon garlic, minced
- 3 tablespoons soy sauce
- 1 tablespoon Worcestershire sauce
- 1/4 cup brown sugar
- Salt and pepper to taste
- 4 chicken breast fillets

Directions:
1. In a bowl, mix all ingredients except chicken.
2. Reserve 1/4 cup of the mixture for later.
3. Marinate the chicken breast in the remaining mixture for 30 minutes.
4. Add grill grate to the Ninja Foodi Grill.
5. Set it to grill and for 25 minutes.
6. Add the chicken breast and close the hood.
7. Cook for 10 minutes.
8. Flip and cook for another 5 minutes.
9. Baste with remaining sauce. Cook for 5 more minutes.
10. Serve with remaining sauce if any.

Nutrition:
Calories: 716 kcal Protein: 63.31 g Fat: 44.04 g Carbohydrates: 13.16

751. Barbecue Chicken Breast
⏱ Prep Time 15 m | ⏱ Cooking Time 50 m | 4 Servings

Ingredients:
- 4 chicken breast fillets
- 2 tablespoons vegetable oil
- Salt and pepper to taste
- 1 cup barbecue sauce

Directions:
1. Add grill grate to the Ninja Foodi Grill.
2. Close the hood.
3. Choose grill setting.
4. Preheat to medium for 25 minutes.
5. Press start.
6. Brush chicken breast with oil.
7. Sprinkle both sides with salt and pepper.
8. Add chicken and cook for 10 minutes.
9. Flip and cook for another 10 minutes.
10. Brush chicken with barbecue sauce.
11. Cook for 5 minutes.
12. Brush the other side and cook for another 5 minutes.

Nutrition:
Calories: 707 kcal Protein: 62.88 g Fat: 35.61 g Carbohydrates: 30.21 g

752. Chicken, Potatoes & Cabbage
⏱ Prep Time 30 m | ⏱ Cooking Time 40 m | 8 Servings

Ingredients:
- 1 cup apple cider vinegar
- 2 lb. chicken thigh fillets
- 6 oz. barbecue sauce
- 2 lb. cabbage, sliced into wedges and steamed
- 1 lb. potatoes, roasted
- Salt and pepper to taste

Directions:
1. Pour apple cider vinegar to the inner pot.
2. Add grill grate to the Ninja Foodi Grill.
3. Place the chicken on top of the grill.
4. Sprinkle both sides with salt and pepper.
5. Grill the chicken for 15 to 20 minutes per side at 350 degrees F.
6. Baste the chicken with the barbecue sauce.
7. Serve chicken with potatoes and cabbage.

Nutrition:
Calories:385 kcal Protein: 22.59 g Fat: 19.97 g Carbohydrates: 28.03 g

753. Roasted Chicken
⏱ Prep Time 30 m | ⏱ Cooking Time 1 h 10 m | 6 Servings

Ingredients:
- 1 whole chicken
- 1/2 teaspoon onion powder
- 1 teaspoon garlic powder
- 1 teaspoon paprika
- Salt and pepper to taste
- 2 drops liquid smoke
- 1 cup water
- 2 tablespoons butter
- 1/4 cup flour
- 2 cups chicken broth
- Basting Butter
- 2 tablespoons butter
- Dash garlic powder

Directions:
1. Season chicken with a mixture of onion powder, garlic powder, paprika, salt and pepper.
2. Add the chicken to the air frying basket.
3. Combine liquid smoke and butter.
4. Pour into the pot of your Ninja Foodi grill.
5. Seal the unit and cook at 350 degrees F for 45 minutes.
6. Drain the pot.
7. Sprinkle chicken with butter and flour.
8. Air fry at 400 degrees F for 15 minutes.
9. Baste with a mixture of the basting butter ingredients.
10. Cook for another 10 minutes.

Nutrition:
Calories: 410 kcal Protein: 51.61 g Fat: 18.64 g Carbohydrates: 6.05 g

754. Sugar Glazed Chicken

⏱ Prep Time 15 m | ⏱ Cooking Time 45 m | 8 Servings

Ingredients:

- 1 tablespoon olive oil
- 1/2 tablespoon apple cider vinegar
- 3 teaspoon garlic, minced
- 1 tablespoon honey
- 1/4 cup light brown sugar
- 1/3 cup soy sauce
- 8 chicken thigh fillets

Directions:

1. Combine all the ingredients except chicken.
2. Reserve 1/4 cup of this mixture for later.
3. Marinate the chicken with the remaining mixture for 30 minutes.
4. Add grill grate to your Ninja Foodi Grill.
5. Select grill button.
6. Set it to 25 minutes.
7. Add chicken to the grill.
8. Close the hood.
9. Cook for 10 minutes.
10. Flip and cook for 5 minutes.
11. Brush with the remaining mixture.
12. Cook for another 5 minutes.

Nutrition:

Calories: 518 kcal Protein: 33.52 g Fat: 36.41 g Carbohydrates: 12.36 g

755. Steamed Pot Stickers
⏲ Prep Time 20 m | ⏱ Cooking Time 10 m | 30 Servings

Ingredients
- ½ cup finely chopped cabbage
- 2 teaspoons low-sodium soy sauce
- 2 tablespoons cocktail sauce
- 30 wonton wrappers
- ¼ cup finely chopped red bell pepper
- 3 tablespoons water, and more for brushing the wrappers
- 2 green onions, finely chopped
- 1 egg, beaten

Directions
1. Combine the cabbage, bell pepper, chives, egg, cocktail sauce in a small bowl, and soy sauce and mix well.
2. Put exactly 1 teaspoon of the mixture in the middle of each wonton wrapper. Fold the wrap in half, covering the filling. wet the edges with water and seal. You can fold the edges of the wrapper with your fingers so they look like the stickers you get at restaurants. Brush them with water.
3. Put 3 tablespoons of water in the skillet under the fryer basket. Cook potstickers in 2 batches for 9 to 10 minutes or until potstickers are hot and the bottom is light.
4. Substitution Tip: Use other veggies in this recipe, like chopped corn, peas, or zucchini, or squash in the summer. You can also add the rest of the cooked meat, such as minced pork or chicken.

Nutrition
Calories 291 | Fat 2g | Saturated Fat 0g | Cholesterol 35mg | Sodium 649mg | Carbohydrates 57g | Fiber 3g | Protein 10g

756. Beef and Mango Skewers
⏲ Prep Time 10 m | ⏱ Cooking Time 5 m | 4 Servings

Ingredients
- 2 tablespoons balsamic vinegar
- 1 tablespoon olive oil
- 1 tablespoon honey
- ½ teaspoon dried marjoram
- A pinch of salt
- Freshly ground black pepper
- 1 mango
- ¾ pound beef sirloin (cut into 1-inch cubes)

Directions
1. Put the meat cubes in a medium bowl and add the balsamic vinegar, olive oil, honey, marjoram, salt, and pepper. Mix well and then massage the marinade into the meat with your hands. Set aside.
2. To prepare the mango, leave it last and cut the skin with a sharp blade.
3. Then gently cut around the oval pit to remove the pulp. Cut the mango into 1-inch cubes.
4. The metal wire skewers alternate with three cubes of meat and two cubes of mango.
5. Bake the skewers in the skillet for 4 to 7 minutes or until the meat is browned and at least 145 ° F.

Nutrition
Calories 242 | Fat 9g | Saturated Fat 3g | Cholesterol 76mg | Sodium 96mg | Carbohydrates 13g | Fiber 1g | Protein 26g

757. Curried Sweet Potato Fries
⏲ Prep Time 5 m | ⏱ Cooking Time 12 m | 4 Servings

Ingredients
- ½ cup sour cream
- ½ cup mango chutney
- 3 teaspoons curry powder, divided
- 4 cups frozen sweet potato fries
- 1 tablespoon olive oil
- A pinch of salt
- Freshly ground black pepper

Directions
1. In a bowl, add together sour cream, chutney, and 1½ teaspoon curry powder. Mix well and let stand.
2. Place the sweet potatoes in a sizeable bowl. Pour over the olive oil and sprinkle with the remaining 1½ teaspoon curry powder, salt, and pepper.
3. Put the potatoes in the fryer basket. Cook 8 to 12 minutes or until crisp, hot and golden, shaking the basket once during cooking.
4. Place the potatoes in a basket and serve with the teaspoon.
5. Substitution Tip: You can choose to use fresh sweet potatoes instead of frozen potatoes. Take one or two sweet potatoes, peel them, and cut them into 1-inch-thick strips with a sharp knife or mandolin. Use according to the recipe instructions. but you will need to increase the time for cooking.

Nutrition
Calories 323 | Fat 10g | Saturated Fat 4g | Cholesterol 13mg | Sodium 138mg | Carbohydrates 58g | Fiber 7g | Protein 3g

758. Spicy Kale Chips with Yogurt Sauce
⏲ Prep Time 10 m | ⏱ Cooking Time 5 m | 4 Servings

Ingredients
- 1 cup Greek yogurt
- 3 tablespoons lemon juice
- 2 tablespoons honey mustard
- ½ teaspoon dried oregano
- 1 bunch curly kale
- 2 tablespoons olive oil
- ½ teaspoon salt
- ⅛ teaspoon pepper

Directions
1. In a bowl, add together the yogurt, lemon juice, honey mustard, and oregano and set aside.
2. Remove the stems and ribs from the cabbage with a sharp knife. Cut the leaves into 2 to 3-inch pieces.
3. Toss the cabbage with olive oil, salt, and pepper. Massage the oil with your hands.
4. Fry the kale in batches until crisp, about 5 minutes, shaking the basket once during cooking. Serve with yogurt sauce.

Ingredient Tip: Kale is available in different varieties. Tuscan (also known as dinosaur or lacinato) is the most powerful and makes excellent marks. Kale, the variety widely found in grocery stores, can be slightly frozen when cooked in the deep fryer, but it's still delicious.

Nutrition
Calories 154 | Fat 8g | Saturated Fat 2g | Cholesterol 3mg | Sodium 378mg | Carbohydrates 13g | Fiber 1g | Protein 8g

759. Phyllo Artichoke Triangles

Prep Time 15 m | Cooking Time 9 m | 18 Servings

Ingredients

- ¼ cup ricotta cheese
- 1 egg white
- ⅓ cup minced drained artichoke hearts
- 3 tablespoons grated mozzarella cheese
- ½ teaspoon dried thyme
- 6 sheets frozen phyllo dough, thawed
- 2 tablespoons melted butter

Directions

1. In a bowl, combine ricotta cheese, egg white, artichoke hearts, mozzarella cheese, and thyme and mix well.
2. Cover the dough with a damp kitchen towel while you work so it doesn't dry out. Using one sheet at a time, lay it out on your work surface and cut into thirds lengthwise.
3. Apply 1½ tsp of filling on each strip at the base. Fold the bottom-right edge of the sheet over the filling to meet the other side in a triangle, then continue folding into a triangle. Brush each angle with butter to seal the edges. Repeat with the remaining dough and filling.
4. Bake, 7 at a time, for about 3 to 4 minutes or until the sex is golden and crisp.
5. Replacement Tip: You can use anything in this filling in place of artichoke hearts. Try spinach, minced shrimp, cooked sausage or keep vegetarian and use all the grated cheese.

Nutrition

Calories 271 | Fat 17g | Saturated Fat 7g | Cholesterol 19mg | Sodium 232mg | Carbohydrates 23g | Fiber 5g | Protein 9g

760. Arancini

Prep Time 15 m | Cooking Time 22 m | 16 Servings

Ingredients

- 2 eggs, beaten
- 1½ cups panko bread crumbs, divided
- ½ cup grated Parmesan cheese
- 2 tablespoons minced fresh basil
- 2 cups cooked rice or leftover risotto
- 16 ¾-inch cubes mozzarella cheese
- 2 tablespoons olive oil

Directions

1. In a medium bowl, add together the rice, eggs, a cup of breadcrumbs, Parmesan, and basil. Shape this mixture into 16 1-inch balls.
2. Create a hole in each of the balls with your finger and place a cube of mozzarella. Glue the rice mixture firmly around the cheese.
3. On a shallow plate, add together the remaining 1 cup of breadcrumbs with the olive oil and mix well. Wrap the rice balls in the breadcrumbs for color.
4. Cook the arancini in batches for 8 to 11 minutes or until golden brown.

Did you know that in Italy, arancini, also called frittata or rice soup, is sold on the street as a snack? They have grown much larger in this country, the size of an orange, and are often cone-shaped.

Nutrition

Calories 378 | Fat: 11g | Saturated Fat 4g | Cholesterol 57mg | Sodium 361mg | Carbohydrates 53g | Fiber 2g | Protein 16g

761. Pesto Bruschetta

Prep Time 10 m | Cooking Time 8 m | 4 Servings

Ingredients

- 8 slices French bread, ½ inch thick
- 2 tablespoons softened butter
- 1 cup shredded mozzarella cheese
- ½ cup basil pesto
- 1 cup chopped grape tomatoes
- 2 green onions, thinly sliced

Directions

1. Butter the bread and place the butter in the deep fryer basket. Bake 3 to 5 minutes or until bread is lightly golden.
2. Take the bread out of the basket and fill each piece with a little cheese. Return to the basket in batches and bake until cheese is melted, for about 1 to 3 minutes.
3. Meanwhile, combine pesto, tomatoes, and chives in a small bowl.
4. When the cheese is melted, remove the bread from the fryer and place it on a plate. Fill each slice with a little pesto mix and serve.

Nutrition

Calories: 462 | Fat 25g | Saturated Fat 10g | Cholesterol 38mg | Sodium 822mg | Carbohydrates 41g | Fiber 3g | Protein 19g

762. Fried Tortellini with Spicy Dipping Sauce

Prep Time 8 m | Cooking Time 20 m | 4 Servings

Ingredients

- ¾ cup mayonnaise
- 2 tablespoons mustard
- 1 egg
- ½ cup flour
- ½ teaspoon dried oregano
- 1½ cups bread crumbs
- 2 tablespoons olive oil
- 2 cups frozen cheese tortellini

Directions

1. In a small bowl, add together the mayonnaise and mustard and mix well. Set aside.
2. In a shallow bowl, beat the egg. In a separate bowl, combine the flour and oregano. In another bowl, combine the breadcrumbs and olive oil and mix well.
3. Add the tortellini, a few at a time, to the egg, then the flour, then the egg again, then the breadcrumbs to coat. Place in the fryer basket, cooking in batches.
4. Air fry for about 10 minutes, stirring halfway through cooking time, or until tortellini are crisp and golden on the outside. Serve with mayonnaise.

Nutrition

Calories 698 | Fat 31g | Saturated Fat 4g | Cholesterol 66mg | Sodium 832mg | Carbohydrates 88g | Fiber 3g | Protein 18g

763. Shrimp Toast

⏲ Prep Time 15 m | ⏲ Cooking Time 12 m | 12 Servings

Ingredients

- 3 slices firm white bread
- ⅔ cup finely chopped peeled and deveined raw shrimp
- 1 egg white
- 2 cloves garlic, minced
- 2 tablespoons cornstarch
- ¼ teaspoon ground ginger
- A pinch of salt
- Freshly ground black pepper
- 2 tablespoons olive oil

Directions

1. Cut the crust from the bread with a sharp knife. crumble the crusts to make breadcrumbs. Set aside.
2. In a small bowl, add together the shrimp, egg white, garlic, cornstarch, ginger, salt, and pepper and mix well.
3. Spread the shrimp mixture evenly over the pan around the edges. With a sharp blade or knife, cut each slice into 4 strips.
4. Mix the breadcrumbs with the olive oil and beat with the shrimp mixture. Arrange the shrimp tostadas in the fryer basket in one layer. You may need to cook in batches.
5. Air fry for 3 to 6 minutes, until crisp and golden.

Substitution Tip: Replace the minced crab with minced shrimp in this recipe or use ground chicken or turkey.

Nutrition

Calories 121 | Fat 6g | Saturated Fat 1g | Cholesterol 72mg | Sodium 158mg | Carbohydrates 7g | Fiber 0g | Protein 9g

764. Bacon Tater Tots

⏲ Prep Time 5 m | ⏲ Cooking Time 17 m | 4 Servings

Ingredients

- 24 frozen tater tots
- 6 slices precooked bacon
- 2 tablespoons maple syrup
- 1 cup shredded Cheddar cheese

Directions

1. Put the tattoos in the fryer basket. Fry for 10 minutes, shaking the fryer basket halfway through the cooking time.
2. Cut the bacon into 1-inch pieces and slice the cheese.
3. Remove the hook from the fryer basket and place it in a 6-by-6-by-2-inch pot. Fill the bacon with the maple syrup. Air fry 5 minutes or until spoons and bacon are crisp.
4. Fill with cheese and air fry for 2 minutes or until cheese is melted.
5. Ingredient Tip: Use only precooked bacon that does not need refrigeration for this recipe. If you use regular bacon, it will emit too much fat and the cookies will end up runny, not crisp.

Nutrition

Calories: 374 | Fat: 22g | Saturated Fat: 9g | Cholesterol: 40mg | Sodium: 857mg | Carbohydrates: 34g | Fiber: 2g | Protein: 13g

765. Hash Brown Bruschetta

⏲ Prep Time 7 m | ⏲ Cooking Time 8 m | 4 Servings

Ingredients

- 4 frozen hash brown patties
- 1 tablespoon olive oil
- ⅓ cup chopped cherry tomatoes
- 3 tablespoons diced fresh mozzarella
- 2 tablespoons grated Parmesan cheese
- 1 tablespoon balsamic vinegar
- 1 tablespoon minced fresh basil

Directions

1. Place the brown cake patties in the air fryer in a single layer. Air fry for 8 minutes or until the potatoes are crisp, hot, and golden.
2. Meanwhile, combine olive oil, tomatoes, mozzarella, Parmesan, vinegar, and basil in a small bowl.
3. When the potatoes are cooked, carefully remove them from the basket and place them on a plate. Fill with tomato mixture and serve.

Nutrition

Calories: 123 | Total Fat: 6g | Saturated Fat: 2g | Cholesterol: 6mg | Sodium: 81mg | Carbohydrates: 14g | Fiber: 2g | Protein: 5g

766. Waffle Fry Poutine

⏲ Prep Time 10 m | ⏲ Cooking Time 17 m | 4 Servings

Ingredients

- 2 cups frozen waffle cut fries
- 2 teaspoons olive oil
- 1 red bell pepper, chopped
- 2 green onions, sliced
- 1 cup shredded Swiss cheese
- ½ cup bottled chicken gravy

Directions

1. Toss the waffle fries with olive oil and place it in the air fryer basket. Air-fry for 10 to 12 minutes or until the fries are crisp and light golden brown, shaking the basket halfway through the cooking time.
2. Transfer the potatoes to a 6-by-6 by 2-inch skillet and top with the bell pepper, green onions, and cheese. Air fry for 3 minutes until vegetables are crisp and soft.
3. Remove the skillet from the fryer and sprinkle the broth over the potatoes. Air fry for 2 minutes or until the broth is lukewarm. Serve immediately.

Substitution Tip: You can also make this recipe with regular frozen fries, but they may take a few more minutes to cook. Use your favorite cheese in this rich recipe.

Nutrition

Calories: 347 | Total Fat: 19g | Saturated Fat: 7g | Cholesterol: 26mg | Sodium: 435mg | Carbohydrates: 33g | Fiber: 4g | Protein: 12g

767. Crispy Beef Cubes
Prep Time 10 m | Cooking Time 16 m | 4 Servings

Ingredients
- 1 cup cheese pasta sauce (from a 16-ounce jar)
- 1½ cups soft bread crumbs
- 2 tablespoons olive oil
- ½ teaspoon dried marjoram
- 1 pound sirloin, cut into 1-inch cubes

Directions
1. In a medium bowl, mix the meat with the pasta sauce to coat.
2. In a shallow bowl, combine the pieces of bread, oil, and marjoram and mix well. Add the meat cubes, one at a time, to the bread mixture to coat well.
3. Cook meat in two batches for 6 to 8 minutes, shaking basket once during cooking, until meat is at least 145 ° F and outside is crisp and golden. Serve with toothpicks or small forks.
4. Cooking Tip: You can use the rest of the pasta sauce to make a quick meal. Just cook one cup or two of pasta while reheating the sauce in a saucepan. Combine and enjoy.

Nutrition
Calories: 554 | Fat: 22g | Saturated Fat: 8g | Cholesterol: 112mg | Sodium: 1,832mg | Carbohydrates: 43g | Fiber: 2g | Protein: 44g

768. Buffalo Chicken Bites
Prep Time 10 m | Cooking Time 18 m | 4 Servings

Ingredients
- ⅔ cup sour cream
- ¼ cup creamy blue cheese salad dressing
- ¼ cup crumbled blue cheese
- 3 tablespoons Buffalo chicken wing sauce
- 1 cup panko bread crumbs
- 2 tbsp. olive oil
- 1 celery stalk, finely chopped
- A pound of chicken tenders, cut into three

Directions
1. In a small bowl, add together salad dressing, sour cream, blue cheese, and celery and set aside.
2. In a medium bowl, combine chicken pieces and chicken wing sauce and toss to coat. Let stand while you prepare the ready breadcrumbs.
3. Combine the breadcrumbs and olive oil on a plate and mix.
4. Top the chicken pieces with the bread mixture, beating each piece so the crumbs stick together.
5. Fry in batches for 7 to 9 minutes, shaking basket once until chicken is cooked to 165 ° F and golden brown. Serve with the blue cheese sauce on the side.
6. Did you know that Buffalo chicken wings were first invented at Anchor Bar in Buffalo, New York, when the owner had to serve many appetizers in a hurry? It became an immediate hit and the flavor, a combination of hot sauce with fresh blue cheese, is now a classic.

Nutrition
Calories: 467 | Fat: 23g | Saturated Fat: 8g | Cholesterol: 119mg | Sodium: 821mg | Carbohydrates: 22g | Fiber: 1g | Protein: 43g

769. Sweet and Hot Chicken Wings
Prep Time 5 m | Cooking Time 25 m | 16 Servings

Ingredients
- 8 chicken wings
- 1 tablespoon olive oil
- ⅓ cup brown sugar
- 2 tablespoons honey
- ⅓ cup apple cider vinegar
- 2 cloves garlic, minced
- ½ teaspoon dried red pepper flakes
- ¼ teaspoon salt

Directions
1. Cut each chicken wing into three pieces. You will have a large piece, a middle piece, and a small tip. Discard the small tip or save it for stock.
2. In a medium bowl, rub the wings with the oil. Transfer to the fryer basket and cook for 20 minutes, shaking the basket twice while cooking.
3. Also, in a small bowl, combine the honey, vinegar, red pepper flakes, sugar, and salt and mix until just combined.
4. Remove the feathers from the fryer basket and place them in a 6-by-6-inch pot. Pour the sauce over the wings and pour.
5. Return to the fryer and cook for 5 minutes or until the wings are polished.
6. Ingredient Tip: You can sometimes buy "chicken drums" in the meat section. They are made from chicken meat. If you want to use these instead of cutting whole feathers, use about 10 in this recipe.

Nutrition
Calories 438 | Fat 16g | Saturated Fat 4g | Cholesterol 151mg | Sodium 299mg | Carbohydrates 21g | Fiber 0g | Protein 49g

770. Steamed Pot Stickers
Prep Time 10 m | Cooking Time 20 m | 30 Servings

Ingredients:
- ½ cup finely chopped cabbage
- 2 teaspoons low-sodium soy sauce
- 2 tablespoons cocktail sauce
- 30 wonton wrappers
- ¼ cup finely chopped red bell pepper
- 3 tablespoons water, and more for brushing the wrappers
- 2 green onions, finely chopped
- 1 egg, beaten

Directions:
1. Combine the cabbage, bell pepper, chives, egg, cocktail sauce in a small bowl, and soy sauce and mix well.
2. Put exactly 1 teaspoon of the mixture in the middle of each wonton wrapper. Fold the wrap in half, covering the filling. Wet the edges with water and seal. You can fold the edges of the wrapper with your fingers so they look like the stickers you get at restaurants. Brush them with water.
3. Put 3 tablespoons of water in the skillet under the fryer basket. Cook pot stickers in 2 batches for 9 to 10 minutes or until pot stickers are hot and bottom is light.
4. Substitution Tip: Use other veggies in this recipe, like chopped corn, peas, or zucchini or squash in the summer. You can also add the rest of the cooked meat, such as minced pork or chicken.

Nutrition:
Calories: 291 | Fat 2g | Cholesterol 35mg | Sodium 649mg | Carbo 57g | Fiber 3g | Protein 10g

771. Beef and Mango Skewers
⏱ Prep Time 10 m | ⏱ Cooking Time 5 m | 4 Servings

Ingredients:

- 2 tablespoons balsamic vinegar
- 1 tablespoon olive oil
- 1 tablespoon honey
- ½ teaspoon dried marjoram

- Pinch salt
- Freshly ground black pepper
- 1 mango
- ¾ pound beef sirloin (cut into 1-inch cubes)

Directions:

1. Put the meat cubes in a medium bowl and add the balsamic vinegar, olive oil, honey, marjoram, salt and pepper. Mix well and then massage the marinade into the meat with your hands. Set aside.
2. To prepare the mango, leave it last and cut the skin with a sharp blade.
3. Then gently cut around the oval pit to remove the pulp. Cut the mango into 1-inch cubes.
4. The metal wire skewers alternate with three cubes of meat and two cubes of mango.
5. Bake the skewers in the skillet for 4 to 7 minutes or until the meat is browned and at least 145 ° F.

Nutrition:

Calories 242 | Fat 9g | Cholesterol 76mg | Sodium 96mg | Carbo 13g | Fiber 1g | Protein 26g

772. Curried Sweet Potato Fries
⏱ Prep Time 5 m | ⏱ Cooking Time 12 m | 4 Servings

Ingredients:

- ½ cup sour cream
- ½ cup mango chutney
- 3 teaspoons curry powder, divided
- 4 cups frozen sweet potato fries

- 1 tablespoon olive oil
- Pinch salt
- Freshly ground black pepper

Directions:

1. In a bowl, add together sour cream, chutney, and 1½ teaspoon curry powder. Mix well and let stand.
2. Place the sweet potatoes in a sizeable bowl. Pour over the olive oil and sprinkle with the remaining 1½ teaspoon curry powder, salt, and pepper.
3. Put the potatoes in the fryer basket. Cook 8 to 12 minutes or until crisp, hot and golden, shaking the basket once during cooking.
4. Place the potatoes in a basket and serve with the teaspoon.
5. Substitution Tip: You can choose to use fresh sweet potatoes instead of frozen potatoes. Take one or two sweet potatoes, peel them, and cut them into 1-inch-thick strips with a sharp knife or mandolin. Use according to the recipe instructions. But you will need to increase the time for cooking.

Nutrition:

Calories: 323 | Fat 10g | Cholesterol: 13mg | Sodium: 138mg | Carbo 58g | Fiber: 7g | Protein: 3g

773. Spicy Kale Chips with Yogurt Sauce
⏱ Prep Time 10 m | ⏱ Cooking Time 5 m | 4 Servings

Ingredients:

- 1 cup Greek yogurt
- 3 tablespoons lemon juice
- 2 tablespoons honey mustard
- ½ teaspoon dried oregano

- 1 bunch curly kale
- 2 tablespoons olive oil
- ½ teaspoon salt
- 1/2 teaspoon pepper

Directions:

1. In a bowl, add together the yogurt, lemon juice, honey mustard, and oregano and set aside. \
2. Remove the stems and ribs from the cabbage with a sharp knife. Cut the leaves into 2 to 3-inch pieces.
3. Toss the cabbage with olive oil, salt, and pepper. Massage the oil with your hands.
4. Fry the kale in batches until crisp, about 5 minutes, shaking the basket once during cooking. Serve with yogurt sauce.
5. Ingredient Tip: Kale is available in different varieties. Tuscan (also known as dinosaur or lacing) is the most powerful and makes excellent marks. Kale, the variety widely found in grocery stores, can be slightly frozen when cooked in the deep fryer, but it's still delicious.

Nutrition:

Calories: 154 | Fat: 8g | Cholesterol: 3mg | Sodium: 378mg | Carbo 13g | Fiber: 1g | Protein: 8g

774. Phyllo Artichoke Triangles

⏲ Prep Time 15 m | ⏲ Cooking Time 9 m | 18 Servings

Ingredients:

- ¼ cup ricotta cheese
- 1 egg white
- 1/3 cup minced drained artichoke hearts
- 3 tablespoons grated mozzarella cheese
- ½ teaspoon dried thyme
- 6 sheets frozen phyllo dough, thawed
- 2 tablespoons melted butter

Directions:

1. In a bowl, combine ricotta cheese, egg white, artichoke hearts, mozzarella cheese, and thyme and mix well.
2. Cover the dough with a damp kitchen towel while you work so it doesn't dry out. Using one sheet at a time, lay it out on your work surface and cut into thirds lengthwise.
3. Apply 1½ tsp of filling on each strip at the base. Fold the bottom right edge of the sheet over the filling to meet the other side in a triangle, then continue folding into a triangle. Brush each angle with butter to seal the edges. Repeat with the remaining dough and filling.
4. Bake, 7 at a time, for about 3 to 4 minutes or until the sex is golden and crisp.
5. Replacement Tip: You can use anything in this filling in place of artichoke hearts. Try spinach, minced shrimp, and cooked sausage or keep vegetarian and use all the grated cheese.

Nutrition: Calories: 271 | Fat: 17g | Cholesterol: 19mg | Sodium: 232mg | Carbo 23g | Fiber: 5g | Protein: 9g

775. Arancini

⏲ Prep Time 15 m | ⏲ Cooking Time 22 m | 16 Servings

Ingredients:

- 2 eggs, beaten
- 1½ cups panko bread crumbs, divided
- ½ cup grated Parmesan cheese
- 2 tablespoons minced fresh basil
- 2 cups cooked rice or leftover risotto
- 16 ¾-inch cubes mozzarella cheese
- 2 tablespoons olive oil

Directions:

1. In a medium bowl, add together the rice, eggs, and a cup of breadcrumbs, Parmesan, and basil. Shape this mixture into 16 1-inch balls.
2. Create a hole in each of the balls with your finger and place a cube of mozzarella. Glue the rice mixture firmly around the cheese.
3. On a shallow plate, add together the remaining 1 cup of breadcrumbs with the olive oil and mix well. Wrap the rice balls in the breadcrumbs for color.
4. Cook the rank in batches for 8 to 11 minutes or until golden brown.
5. You knew that? In Italy, arancini, also called frittata or rice soup, is sold on the street as a snack. They have grown much larger in this country, the size of an orange, and are often cone-shaped.

Nutrition:

Calories: 378 | Fat: 11g | Cholesterol: 57mg | Sodium: 361mg | Carbo 53g | Fiber: 2g | Protein: 16g

776. Fried Tortellini with Spicy Dipping Sauce

⏲ Prep Time 8 m | ⏲ Cooking Time 20 m | 4 Servings

Ingredients:

- ¾ cup mayonnaise
- 2 tablespoons mustard
- 1 egg
- ½ cup flour
- ½ teaspoon dried oregano
- 1½ cups bread crumbs
- 2 tablespoons olive oil
- 2 cups frozen cheese tortellini

Directions:

1. In a small bowl, add together the mayonnaise and mustard and mix well. Set aside.
2. In a shallow bowl, beat the egg. In a separate bowl, combine the flour and oregano. In another bowl, combine the breadcrumbs and olive oil and mix well.
3. Add the tortellini, a few at a time, to the egg, then the flour, then the egg again, then the breadcrumbs to coat. Place in the fryer basket, cooking in batches.
4. Air fry for about 10 minutes, stirring halfway through cooking time, or until tortellini are crisp and golden on the outside. Serve with mayonnaise.

Nutrition:

Calories: 698 | Fat: 31g | Cholesterol: 66mg | Sodium: 832mg | Carbo 88g | Fiber: 3g | Protein: 18g

777. Sweet and Hot Chicken Wings

⏰ Prep Time 5 m | ⏰ Cooking Time 25 m | 16 Servings

Ingredients:

- 8 chicken wings
- 1 tablespoon olive oil
- 1/3 cup brown sugar
- 2 tablespoons honey
- 1/3 cup apple cider vinegar
- 2 cloves garlic, minced
- ½ teaspoon dried red pepper flakes
- ¼ teaspoon salt

Directions:

1. Cut each chicken wing into three pieces. You will have a large piece, a middle piece, and a small tip. Discard the small tip or save it for stock.
2. In a medium bowl, rub the wings with the oil. Transfer to the fryer basket and cook for 20 minutes, shaking the basket twice while cooking.
3. Also, in a small bowl, combine the honey, vinegar, red pepper flakes, sugar, and salt and mix until just combined.
4. Remove the feathers from the fryer basket and place them in a 6-by-6-inch pot. Pour the sauce over the wings and pour.
5. Return to the fryer and cook for 5 minutes or until the wings are polished.
6. Ingredient Tip: You can sometimes buy "chicken drums" in the meat section. They are made from chicken meat. If you want to use these instead of cutting whole feathers, use about 10 in this recipe.

Nutrition: Calories: 438| Fat: 16g |Cholesterol: 151mg |Sodium: 299mg| Carbo 21g| Fiber: 0g

778. Shrimp Toast

⏰ Prep Time 15 m | ⏰ Cooking Time 12 m | 12 Servings

Ingredients:

- 3 slices firm white bread
- 2/3 cup finely chopped peeled and deveined raw shrimp
- 1 egg white
- 2 cloves garlic, minced
- 2 tablespoons cornstarch
- ¼ teaspoon ground ginger
- Pinch salt
- Freshly ground black pepper
- 2 tablespoons olive oil

Directions:

1. Cut the crust from the bread with a sharp knife. Crumble the crusts to make breadcrumbs. Set aside.
2. In a small bowl, add together the shrimp, egg white, garlic, cornstarch, ginger, salt, and pepper and mix well.
3. Spread the shrimp mixture evenly over the pan around the edges. With a sharp blade or knife, cut each slice into 4 strips.
4. Mix the breadcrumbs with the olive oil and beat with the shrimp mixture. Arrange the shrimp tostadas in the fryer basket in one layer. You may need to cook in batches.
5. Air fry for 3 to 6 minutes, until crisp and golden.
6. Substitution Tip: Replace the minced crab with minced shrimp in this recipe or use ground chicken or turkey.

Nutrition:
Calories: 121 Fat: 6g Cholesterol: 72mg Sodium: 158mg Carbohydrates: 7g Fiber: 0g Protein: 9g

779. Bacon Tater Tots

⏰ Prep Time 5 m | ⏰ Cooking Time 17 m | 4 Servings

Ingredients:

- 24 frozen tater tots
- 6 slices precooked bacon
- 2 tablespoons maple syrup
- 1 cup shredded Cheddar cheese

Directions:

1. Put the tattoos in the fryer basket. Fry for 10 minutes, shaking the fryer basket halfway through the cooking time.
2. Cut the bacon into 1-inch pieces and slice the cheese.
3. Remove the hook from the fryer basket and place in a 6-by-6-by-2-inch pot. Fill the bacon with the maple syrup. Air fry 5 minutes or until spoons and bacon are crisp.
4. Fill with cheese and air fry for 2 minutes or until cheese is melted.
5. Ingredient Tip: Use only precooked bacon that does not need refrigeration for this recipe. If you use regular bacon, it will emit too much fat and the cookies will end up runny, not crisp.

Nutrition:
Calories: 374|Fat: 22g| Cholesterol: 40mg |Sodium: 857mg| Carbo 34g |Fiber: 2g| Protein: 13g

780. Pesto Bruschetta

⏰ Prep Time 10 m | ⏰ Cooking Time 8 m | 4 Servings

Ingredients:

- 8 slices French bread, ½ inch thick
- 2 tablespoons softened butter
- 1 cup shredded mozzarella cheese
- ½ cup basil pesto
- 1 cup chopped grape tomatoes
- 2 green onions, thinly sliced

Directions:

1. Butter the bread and place the butter in the deep fryer basket. Bake 3 to 5 minutes or until bread is lightly golden.
2. Take the bread out of the basket and fill each piece with a little cheese. Return to basket in batches and bake until cheese is melted, about 1 to 3 minutes.
3. Meanwhile, combine pesto, tomatoes, and chives in a small bowl.
4. When the cheese is melted, remove the bread from the fryer and place it on a plate. Fill each slice with a little pesto mix and serve.

Nutrition:
Calories: 462 |Fat: 25g| Cholesterol: 38mg| Sodium: 822mg| Carbo 41g |Fiber: 3g |Protein: 19g

781. Hash Brown Bruschetta

⏱ Prep Time 7 m | ⏱ Cooking Time 8 m | 4 Servings

Ingredients:

- 4 frozen hash brown patties
- 1 tablespoon olive oil
- 1/3 cup chopped cherry tomatoes
- 3 tablespoons diced fresh mozzarella
- 2 tablespoons grated Parmesan cheese
- 1 tablespoon balsamic vinegar
- 1 tablespoon minced fresh basil

Directions:

1. Place the brown cake patties in the air fryer in a single layer. Air fry for 8 minutes or until the potatoes are crisp, hot and golden.
2. Meanwhile, combine olive oil, tomatoes, mozzarella, Parmesan, vinegar, and basil in a small bowl.
3. When the potatoes are cooked, carefully remove them from the basket and place them on a plate. Fill with tomato mixture and serve.

Nutrition:

Calories: 123 | Fat: 6g | Cholesterol: 6mg | Sodium: 81mg | Carbo 14g | Fiber: 2g | Protein: 5g

782. Waffle Fry Poutine

⏱ Prep Time 10 m | ⏱ Cooking Time 17 m | 4 Servings

Ingredients:

- 2 cups frozen waffle cut fries
- 2 teaspoons olive oil
- 1 red bell pepper, chopped
- 2 green onions, sliced
- 1 cup shredded Swiss cheese
- ½ cup bottled chicken gravy

Directions:

1. Toss the waffle fries with olive oil and place in the air fryer basket. Air-fry for 10 to 12 minutes or until the fries are crisp and light golden brown, shaking the basket halfway through the cooking time.
2. Transfer the potatoes to a 6-by-6 by 2-inch skillet and top with the bell pepper, green onions, and cheese. Air fry for 3 minutes until vegetables are crisp and soft.
3. Remove the skillet from the fryer and sprinkle the broth over the potatoes. Air fry for 2 minutes or until the broth is lukewarm. Serve immediately.
4. Substitution Tip: You can also make this recipe with regular frozen fries, but they may take a few more minutes to cook. Use your favorite cheese in this rich recipe.

Nutrition:

Calories: 347 | Fat: 19g | Cholesterol: 26mg | Sodium: 435mg | Carbo 33g | Fiber: 4g | Protein: 12g

783. Crispy Beef Cubes

⏱ Prep Time 10 m | ⏱ Cooking Time 16 m | 4 Servings

Ingredients:

- 1 cup cheese pasta sauce (from a 16-ounce jar)
- 1½ cups soft bread crumbs
- 2 tablespoons olive oil
- ½ teaspoon dried marjoram
- 1 pound sirloin, cut into 1-inch cubes

Directions:

1. In medium bowl, mix meat with pasta sauce to coat.
2. In a shallow bowl, combine the breads, oil, and marjoram and mix well. Add the meat cubes, one at a time, to the bread mixture to coat well.
3. Cook meat in two batches for 6 to 8 minutes, shaking basket once during cooking, until meat is at least 145 ° F and outside is crisp and golden. Serve with toothpicks or small forks.
4. Cooking Tip: You can use the rest of the pasta sauce to make a quick meal. Just cook one cup or two of pasta while reheating the sauce in a saucepan. Combine and enjoy.

Nutrition:

Calories 554 | Fat 22g | Cholesterol 112mg | Sodium: 1,83mg | Carbo 43g | Fiber: 2g | Protein: 44g

784. Buffalo Chicken Bites

⏱ Prep Time 10 m | ⏱ Cooking Time 18 m | 4 Servings

Ingredients:

- 2/3 cup sour cream
- ¼ cup creamy blue cheese salad dressing
- ¼ cup crumbled blue cheese
- 3 tablespoons Buffalo chicken wing sauce
- 1 cup panko bread crumbs
- 2 tbsp. olive oil
- 1 celery stalk, finely chopped
- A pound of chicken tenders, cut into three

Directions:

1. In a small bowl, add together salad dressing, sour cream, blue cheese, and celery and set aside.
2. In a medium bowl, combine chicken pieces and chicken wing sauce and toss to coat. Let stand while you prepare the ready breadcrumbs.
3. Combine the breadcrumbs and olive oil on a plate and mix.
4. Top the chicken pieces with the bread mixture, beating each piece so the crumbs stick together.
5. Fry in batches for 7 to 9 minutes, shaking basket once, until chicken is cooked to 165 ° F and golden brown. Serve with the blue cheese sauce on the side.
6. You knew that? Buffalo chicken wings were first invented at Anchor Bar in Buffalo, New York, when the owner had to serve many appetizers in a hurry. It became an immediate hit and the flavor, a combination of hot sauce with fresh blue cheese, is now a classic.

Nutrition:

Calories: 467 | Fat: 23g | Cholesterol: 119mg | Sodium: 821mg | Carbo 22g | Fiber: 1g | Protein: 43g

785. Peanut Butter Banana Bread

⏱ Prep Time 15 m | ⏱ Cooking Time 40 m | 6 Servings

Ingredients:

- 1 cup plus 1 tablespoon all-purpose flour
- ¼ teaspoon baking soda
- 1 teaspoon baking powder
- ¼ teaspoon salt
- 1 large egg
- 1/3 cup granulated sugar
- ¼ cup canola oil
- 2 tablespoons creamy peanut butter
- 2 tablespoons sour cream
- 1 teaspoon vanilla extract
- 2 medium ripe bananas, peeled and mashed
- ¾ cup walnuts, roughly chopped

Directions:

1. In a bowl and mix the flour, baking powder, baking soda, and salt together.
2. In another large bowl, add the egg, sugar, oil, peanut butter, sour cream, and vanilla extract and beat until well combined.
3. Add the bananas and beat until well combined.
4. Add the flour mixture and mix until just combined.
5. Gently, fold in the walnuts.
6. Place the mixture into a lightly greased pan.
7. Press "Power Button" of Air Fry Oven and turn the dial to select the "Air Crisp" mode.
8. Press the Time button and again turn the dial to set the cooking time to 40 minutes
9. Now push the Temp button and rotate the dial to set the temperature at 330 degrees F.
10. Press "Start/Pause" button to start.
11. When the unit beeps to show that it is preheated, open the lid.
12. Arrange the pan in "Air Fry Basket" and insert in the oven.
13. Place the pan onto a wire rack to cool for about 10 minutes
14. Carefully, invert the bread onto wire rack to cool completely before slicing.
15. Cut the bread into desired-sized slices and serve.

Nutrition:

Calories 384 Fat 23 g Carbs 39.3 g Protein 8.9 g

786. Chocolate Banana Bread

⏱ Prep Time 15 m | ⏱ Cooking Time 20 m | 8 Servings

Ingredients:

- 2 cups flour
- ½ teaspoon baking soda
- ½ teaspoon baking powder
- ½ teaspoon salt
- ¾ cup sugar
- 1/3 cup butter, softened
- 3 eggs
- 1 tablespoon vanilla extract
- 1 cup milk
- ½ cup bananas, peeled and mashed
- 1 cup chocolate chips

Directions:

1. In a bowl, mix together the flour, baking soda, baking powder, and salt.
2. In another large bowl, add the butter, and sugar and beat until light and fluffy.
3. Add the eggs, and vanilla extract and whisk until well combined.
4. Add the flour mixture and mix until well combined.
5. Add the milk, and mashed bananas and mix well.
6. Gently, fold in the chocolate chips. Place the mixture into a lightly greased loaf pan.
7. Press "Power Button" of Air Fry Oven and turn the dial to select the "Air Crisp" mode.
8. Press the Time button and again turn the dial to set the cooking time to 20 minutes
9. Now push the Temp button and rotate the dial to set the temperature at 360 degrees F.
10. Press "Start/Pause" button to start.When the unit beeps to show that it is preheated, open the lid.
11. Arrange the pan in "Air Fry Basket" and insert in the oven.
12. Place the pan onto a wire rack to cool for about 10 minutesCarefully, invert the bread onto wire rack to cool completely before slicing.
13. Cut the bread into desired-sized slices and serve.

Nutrition:

Calories 416 Fat 16.5 g Carbs 59.2 g Protein 8.1 g

787. Allspice Chicken Wings

⏱ Prep Time 10 m | ⏱ Cooking Time 45 m | 8 Servings

Ingredients:

- ½ tsp celery salt
- ½ tsp bay leaf powder
- ½ tsp ground black pepper
- ½ tsp paprika
- ¼ tsp dry mustard
- ¼ tsp cayenne pepper
- ¼ tsp allspice
- 2 pounds chicken wings

Directions:

1. Grease the air fryer basket and preheat to 340 F. In a bowl, mix celery salt, bay leaf powder, black pepper, paprika, dry mustard, cayenne pepper, and allspice. Coat the wings thoroughly in this mixture.
2. Arrange the wings in an even layer in the basket of the air fryer. Cook the chicken until it's no longer pink around the bone, for 30 minutes then, increase the temperature to 380 F and cook for 6 minutes more, until crispy on the outside.

Nutrition:

Calories 332 Fat 10.1 g Carbs 31.3 g Protein 12 g

788. Friday Night Pineapple Sticky Ribs

⏱ Prep Time 10 m | ⏱ Cooking Time 20 m | 4 Servings

Ingredients:

- 2 lb. cut spareribs
- 7 oz salad dressing
- 1 (5-oz) can pineapple juice
- 2 cups water
- Garlic salt to taste
- Salt and black pepper

Directions:

1. Sprinkle the ribs with salt and pepper, and place them in a saucepan. Pour water and cook the ribs for 12 minutes on high heat.
2. Dry out the ribs and arrange them in the fryer; sprinkle with garlic salt. Cook it for 15minutes at 390 F.
3. Prepare the sauce by combining the salad dressing and the pineapple juice. Serve the ribs drizzled with the sauce.

Nutrition:

Calories 316 Fat 3.1 g Carbs 1.9 g Protein 5 g

789. Egg Roll Wrapped With Cabbage And Prawns

⏱ Prep Time 10 m | ⏱ Cooking Time 40 m | 4 Servings

Ingredients:

- 2 tbsp vegetable oil
- 1-inch piece fresh ginger, grated
- 1 tbsp minced garlic
- 1 carrot, cut into strips
- ¼ cup chicken broth
- 2 tbsp reduced-sodium soy sauce
- 1 tbsp sugar
- 1 cup shredded Napa cabbage
- 1 tbsp sesame oil
- 8 cooked prawns, minced
- 1 egg
- 8 egg roll wrappers

Directions:

1. In a skillet over high heat, heat vegetable oil, and cook ginger and garlic for 40 seconds, until fragrant. Stir in carrot and cook for another 2 minutes Pour in chicken broth, soy sauce, and sugar and bring to a boil.
2. Add cabbage and let simmer until softened, for 4 minutes Remove skillet from the heat and stir in sesame oil. Let cool for 15 minutes Strain cabbage mixture, and fold in minced prawns. Whisk an egg in a small bowl. Fill each egg roll wrapper with prawn mixture, arranging the mixture just below the center of the wrapper.
3. Fold the bottom part over the filling and tuck under. Fold in both sides and tightly roll up. Use the whisked egg to seal the wrapper. Repeat until all egg rolls are ready. Place the rolls into a greased air fryer basket, spray them with oil and cook for 12 minutes at 370 F, turning once halfway through.

Nutrition:

Calories 215 Fat 7.9 g Carbs 6.7 g Protein 8 g

790. Sesame Garlic Chicken Wings

⏱ Prep Time 10 m | ⏱ Cooking Time 40 m | 4 Servings

Ingredients:

- 1-pound chicken wings
- 1 cup soy sauce, divided
- ½ cup brown sugar
- ½ cup apple cider vinegar
- 2 tbsp fresh ginger, minced
- 2 tbsp fresh garlic, minced
- 1 tsp finely ground black pepper
- 2 tbsp cornstarch
- 2 tbsp cold water
- 1 tsp sesame seeds

Directions:

1. In a bowl, add chicken wings, and pour in half cup soy sauce. Refrigerate for 20 minutes; Dry out and pat dry. Arrange the wings in the air fryer and cook for 30 minutes at 380 F, turning once halfway through. Make sure you check them towards the end to avoid overcooking.
2. In a skillet and over medium heat, stir sugar, half cup soy sauce, vinegar, ginger, garlic, and black pepper. Cook until sauce has reduced slightly, about 4 to 6 minutes
3. Dissolve 2 tbsp of cornstarch in cold water, in a bowl, and stir in the slurry into the sauce, until it thickens, for 2 minutes Pour the sauce over wings and sprinkle with sesame seeds.

Nutrition:

Calories 413 Fat 8.3 g Carbs 7 g Protein 8.3 g

791. Savory Chicken Nuggets With Parmesan Cheese

⏱ Prep Time 5 m | ⏱ Cooking Time 20 m | 4 Servings

Ingredients:

- 1 lb. chicken breast, boneless, skinless, cubed
- ½ tsp ground black pepper
- ¼ tsp kosher salt
- ¼ tsp seasoned salt
- 2 tbsp olive oil
- 5 tbsp plain breadcrumbs
- 2 tbsp panko breadcrumbs
- 2 tbsp grated Parmesan cheese

Directions:

1. Preheat the air fryer to 380 F and grease. Season the chicken with pepper, kosher salt, and seasoned salt; set aside. In a bowl, pour olive oil. In a separate bowl, add crumb, and Parmesan cheese.
2. Place the chicken pieces in the oil to coat, then dip into breadcrumb mixture, and transfer to the air fryer. Work in batches if needed. Lightly spray chicken with cooking spray.
3. Cook the chicken for 10 minutes, flipping once halfway through. Cook until golden brown on the outside and no more pink on the inside.

Nutrition:

Calories 312 Fat 8.9 g Carbs 7 g Protein 10 g

792. Butternut Squash With Thyme
⏱ Prep Time 5 m | ⏱ Cooking Time 20 m | 4 Servings

Ingredients:
- 2 cups peeled, butternut squash, cubed
- 1 tbsp olive oil
- ¼ tsp salt
- ¼ tsp black pepper
- ¼ tsp dried thyme
- 1 tbsp finely chopped fresh parsley

Directions:
1. In a bowl, add squash, oil, salt, pepper, and thyme, and toss until squash is well-coated.
2. Place squash in the air fryer and cook for 14 minutes at 360 F.
3. When ready, sprinkle with freshly chopped parsley and serve chilled.

Nutrition:
Calories 219 Fat 4.3 g Carbs 9.4 g Protein 7.8 g

793. Chicken Breasts In Golden Crumb
⏱ Prep Time 10 m | ⏱ Cooking Time 25 m | 4 Servings

Ingredients:
- 1 ½ lb. chicken breasts, boneless, cut into strips
- 1 egg, lightly beaten
- 1 cup seasoned breadcrumbs
- Salt and black pepper to taste
- ½ tsp dried oregano

Directions:
1. Preheat the air fryer to 390 F. Season the chicken with oregano, salt, and black pepper. In a small bowl, whisk in some salt and pepper to the beaten egg. In a separate bowl, add the crumbs. Dip chicken tenders in the egg wash, then in the crumbs.
2. Roll the strips in the breadcrumbs and press firmly, so the breadcrumbs stick well. Spray the chicken tenders with cooking spray and arrange them in the air fryer. Cook for 14 minutes, until no longer pink in the center, and nice and crispy on the outside.

Nutrition:
Calories 223 Fat 3.2 g Carbs 4.3 g Protein 5 g

794. Yogurt Chicken Tacos
⏱ Prep Time 5 m | ⏱ Cooking Time 20 m | 4 Servings

Ingredients:
- 1 cup cooked chicken, shredded
- 1 cup shredded mozzarella cheese
- ¼ cup salsa
- ¼ cup Greek yogurt
- Salt and ground black pepper
- 8 flour tortillas

Directions:
1. In a bowl, mix chicken, cheese, salsa, and yogurt, and season with salt and pepper. Spray one side of the tortilla with cooking spray. Lay 2 tbsp of the chicken mixture at the center of the non-oiled side of each tortilla.
2. Roll tightly around the mixture. Arrange taquitos into your air fryer basket, without overcrowding. Cook in batches if needed. Place the seam side down, or it will unravel during cooking crisps.
3. Cook it for 12 to 14 minutes, or until crispy, at 380 F.

Nutrition:
Calories 312 Fat 3 g Carbs 6.5 g Protein 6.2 g

795. Flawless Kale Chips
⏱ Prep Time 5 m | ⏱ Cooking Time 20 m | 4 Servings

Ingredients:
- 4 cups chopped kale leaves; stems removed
- 2 tbsp olive oil
- 1 tsp garlic powder
- ½ tsp salt
- ¼ tsp onion powder
- ¼ tsp black pepper

Directions:
1. In a bowl, mix kale and oil together, until well-coated. Add in garlic, salt, onion, and pepper and toss until well-coated. Arrange half the kale leaves to air fryer, in a single layer.
2. Cook for 8 minutes at 350 F, shaking once halfway through. Remove chips to a sheet to cool; do not touch.

Nutrition:
Calories 312 Fat 5.3 g Carbs 5 g Protein 7 g

796. Cheese Fish Balls
⏱ Prep Time 5 m | ⏱ Cooking Time 40 m | 6 Servings

Ingredients:
- 1 cup smoked fish, flaked
- 2 cups cooked rice
- 2 eggs, lightly beaten
- 1 cup grated Grana Padano cheese
- ¼ cup finely chopped thyme
- Salt and black pepper to taste
- 1 cup panko crumbs

Directions:
1. In a bowl, add fish, rice, eggs, Parmesan cheese, thyme, salt and pepper into a bowl; stir to combine. Shape the mixture into 12 even-sized balls. Roll the balls in the crumbs then spray with oil.
2. Arrange the balls into the fryer and cook for 16 minutes at 400 F, until crispy.

Nutrition:
Calories 234 Fat 5.2 g Carbs 4.3 g Protein 6.2 g

797. Baguette Bread

⏰ Prep Time 15 m | ⏱ Cooking Time 20 m | 8 Servings

Ingredients:

- ¾ cup warm water
- ¾ teaspoon quick yeast
- ½ teaspoon demerara sugar
- 1 cup bread flour
- ½ cup whole-wheat flour
- ½ cup oat flour
- 1¼ teaspoons salt

Directions:

1. In a large bowl, place the water and sprinkle with yeast and sugar.
2. Set aside for 5 minutes or until foamy.
3. Add the bread flour and salt mix until a stiff dough form.
4. Put the dough onto a floured surface and with your hands, knead until smooth and elastic.
5. Now, shape the dough into a ball.
6. Place the dough into a slightly oiled bowl and turn to coat well.
7. With a plastic wrap, cover the bowl and place in a warm place for about 1 hour or until doubled in size.
8. With your hands, punch down the dough and form into a long slender loaf.
9. Place the loaf onto a lightly greased baking sheet and set aside in warm place, uncovered, for about 30 minutes
10. Press "Power Button" of Air Fry Oven and turn the dial to select the "Air Bake" mode.
11. Press the Time button and again turn the dial to set the cooking time to 20 minutes
12. Now push the Temp button and rotate the dial to set the temperature at 450 degrees F.
13. Press "Start/Pause" button to start.
14. When the unit beeps to show that it is preheated, open the lid.
15. Carefully, arrange the dough onto the "Wire Rack" and insert in the oven.
16. Carefully, invert the bread onto wire rack to cool completely before slicing.
17. Cut the bread into desired-sized slices and serve.

Nutrition:
Calories 114 Fat 0.8 g Carbs 22.8 g Protein 3.8 g

798. Soda Bread

⏰ Prep Time 15 m | ⏱ Cooking Time 30 m | 10 Servings

Ingredients:

- 3 cups whole-wheat flour
- 1 tablespoon sugar
- 2 teaspoon caraway seeds
- 1 teaspoon baking soda
- 1 teaspoon sea salt
- ¼ cup chilled butter, cubed into small pieces
- 1 large egg, beaten
- 1½ cups buttermilk

Directions:

1. In a large bowl, mix together the flour, sugar, caraway seeds, baking soda and salt and mix well.
2. With a pastry cutter, cut in the butter flour until coarse crumbs like mixture is formed.
3. Make a well in the center of flour mixture.
4. In the well, add the egg, followed by the buttermilk and with a spatula, mix until well combined.
5. With floured hand, shape the dough into a ball.
6. Place the dough onto a floured surface and lightly need it.
7. Shape the dough into a 6-inch ball.
8. With a serrated knife, score an X on the top of the dough.
9. Press "Power Button" of Air Fry Oven and turn the dial to select the "Air Crisp" mode.
10. Press the Time button and again turn the dial to set the cooking time to 30 minutes
11. Now push the Temp button and rotate the dial to set the temperature at 350 degrees F.
12. Press "Start/Pause" button to start.
13. When the unit beeps to show that it is preheated, open the lid.
14. Arrange the dough in lightly greased "Air Fry Basket" and insert in the oven.
15. Place the pan onto a wire rack to cool for about 10 minutes
16. Carefully, invert the bread onto wire rack to cool completely before slicing.
17. Cut the bread into desired-sized slices and serve.

Nutrition:
Calories 205 Fat 5.9 g Carbs 31.8 g Protein 5.9 g

799. Yogurt Bread

⏰ Prep Time 20 m | ⏱ Cooking Time 40 m | 10 Servings

Ingredients:

- 1½ cups warm water, divided
- 1½ teaspoons active dry yeast
- 1 teaspoon sugar
- 3 cups all-purpose flour
- 1 cup plain Greek yogurt
- 2 teaspoons kosher salt

Directions:

1. Add ½ cup of the warm water, yeast and sugar in the bowl of a stand mixer, fitted with the dough hook attachment and mix well.
2. Set aside for about 5 minutes
3. Add the flour, yogurt, and salt and mix on medium-low speed until the dough comes together.
4. Then, mix on medium speed for 5 minutes
5. Place the dough into a bowl.
6. With a plastic wrap, cover the bowl and place in a warm place for about 2-3 hours or until doubled in size.
7. Transfer the dough onto a lightly floured surface and shape into a smooth ball.
8. Place the dough onto a greased parchment paper-lined rack.
9. With a kitchen towel, cover the dough and let rest for 15 minutes
10. With a very sharp knife, cut a 4x½-inch deep cut down the center of the dough.
11. Press "Power Button" of Air Fry Oven and turn the dial to select the "Air Roast" mode.
12. Press the Time button and again turn the dial to set the cooking time to 40 minutes
13. Now push the Temp button and rotate the dial to set the temperature at 325 degrees F.
14. Press "Start/Pause" button to start.
15. When the unit beeps to show that it is preheated, open the lid.
16. Carefully, arrange the dough onto the "Wire Rack" and insert in the oven.
17. Carefully, invert the bread onto wire rack to cool completely before slicing.
18. Cut the bread into desired-sized slices and serve.

Nutrition:
Calories 157 Fat 0.7 g Carbs 31 g Protein 5.5 g

800. Sunflower Seed Bread

Prep Time 15 m | Cooking Time 18 m | 6 Servings

Ingredients:
- 2/3 cup whole-wheat flour
- 2/3 cup plain flour
- 1/3 cup sunflower seeds
- ½ sachet instant yeast
- 1 teaspoon salt
- 2/3-1 cup lukewarm water

Directions:
1. In a bowl, mix together the flours, sunflower seeds, yeast, and salt.
2. Slowly, add in the water, stirring continuously until a soft dough ball form.
3. Now, move the dough onto a lightly floured surface and knead for about 5 minutes using your hands.
4. Make a ball from the dough and place into a bowl.
5. With a plastic wrap, cover the bowl and place at a warm place for about 30 minutes
6. Grease a cake pan.
7. Coat the top of dough with water and place into the prepared cake pan.
8. Press "Power Button" of Air Fry Oven and turn the dial to select the "Air Crisp" mode.
9. Press the Time button and again turn the dial to set the cooking time to 18 minutes
10. Now push the Temp button and rotate the dial to set the temperature at 390 degrees F.
11. Press "Start/Pause" button to start.
12. When the unit beeps to show that it is preheated, open the lid.
13. Arrange the pan in "Air Fry Basket" and insert in the oven.
14. Place the pan onto a wire rack to cool for about 10 minutes
15. Carefully, invert the bread onto wire rack to cool completely before slicing.
16. Cut the bread into desired-sized slices and serve.

Nutrition:
Calories 132 Fat 1.7 g Carbs 24.4 g Protein 4.9 g

801. Date Bread

Prep Time 15 m | Cooking Time 22 m | 10 Servings

Ingredients:
- 2½ cup dates, pitted and chopped
- ¼ cup butter
- 1 cup hot water
- 1½ cups flour
- ½ cup brown sugar
- 1 teaspoon baking powder
- 1 teaspoon baking soda
- ½ teaspoon salt
- 1 egg

Directions:
1. In a large bowl, add the dates, butter and top with the hot water.
2. Set aside for about 5 minutes
3. In another bowl, mix together the flour, brown sugar, baking powder, baking soda, and salt.
4. In the same bowl of dates, mix well the flour mixture, and egg.
5. Grease a baking pan.
6. Place the mixture into the prepared pan.
7. Press "Power Button" of Air Fry Oven and turn the dial to select the "Air Crisp" mode.
8. Press the Time button and again turn the dial to set the cooking time to 22 minutes
9. Now push the Temp button and rotate the dial to set the temperature at 340 degrees F.
10. Press "Start/Pause" button to start.
11. When the unit beeps to show that it is preheated, open the lid.
12. Arrange the pan in "Air Fry Basket" and insert in the oven.
13. Place the pan onto a wire rack to cool for about 10 minutes
14. Carefully, invert the bread onto wire rack to cool completely before slicing.
15. Cut the bread into desired-sized slices and serve.

Nutrition:
Calories 269 Fat 5.4 g Carbs 55.1 g Protein 3.6 g

802. Date & Walnut Bread

Prep Time 15 m | Cooking Time 35 m | 5 Servings

Ingredients:
- 1 cup dates, pitted and sliced
- ¾ cup walnuts, chopped
- 1 tablespoon instant coffee powder
- 1 tablespoon hot water
- 1¼ cups plain flour
- ¼ teaspoon salt
- ½ teaspoon baking powder
- ½ teaspoon baking soda
- ½ cup condensed milk
- ½ cup butter, softened
- ½ teaspoon vanilla essence

Directions:
1. In a large bowl, add the dates, butter and top with the hot water.
2. Set aside for about 30 minutes
3. Dry out well and set aside.
4. In a small bowl, add the coffee powder and hot water and mix well.
5. In a large bowl, mix together the flour, baking powder, baking soda and salt.
6. In another large bowl, add the condensed milk and butter and beat until smooth.
7. Add the flour mixture, coffee mixture and vanilla essence and mix until well combined.
8. Fold in dates and ½ cup of walnut.
9. Line a baking pan with a lightly greased parchment paper.
10. Place the mixture into the prepared pan and sprinkle with the remaining walnuts.
11. Press "Power Button" of Air Fry Oven and turn the dial to select the "Air Crisp" mode.
12. Press the Time button and again turn the dial to set the cooking time to 35 minutes
13. Now push the Temp button and rotate the dial to set the temperature at 320 degrees F.
14. Press "Start/Pause" button to start.
15. When the unit beeps to show that it is preheated, open the lid.
16. Arrange the pan in "Air Fry Basket" and insert in the oven.
17. Place the pan onto a wire rack to cool for about 10 minutes
18. Carefully, invert the bread onto wire rack to cool completely before slicing.
19. Cut the bread into desired-sized slices and serve.

Nutrition:
Calories 593 Fat 32.6 g Carbs 69.4 g Protein 11.2 g

803. Brown Sugar Banana Bread

☉ Prep Time 15 m | ☉ Cooking Time 30 m | 4 Servings

Ingredients:
- 1 egg
- 1 ripe banana, peeled and mashed
- ¼ cup milk
- 2 tablespoons canola oil
- 2 tablespoons brown sugar
- ¾ cup plain flour
- ½ teaspoon baking soda

Directions:
1. Line a very small baking pan with a greased parchment paper.
2. In a small bowl, add the egg and banana and beat well.
3. Add the milk, oil and sugar and beat until well combined.
4. Add the flour and baking soda and mix until just combined.
5. Place the mixture into prepared pan.
6. Press "Power Button" of Air Fry Oven and turn the dial to select the "Air Crisp" mode.
7. Press the Time button and again turn the dial to set the cooking time to 30 minutes
8. Now push the Temp button and rotate the dial to set the temperature at 320 degrees F.
9. Press "Start/Pause" button to start.
10. When the unit beeps to show that it is preheated, open the lid.
11. Arrange the pan in "Air Fry Basket" and insert in the oven.
12. Place the pan onto a wire rack to cool for about 10 minutes
13. Carefully, invert the bread onto wire rack to cool completely before slicing.
14. Cut the bread into desired-sized slices and serve.

Nutrition:
Calories 214 Fat 8.7 g Carbs 29.9 g Protein 4.6 g

804. Cinnamon Banana Bread

☉ Prep Time 15 m | ☉ Cooking Time 20 m | 8 Servings

Ingredients:
- 1 1/3 cups flour
- 2/3 cup sugar
- 1 teaspoon baking soda
- 1 teaspoon baking powder
- 1 teaspoon ground cinnamon
- 1 teaspoon salt
- ½ cup milk
- ½ cup olive oil
- 3 bananas, peeled and sliced

Directions:
1. In the bowl of a stand mixer, add all the ingredients and mix well.
2. Grease a loaf pan.
3. Place the mixture into the prepared pan.
4. Press "Power Button" of Air Fry Oven and turn the dial to select the "Air Crisp" mode.
5. Press the Time button and again turn the dial to set the cooking time to 20 minutes
6. Now push the Temp button and rotate the dial to set the temperature at 330 degrees F.
7. Press "Start/Pause" button to start.
8. When the unit beeps to show that it is preheated, open the lid.
9. Arrange the pan in "Air Fry Basket" and insert in the oven.
10. Place the pan onto a wire rack to cool for about 10 minutes
11. Carefully, invert the bread onto wire rack to cool completely before slicing.
12. Cut the bread into desired-sized slices and serve.

Nutrition:
Calories 295 Fat 13.3g Carbs 44 g Protein 3.1 g

805. Banana & Walnut Bread

☉ Prep Time 15 m | ☉ Cooking Time 25 m | 10 Servings

Ingredients:
- 1½ cups self-rising flour
- ¼ teaspoon bicarbonate of soda
- 5 tablespoons plus 1 teaspoon butter
- 2/3 cup plus ½ tablespoon caster sugar
- 2 medium eggs
- 3½ oz. walnuts, chopped
- 2 cups bananas, peeled and mashed

Directions:
1. In a bowl, mix together the flour and bicarbonate of soda.
2. In another bowl, add the butter, and sugar and beat until pale and fluffy.
3. Add the eggs, one at a time along with a little flour and mix well.
4. Stir in the remaining flour and walnuts.
5. Add the bananas and mix until well combined.
6. Grease a loaf pan.
7. Place the mixture into the prepared pan.
8. Press "Power Button" of Air Fry Oven and turn the dial to select the "Air Crisp" mode.
9. Press the Time button and again turn the dial to set the cooking time to 10 minutes
10. Now push the Temp button and rotate the dial to set the temperature at 355 degrees F.
11. Press "Start/Pause" button to start.
12. When the unit beeps to show that it is preheated, open the lid.
13. Arrange the pan in "Air Fry Basket" and insert in the oven.
14. After 10 minutes of cooking, set the temperature at 338 degrees F for 15 minutes
15. Place the pan onto a wire rack to cool for about 10 minutes
16. Carefully, invert the bread onto wire rack to cool completely before slicing.
17. Cut the bread into desired-sized slices and serve.

Nutrition:
Calories 270 Fat 12.8 g Carbs 35.5 g Protein 5.8 g

806. Banana & Raisin Bread

⏲ Prep Time 15 m | ⏲ Cooking Time 40 m | 6 Servings

Ingredients:

- 1½ cups cake flour
- 1 teaspoon baking soda
- ½ teaspoon ground cinnamon
- Salt, to taste
- ½ cup vegetable oil
- 2 eggs
- ½ cup sugar
- ½ teaspoon vanilla extract
- 3 medium bananas, peeled and mashed
- ½ cup raisins, chopped finely

Directions:

1. In a large bowl, mix together the flour, baking soda, cinnamon, and salt.
2. In another bowl, beat well eggs and oil.
3. Add the sugar, vanilla extract, and bananas and beat until well combined.
4. Add the flour mixture and stir until just combined.
5. Place the mixture into a lightly greased baking pan and sprinkle with raisins.
6. With a piece of foil, cover the pan loosely.
7. Press "Power Button" of Air Fry Oven and turn the dial to select the "Air Bake" mode.
8. Press the Time button and again turn the dial to set the cooking time to 30 minutes
9. Now push the Temp button and rotate the dial to set the temperature at 300 degrees F.
10. Press "Start/Pause" button to start.
11. When the unit beeps to show that it is preheated, open the lid.
12. Arrange the pan in "Air Fry Basket" and insert in the oven.
13. After 30 minutes of cooking, set the temperature to 285 degrees F for 10 minutes
14. Place the pan onto a wire rack to cool for about 10 minutes
15. Carefully, invert the bread onto wire rack to cool completely before slicing.
16. Cut the bread into desired-sized slices and serve.

Nutrition:

Calories 448 Fat 20.2 g Carbs 63.9 g Protein 6.1 g

807. 3-Ingredients Banana Bread

⏲ Prep Time 10 m | ⏲ Cooking Time 20 m | 6 Servings

Ingredients:

2 (6.4-oz.) banana muffin mix
1 cup water

1 ripe banana, peeled and mashed

Directions:

1. In a bowl, add all the ingredients and with a whisk, mix until well combined.
2. Place the mixture into a lightly greased loaf pan.
3. Press "Power Button" of Air Fry Oven and turn the dial to select the "Air Bake" mode.
4. Press the Time button and again turn the dial to set the cooking time to 20 minutes
5. Now push the Temp button and rotate the dial to set the temperature at 360 degrees F.
6. Press "Start/Pause" button to start.
7. When the unit beeps to show that it is preheated, open the lid.
8. Arrange the pan in "Air Fry Basket" and insert in the oven.
9. Place the pan onto a wire rack to cool for about 10 minutes
10. Carefully, invert the bread onto wire rack to cool completely before slicing.
11. Cut the bread into desired-sized slices and serve.

Nutrition:

Calories 144 Fat 3.8 g Carbs 25.5 g Protein 1.9 g

808. Yogurt Banana Bread

⏲ Prep Time 15 m | ⏲ Cooking Time 18 m | 5 Servings

Ingredients:

- 1 medium very ripe banana, peeled and mashed
- 1 large egg
- 1 tablespoon canola oil
- 1 tablespoon plain Greek yogurt
- ¼ teaspoon pure vanilla extract
- ½ cup all-purpose flour
- ¼ cup granulated white sugar
- ¼ teaspoon ground cinnamon
- ¼ teaspoon baking soda
- 1/8 teaspoon sea salt

Directions:

1. In a bowl, add the mashed banana, egg, oil, yogurt and vanilla and beat until well combined.
2. Add the flour, sugar, baking soda, cinnamon and salt and mix until just combined.
3. Place the mixture into a lightly greased mini loaf pan.
4. Press "Power Button" of Air Fry Oven and turn the dial to select the "Air Bake" mode.
5. Press the Time button and again turn the dial to set the cooking time to 28 minutes
6. Now push the Temp button and rotate the dial to set the temperature at 350 degrees F.
7. Press "Start/Pause" button to start.
8. When the unit beeps to show that it is preheated, open the lid.
9. Arrange the pan in "Air Fry Basket" and insert in the oven.
10. Place the pan onto a wire rack to cool for about 10 minutes
11. Carefully, invert the bread onto wire rack to cool completely before slicing.
12. Cut the bread into desired-sized slices and serve.

Nutrition:

Calories 145 Fat 4 g Carbs 25 g Protein 3 g

809. Sour Cream Banana Bread

⏱ Prep Time 15 m | ⏱ Cooking Time 37 m | 8 Servings

Ingredients:

- ¾ cup all-purpose flour
- ¼ teaspoon baking soda
- ¼ teaspoon salt
- 2 ripe bananas, peeled and mashed
- ½ cup granulated sugar

- ¼ cup sour cream
- ¼ cup vegetable oil
- 1 large egg
- ½ teaspoon pure vanilla extract

Directions:

1. In a large bowl, mix together the flour, baking soda and salt.
2. In another bowl, add the bananas, egg, sugar, sour cream, oil and vanilla and beat until well combined.
3. Add the flour mixture and mix until just combined.
4. Place the mixture into a lightly greased pan. Press "Power Button" of Air Fry Oven and turn the dial to select the "Air Crisp" mode.
5. Press the Time button and again turn the dial to set the cooking time to 37 minutes

6. Now push the Temp button and rotate the dial to set the temperature at 310 degrees F. Press "Start/Pause" button to start.
7. When the unit beeps to show that it is preheated, open the lid. Arrange the pan in "Air Fry Basket" and insert in the oven.
8. Place the pan onto a wire rack to cool for about 10 minutes
9. Carefully, invert the bread onto wire rack to cool completely before slicing.
10. Cut the bread into desired-sized slices and serve.

Nutrition:
Calories 201 Fat 9.2g Carbs 28.6g Protein 2.6g

810. Cool Crab Sticks

⏱ Prep Time 10 m | ⏱ Cooking Time 20 m | 4 Servings

Ingredients:

- 20 ounces crabsticks, sliced into thin strips
- 1 teaspoon Cajun seasoning

- 2 teaspoons sesame oil

Directions:

1. Season the crabsticks with sesame oil and Cajun seasoning
2. Cook for 10-12 minutes at 320 degrees F in "AIR FRY" mode

3. Serve and enjoy!

Nutrition:
Calories 105 Fat 5 g Carbs 15 g Protein 9g

811. Curly Fries

⏱ Prep Time 10 m | ⏱ Cooking Time 15 m | 4 Servings

Ingredients:

- 2 potatoes
- 1 tablespoon extra-virgin olive oil
- 1 teaspoon pepper

- 1 teaspoon salt
- 1 teaspoon paprika

Directions:

1. Preheat your Air Fryer to 350 degrees F in "AIR FRY" mode. Wash potatoes thoroughly and pass them through a spiralizer to get curly shapes

2. Take a bowl and add potatoes to the bowl, toss, and coat well with pepper, salt, oil, and paprika Transfer the curly fries to Air Fryer cooking basket and cook for 15 minutes
3. Sprinkle more salt and paprika, serve and enjoy!

Nutrition:
Calories 150 Fat 5 g Carbs 20 g Protein 5 g.

812. Garlic Prawn

⏱ Prep Time 10 m | ⏱ Cooking Time 8 m | 4 Servings

Ingredients:

- 15 fresh prawns
- 1 tablespoon olive oil
- 1 teaspoon chili powder
- 1 tablespoon black pepper

- 1 tablespoon chili sauce
- 1 garlic clove, minced
- Salt as needed

Directions:

1. Preheat your Air Fryer to 356 degrees F in "AIR FRY" mode
2. Wash prawns thoroughly and rinse them
3. Take a mixing bowl and add washed prawn, chili powder, oil, garlic, pepper, chili sauce and stir the mix

4. Transfer prawn to Air Fryer and cook for 8 minutes
5. Serve and enjoy!

Nutrition: Calories 140 Fat 10 g Carbs 5 g Protein 8g

813. Beef Tomato Meatballs

⏱ Prep Time 10 m | ⏱ Cooking Time 5 m | 4 Servings

Ingredients:

- 1 small onion, chopped
- 3/4 pounds ground beef
- 1 tablespoon fresh parsley, chopped
- 1/2 tablespoon fresh thyme leaves, chopped

- 1 whole egg
- 3 tablespoons breadcrumbs
- Salt and pepper to taste

Directions:

1. Chop onion and keep them on the side
2. Take a bowl and add listed ingredients, mix well (including onions)
3. Make 12 balls
4. Preheat your Air Fryer to 390 degrees F, transfer balls to the fryer in "AIR FRY" mode
5. Cook for 8 minutes (in batches if needed) and transfer the balls to oven

6. Add tomatoes sauce and drown the balls
7. Transfer the dish to your Air Fryer and cook for 5 minutes at 300 degrees F
8. Stir and serve
9. Enjoy!

Nutrition: Calories 270 Fat 25 g Carbs 8 g Protein 15g

814. Steamed Pot Stickers

⏱ Prep Time 20 m | ⏱ Cooking Time 10 m | 10 Servings

Ingredients:

- ½ cup finely chopped cabbage
- ¼ cup finely chopped red bell pepper
- 2 green onions, finely chopped
- 1 egg, beaten
- 2 tablespoons cocktail sauce
- 2 teaspoons low-sodium soy sauce
- 30 wonton wrappers
- 3 tablespoons water, plus more for brushing the wrappers

Directions:

1. In a small bowl, combine the cabbage, pepper, green onions, egg, cocktail sauce, and soy sauce, and mix well.
2. Put about 1 teaspoon of the mixture in the center of each wonton wrapper. Fold the wrapper in half, covering the filling dampen the edges with water, and seal. You can crimp the edges of the wrapper with your fingers so they look like the pot stickers you get in restaurants. Brush them with water.
3. Put 3 tablespoons water in the pan under the air fryer basket. Cook the pot stickers in 2 batches for 9 to 10 minutes or until the pot stickers are hot and the bottoms are lightly browned.
4. Substitution tip: Use other vegetables in this recipe, such as corn, baby peas, or chopped zucchini or summer squash. You could also add leftover cooked meat such as pork or chicken, finely chopped.

Nutrition:

Calories 291 Fat 2g Carbs 57g Protein 10g

815. Beef And Mango Skewers

⏱ Prep Time 10 m | ⏱ Cooking Time 5 m | 4 Servings

Ingredients:

- ¾ pound beef sirloin tip, cut into 1-inch cubes
- 2 tablespoons balsamic vinegar
- 1 tablespoon olive oil
- 1 tablespoon honey
- ½ teaspoon dried marjoram
- Pinch salt
- Freshly ground black pepper
- 1 mango

Directions:

1. Put the beef cubes in a medium bowl and add the balsamic vinegar, olive oil, honey, marjoram, salt, and pepper. Mix well, and then massage the marinade into the beef with your hands. Set aside.
2. To prepare the mango, stand it on end and cut the skin off, using a sharp knife. Then carefully cut around the oval pit to remove the flesh. Cut the mango into 1-inch cubes.
3. Thread metal skewers alternating with three beef cubes and two mango cubes.
4. Grill the skewers in the air fryer basket for 4 to 7 minutes or until the beef is browned and at least 145°F.

Nutrition:

Calories 242 Fat 9g Carbs 13g Protein 26g

816. Curried Sweet Potato Fries

⏱ Prep Time 5 m | ⏱ Cooking Time 12 m | 4 Servings

Ingredients:

- ½ cup sour cream
- ½ cup mango chutney
- 3 teaspoons curry powder, divided
- 4 cups frozen sweet potato fries
- 1 tablespoon olive oil
- Pinch salt
- Freshly ground black pepper

Directions:

1. In a small bowl, combine sour cream, chutney, and 1½ teaspoons of the curry powder. Mix well and set aside. Put the sweet potatoes in a medium bowl. Drizzle with the olive oil and sprinkle with remaining 1½ teaspoons curry powder, salt, and pepper.
2. Put the potatoes in the air fryer basket. Cook for 8 to 12 minutes or until crisp, hot, and golden brown, shaking the basket once during cooking time. Place the fries in a serving basket and serve with the chutney dip.
3. Substitution tip: You can use fresh sweet potatoes in place of the frozen precut fries. Use one or two sweet potatoes, peel them, and cut into ⅓-inch thick strips using a sharp knife or mandoline. Use as directed in recipe; but you will need to increase the cooking time.

Nutrition:

Calories 323 Fat 10g Carbs 58g Protein 3g

817. Spicy Kale Chips With Yogurt Sauce

⏱ Prep Time 10 m | ⏱ Cooking Time 5 m | 4 Servings

Ingredients:

- 1 cup Greek yogurt
- 3 tablespoons lemon juice
- 2 tablespoons honey mustard
- ½ teaspoon dried oregano
- 1 bunch curly kale
- 2 tablespoons olive oil
- ½ teaspoon salt
- ⅛ Teaspoon pepper

Directions:

1. In a small bowl, combine the yogurt, lemon juice, honey mustard, and oregano, and set aside.
2. Remove the stems and ribs from the kale with a sharp knife. Cut the leaves into 2- to 3-inch pieces.
3. Toss the kale with olive oil, salt, and pepper. Massage the oil into the leaves with your hands.
4. Air-fry the kale in batches until crisp, about 5 minutes, shaking the basket once during cooking time. Serve with the yogurt sauce.
5. Ingredient tip: Kale comes in several different varieties. Tuscan (also known as dinosaur or lacinato) kale is the sturdiest and makes excellent chips. Curly kale, the variety most widely found in grocery stores, can become slightly frizzy when cooked in the air fryer, but is still delicious.

Nutrition:

Calories 154 Fat 8g Carbs 13g Protein 8g

818. Phyllo Artichoke Triangles

⏲ Prep Time 15 m | ⏲ Cooking Time 10 m | 14 Servings

Ingredients:

- ¼ cup ricotta cheese
- 1 egg white
- ⅓ Cup minced Dry-out artichoke hearts
- 3 tablespoons grated mozzarella cheese
- ½ teaspoon dried thyme
- 6 sheets frozen phyllo dough, thawed
- 2 tablespoons melted butter

Directions:

1. In a small bowl, combine ricotta cheese, egg white, artichoke hearts, mozzarella cheese, and thyme, and mix well. Cover the phyllo dough with a damp kitchen towel while you work so it doesn't dry out. Place on the work surface and cut into thirds lengthwise using one sheet at a time.
2. Put about 1½ teaspoons of the filling on each strip at the base. Fold the bottom right-hand tip of phyllo over the filling to meet the other side in a triangle, and then continue folding in a triangle.

Brush each triangle with butter to seal the edges. Repeat with remaining phyllo dough and filling.

3. Bake, 6 at a time, for about 3 to 4 minutes or until the phyllo is golden brown and crisp.
4. Substitution tip: You can use anything in this filling in place of the artichoke hearts. Try spinach, chopped cooked shrimp, cooked sausage, or keep it vegetarian and use all grated cheese.

Nutrition:

Calories 271 Fat 17g Carbs 23g Protein 9g

819. Spinach Dip With Bread Knots

⏲ Prep Time 12 m | ⏲ Cooking Time 20 m | 6 Servings

Ingredients:

- Nonstick cooking spray
- 1 (8-ounce) package cream cheese, cut into cubes
- ¼ cup sour cream
- ½ cup frozen chopped spinach, thawed and Dry-out
- ½ cup grated Swiss cheese
- 2 green onions, chopped
- ½ (11-ounce) can refrigerated breadstick dough
- 2 tablespoons melted butter
- 3 tablespoons grated Parmesan cheese

Directions:

1. Spray a 6-by-6-by-2-inch pan with nonstick cooking spray.
2. In a medium bowl, combine the cream cheese, sour cream, spinach, Swiss cheese, and green onions, and mix well. Spread into the prepared pan and Bake it for 8 minutes or until hot. While the dip is baking, unroll six of the breadsticks and cut them in half crosswise to make 12 pieces.
3. Gently stretch each piece of dough and tie into a loose knot; tuck in the ends.
4. When the dip is hot, remove from the air fryer and carefully place each bread knot on top of the dip, covering the surface of the dip. Brush each knot with melted butter and sprinkle Parmesan cheese on top.
5. Bake it for 8 to 13 minutes or until the bread knots are golden brown and cooked through.

Nutrition:

Calories 264 Fat 23g Carbs 7g Protein 8g

820. Arancini

⏲ Prep Time 15 m | ⏲ Cooking Time 20 m | 16 Servings

Ingredients:

- 2 cups cooked and cooled rice or leftover risotto
- 2 eggs, beaten
- 1½ cups panko bread crumbs, divided
- ½ cup grated Parmesan cheese
- 2 tablespoons minced fresh basil
- 16 ¾-inch cubes mozzarella cheese
- 2 tablespoons olive oil

Directions:

1. In a medium bowl, combine the rice, eggs, ½ cup of the bread crumbs, Parmesan cheese, and basil. Form this mixture into 16 1½-inch balls.
2. Poke a hole in each of the balls with your finger and insert a mozzarella cube. Form the rice mixture firmly around the

cheese. On a shallow plate, combine the remaining 1 cup bread crumbs with the olive oil and mix well. Roll the rice balls in the bread crumbs to coat.

3. Cook the arancini in batches for 8 to 11 minutes or until golden brown.

Nutrition:

Calories 378 Fat 11g Carbs 53g Protein 16g

821. Pesto Bruschetta

⏲ Prep Time 10 m | ⏲ Cooking Time 10 m | 4 Servings

Ingredients:

- 8 slices French bread, ½ inch thick
- 2 tablespoons softened butter
- 1 cup shredded mozzarella cheese
- ½ cup basil pesto
- 1 cup chopped grape tomatoes
- 2 green onions, thinly sliced

Directions:

1. Spread the bread with the butter and place butter-side up in the air fryer basket. Bake it for 3 to 5 minutes or until the bread is light golden brown.
2. Remove the bread from the basket and top each piece with some of the cheese. Return to the basket in batches and bake until the

cheese melts, about 1 to 3 minutes. Meanwhile, combine the pesto, tomatoes, and green onions in a small bowl.

3. When the cheese has melted, remove the bread from the air fryer and place on a serving plate. Top each slice with some of the pesto mixture and serve.

Nutrition:

Calories 462 Fat 25g Carbs 41g Protein 19g

822. Soda Bread
⏱ Prep Time 15 m | ⏱ Cooking Time 30 m | 10 Servings

Ingredients:

- cups whole-wheat flour
- 1 tablespoon sugar
- teaspoon caraway seeds
- 1 teaspoon baking soda

- 1 teaspoon sea salt
- ¼ cup chilled butter, cubed into small pieces
- 1 large egg, beaten
- 1½ cups buttermilk

Directions:

1. In a large bowl, mix together the flour, sugar, caraway seeds, baking soda and salt and mix well.
2. With a pastry cutter, cut in the butter flour until coarse crumbs like mixture is formed.
3. Make a well in the center of flour mixture.
4. In the well, add the egg, followed by the buttermilk and with a spatula, mix until well combined.
5. With floured hand, shape the dough into a ball.
6. Place the dough onto a floured surface and lightly need it.
7. Shape the dough into a 6-inch ball.
8. With a serrated knife, score an X on the top of the dough.
9. Press "Power Button" of Air Fry Oven and turn the dial to select the "Air Crisp" mode.
10. Press the Time button and again turn the dial to set the cooking time to 30 minutes
11. Now push the Temp button and rotate the dial to set the temperature at 350 degrees F.
12. Press "Start/Pause" button to start.
13. When the unit beeps to show that it is preheated, open the lid.
14. Arrange the dough in lightly greased "Air Fry Basket" and insert in the oven.
15. Place the pan onto a wire rack to cool for about 10 minutes
16. Carefully, invert the bread onto wire rack to cool completely before slicing.
17. Cut the bread into desired-sized slices and serve.

Nutrition:
Calories 205 | Fat 5.9 g | Carbs 31.8 g | Protein 5.9 g

823. Baguette Bread
⏱ Prep Time 15 m | ⏱ Cooking Time 20 m | 8 Servings

Ingredients:

¾ cup warm water
¾ teaspoon quick yeast
½ teaspoon demerara sugar
1 cup bread flour

½ cup whole-wheat flour
½ cup oat flour
1¼ teaspoons salt

Directions:

1. In a large bowl, place the water and sprinkle with yeast and sugar.
2. Set aside for 5 minutes or until foamy.
3. Add the bread flour and salt mix until a stiff dough form.
4. Put the dough onto a floured surface and with your hands, knead until smooth and elastic.
5. Now, shape the dough into a ball.
6. Place the dough into a slightly oiled bowl and turn to coat well.
7. With a plastic wrap, cover the bowl and place in a warm place for about 1 hour or until doubled in size.
8. With your hands, punch down the dough and form into a long slender loaf.
9. Place the loaf onto a lightly greased baking sheet and set aside in warm place, uncovered, for about 30 minutes
10. Press "Power Button" of Air Fry Oven and turn the dial to select the "Air Bake" mode.
11. Press the Time button and again turn the dial to set the cooking time to 20 minutes
12. Now push the Temp button and rotate the dial to set the temperature at 450 degrees F.
13. Press "Start/Pause" button to start.
14. When the unit beeps to show that it is preheated, open the lid.
15. Carefully, arrange the dough onto the "Wire Rack" and insert in the oven.
16. Carefully, invert the bread onto wire rack to cool completely before slicing.
17. Cut the bread into desired-sized slices and serve.

Nutrition:
Calories 114 | Fat 0.8 g | Carbs 22.8 g | Protein 3.8 g

824. Yogurt Bread

⏱ Prep Time 20 m | ⏱ Cooking Time 40 m | 10 Servings

Ingredients:

- 1½ cups warm water, divided
- 1½ teaspoons active dry yeast
- 1 teaspoon sugar

- cups all-purpose flour
- 1 cup plain Greek yogurt
- teaspoons kosher salt

Directions:

1. Add ½ cup of the warm water, yeast and sugar in the bowl of a stand mixer, fitted with the dough hook attachment and mix well.
2. Set aside for about 5 minutes
3. Add the flour, yogurt, and salt and mix on medium-low speed until the dough comes together.
4. Then, mix on medium speed for 5 minutes
5. Place the dough into a bowl.
6. With a plastic wrap, cover the bowl and place in a warm place for about 2-3 hours or until doubled in size.
7. Transfer the dough onto a lightly floured surface and shape into a smooth ball.
8. Place the dough onto a greased parchment paper-lined rack.
9. With a kitchen towel, cover the dough and let rest for 15 minutes

10. With a very sharp knife, cut a 4x½-inch deep cut down the center of the dough.
11. Press "Power Button" of Air Fry Oven and turn the dial to select the "Air Roast" mode.
12. Press the Time button and again turn the dial to set the cooking time to 40 minutes
13. Now push the Temp button and rotate the dial to set the temperature at 325 degrees F.
14. Press "Start/Pause" button to start.
15. When the unit beeps to show that it is preheated, open the lid.
16. Carefully, arrange the dough onto the "Wire Rack" and insert in the oven.
17. Carefully, invert the bread onto wire rack to cool completely before slicing.
18. Cut the bread into desired-sized slices and serve.

Nutrition:

Calories 157| Fat 0.7 g |Carbs 31 g |Protein 5.5 g

825. Sunflower Seed Bread

⏱ Prep Time 15 m | ⏱ Cooking Time 18 m | 6 Servings

Ingredients:

- 2/3 cup whole-wheat flour
- 2/3 cup plain flour
- 1/3 cup sunflower seeds

- ½ sachet instant yeast
- 1 teaspoon salt
- 2/3-1 cup lukewarm water

Directions:

1. In a bowl, mix together the flours, sunflower seeds, yeast, and salt.
2. Slowly, add in the water, stirring continuously until a soft dough ball form.
3. Now, move the dough onto a lightly floured surface and knead for about 5 minutes using your hands.
4. Make a ball from the dough and place into a bowl.
5. With a plastic wrap, cover the bowl and place at a warm place for about 30 minutes
6. Grease a cake pan.
7. Coat the top of dough with water and place into the prepared cake pan.
8. Press "Power Button" of Air Fry Oven and turn the dial to select the "Air Crisp" mode.

9. Press the Time button and again turn the dial to set the cooking time to 18 minutes
10. Now push the Temp button and rotate the dial to set the temperature at 390 degrees F.
11. Press "Start/Pause" button to start.
12. When the unit beeps to show that it is preheated, open the lid.
13. Arrange the pan in "Air Fry Basket" and insert in the oven.
14. Place the pan onto a wire rack to cool for about 10 minutes
15. Carefully, invert the bread onto wire rack to cool completely before slicing.
16. Cut the bread into desired-sized slices and serve.

Nutrition:

Calories 132| Fat 1.7 g |Carbs 24.4 g |Protein 4.9 g

826. Easy Sweet Potato Fries

⏱ Prep Time 10 m | ⏱ Cooking Time 16 m | 2 Servings

Ingredients:

- sweet potatoes, peeled and cut into fries shape
- 1 tbsp olive oil

- Salt

Directions:

1. Fit the cuisinart oven with the rack in position 2.
2. Toss sweet potato fries with oil and salt and place in the air fryer basket then place the air fryer basket in the baking pan.

3. Place a baking pan on the oven rack. Set to air fry at 375 f for 16 minutes.
4. Serve and enjoy.

Nutrition:

Calories 178 |Fat 7.2 g |Carbohydrates 27.9 g| Sugar 0.5 g |Protein 1.5 g| Cholesterol 0 mg

827. Date Bread

Ingredients:

- 2½ cup dates, pitted and chopped
- ¼ cup butter
- 1 cup hot water
- 1½ cups flour
- ½ cup brown sugar
- 1 teaspoon baking powder
- 1 teaspoon baking soda
- ½ teaspoon salt
- 1 egg

Directions:

1. In a large bowl, add the dates, butter and top with the hot water.
2. Set aside for about 5 minutes
3. In another bowl, mix together the flour, brown sugar, baking powder, baking soda, and salt.
4. In the same bowl of dates, mix well the flour mixture, and egg.
5. Grease a baking pan.
6. Place the mixture into the prepared pan.
7. Press "Power Button" of Air Fry Oven and turn the dial to select the "Air Crisp" mode.
8. Press the Time button and again turn the dial to set the cooking time to 22 minutes
9. Now push the Temp button and rotate the dial to set the temperature at 340 degrees F.
10. Press "Start/Pause" button to start.
11. When the unit beeps to show that it is preheated, open the lid.
12. Arrange the pan in "Air Fry Basket" and insert in the oven.
13. Place the pan onto a wire rack to cool for about 10 minutes
14. Carefully, invert the bread onto wire rack to cool completely before slicing.
15. Cut the bread into desired-sized slices and serve.

Nutrition:

Calories 269| Fat 5.4 g| Carbs 55.1 g | Protein 3.6 g

828. Salsa Cheese Dip

Ingredients:

- oz cream cheese, softened
- cups cheddar cheese, shredded
- 1 cup sour cream
- 1/2 cup hot salsa

Directions:

1. Fit the cuisinart oven with the rack in position 1.
2. In a bowl, mix all ingredients until just combined and pour into the baking dish.
3. Set to bake at 350 f for 35 minutes. After 5 minutes place the baking dish in the preheated oven.
4. Serve and enjoy.

Nutrition:

Calories 348 |Fat 31.9 g |Carbohydrates 3.4 g| Sugar 0.7 g |Protein 12.8 g |Cholesterol 96 mg

829. Perfect Ranch Potatoes

Ingredients:

- 1/2 lb baby potatoes, wash and cut in half
- 1/4 tsp parsley
- 1/2 tbsp olive oil
- 1/4 tsp dill
- 1/4 tsp paprika
- 1/4 tsp onion powder
- 1/4 tsp garlic powder
- 1/4 tsp chives
- Salt

Directions:

1. Fit the cuisinart oven with the rack in position 2.
2. Add all ingredients into the bowl and toss well.
3. Spread potatoes in the air fryer basket then place an air fryer basket in the baking pan.
4. Place a baking pan on the oven rack. Set to air fry at 400 f for 20 minutes.
5. Serve and enjoy.

Nutrition:

Calories 99 |Fat 3.7 g |Carbohydrates 14.8 g | Sugar 0.2 g |Protein 3.1 g |Cholesterol 0 mg

830. Tasty Potato Wedges

Ingredients:

- medium potatoes, cut into wedges
- 1/4 tsp garlic powder
- 1/4 tsp pepper
- 1/2 tsp paprika
- 1 1/2 tbsp olive oil
- 1/8 tsp cayenne
- 1 tsp sea salt

Directions:

1. Fit the cuisinart oven with the rack in position 2.
2. Soak potato wedges into the water for 30 minutes.
3. Drain well and pat dry with a paper towel.
4. In a bowl, toss potato wedges with remaining ingredients.
5. Place potato wedges in the air fryer basket then place an air fryer basket in the baking pan.
6. Place a baking pan on the oven rack. Set to air fry at 400 f for 15 minutes.

Nutrition:

Calories 120 |Fat 5.4 g |Carbohydrates 17.1 g | Sugar 1.3 g |Protein 1.9 g |Cholesterol 0 mg

831. Delicious Cauliflower Hummus

Prep Time 10 m | Cooking Time 35 m | 8 Servings

Ingredients:

- 1 cauliflower head, cut into florets
- tbsp olive oil
- 1/2 tsp ground cumin
- tbsp fresh lemon juice
- 1/3 cup tahini
- 1 tsp garlic, chopped
- Pepper
- Salt

Directions:

1. Fit the cuisinart oven with the rack in position 1.
2. Spread cauliflower florets in baking pan.
3. Set to bake at 400 f for 40 minutes. After 5 minutes place the baking dish in the preheated oven.
4. Transfer roasted cauliflower into the food processor along with remaining ingredients and process until smooth.
5. Serve and enjoy.

Nutrition:

Calories 115| Fat 10.7 g| Carbohydrates 4.2 g| Sugar 0.9 g |Protein 2.4 g |Cholesterol 0 mg

832. Brown Sugar Banana Bread

Prep Time 15 m | Cooking Time 30 m | 4 Servings

Ingredients:

- 1 egg
- 1 ripe banana, peeled and mashed
- ¼ cup milk
- tablespoons canola oil
- tablespoons brown sugar
- ¾ cup plain flour
- ½ teaspoon baking soda

Directions:

1. Line a very small baking pan with a greased parchment paper.
2. In a small bowl, add the egg and banana and beat well.
3. Add the milk, oil and sugar and beat until well combined.
4. Add the flour and baking soda and mix until just combined.
5. Place the mixture into prepared pan.
6. Press "Power Button" of Air Fry Oven and turn the dial to select the "Air Crisp" mode.
7. Press the Time button and again turn the dial to set the cooking time to 30 minutes
8. Now push the Temp button and rotate the dial to set the temperature at 320 degrees F.
9. Press "Start/Pause" button to start.
10. When the unit beeps to show that it is preheated, open the lid.
11. Arrange the pan in "Air Fry Basket" and insert in the oven.
12. Place the pan onto a wire rack to cool for about 10 minutes
13. Carefully, invert the bread onto wire rack to cool completely before slicing.
14. Cut the bread into desired-sized slices and serve.

Nutrition:

Calories 214 |Fat 8.7 g |Carbs 29.9 g |Protein 4.6 g

833. Date & Walnut Bread

Prep Time 15 m | Cooking Time 35 m | 5 Servings

Ingredients:

- 1 cup dates, pitted and sliced
- ¾ cup walnuts, chopped
- 1 tablespoon instant coffee powder
- 1 tablespoon hot water
- 1¼ cups plain flour
- ¼ teaspoon salt
- ½ teaspoon baking powder
- ½ teaspoon baking soda
- ½ cup condensed milk
- ½ cup butter, softened
- ½ teaspoon vanilla essence

Directions:

1. In a large bowl, add the dates, butter and top with the hot water.
2. Set aside for about 30 minutes
3. Dry out well and set aside.
4. In a small bowl, add the coffee powder and hot water and mix well.
5. In a large bowl, mix together the flour, baking powder, baking soda and salt.
6. In another large bowl, add the condensed milk and butter and beat until smooth.
7. Add the flour mixture, coffee mixture and vanilla essence and mix until well combined.
8. Fold in dates and ½ cup of walnut.
9. Line a baking pan with a lightly greased parchment paper.
10. Place the mixture into the prepared pan and sprinkle with the remaining walnuts.
11. Press "Power Button" of Air Fry Oven and turn the dial to select the "Air Crisp" mode.
12. Press the Time button and again turn the dial to set the cooking time to 35 minutes
13. Now push the Temp button and rotate the dial to set the temperature at 320 degrees F.
14. Press "Start/Pause" button to start.
15. When the unit beeps to show that it is preheated, open the lid.
16. Arrange the pan in "Air Fry Basket" and insert in the oven.
17. Place the pan onto a wire rack to cool for about 10 minutes
18. Carefully, invert the bread onto wire rack to cool completely before slicing.
19. Cut the bread into desired-sized slices and serve.

Nutrition:

Calories 593 |Fat 32.6 g |Carbs 69.4 g | Protein 11.2 g

834. Cinnamon Banana Bread
⏰ Prep Time 15 m | ⏰ Cooking Time 20 m | 8 Servings

Ingredients:

- 1 1/3 cups flour
- 2/3 cup sugar
- 1 teaspoon baking soda
- 1 teaspoon baking powder
- 1 teaspoon ground cinnamon
- 1 teaspoon salt
- ½ cup milk
- ½ cup olive oil
- bananas, peeled and sliced

Directions:

1. In the bowl of a stand mixer, add all the ingredients and mix well.
2. Grease a loaf pan.
3. Place the mixture into the prepared pan.
4. Press "Power Button" of Air Fry Oven and turn the dial to select the "Air Crisp" mode.
5. Press the Time button and again turn the dial to set the cooking time to 20 minutes
6. Now push the Temp button and rotate the dial to set the temperature at 330 degrees F.
7. Press "Start/Pause" button to start.
8. When the unit beeps to show that it is preheated, open the lid.
9. Arrange the pan in "Air Fry Basket" and insert in the oven.
10. Place the pan onto a wire rack to cool for about 10 minutes
11. Carefully, invert the bread onto wire rack to cool completely before slicing.
12. Cut the bread into desired-sized slices and serve.

Nutrition:

Calories 295| Fat 13.3g| Carbs 44 g | Protein 3.1 g

835. Banana & Walnut Bread
⏰ Prep Time 15 m | ⏰ Cooking Time 25 m | 10 Servings

Ingredients:

- 1½ cups self-rising flour
- ¼ teaspoon bicarbonate of soda
- tablespoons plus 1 teaspoon butter
- 2/3 cup plus ½ tablespoon caster sugar
- medium eggs
- 3½ oz. walnuts, chopped
- cups bananas, peeled and mashed

Directions:

1. In a bowl, mix together the flour and bicarbonate of soda.
2. In another bowl, add the butter, and sugar and beat until pale and fluffy.
3. Add the eggs, one at a time along with a little flour and mix well.
4. Stir in the remaining flour and walnuts.
5. Add the bananas and mix until well combined.
6. Grease a loaf pan.
7. Place the mixture into the prepared pan.
8. Press "Power Button" of Air Fry Oven and turn the dial to select the "Air Crisp" mode.
9. Press the Time button and again turn the dial to set the cooking time to 10 minutes
10. Now push the Temp button and rotate the dial to set the temperature at 355 degrees F.
11. Press "Start/Pause" button to start.
12. When the unit beeps to show that it is preheated, open the lid.
13. Arrange the pan in "Air Fry Basket" and insert in the oven.
14. After 10 minutes of cooking, set the temperature at 338 degrees F for 15 minutes
15. Place the pan onto a wire rack to cool for about 10 minutes
16. Carefully, invert the bread onto wire rack to cool completely before slicing.
17. Cut the bread into desired-sized slices and serve.

Nutrition:

Calories 270 |Fat 12.8 g |Carbs 35.5 g |Protein 5.8 g

836. 3-Ingredients Banana Bread
⏰ Prep Time 10 m | ⏰ Cooking Time 20 m | 6 Servings

Ingredients:

- (6.4-oz.) banana muffin mix
- 1 cup water
- 1 ripe banana, peeled and mashed

Directions:

1. In a bowl, add all the ingredients and with a whisk, mix until well combined.
2. Place the mixture into a lightly greased loaf pan.
3. Press "Power Button" of Air Fry Oven and turn the dial to select the "Air Bake" mode.
4. Press the Time button and again turn the dial to set the cooking time to 20 minutes
5. Now push the Temp button and rotate the dial to set the temperature at 360 degrees F.
6. Press "Start/Pause" button to start.
7. When the unit beeps to show that it is preheated, open the lid.
8. Arrange the pan in "Air Fry Basket" and insert in the oven.
9. Place the pan onto a wire rack to cool for about 10 minutes
10. Carefully, invert the bread onto wire rack to cool completely before slicing.
11. Cut the bread into desired-sized slices and serve.

Nutrition:

Calories 144 |Fat 3.8 g| Carbs 25.5 g| Protein 1.9 g

837. Banana & Raisin Bread

⏱ Prep Time 15 m | ⏱ Cooking Time 40 m | 6 Servings

Ingredients:

- 1½ cups cake flour
- 1 teaspoon baking soda
- ½ teaspoon ground cinnamon
- Salt, to taste
- ½ cup vegetable oil

- eggs
- ½ cup sugar
- ½ teaspoon vanilla extract
- medium bananas, peeled and mashed
- ½ cup raisins, chopped finely

Directions:

1 In a large bowl, mix together the flour, baking soda, cinnamon, and salt.
2 In another bowl, beat well eggs and oil.
3 Add the sugar, vanilla extract, and bananas and beat until well combined.
4 Add the flour mixture and stir until just combined.
5 Place the mixture into a lightly greased baking pan and sprinkle with raisins.
6 With a piece of foil, cover the pan loosely.
7 Press "Power Button" of Air Fry Oven and turn the dial to select the "Air Bake" mode.
8 Press the Time button and again turn the dial to set the cooking time to 30 minutes

9 Now push the Temp button and rotate the dial to set the temperature at 300 degrees F.
10 Press "Start/Pause" button to start.
11 When the unit beeps to show that it is preheated, open the lid.
12 Arrange the pan in "Air Fry Basket" and insert in the oven.
13 After 30 minutes of cooking, set the temperature to 285 degrees F for 10 minutes
14 Place the pan onto a wire rack to cool for about 10 minutes
15 Carefully, invert the bread onto wire rack to cool completely before slicing.
16 Cut the bread into desired-sized slices and serve.

Nutrition:

Calories 448 |Fat 20.2 g| Carbs 63.9 g | Protein 6.1 g

838. Yogurt Banana Bread

⏱ Prep Time 15 m | ⏱ Cooking Time 28 m | 5 Servings

Ingredients:

- 1 medium very ripe banana, peeled and mashed
- 1 large egg
- 1 tablespoon canola oil
- 1 tablespoon plain Greek yogurt
- ¼ teaspoon pure vanilla extract

- ½ cup all-purpose flour
- ¼ cup granulated white sugar
- ¼ teaspoon ground cinnamon
- ¼ teaspoon baking soda
- 1/8 teaspoon sea salt

Directions:

1 In a bowl, add the mashed banana, egg, oil, yogurt and vanilla and beat until well combined.
2 Add the flour, sugar, baking soda, cinnamon and salt and mix until just combined.
3 Place the mixture into a lightly greased mini loaf pan.
4 Press "Power Button" of Air Fry Oven and turn the dial to select the "Air Bake" mode.
5 Press the Time button and again turn the dial to set the cooking time to 28 minutes

6 Now push the Temp button and rotate the dial to set the temperature at 350 degrees F.
7 Press "Start/Pause" button to start.
8 When the unit beeps to show that it is preheated, open the lid.
9 Arrange the pan in "Air Fry Basket" and insert in the oven.
10 Place the pan onto a wire rack to cool for about 10 minutes
11 Carefully, invert the bread onto wire rack to cool completely before slicing.
12 Cut the bread into desired-sized slices and serve.

Nutrition:

Calories 145 |Fat 4 g| Carbs 25 g | Protein 3 g

839. Sour Cream Banana Bread
⏱ Prep Time 15 m | ⏱ Cooking Time 37 m | 8 Servings

Ingredients:

- ¾ cup all-purpose flour
- ¼ teaspoon baking soda
- ¼ teaspoon salt
- ripe bananas, peeled and mashed
- ½ cup granulated sugar
- ¼ cup sour cream
- ¼ cup vegetable oil
- 1 large egg
- ½ teaspoon pure vanilla extract

Directions:

1. In a large bowl, mix together the flour, baking soda and salt.
2. In another bowl, add the bananas, egg, sugar, sour cream, oil and vanilla and beat until well combined.
3. Add the flour mixture and mix until just combined.
4. Place the mixture into a lightly greased pan. Press "Power Button" of Air Fry Oven and turn the dial to select the "Air Crisp" mode.
5. Press the Time button and again turn the dial to set the cooking time to 37 minutes
6. Now push the Temp button and rotate the dial to set the temperature at 310 degrees F. Press "Start/Pause" button to start.
7. When the unit beeps to show that it is preheated, open the lid. Arrange the pan in "Air Fry Basket" and insert in the oven.
8. Place the pan onto a wire rack to cool for about 10 minutes
9. Carefully, invert the bread onto wire rack to cool completely before slicing.
10. Cut the bread into desired-sized slices and serve.

Nutrition:
Calories 201 | Fat 9.2g | Carbs 28.6g | Protein 2.6g

840. Peanut Butter Banana Bread
⏱ Prep Time 15 m | ⏱ Cooking Time 40 m | 6 Servings

Ingredients:

- 1 cup plus 1 tablespoon all-purpose flour
- ¼ teaspoon baking soda
- 1 teaspoon baking powder
- ¼ teaspoon salt
- 1 large egg
- 1/3 cup granulated sugar
- ¼ cup canola oil
- tablespoons creamy peanut butter
- tablespoons sour cream
- 1 teaspoon vanilla extract
- medium ripe bananas, peeled and mashed
- ¾ cup walnuts, roughly chopped

Directions:

1. In a bowl and mix the flour, baking powder, baking soda, and salt together.
2. In another large bowl, add the egg, sugar, oil, peanut butter, sour cream, and vanilla extract and beat until well combined.
3. Add the bananas and beat until well combined.
4. Add the flour mixture and mix until just combined.
5. Gently, fold in the walnuts.
6. Place the mixture into a lightly greased pan.
7. Press "Power Button" of Air Fry Oven and turn the dial to select the "Air Crisp" mode.
8. Press the Time button and again turn the dial to set the cooking time to 40 minutes
9. Now push the Temp button and rotate the dial to set the temperature at 330 degrees F.
10. Press "Start/Pause" button to start.
11. When the unit beeps to show that it is preheated, open the lid.
12. Arrange the pan in "Air Fry Basket" and insert in the oven.
13. Place the pan onto a wire rack to cool for about 10 minutes
14. Carefully, invert the bread onto wire rack to cool completely before slicing.
15. Cut the bread into desired-sized slices and serve.

Nutrition:
Calories 384 | Fat 23 g | Carbs 39.3 g | Protein 8.9 g

841. Sticky Barbecued Drumettes
⏱ Prep Time 5 m | ⏱ Cooking Time 24 m | 4 Servings

Ingredients:

- 2 pound Chicken Drumettes, bone in and skin in
- ½ cup Chicken Broth
- ½ teaspoon Dry Mustard
- ½ teaspoon Sweet Paprika
- ½ tablespoon Cumin Powder
- ½ teaspoon Onion Powder
- ¼ teaspoon Cayenne Powder
- Salt and Pepper, to taste
- 1 stick Butter, sliced in 5 to 7 pieces
- BBQ Sauce to taste

Directions:

1. Pour the chicken broth into the inner pot of cooker P and insert the reversible rack. In a zipper bag, pour in dry mustard, cumin powder, onion powder, cayenne powder, salt, and pepper. Add chicken, close the bag and shake to coat the chicken well with the spices.
2. Then, remove the chicken from the bag and place on the rack. Spread the butter slices on the drumsticks. Close the lid, secure the pressure valve, and select Pressure mode on High pressure for 10 minutes. Press Start.
3. Once the timer has ended, do a quick pressure release, and open the lid.
4. Remove the chicken onto a clean flat surface like a cutting board and brush them with the barbecue sauce using the brush. Return to the rack and close the crisping lid. Cook for 10 minutes at 400 F on Air Fry mode. Serve immediately.

Nutrition:
Calories 374 Fat 11.3g Carbs 2.85g Protein 38.3g

842. Tasty Chicken Wings

🕙 Prep Time 5 m | 🕙 Cooking Time 25 m | 6 Servings

Ingredients:

- 3 pounds Chicken Wingettes
- 3 tablespoons Cajun Garlic Powder
- Salt to taste
- ¼ cup Barbecue Sauce
- ½ cup Hot Sauce
- ¼ cup Butter, melted
- ½ cup Water

Directions:

1. Pat the wingettes dry with a paper towel and put them in a bowl. Season them with Cajun garlic powder and salt.
2. Open the cooker, pour in the water, and fit in the reversible rack. Arrange the wingettes on top, close the lid, secure the pressure valve, and select Pressure mode for 5 minutes. Press Start to start cooking.
3. Once the timer has ended, do a natural pressure release for 10 minutes, and then a quick pressure release to let out any more steam. Open the lid.
4. Remove the wings with tongs to a crisp basket and add the butter, half of the hot sauce and half of the barbecue sauce. Stir the chicken until well coated in the sauce.
5. Insert the basket in the pot and close the crisping lid. Select Air Fry, set to 380 F, and cook for 10 minutes. Select Start.
6. Once nice and crispy, remove them to a bowl, and top with the remaining barbecue and hot sauces. Stir and serve the chicken with a cheese dip.

Nutrition:

Calories 361 Fat 13.7g Carbs 9g Protein 35.7g

843. Traditional Italian Rice & Parmesan Balls

🕙 Prep Time 15 m | 🕙 Cooking Time 27 m | 6 Servings

Ingredients:

- ½ cup olive oil + 1 tablespoon
- 1 onion, diced
- 2 garlic cloves, minced
- 5 cups chicken stock
- ½ cup apple vinegar
- 2 cups rice
- 1½ cups grated Parmesan cheese
- 1 cup chopped green beans
- Salt and black pepper to taste
- 2 cups fresh panko breadcrumbs
- 2 eggs

Directions:

1. Choose Sear/Sauté on the pot and add in 1 tablespoon of oil and onion. Sauté the onion until translucent, add the garlic and cook further for 2 minutes or until the garlic starts getting fragrant. Stir in the stock, vinegar, and rice. Seal the pressure lid, choose Pressure, set to High, and set the time to 7 minutes. Press Start.
2. After cooking, perform a natural pressure release for 10 minutes.
3. Stir in the Parmesan cheese, green beans, salt, and pepper to mash the rice until a risotto forms. Spoon the mixture into a bowl and set aside to cool completely.
4. Clean the pot and in a bowl, combine the breadcrumbs and the remaining olive oil. In another bowl, lightly beat the eggs.
5. Form 12 croquettes out of the rice mixture or as many as you can get. Dip each into the beaten eggs, and coat in the breadcrumb mixture.
6. Put the rice balls in the Cook & Crisp basket in a single layer.
7. Close the crisping lid, choose Air Fry, set the temperature to 390 F, and set the time to 12 minutes. Choose Start to begin frying or until the balls are crisp and golden brown. At the 6-minute mark, turn the croquettes.
8. Allow cooling before serving. Serve with tangy relish.

Nutrition:

Calories 769 Fat 32g Carbs 91g Protein 27g

844. Herby Chicken Thighs

🕙 Prep Time 10 m | 🕙 Cooking Time 25 m | 4 Servings

Ingredients:

- 2 pounds Chicken Thighs, bone in and skin on
- 2 tablespoons Olive Oil
- Salt and Pepper, to taste
- 1 ½ cups diced Tomatoes
- ¾ cup Yellow Onion
- 2 teaspoons minced Garlic
- ½ cup Balsamic Vinegar
- 3 teaspoons chopped fresh Thyme
- 1 cup Chicken Broth
- 2 tablespoons chopped Parsley

Directions:

1. With paper towels, pat dry the chicken and season with salt and pepper.
2. Select Sear/Sauté mode. Warm the olive and add the chicken with skin side down. Cook to golden brown on each side, for about 9 minutes.
3. Remove onto a clean plate.
4. Then, add onions and tomatoes to the pot and sauté for 3 minutes, stirring occasionally with a spoon. Add in garlic and cook for 30 seconds, until fragrant.
5. Pour the chicken broth, and add some salt, thyme, and balsamic vinegar. Stir them using a spoon. Add the chicken back to the pot.
6. Close the lid, secure the pressure valve, and select Pressure mode on High pressure for 15 minutes. Press Start to start cooking.
7. When ready, do a quick pressure release.
8. Close the crisping lid and cook on Air Fry mode for 5 minutes at 400 F.
9. Garnish with parsley and serve with thyme roasted tomatoes, carrots, and sweet potatoes.

Nutrition:

Calories 412 Fat 16g Carbs 13g Protein 39g

845. Mexican Chicken Fajitas with Guacamole
⏱ Prep Time 10 m | ⏱ Cooking Time 20 m | 4 Servings

Ingredients:
- 2 pounds Chicken Breasts, skinless and cut in 1-inch slices
- ½ cup Chicken Broth
- 1 Yellow Onion, sliced
- 1 Green Bell Pepper, seeded and sliced
- 1 Yellow Bell Pepper, seeded and sliced
- 1 Red Bell Pepper, seeded and sliced
- 2 tablespoons Cumin Powder
- 2 tablespoons Chili Powder
- Salt to taste
- Half a Lime
- Cooking Spray
- Fresh cilantro, to garnish
- Assembling:
- Tacos, Guacamole, Sour Cream, Salsa, Cheese

Directions:
1. Grease the inner pot with cooking spray and line the bottom with the peppers and onion. Lay the chicken on the bed of peppers.
2. Sprinkle with salt, chili powder, and cumin powder. Squeeze some lime juice and pour in chicken broth. Close the lid, secure the pressure valve, and select Pressure mode on High pressure for 15 minutes. Press Start.
3. Once the timer has ended, do a quick pressure release, and open the lid.
4. Close the crisping lid and cook for 5 minutes on Roast mode at 370 F.
5. Dish the chicken with the vegetables and juice onto a large serving platter.
6. Add sour cream, cheese, guacamole, salsa, and tacos in one layer on the side of the chicken.

Nutrition:
Calories 423 Fat 22.1g Carbs 9g Protein 39.7g

846. Kale & Artichoke Bites
⏱ Prep Time 15 m | ⏱ Cooking Time 15 m | 8 Servings

Ingredients:
- ¼ cup chopped kale
- ¼ cup chopped artichoke hearts
- ¼ cup ricotta cheese
- 2 tablespoon grated Parmesan cheese
- ¼ cup goat cheese
- 1 large egg white
- 1 lemon, zested
- Salt and black pepper to taste
- 4 sheets frozen phyllo dough, thawed
- 1 tablespoon olive oil

Directions:
1. In a bowl, mix the kale, artichoke hearts, ricotta cheese, parmesan cheese, goat cheese, egg white, lemon zest, salt, and pepper.
2. Close the crisping lid, choose Air Fry, set the temperature to 370 F, and the time to 5 minutes. Press Start.
3. Then, place a phyllo sheet on a clean flat surface. Brush with olive oil, place a second phyllo sheet on the first, and brush with oil. Continue layering to form a pile of four oiled sheets.
4. Working from the short side, cut the phyllo sheets into 8 strips. Cut the strips in half to form 16 strips.
5. Spoon 1 tablespoon of filling onto one short side of every strip. Fold a corner to cover the filling to make a triangle; continue folding repeatedly to the end of the strip, creating a triangle-shaped phyllo packet. Repeat the process with the other phyllo bites.
6. Open the Crisping lid and place the bites in the basket in one layer. Close the lid, choose Air Fry, set the temperature to 350 F, and the timer to 10 minutes. Press Start to begin baking.
7. At the 5-minute mark, open the lid, and flip the bites. Return the basket to the pot and close the lid to continue baking. Once the timer beeps, check to ensure the bites are cooked all the way through.

Nutrition:
Calories 75 Fat 4g Carbs 7g Protein 3g

847. Panko Chicken Croquettes
⏱ Prep Time 10 m | ⏱ Cooking Time 25 m | 6 Servings

Ingredients:
- 1 pound ground chicken
- 1 green bell pepper, minced
- 2 celery stalks, minced
- ¼ cup crumbled queso fresco
- ¼ cup hot sauce
- ¼ cup panko breadcrumbs
- 1 egg
- 2 tablespoons melted butter
- ½ cup water

Directions:
1. In a bowl, combine the chicken, bell pepper, celery, queso fresco, hot sauce, breadcrumbs, and egg. Form balls (approximately the size of golf balls) out of the mixture.
2. Choose Sear/Sauté on the pot and set to High. Pour in the melted butter and fry the meatballs in batches until lightly browned on all sides. Use a slotted spoon to remove the meatballs onto a plate.
3. Put the Cook & Crisp basket in the pot. Pour in the water and put all the meatballs in the basket.
4. Seal the pressure lid, choose Pressure, set to High, and set the timer to 5 minutes. Hit Start.
5. When done cooking, perform a quick pressure release and carefully open the lid.
6. Close the crisping lid, press Air Fry button set the temperature to 360 F and set the time to 10 minutes. Choose Start.
7. At the 5-minute mark, shake the meatballs. Serve.

Nutrition:
Calories 204 Fat 13g Carbs 5g Protein 16g

848. Mini Buffalo Chicken Balls with Roquefort Sauce

Prep Time 10 m | Cooking Time 24 m | 4 Servings

Ingredients:

- 1 pound Ground Chicken
- 2 tablespoons Buffalo wing sauce
- 1 Egg, beaten
- Salt and Pepper to taste
- 2 tablespoons Minced Garlic
- 2 tablespoons Olive Oil
- 5 tablespoons Hot Sauce
- 2 tablespoons chopped Green Onions + extra for garnish
- For the sauce:
- ½ cup Roquefort Cheese, crumbled
- ¼ tablespoon Heavy Cream
- 2 tablespoons Mayonnaise
- Juice from ½ Lemon
- 2 tablespoons Olive Oil

Directions:

1. Mix all salsa ingredients in a bowl until uniform and creamy. Add ground chicken, salt, garlic, and two tablespoons of green onions. Mix well. Form bite-size balls out of the mixture. Lay onto crisp basket. Spray with cooking spray.
2. Select Air Fry, set the temperature to 385 F and the time to 14 minutes. At the 7-minute mark, turn the meatballs.
3. Meanwhile, add the hot sauce and butter to a bowl and microwave them until the butter melts. Mix the sauce with a spoon. Pour the hot sauce mixture and a half cup of water over the meatballs. Close the lid, secure the pressure valve, and select Sear/Sauté mode on High Pressure for 10 minutes. Press Start.
4. Once the timer has ended, do a quick pressure release. Dish the meatballs.
5. Garnish with green onions, and serve with Roquefort sauce.

Nutrition:
Calories 424 Fat 38g Carbs 7g Protein 26g

849. Wrapped in Prosciutto Asparagus with Bean Dip

Prep Time 5 m | Cooking Time 10 m | 6 Servings

Ingredients:

- 1 pound Asparagus, stalks trimmed
- 10 ounces Prosciutto, thinly sliced
- For the Dip:
- 1 cup canned white beans
- 1 medium onion, diced
- 2 cloves of garlic, minced
- 2 medium jalapeños, chopped
- 1 cup crushed Tomatoes
- 1 cup vegetable broth
- 1 ½ tablespoon olive oil
- 1 teaspoon paprika
- ¾ teaspoon sea salt
- ½ teaspoon chili powder

Directions:

1. Open the cooker and add the white beans, onion, jalapeños, garlic, tomatoes, broth, oil, paprika, chili powder, and salt.
2. Close the lid, secure the pressure valve, and select Pressure mode on High for 8 minutes. Press Start.
3. Once the timer has ended, do a quick pressure release, and open the pot.
4. Transfer the ingredients to a food processor, and blend until creamy and smooth. Set aside. Wrap each asparagus with a slice of prosciutto from top to bottom.
5. Grease the crisp basket with cooking spray, and add in the wrapped asparagus. Close the crisping lid, select Air Fry mode at 370 F and set the time to 8 minutes. Press Start. At the 4-minute mark, turn the bombs. Serve.

Nutrition:
Calories 154 Fat 12.4g Carbs 3g Protein 9.4g

850. Ground Beef & Cabbage Dumplings

Prep Time 20 m | Cooking Time 12 m | 8 Servings

Ingredients:

- 8 ounces ground beef
- ½ cup grated cabbage
- 1 carrot, grated
- 1 large egg, beaten
- 1 garlic clove, minced
- 2 tablespoons coconut amino
- ½ tablespoon melted ghee
- ½ tablespoon ginger powder
- ½ teaspoon salt
- ½ teaspoon freshly ground black pepper
- 20 wonton wrappers
- 2 tablespoons olive oil

Directions:

1. Close crisping lid. Preheat your cooker by choosing Air Fry at 390 F for 5 minutes.
2. In a large bowl, mix beef, cabbage, carrot, egg, garlic, coconut aminos, ghee, ginger, salt, and pepper. Put wonton wrappers on a clean flat surface and spoon 1 tbsp. of the beef mixture into the middle of each wrapper. Run the edges of the wrapper with a little water; fold the wrapper to cover the filling into a semi-circle shape and pinch the edges to seal. Brush the dumplings with olive oil.
3. Lay the dumplings in the preheated basket, choose Air Fry, set the temperature to 390 F, and set the time to 12 minutes. Choose Start.
4. At the 6-minute mark, open the lid, pull out the basket and shake the dumplings. Return the basket to the pot and close the lid to continue frying until the dumplings are crispy to your desire.

Nutrition:
Calories 186 Fat 11g Carbs 13g Protein 8g

851. Paprika Crispy Wings

⏱ Prep Time 10 m | ⏱ Cooking Time 20 m | 4 Servings

Ingredients:
- ½ cup water
- ½ cup sriracha sauce
- 2 tablespoons butter, melted
- 1 tablespoon lemon juice
- 8 chicken wings
- ½ teaspoon hot paprika
- Cooking spray

Directions:
1. Mix the water, sriracha, butter and lemon juice in the pot. In the Cook & Crisp basket, put the wings, and then the basket into the pot. Seal the pressure lid.
2. Choose Pressure, set to High, set the timer at 5 minutes, and choose Start.
3. When the timer is done reading, perform a quick pressure release, and carefully open the lid.
4. Pour the paprika all over the chicken and oil with cooking spray. Cover the crisping lid. Choose Air Fry, set the temperature to 375 F, and the timer to 15 minutes. Choose Start to commence frying.
5. After half the Cook Time, open the crisping lid, shake the wings. Oil the chicken again with cooking spray and return the basket to the pot. Close the lid and continue cooking until the wingettes are crispy.

Nutrition: Calories 405 Fat 30g Carbs 4g Protein 28g

852. Cheese & Bacon Filled Sweet Potatoes

⏱ Prep Time 10 m | ⏱ Cooking Time 30 m | 4 Servings

Ingredients:
- 12 ounces sweet potatoes
- 1 teaspoon melted butter
- ¼ cup shredded Monterey Jack cheese
- ¼ cup buttermilk
- 2 slices bacon, cooked and crumbled
- 1 tablespoon chopped scallions
- Salt to taste

Directions:
1. Close crisping lid. Preheat your cooker by choosing Air Fry at 390 F for 5 minutes.
2. Toss the sweet potatoes with the melted butter until evenly coated.
3. Add to the Cook & Crisp basket. Close the lid, choose Air Fry, set the temperature to 345 F, and set the time to 30 minutes. Press Start.
4. After 15 minutes, open the lid, pull out the basket and shake the potatoes.
5. At the 15-minute mark, check the potatoes to see if they're crisped to your liking. In a bowl, mix cheese, buttermilk, and bacon, and scallions, season with salt and set aside.
6. Take out the potatoes from the basket and halve the potatoes lengthways. Top with the bacon-cheese filling and serve.

Nutrition: Calories 154 Fat 8g Carbs 16g Protein 5g

853. Cheesy Bombs in Bacon

⏱ Prep Time 10 m | ⏱ Cooking Time 10 m | 8 Servings

Ingredients:
- 8 Bacon Slices, cut in half
- 16 ounces Mozzarella Cheese, cut into 8 pieces
- 3 tablespoons Butter, melted

Directions:
1. Wrap each cheese string with a slice of bacon and secure the ends with toothpicks. Set aside.
2. Grease the crisp basket with the melted butter and add in the bombs. Close the crisping lid, select Air Fry mode, and set the temperature to 370 F and set the time to 10 minutes.
3. At the 5-minute mark, turn the bombs. When ready, remove to a paper-lined plate to drain the excess oil. Serve on a platter with toothpicks.

Nutrition: Calories 230 Fat 13.5g Carbs 2g Protein 24g

854. Goddess Tomato-Basil Dip

⏱ Prep Time 5 m | ⏱ Cooking Time 13 m | 6 Servings

Ingredients:
- 1 cup chopped Tomatoes
- ¼ cup chopped Basil
- 10 ounces shredded Parmesan Cheese
- 10 ounces Cream Cheese
- ½ cup Heavy Cream
- 1 cup Water

Directions:
1. Open the cooker and pour in the tomatoes, basil, heavy cream, cream cheese, and water. Close the lid, secure the pressure valve, and select Pressure for 3 minutes at High. Press Start.
2. Once the timer has ended, do a natural pressure release for 10 minutes. Stir the mixture with a spoon while mashing the tomatoes with the back of the spoon.
3. Add the Parmesan cheese and Close the crisping lid. Select Bake mode, set the temperature to 370 F and the time to 3 minutes. Serve with chips.

Nutrition: Calories 350 Fat 28g Carbs 10g Protein 13g

855. Nutty Asparagus

⏱ Prep Time 2 m | ⏱ Cooking Time 11 m | 4 Servings

Ingredients
- 1 ½ pound Asparagus, ends trimmed
- Salt and Pepper, to taste
- 1 cup Water
- 1 tablespoon butter
- ½ cup chopped Pine Nuts
- 1 tablespoon Olive Oil to garnish

Directions:
1. Open the cooker, pour the water in, and fit the reversible rack at the bottom.
2. Place the asparagus on the rack, close the crisping lid, select Air Fry mode, and set the time to 8 minutes on 380 F. Press Start.
3. At the 4-minute mark, carefully turn the asparagus over.
4. When ready, remove to a plate, sprinkle with salt and pepper, and set aside.
5. Select Sear/Sauté on your cooker, set to Medium and melt the butter.
6. Add the pine nuts and cook for 2-3 minutes until golden. Scatter over the asparagus the pine nuts, and drizzle olive oil.

Nutrition: Calories 182 Fat 15g Carbs 13g Protein 7g

856. Cheesy Spinach Dip with Pita Chips

⏰ Prep Time 15 m | ⏱ Cooking Time 40 m | 6-8 Servings

Ingredients:

- Pita Chips:
- 4 pita breads
- 1 tablespoon olive oil
- ½ teaspoon paprika
- Salt and freshly ground black pepper to taste
- Cooking spray
- Spinach Dip:
- 8 ounces cream cheese, softened at room temperature
- 1 cup ricotta cheese
- 1 cup grated Fontina cheese
- ½ teaspoon Italian seasoning
- ½ teaspoon garlic powder
- ¾ teaspoon salt
- Freshly ground black pepper to taste
- 16 ounces frozen chopped spinach, thawed and squeezed dry
- ¼ cup grated Parmesan cheese
- ½ tomato, finely diced
- ¼ teaspoon dried oregano

Directions:

1. On a clean work surface, cut each pita bread into 8 wedges and place them in a large bowl. Add the olive oil and toss until the bread is coated evenly. Sprinkle the paprika, salt, and pepper to season.
2. Spray the air fryer basket with cooking spray. Arrange the oiled pita wedges in the air fryer basket.
3. Put the air fryer lid on and cook in batches in the preheated instant pot at 400°F for 5 minutes. Shake the basket once when the lid screen indicates 'TURN FOOD' during cooking time.
4. Meanwhile, to make the spinach dip, combine the ricotta cheese, cream cheese, Fontina cheese, Italian seasoning, garlic powder, salt and pepper in a separate bowl. Add the spinach and toss well.
5. Remove the pita chips from the basket and keep warm.
6. Pour the spinach-cheese mixture into a 7-inch cake pan and spread it evenly. Scatter the Parmesan cheese on top. Cover the pan with aluminum foil, then transfer the pan to the air fryer basket.
7. Put the air fryer lid on and cook in the preheated instant pot at 400°F for 20 minutes. Remove the aluminum foil and allow the cheese on top to brown for 4 minutes.
8. Remove the pan from the basket. Top with the diced tomato and oregano. Serve the spinach dip alongside the pita chips.

Nutrition:
Calories: 302 Fat: 21.24g Carbs: 13.51g Protein: 15.4g

857. Crunchy Spiced Nuts

⏰ Prep Time 10 m | ⏱ Cooking Time 25 m | 3 Servings

Ingredients:

- 1 egg white, lightly beaten
- ¼ cup sugar
- 1 teaspoon salt
- ½ teaspoon ground cinnamon
- ¼ teaspoon ground cloves
- ¼ teaspoon ground allspice
- Pinch ground cayenne pepper
- 1 cup pecan halves
- 1 cup cashews
- 1 cup almonds
- Cooking spray

Directions:

1. In a large bowl, mix together the egg white, sugar, salt, cinnamon, cloves, allspice, and cayenne pepper. Add the nuts and toss until well coated.
2. Spray the air fryer basket with cooking spray, then transfer the nuts to the basket.
3. Put the air fryer lid on and cook in the preheated instant pot at 300 degree for 25 minutes. Stir the nuts constantly during cooking time. To test doneness, the nuts should be nicely browned, inside and out (you can cut one open to see if it's browned inside).
4. Remove from the basket to a serving bowl. Serve warm or at room temperature.

Nutrition:
Calories: 482 Fat: 27.83g Carbs: 42.88g Protein: 28.35g

858. Panko and Cheese Arancini

⏰ Prep Time 10 m | ⏱ Cooking Time 25 m | 10 Servings

Ingredients:

- 1½ cups panko bread crumbs
- ½ cup Parmesan cheese, grated
- 16 cubes (¾-inch) Mozzarella cheese
- 2 cups cooked and cooled rice or leftover risotto
- 2 eggs, beaten
- 2 tablespoons olive oil
- 2 tablespoons minced fresh basil

Directions:

1. In a medium bowl, mix together the egg, rice, Parmesan, basil and ½ cup bread crumbs, and stir well.
2. To make the arancini, scoop out the mixture and shape into 16 bite-sized meatballs on a clean work surface. Using your thumb to make a well in the center of each meatball and fill in a Mozzarella cube.
3. In a separate bowl, mix the remaining bread crumbs and oil. Dip each arancini in the bread crumbs, shaking off any excess. Arrange each arancini in the air fryer basket.
4. Put the air fryer lid on and cook in batches in the preheated instant pot at 400°F for 8 to 10 minutes, or until cooked through.
5. Remove from the basket and serve on a plate.

Nutrition:
Calories: 177 Fat: 11.78g Carbs: 18.5g Protein: 5.91g

859. Crispy Fries

⏱ Prep Time 5 m | ⏱ Cooking Time 30 m | 2 Servings

Ingredients:

- 2 to 3 russet potatoes, peeled and cut into ¼-inch sticks
- 2 to 3 teaspoons olive oil

Directions:

1. On your cutting board, slice the potatoes into ¼-inch sticks or by using a mandolin with a julienne blade. Soak the potato sticks in cold water for at least 10 minutes or rinse them under cold water to remove the excess starch. Drain and thoroughly dry the potato sticks with paper towels.
2. In a bowl, mix the potato sticks with the olive oil. Toss well.
3. Transfer them to the air fryer basket. You may need to work in batches to avoid overcrowding.

Nutrition:

Calories: 425 Fat: 9.74g Carbs: 71.12g Protein: 15.65g

- Salt to taste
- Ketchup, for dipping (optional)

4. Put the air fryer lid on and cook in the preheated instant pot at 375°F for 15 minutes. Shake the basket twice halfway through the cooking time.
5. When ready to serve, season the fries as needed with salt.
6. Remove from the basket to a plate and repeat with remaining sticks.
7. Serve warm with the ketchup on the side, if desired.

860. Steamed Chinese Pot Stickers

⏱ Prep Time 10 m | ⏱ Cooking Time 30 m | 10 Servings

Ingredients:

- 30 wonton wrappers
- 3 tablespoons water, plus more for brushing the wrappers
- Filling:
- 1 egg, beaten
- ½ cup cabbage, finely chopped

Directions:

1. To make the filling, in a large bowl, mix together the egg, cabbage, green onions, cocktail sauce, soy sauce and pepper. Stir to combine well.
2. Start the pot stickers by using a cookie scoop to measure out equal-sized portions of the filling onto the center of each wrapper. Brush the edges of wrappers with a little water and fold each wrapper diagonally, then pinch the edges together to seal.

Nutrition:

Calories: 794 Fat: 6.36g Carbs: 52.43g Protein: 28.33g

- 2 green onions, finely chopped
- 2 tablespoons cocktail sauce
- 2 teaspoons low-sodium soy sauce
- ¼ cup red bell pepper, finely chopped

3. Arrange the pot stickers in the 6×6×2-inch baking pan and place the pan into the air fryer basket. Add 3 tablespoons water into the pan.
4. Put the air fryer lid on and cook in the preheated instant pot at 350°F, until the bottoms of pot stickers are golden brown, about 9 to 10 minutes.
5. Remove from the pan and allow to cool for 5 minutes before serving.

861. Mango-Spiced Beef Skewers

⏱ Prep Time 10 m | ⏱ Cooking Time 15 m | 4 Servings

Ingredients:

- 1 mango
- ¾ pound beef sirloin tip, cut into 1-inch cubes
- 1 tablespoon honey
- ½ teaspoon dried marjoram

Directions:

1. In a bowl, mix together the olive oil, balsamic vinegar, marjoram, honey, salt, and pepper. Rub the marinade all over the beef cubes. Set aside.
2. On your cutting board, peel the mango and cut the flesh into 1-inch cubes.
3. Alternately thread beef and mango cubes onto bamboo skewers.

Nutrition:

Calories: 972 Fat: 53g Carbs: 5.73g Protein: 24.25g

- 2 tablespoons balsamic vinegar
- 1 tablespoon olive oil
- 4 bamboo skewers
- Freshly ground black pepper and salt to taste

4. Arrange the skewers in the air fryer basket. Put the air fryer lid on and cook in the preheated instant pot at 400°F for 4 to 7 minutes. Flip the skewers when it shows 'TURN FOOD' on the lid screen halfway through cooking time, or until the beef reaches at least 145°F on a meat thermometer.
5. Transfer to a plate and allow to cool for 5 minutes before serving.

862. Delicious Shrimp Toast

⏱ Prep Time 10 m | ⏱ Cooking Time 20 m | 12 Servings

Ingredients:

- 2/3 Cup raw shrimp, peeled and deveined; finely chopped
- 2 tablespoons cornstarch
- 1 egg white
- 3 slices firm white bread

Directions:

1. On a clean work surface, cut the crusts off the bread with a sharp knife. Make bread crumbs by crumbling the crust and set aside.
2. In a large bowl, mix together the shrimp, cornstarch, egg white, garlic, ginger, salt and pepper.
3. To make the shrimp toasts, spoon the shrimp mixture onto the slices of bread and spread evenly, then cut each slice into four strips.
4. In a small bowl, combine the bread crumbs with the olive oil. Evenly spread the bread crumbs on top of the shrimp mixture.

Nutrition:

Calories: 57 Fat: 3.49g Carbs: 3.71g Protein: 3.15g

- 2 tablespoons olive oil
- ¼ teaspoon ground ginger
- 2 cloves garlic, minced
- Freshly ground black pepper and salt to taste

5. Arrange the shrimp toasts in the air fryer basket. You may need to work in batches to avoid overcrowding.
6. Put the air fryer lid on and air fry in the preheated instant pot at 350°F for 3 to 6 minutes, or until golden brown and crisp.
7. Transfer to a serving dish and repeat with remaining shrimp toasts.
8. Allow to cool for 3 minutes before serving.

863. Poutine

Prep Time 15 m | Cooking Time 25 m | 2 Servings

Ingredients:

- 2 russet potatoes, peeled and cut into ½-inch sticks
- 6 cups water

Gravy:

- 2 tablespoons butter
- 1 clove garlic, smashed
- ¼ onion, minced (about ¼ cup)
- ¼ teaspoon dried thyme
- 3 tablespoons flour

- 2 teaspoons vegetable oil
- 2/3 cup chopped cheese curds
- 1 teaspoon tomato paste
- 1½ cups strong beef stock
- Salt and freshly ground black pepper to taste
- A few dashes of Worcestershire sauce

Directions:

1. Put the potato sticks in a large saucepan of salted water and bring them to a boil. Blanch the potato sticks in the boiling, salted water for 4 minutes or until they start to soften.
2. Rinse the potato sticks under cold water in a colander for 2 minutes, then dry them with paper towels.
3. Toss the dried potato sticks with the oil in a bowl, then transfer to the air fryer basket.
4. Put the air fryer lid on and air fry in the preheated instant pot at 375ºF for 20 minutes. Shake the basket a few times during the cooking time for more even browning.
5. Meanwhile, to make the gravy, put the butter in the saucepan over medium heat. When the butter melts, tilt the pan so the butter covers the bottom evenly. Add the garlic, onion, and thyme to cook for 5 minutes until the garlic is fragrant. Mix in the flour and cook for 2 minutes more, stirring occasionally. Add the tomato paste and cook for an additional 2 minutes. Pour in the beef stock and simmer until the mixture is thickened. Season as desired with the salt, pepper, and a few dashes of Worcestershire sauce. Remove from the heat and keep warm.
6. When the fries are ready to serve, season with salt to taste.
7. Remove from the basket to a plate. Generously sprinkle the cheese curds on top, then pour the warm gravy over the fries. Serve immediately.

Nutrition:
Calories: 862 Fat: 22.75g Carbs: 136.66g Protein: 31.74g

864. Hash Brown Cheese Bruschetta

Prep Time 10 m | Cooking Time 15 m | 4 Servings

Ingredients:

- 4 frozen hash brown patties
- 2 tablespoons grated Parmesan cheese
- 1/3 Cup chopped cherry tomatoes

- 1 tablespoon balsamic vinegar
- 1 tablespoon olive oil
- 1 tablespoon minced fresh basil

Directions:

1. Arrange the hash brown patties in a single layer in the air fryer basket.
2. Put the air fryer lid on and air fry in the preheated instant pot at 400ºF until the patties are lightly browned, about 6 to 8 minutes.
3. In a medium bowl, mix the tomatoes, olive oil, Parmesan, mozzarella, basil and vinegar, and toss well.
4. Remove from the basket to a serving plate. Pour the tomato mixture over the cooked hash brown patties and serve.

Nutrition:
Calories: 247 Fat: 15.43g Carbs: 21.12g Protein: 7.18g

865. Cheesy Waffle Fries

Prep Time 10 m | Cooking Time 20 m | 4 Servings

Ingredients:

- 1 cup Swiss cheese, shredded
- 2 cups frozen waffle fries
- 2 green onions, sliced

- 2 teaspoons olive oil
- 1 red bell pepper, chopped
- ½ cup bottled chicken gravy

Directions:

1. In a bowl, combine the waffle fries with olive oil. Toss well.
2. Arrange the waffle fries in the air fryer basket. Put the air fryer lid on and air fry in the preheated instant pot at 375ºF for 10 to 12 minutes. Shake the basket once when it shows 'TURN FOOD' on the air fryer lid screen during cooking time.
3. Transfer the fries into a 6×6×2-inch baking pan and sprinkle the pepper, green onions and cheese on top. Put the pan into the air fryer basket and put the air fryer lid on. Air fry for 3 minutes until the vegetables are tender.
4. Remove the pan from the basket and pour the gravy over the fries. Return the pan to the basket and air fry for 2 minutes more or until the gravy is hot.
5. Allow to cool for 5 minutes before serving.

Nutrition:
Calories: 283 Fat: 18.36g Carbs: 5.46g Protein: 22.76g

866. Beef Cubes with Pasta Sauce

Prep Time 7 m | Cooking Time 25 m | 4 Servings

Ingredients:

- 1 pound sirloin tip, cut into 1-inch cubes
- 1 cup cheese pasta sauce (from a 16-ounce jar)
- 1½ cups soft bread crumbs

- ½ teaspoon dried marjoram
- 2 tablespoons olive oil

Directions:

1. In a medium bowl, combine the beef and pasta sauce. Toss to coat well.
2. In a shallow bowl, mix together the bread crumbs, oil, and marjoram. Dunk beef cubes into the bread crumb mixture to coat, shaking off excess.
3. Place the breaded beef cubes into the air fryer basket. Put the air fryer lid on and cook in batches in the preheated instant pot at 350ºF for 6 to 8 minutes. Shake the basket when it shows 'TURN FOOD' on the air fryer lid screen halfway through cooking time, or until the beef registers at least 145ºF.
4. Transfer to a serving dish and serve warm.

Nutrition:
Calories: 255 Fat: 10.45g Carbs: 11.51g Protein: 26.65g

867. Crunchy Zucchini Fries
⏱ Prep Time 15 m | ⏱ Cooking Time 30 m | 6 Servings

Ingredients:
- 2 medium zucchinis
- 2 eggs
- 1/3 Cup bread crumbs

Aioli:
- ½ tablespoon olive oil
- ½ cup mayonnaise
- 1 teaspoon minced garlic
- 1/3 Cup grated Parmesan cheese
- Salt and pepper to taste
- Cooking spray
- Juice of ½ lemon
- Salt and pepper to taste

Directions:
1. On your cutting board, cut the zucchini lengthwise in half and slice into strips with a mandolin.
2. In a small bowl, whisk the eggs until frothy. In a separate bowl, add the Parmesan cheese, bread crumbs, salt and pepper. Stir well.
3. Dredge the zucchini strips in the eggs one at a time, and then in the bread crumb mixture.
4. Lightly spray the air fryer basket with cooking spray. Arrange the breaded zucchini strips in the air fryer basket, making sure they are not stacked. Spritz them with cooking spray.
5. Put the air fryer lid on and cook in batches in the preheated instant pot at 350ºF for 10 minutes.
6. To make the lemon aioli, add the olive oil, mayonnaise, garlic and lemon juice to a bowl, then season with salt and pepper to taste. Stir well until completely combined.
7. Transfer the zucchini fries to a plate lined with paper towels. Dip into the aioli and serve.

Nutrition:
Calories: 208 Fat: 20g Carbohydrates: 2g Protein: 8g

868. Fried Dill Pickles
⏱ Prep Time 5 m | ⏱ Cooking Time 15 m | 4 Servings

Ingredients:
- 1 pound whole dill pickles
- 1/3 Cup bread crumbs
- 2 eggs
- 1/3 Cup all-purpose flour
- Cooking spray

Directions:
1. On a flat work surface, cut the pickles into ½-inch slices. Dry them thoroughly with paper towels.
2. In a small bowl, whisk the eggs until frothy. In another bowl, pour the flour. Place the bread crumbs onto a platter.
3. Dredge the pickle slices in the flour, then in the whisked egg, and finally in the bread crumbs to coat.
4. Spritz the air fryer basket with cooking spray. Arrange the breaded pickle slices in the basket and spritz with cooking spray.
5. Put the air fryer lid on and cook in the preheated instant pot at 375ºF for 8 minutes. Shake the basket when the lid screen indicates 'TURN FOOD' during cooking time.
6. Transfer to a plate and let cool for 5 minutes before serving.

Nutrition:
Calories: 168 Fat: 13g Carbohydrates: 10g Protein: 7g

869. Baked Candied Nuts
⏱ Prep Time 10 m | ⏱ Cooking Time 20 m | 4 Servings

Ingredients:
- 1 cup nuts (walnuts, pecans, and almonds work well)
- ½ teaspoon cinnamon
- ½ tablespoon stevia
- 1 egg white
- Pepper to taste
- Cooking spray

Directions:
1. In a bowl, mix the stevia, cinnamon and pepper together.
2. In another bowl, combine the nuts with the egg white, then add into the stevia mixture. Stir well.
3. Spritz the air fryer basket with cooking spray. Transfer the nuts into the air fryer basket and spray with cooking spray.
4. Put the air fryer lid on and cook in the preheated instant pot at 300ºF for 13 minutes, shaking the air fryer basket when it shows 'TURN FOOD' on the air fryer lid screen during cooking time.
5. Transfer to a serving dish and cool for 5 minutes before serving.

Nutrition:
Calories: 140 Fat: 21g Carbohydrates: 4g Protein: 5g

870. Crips Artichoke Bites
⏱ Prep Time 10 m | ⏱ Cooking Time 20 m | 6 Servings

Ingredients:
- 14 whole artichoke hearts packed in water
- 1 egg
- 1/3 Cup panko bread crumbs
- ½ cup all-purpose flour
- 1 teaspoon Italian seasoning
- Cooking spray

Directions:
1. Drain and dry the artichoke hearts thoroughly with paper towels.
2. In a small bowl, whisk the egg until foamy. In another bowl, pour the flour. Combine the bread crumbs with Italian seasoning in a third bowl. Stir well.
3. Dredge the artichoke hearts in the flour, then in the whisked egg, and finally in the bread crumbs mixture to coat.
4. Arrange the breaded artichoke hearts in the air fryer basket and spritz with cooking spray.
5. Put the air fryer lid on and cook in the preheated instant pot at 375ºF for 8 minutes, flipping the artichoke hearts when it shows 'TURN FOOD' on the air fryer lid screen during cooking time, or until nicely browned.
6. Transfer to a serving dish lined with paper towels. Allow to cool for 5 minutes before serving.

Nutrition:
Calories: 67 Fat: 4g Carbohydrates: 7g Protein: 2g

871. Salmon Crisps

Prep Time 5-12 m | Cooking Time 10 m | 2-4 Servings

Ingredients:

- 2 tablespoons dill, chopped
- ½ cup panko breadcrumbs
- ¼ teaspoon ground black pepper
- 2 teaspoons mustard, Dijon
- 2 tablespoons of canola mayonnaise
- 2 cans (5 ounces) salmon, unsalted, with bones and skin
- 2 lemon wedges
- 1 egg, large

Directions:

1. In a mixing bowl, add the salmon, dill, panko, mayonnaise, pepper, and mustard. Combine the ingredients to mix well with each other. Prepare cakes from the mixture.
2. Grease Air Fryer Basket with some cooking spray.
3. Place Instant Pot Air Fryer Crisp over kitchen platform. Press Air Fry, set the temperature to 400°F and set the timer to 5 minutes to preheat. Press "Start" and allow it to preheat for 5 minutes.
4. In the inner pot, place the Air Fryer basket. In the basket, add the salmon cakes.
5. Close the Crisp Lid and press the "Bake" setting. Set temperature to 400°F and set the timer to 12 minutes. Press "Start." Flip the cakes halfway down.
6. Open the Crisp Lid after cooking time is over. Serve with your choice of dip or tomato ketchup.

Nutrition:
Calories: 287 Fat: 15g Carbohydrates: 16g Protein: 26g

872. Wholesome Asparagus

Prep Time 5-10 m | Cooking Time 10 m | 4 Servings

Ingredients:

- Pound (½ bunch) asparagus, washed and trimmed
- ½ teaspoon Himalayan salt
- 1 olive oil spray
- 1/4 teaspoon garlic powder
- 1 tablespoons sherry vinegar or red-wine vinegar
- 1 teaspoon chili powder or 1/2 teaspoon smoked paprika

Directions:

1. Add the asparagus in the frying basket, coat with the oil spray, add the chili powder/paprika, garlic powder and salt on top. Stir well to coat evenly.
2. Place Instant Pot Air Fryer Crisp over kitchen platform. Press Air Fry, set temperature to 400°F and set timer to 5 minutes to preheat. Press "Start" and allow it to preheat for 5 minute.
3. In the inner pot, place the Air Fryer basket. In the basket, add the asparagus mixture.
4. Close the Crisp Lid and press "Air Fry" setting. Set temperature to 400°F and set timer to 10 minutes. Press "Start".
5. Half way down, open the Crisp Lid, shake the basket and close the lid to continue cooking for remaining time.
6. Open the Crisp Lid after cooking time is over. Drizzle with the vinegar on top and serve with your choice of dip or ketchup.

Nutrition:
Calories: 62 Fat: 4g Carbohydrates: 6g Protein: 3g

873. Apple Sweet Chips

Prep Time 5-10 m | Cooking Time 12 m | 2-3 Servings

Ingredients:

- 2 teaspoons sugar
- ½ teaspoon ground cinnamon
- 2 large apples, cored and sliced

Directions:

1. In a bowl, mix the apple pieces with sugar and cinnamon. Place Instant Pot Air Fryer Crisp over kitchen platform. Press Air Fry, set the temperature to 400°F and set the timer to 5 minutes to preheat. Press "Start" and allow it to preheat for 5 minutes. In the inner pot, place the Air Fryer basket. In the basket, add the coated apples. Do not overlap. Close the Crisp Lid and press the "Roast" setting. Set temperature to 350°F and set the timer to 12 minutes. Press "Start." Halfway down, open the Crisp Lid, shake the basket and close the lid to continue cooking for the remaining time. Open the Crisp Lid after cooking time is over. Serve warm.

Nutrition:
Calories: 132 Fat: 5g Carbohydrates: 35g Protein: 1g

874. Classic French Fries

Prep Time 5-10 m | Cooking Time 24 m | 4 Servings

Ingredients:

- 1 pound sweet potatoes, cut into French Fries size
- ¼ teaspoon garlic powder
- Salt to taste
- Olive oil

Directions:

1. In a mixing bowl, add the olive oil, potatoes, salt, and garlic powder. Combine the ingredients to mix well with each other. Place Instant Pot Air Fryer Crisp over kitchen platform. Press Air Fry, set the temperature to 400°F and set the timer to 5 minutes to preheat. Press "Start" and allow it to preheat for 5 minutes. In the inner pot, place the Air Fryer basket. In the basket, add the potato mixture. Close the Crisp Lid and press the "Air Fry" setting. Set temperature to 380°F and set the timer to 18-20 minutes. Press "Start." Halfway down, open the Crisp Lid, shake the basket and close the lid to continue cooking for the remaining time. Open the Crisp Lid after cooking time is over. Season to taste and serve warm.

Nutrition:
Calories: 156 Fat: 5g Carbohydrates: 22g Protein: 5g

875. Crunchy Zucchini Chips
🕐 Prep Time 5 m | 🕐 Cooking Time 12 m | 4 Servings

Ingredients:
- 1 medium zucchini, thinly sliced
- 3/4 cup Parmesan cheese, grated
- 1 cup Panko breadcrumbs
- 1 large egg, beaten

Directions:
1. In a mixing bowl, add the Parmesan cheese and panko breadcrumbs. Combine the ingredients to mix well with each other.
2. In a mixing bowl, beat the eggs. Coat the zucchini slices with the eggs and then with the crumb mixture. Spray the slices with some cooking spray.
3. Place Instant Pot Air Fryer Crisp over kitchen platform. Press Air Fry, set the temperature to 400°F and set the timer to 5 minutes to preheat. Press "Start" and allow it to preheat for 5 minutes.
4. In the inner pot, place the Air Fryer basket. Line it with a parchment paper, add the zucchini slices.
5. Close the Crisp Lid and press the "Air Fry" setting. Set temperature to 350°F and set the timer to 10-12 minutes. Press "Start."
6. Halfway down, open the Crisp Lid, shake the basket and close the lid to continue cooking for the remaining time.
7. Open the Crisp Lid after cooking time is over. Serve warm.

Nutrition:
Calories: 132 Carbs: 14g Fat: 7g Protein: 6g

876. Cauliflower Fritters
🕐 Prep Time 5-10 m | 🕐 Cooking Time 8 m | 6-8 Servings

Ingredients:
- 1/3 cup shredded mozzarella cheese
- 1/3 cup shredded sharp cheddar cheese
- ½ cup chopped parsley
- 1 cup Italian breadcrumbs
- 3 chopped scallions
- 1 head of cauliflower, cut into florets
- 1 egg
- 2 minced garlic cloves

Directions:
1. Blend the florets into a blender to make the rice like structure. Add in a bowl. Mix in the pepper, salt, egg, cheeses, breadcrumbs, garlic, and scallions. Prepare 15 patties from the mixture. Coat them with some cooking spray.
2. Place Instant Pot Air Fryer Crisp over kitchen platform. Press Air Fry, set the temperature to 400°F and set the timer to 5 minutes to preheat. Press "Start" and allow it to preheat for 5 minutes.
3. In the inner pot, place the Air Fryer basket. In the basket, add the patties.
4. Close the Crisp Lid and press the "Air Fry" setting. Set temperature to 390°F and set the timer to 8 minutes. Press "Start."
5. Halfway down, open the Crisp Lid, shake the basket and close the lid to continue cooking for the remaining time.
6. Open the Crisp Lid after cooking time is over. Serve warm.

Nutrition:
Calories: 235 Fat: 19g Carbohydrates: 31g Protein: 6g

877. Paneer Cheese Balls
🕐 Prep Time 10 m | 🕐 Cooking Time 15 m | 6 Servings

Ingredients:
- 1 cup paneer, crumbled
- 1 cup cheese, grated
- 1 potato, boiled and mashed
- 1 onion, chopped finely
- 1 green chili, chopped finely
- 1 teaspoon red chili flakes
- Salt to taste
- 4 tablespoons coriander leaves, chopped finely
- ½ cup all-purpose flour
- ¾ cup of water
- Breadcrumbs as needed

Directions:
1. Mix flour with water in a bowl and spread the breadcrumbs in a tray.
2. Add the rest of the ingredients to make the paneer mixture.
3. Make golf ball-sized balls out of this mixture.
4. Dip each ball in the flour liquid then coat with the breadcrumbs.
5. Place the cheese balls in the Instant Pot Duo and spray it with cooking spray.
6. Put on the Air Fryer lid and seal it.
7. Hit the "Air fry Button" and select 15 minutes of cooking time, then press "Start."
8. Once the Instant Pot Duo beeps, remove its lid. Serve.

Nutrition:
Calories 227 Fat 16g Carbohydrate 24g Protein 9g

878. Russet Potato Hay
🕐 Prep Time 10 m | 🕐 Cooking Time 15 m | 4 Servings

Ingredients:
- 2 russet potatoes
- 1 tablespoon olive oil
- Salt and black pepper to taste

Directions:
1. Pass the potatoes through a spiralizer to get potato spirals.
2. Soak these potato spirals in a bowl filled with water for about 20 minutes.
3. Drain and rinse the soaked potatoes then pat them dry.
4. Toss the potato spirals with salt, black pepper, and oil in a bowl.
5. Spread the seasoned potato spirals in the Air Fryer Basket.
6. Set this Air Fryer Basket in the Instant Pot duo.
7. Put on the Air Fryer lid and seal it.
8. Hit the "Air fry Button" and select 15 minutes of cooking time, then press "Start."
9. Toss the potato spiral when halfway cooked then resume cooking.
10. Once the Instant Pot Duo beeps, remove its lid. Serve.

Nutrition:
Calories 104 Fat 6g Carbohydrate 17g Protein 8g

879. Onion Rings
⏱ Prep Time 10 m | ⏱ Cooking Time 10 m | 4 Servings

Ingredients:

- 3/4 cup flour
- 1 large yellow onion, sliced and rings separated
- ¼ teaspoon garlic powder
- ¼ teaspoon paprika
- 1 cup almond milk
- 1 large egg

- 1/2 cup cornstarch
- 1 ½ teaspoons of baking powder
- 1 teaspoon salt
- 1 cup bread crumbs
- Cooking spray

Directions:

1. Whisk flour with baking powder, salt, and cornstarch in a bowl.
2. Coat the onion rings with this dry flour mixture and keep them aside.
3. Beat egg with milk in a bowl and dip the rings in this mixture.
4. Place the coated rings in the Air Fryer Basket and set it inside the Instant Pot Duo.
5. Spray the onion rings with cooking oil. Put on the Air Fryer lid and seal it.
6. Hit the "Air fry Button" and select 10 minutes of cooking time, then press "Start."
7. Flip the rings when cooked halfway through.
8. Once the Instant Pot Duo beeps, remove its lid. Serve.

Nutrition:
Calories 319 Fat 2g Carbohydrate 59g Protein 9g

880. Breaded Avocado Fries
⏱ Prep Time 10 m | ⏱ Cooking Time 7 m | 4 Servings

Ingredients:

- 1/4 cup all-purpose flour
- 1/2 teaspoon ground black pepper
- 1/4 teaspoon salt
- 1 egg

- 1 teaspoon water
- 1 ripe avocado, peeled, pitted and sliced
- 1/2 cup panko bread crumbs
- Cooking spray

Directions:

1. Whisk flour with salt and black pepper in one bowl.
2. Beat egg with water in another and spread the crumbs in a shallow tray.
3. First coat the avocado slices with the flour mixture then dip them into the egg.
4. Drop off the excess and coat the avocado with panko crumbs liberally.
5. Place all the coated slices in the Air Fryer Basket and spray them with cooking oil.
6. Set the Air Fryer Basket inside the Instant Pot Duo.
7. Put on the Air Fryer lid and seal it.
8. Hit the "Air fry Button" and select 7 minutes of cooking time, then press "Start."
9. Flip the fries after 4 minutes of cooking and resume cooking.
10. Once the Instant Pot Duo beeps, remove its lid. Serve fresh.

Nutrition:
Calories 201 Fat 17g Carbohydrate 23g Protein 5g

881. Buffalo Chicken Strips
⏱ Prep Time 10 m | ⏱ Cooking Time 8 m | 4 Servings

Ingredients:

- 1/2 cup Greek yogurt
- 1/4 cup egg
- 1 ½ tablespoon hot sauce
- 1 cup panko bread crumbs

- 1 tablespoon sweet paprika
- 1 tablespoon garlic pepper seasoning
- 1 tablespoon cayenne pepper
- 1-pound chicken breasts, cut into strips

Directions:

1. Mix Greek yogurt with hot sauce and egg in a bowl.
2. Whisk bread crumbs with garlic powder, cayenne pepper, and paprika in another bowl.
3. First, dip the chicken strips in the yogurt sauce then coat them with the crumb's mixture.
4. Place the coated strips in the Air Fryer Basket and spray them with cooking oil.
5. Set the Air Fryer Basket inside the Instant Pot Duo.
6. Put on the Air Fryer lid and seal it.
7. Hit the "Air fry Button" and select 16 minutes of cooking time, then press "Start."
8. Flip the chicken strips after 8 minutes of cooking then resume Air fearing.
9. Once the Instant Pot Duo beeps, remove its lid. Serve.

Nutrition:
Calories 368 Fat 18g Carbohydrate 25g Protein 44g

882. Buffalo Chicken Tenders
⏱ Prep Time 10 m | ⏱ Cooking Time 30 m | 4 Servings

Ingredients

- 1-pound chicken breasts, cut into thick strips
- Salt and pepper to taste
- 1 cup almond flour
- 1 large egg, beaten
- 3 tablespoons butter

- ¼ cup Sugar-free hot sauce
- 1 clove of garlic, minced
- ¼ teaspoon paprika
- ¼ teaspoon cayenne pepper
- 1 teaspoon stevia powder

Directions:

1. Preheat the air fryer at 3500F for 5 minutes.
2. Season the chicken breasts with salt and pepper to taste.
3. Dredge first in beaten egg then in flour mixture.
4. Arrange neatly in the air fryer basket.
5. Close and cook for 30 minutes at 3500F.
6. Halfway through the cooking time, shake the air fryer basket to cook evenly.
7. Meanwhile, prepare the sauce by combine the rest of the ingredients Season the sauce with salt and pepper to taste. Set aside.
8. Once the chicken tenders are cooked, place in a bowl with the sauce and toss to coat. Serve and enjoy!

Nutrition:
Calories 249 Fat 3g Carbs: 11g Protein 2g

883. Hassel back Zucchini
⏰ Prep Time 10 m | ⏰ Cooking Time 20 m | 3 Servings

Ingredients:
- 3 medium zucchinis
- 3 tablespoons olive oil
- 4 tablespoons coconut cream
- 1 tablespoon lemon juice
- Salt and pepper to taste
- 3 slices bacon, fried and crumbled

Directions:
1. Preheat the air fryer at 3500F for 5 minutes.
2. Line up chopsticks on both sides of the zucchini and slice thinly until you hit the stick. Brush the zucchinis with olive oil.
3. Place the zucchini in the air fryer. Bake for 20 minutes at 3500F.
4. Meanwhile, combine the coconut cream and lemon juice in a mixing bowl. Season with salt and pepper to taste.
5. Once the zucchini is cooked, scoop the coconut cream mixture and drizzle on top.
6. Sprinkle with bacon bits. Serve and enjoy!

Nutrition:
Calories 256 Fat 5g Carbs 11g Protein 2g

884. Pesto Stuffed Mushrooms
⏰ Prep Time 10 m | ⏰ Cooking Time 15 m | 5 Servings

Ingredients:
- 1 cup basil leaves
- 1 tablespoon lemon juice, freshly squeezed
- ½ cup pine nuts
- ¼ cup olive oil
- Salt to taste
- ½ cup cream cheese
- 1-pound cremini mushrooms, stalks removed

Directions:
1. Preheat the air fryer at 3500F for 5 minutes.
2. Place all ingredients except the mushrooms in a food processor.
3. Pulse until fine.
4. Scoop the mixture and place on the side where the stalks were removed.
5. Place the mushrooms in the fryer basket.
6. Close and cook for 15 minutes at 3500F. Serve and enjoy!

Nutrition:
Calories 289 Fat 3g Carbs 15g Protein 2g

885. Asparagus Fries
⏰ Prep Time 10 m | ⏰ Cooking Time 15 m | 5 Servings

Ingredients:
- 2 tablespoons parsley, chopped
- ½ teaspoon garlic powder
- ¼ cup almond flour
- ½ teaspoon smoked paprika
- Salt and pepper to taste
- 10 medium asparagus, stems trimmed
- 2 large eggs, beaten

Directions:
1. Preheat the air fryer at 3500F for 5 minutes.
2. In a mixing bowl, combine the parsley, garlic powder, almond flour, and smoked paprika. Season with salt and pepper to taste.
3. Soak the asparagus in the beaten eggs and then dredge in the almond flour mixture.
4. Place in the air fryer basket.
5. Cook for 15 minutes at 3500F. Serve and enjoy!

Nutrition:
Calories 79 Fat 8g Carbs 10g Protein 5g

886. Fat Burger Bombs
⏰ Prep Time 2 h | ⏰ Cooking Time 20 m | 6 Servings

Ingredients:
- 12 slices uncured bacon, chopped
- 1 cup almond flour
- 2 eggs, beaten
- ½ pound ground beef
- Salt and pepper to taste
- 3 tablespoons olive oil

Directions:
1. In a mixing bowl, combine all ingredients except for the olive oil.
2. Use your hands to form small balls with the mixture. Place in a baking sheet and allow it to set in the fridge for at least 2 hours.
3. Preheat the air fryer at 3500F for 5 minutes.
4. Brush the meatballs with olive oil on all sides.
5. Place in the air fryer basket.
6. Cook for 20 minutes at 3500F.
7. Halfway through the cooking time, shake the fryer basket for a more even cooking. Serve and enjoy!

Nutrition:
Calories 402 Fat 3g Carbs 15g Protein 8g

887. Crispy Keto Pork Bites
⏰ Prep Time 2 h | ⏰ Cooking Time 25 m | 3 Servings

Ingredients:
- ½-pound pork belly, sliced to thin strips
- 1 tablespoon butter
- 1 medium onion, diced
- 4 tablespoons coconut cream
- Salt and pepper to taste

Directions:
1. Place all ingredients in a mixing bowl and marinate in the fridge for 2 hours.
2. Preheat the air fryer at 3500F for 5 minutes.
3. Place the pork strips in the air fryer and bake for 25 minutes at 3500F. Serve and enjoy!

Nutrition:
Calories 307 Fat 3g Carbs 7g

888. Angel Food Cake
⏰ Prep Time 10 m | ⏱ Cooking Time 30 m | 12 Servings

Ingredients

- ¼ cup butter, melted
- 1 cup powdered erythritol
- 1 teaspoon strawberry extract
- 12 egg whites
- 2 teaspoons cream of tartar
- A pinch of salt

Directions

1. Preheat the air fryer for 5 minutes.
2. Mix the egg whites together with the cream of tartar.
3. Use a hand mixer and whisk until white and fluffy.
4. Add the rest of the ingredients except for the butter and whisk for another minute.
5. Pour into a baking dish.
6. Place in the oven basket and cook for 30 minutes at 4000F or if a toothpick inserted in the middle comes out clean.
7. Drizzle with melted butter once cooled.

Nutrition

Calories 65 | Carbohydrates 1.8g | Protein 3.1g | Fat 5g

889. Apple Pie in Air Fryer
⏰ Prep Time 15 m | ⏱ Cooking Time 35 m | 4 Servings

Ingredients

- ½ teaspoon vanilla extract
- 1 beaten egg
- 1 large apple, chopped
- 1 Pillsbury Refrigerator pie crust
- 1 tablespoon butter
- 1 tablespoon ground cinnamon
- 1 tablespoon raw sugar
- 2 tablespoon sugar
- 2 teaspoons lemon juice
- Baking spray

Directions

1. Lightly grease baking pan of the air fryer with cooking spray. Spread the pie crust on the rare part of the pan up to the sides.
2. In a bowl, make a mixture of vanilla, sugar, cinnamon, lemon juice, and apples. Pour on top of pie crust. Top apples with butter slices.
3. Cover apples with the other pie crust. Pierce with a knife the tops of the pie.
4. Spread whisked egg on top of crust and sprinkle sugar.
5. Cover with foil.
6. For 25 minutes, cook on 390oF.
7. Remove foil cook for 10 minutes at 330oF until tops are browned.
8. Serve and enjoy.

Nutrition

Calories 372 | Carbs 44.7g | Protein 4.2g | Fat 19.6g

890. Apple-Toffee Upside-Down Cake
⏰ Prep Time 10 m | ⏱ Cooking Time 30 m | 9 Servings

Ingredients

- ¼ cup almond butter
- ¼ cup sunflower oil
- ½ cup walnuts, chopped
- ¾ cup + 3 tablespoon coconut sugar
- ¾ cup water
- 1 ½ teaspoon mixed spice
- 1 cup plain flour
- 1 lemon, zest
- 1 teaspoon baking soda
- 1 teaspoon vinegar
- 3 baking apples, cored and sliced

Directions

1. Preheat the air fryer to 3900F.
2. In a skillet, melt the almond butter and 3 tablespoons sugar. Pour the mixture over a baking dish that will fit in the air fryer. Arrange the slices of apples on top. Set aside.
3. In a mixing bowl, combine flour, ¾ cup sugar, and baking soda. Add the mixed spice.
4. In a different bowl, mix the water, oil, vinegar, and lemon zest. Stir in the chopped walnuts.
5. Combine the wet ingredients to the dry ingredients until well combined.
6. Pour over the tin with apple slices.
7. Bake for 30 minutes or until a toothpick inserted comes out clean.

Nutrition

Calories 335 | Carbohydrates 39.6g | Protein 3.8g | Fat 17.9g

891. Banana-Choco Brownies
⏰ Prep Time 15 m | ⏱ Cooking Time 30 m | 12 Servings

Ingredients

- 2 cups almond flour
- 2 teaspoons baking powder
- ½ teaspoon baking powder
- ½ teaspoon baking soda
- ½ teaspoon salt
- 1 over-ripe banana
- 3 large eggs
- ½ teaspoon stevia powder
- ¼ cup coconut oil
- 1 tablespoon vinegar
- 1/3 cup almond flour
- 1/3 cup cocoa powder

Directions

1. Preheat the air fryer for 5 minutes.
2. Add together all ingredients in a food processor and pulse until well combined.
3. Pour into a skillet that will fit in the deep fryer.
4. Place in the fryer basket and cook for 30 minutes at 3500F or if a toothpick inserted in the middle comes out clean.

Nutrition

Calories 75 | Carbohydrates 2.1g | Protein 1.7g | Fat 6.6g

892. Blueberry & Lemon Cake
Prep Time 10 m | Cooking Time 17 m | 4 Servings

Ingredients
- 2 eggs
- 1 cup blueberries
- zest from 1 lemon
- juice from 1 lemon
- 1 tsp. vanilla
- brown sugar for topping (a little sprinkling on top of each muffin-less than a teaspoon)
- 2 1/2 cups self-rising flour
- 1/2 cup Monk Fruit (or use your preferred sugar)
- 1/2 cup cream
- 1/4 cup avocado oil (any light cooking oil)

Directions
1. In mixing bowl, beat well the wet ingredients. Stir in dry ingredients and mix thoroughly.
2. Lightly grease baking pan of the air fryer with cooking spray. Pour in batter.
3. For 12 minutes, cook on 330F.
4. Let it stand in the air fryer for 5 minutes.
5. Serve and enjoy.

Nutrition
Calories 589 | Carbs 76.7g | Protein 13.5g | Fat 25.3g

893. Bread Pudding with Cranberry
Prep Time 20 m | Cooking Time 45 m | 4 Servings

Ingredients
- 1-1/2 cups milk
- 2-1/2 eggs
- 1/2 cup cranberries 1 teaspoon butter
- 1/4 cup golden raisins
- 1/8 teaspoon ground cinnamon
- 3/4 cup heavy whipping cream
- 3/4 teaspoon lemon zest
- 3/4 teaspoon kosher salt
- 2 tbsp. and 1/4 cup white sugar
- 3/4 French baguettes, cut into 2-inch slices
- 3/8 vanilla bean, split and seeds scraped away

Directions
1. Lightly grease baking pan of the air fryer with cooking spray. Spread baguette slices, cranberries, and raisins.
2. In a blender, blend well vanilla bean, cinnamon, salt, lemon zest, eggs, sugar, and cream. Pour over baguette slices. Let it soak for an hour.
3. Cover pan with foil.
4. For 35 minutes, cook on 330F.
5. Let it rest for 10 minutes.
6. Serve and enjoy.

Nutrition
Calories 581 | Carbs 76.1g | Protein 15.8g | Fat 23.7g

894. Cherries 'n Almond Flour Bars
Prep Time 15 m | Cooking Time 35 m | 12 Servings

Ingredients
- ¼ cup of water
- ½ cup butter softened
- ½ teaspoon salt
- ½ teaspoon vanilla
- 1 ½ cups almond flour
- 1 cup erythritol
- 1 cup fresh cherries, pitted
- 1 tablespoon xanthan gum
- 2 eggs

Directions
1. In a medium bowl, make a mixture of the first 6 ingredients to form a dough.
2. Press the batter onto a baking sheet that will fit in the air fryer.
3. Place in the fryer and bake for 10 minutes at 375F.
4. Meanwhile, mix the cherries, water, and xanthan gum in a bowl.
5. Scoop out the dough and pour over the cherry.
6. Return to the fryer and cook for another 25 minutes at 3750F.

Nutrition
Calories 99 | Carbohydrates 2.1g | Protein 1.8g | Fat 9.3g

895. Cherry-Choco Bars
Prep Time 5 m | Cooking Time 15 m | 8 Servings

Ingredients
- ¼ teaspoon salt
- ½ cup almonds, sliced
- ½ cup chia seeds
- ½ cup dark chocolate, chopped
- ½ cup dried cherries, chopped
- ½ cup prunes, pureed
- ½ cup quinoa, cooked
- ¾ cup almond butter
- 1/3 cup honey
- 2 cups old-fashioned oats
- 2 tablespoon coconut oil

Directions
1. Preheat the air fryer to 3750F.
2. In a bowl, combine the oats, quinoa, chia seeds, almond, cherries, and chocolate.
3. In a saucepan, heat the almond butter, honey, and coconut oil.
4. Pour the butter mixture over the dry mixture. Add salt and prunes.
5. Mix until well combined.
6. Pour over a baking dish that can fit inside the air fryer.
7. Cook for 15 minutes.
8. Allow settling for an hour before slicing into bars.

Nutrition
Calories 321 | Carbohydrates 35g | Protein 7g | Fat 17g

896. Chocolate Chip in a Mug
⏰ Prep Time 10 m | ⏰ Cooking Time 20 m | 6 Servings

Ingredients
- ¼ cup walnuts, shelled and chopped
- ½ cup butter, unsalted
- ½ cup dark chocolate chips
- ½ cup erythritol
- ½ teaspoon baking soda
- ½ teaspoon salt
- 1 tablespoon vanilla extract
- 2 ½ cups almond flour
- 2 large eggs, beaten

Directions
1. Preheat the air fryer for 5 minutes.
2. Combine all ingredients in a mixing bowl.
3. Place in greased mugs.
4. Bake in the air fryer oven for 20 minutes at 3750F.

Nutrition
Calories 234 | Carbohydrates 4.9g | Protein 2.3g | Fat 22.8g

897. Choco-Peanut Mug Cake
⏰ Prep Time 10 m | ⏰ Cooking Time 20 m | 6 Servings

Ingredients
- ¼ teaspoon baking powder
- ½ teaspoon vanilla extract
- 1 egg
- 1 tablespoon heavy cream
- 1 tablespoon peanut butter
- 1 teaspoon butter, softened
- 2 tablespoon erythritol
- 2 tablespoons cocoa powder, unsweetened

Directions
1. Preheat the air fryer for 5 minutes.
2. Combine all ingredients in a mixing bowl.
3. Pour into a greased mug.
4. Place in the air fryer oven basket and cook for 20 minutes at 4000F or if a toothpick inserted in the middle comes out clean.

Nutrition
Calories 293 | Carbohydrates 8.5g | Protein 12.4g | Fat 23.3g

898. Coco-Lime Bars
⏰ Prep Time 10 m | ⏰ Cooking Time 20 m | 3 Servings

Ingredients
- ¼ cup almond flour
- ¼ cup coconut oil
- ¼ cup dried coconut flakes
- ¼ teaspoon salt
- ½ cup lime juice
- ¾ cup coconut flour
- 1 ¼ cup erythritol powder
- 1 tablespoon lime zest
- 4 eggs

Directions
1. Preheat the air fryer for 5 minutes.
2. Combine all ingredients in a mixing bowl.
3. Place in the greased mug.
4. Bake in the air fryer oven for 20 minutes at 375F.

Nutrition
Calories 506 | Carbohydrates 21.9g | Protein 19.3g | Fat 37.9g

899. Coconut 'n Almond Fat Bombs
⏰ Prep Time 5 m | ⏰ Cooking Time 15 m | 12 Servings

Ingredients
- ¼ cup almond flour
- ½ cup shredded coconut
- 1 tablespoon coconut oil
- 1 tablespoon vanilla extract
- 2 tablespoons liquid stevia
- 3 egg whites

Directions
1. Preheat the air fryer for 5 minutes.
2. Combine all ingredients in a mixing bowl.
3. Form small balls using your hands.
4. Place in the air fryer oven basket and cook for 15 minutes at 4000F.

Nutrition
Calories 23 | Carbohydrates 0.7g | Protein 1.1g | Fat 1.8g

900. Coconutty Lemon Bars
⏰ Prep Time 10 m | ⏰ Cooking Time 25 m | 12 Servings

Ingredients
- ¼ cup cashew
- ¼ cup fresh lemon juice, freshly squeezed
- ¾ cup coconut milk
- ¾ cup erythritol
- 1 cup desiccated coconut
- 1 teaspoon baking powder
- 2 eggs, beaten
- 2 tablespoons coconut oil
- A dash of salt

Directions
1. Preheat the air fryer for 5 minutes.
2. In a mixing bowl, combine all ingredients.
3. Use a hand mixer to mix everything.
4. Pour into a baking bowl that will fit in the air fryer.
5. Bake for 25 minutes at 350F or until a toothpick inserted in the middle comes out clean.

Nutrition
Calories 118 | Carbohydrates 3.9g | Protein 2.6g | Fat 10.2g

901. Coffee 'n Blueberry Cake
Prep Time 15 m | Cooking Time 35 m | 6 Servings

Ingredients
- 1 cup white sugar
- 1 egg
- 1/2 cup butter, softened
- 1/2 cup fresh or frozen blueberries
- 1/2 cup sour cream
- 1/2 teaspoon baking powder
- 1/2 teaspoon ground cinnamon
- 1/2 teaspoon vanilla extract
- 1/4 cup brown sugar
- 1/4 cup chopped pecans
- 1/8 teaspoon salt
- 1-1/2 teaspoons confectioners' sugar for dusting
- 3/4 cup and 1 tablespoon all-purpose flour

Directions
1. In a small bowl, whisk well pecans, cinnamon, and brown sugar.
2. In a blender, blend well all wet ingredients. Add dry ingredients except for confectioner's sugar and blueberries. Blend well until smooth and creamy.
3. Lightly grease baking pan of the air fryer with cooking spray.
4. Pour half of the batter in pan. Sprinkle a little of the pecan mixture on top. Pour the remaining batter and then top with the remaining pecan mixture.
5. Cover pan with foil.
6. For 35 minutes, cook on 330oF.
7. Serve and enjoy with a dusting of confectioner's sugar.

Nutrition
Calories 471 | Carbs 59.5g | Protein 4.1g | Fat 24.0g

902. Coffee Flavored Cookie Dough
Prep Time 10 m | Cooking Time 20 m | 12 Servings

Ingredients
- ¼ cup butter
- ¼ teaspoon xanthan gum
- ½ teaspoon coffee espresso powder
- ½ teaspoon stevia powder
- ¾ cup almond flour
- 1 egg
- 1 teaspoon vanilla
- 1/3 cup sesame seeds
- 2 tablespoons cocoa powder
- 2 tablespoons cream cheese, softened

Directions
1. Preheat the air fryer for 5 minutes.
2. Combine all ingredients in a mixing bowl.
3. Press into a baking dish that will fit in the air fryer.
4. Place in the air fryer oven basket and cook for 20 minutes at 4000F or if a toothpick inserted in the middle comes out clean.

Nutrition
Calories 88 | Carbohydrates 1.3g | Protein 1.9g | Fat 8.3g

903. Angel Food Cake
Prep Time 10 m | Cooking Time 30 m | 12 Servings

Ingredients:
- ¼ cup butter, melted
- 1 cup powdered erythritol
- 1 teaspoon strawberry extract
- egg whites
- teaspoons cream of tartar
- A pinch of salt

Directions:
1. Preheat the air fryer for 5 minutes.
2. Mix the egg whites together with the cream of tartar.
3. Use a hand mixer and whisk until white and fluffy.
4. Add the rest of the ingredients except for the butter and whisk for another minute.
5. Pour into a baking dish.
6. Place in the oven basket and cook for 30 minutes at 4000F or if a toothpick inserted in the middle comes out clean.
7. Drizzle with melted butter once cooled.

Nutrition:
Calories: 65 | Carbohydrates: 1.8g | Protein: 3.1g | Fat: 5g

904. Apple Pie in Air Fryer
Prep Time 15 m | Cooking Time 35 m | 4 Servings

Ingredients:
- ½ teaspoon vanilla extract
- 1 beaten egg
- 1 large apple, chopped
- 1 Pillsbury Refrigerator pie crust
- 1 tablespoon butter
- 1 tablespoon ground cinnamon
- 1 tablespoon raw sugar
- tablespoon sugar
- teaspoons lemon juice
- Baking spray

Directions:
1. Lightly grease baking pan of air fryer with cooking spray. Spread pie crust on rare part of the pan up to the sides.
2. In a bowl, make a mixture of vanilla, sugar, cinnamon, lemon juice, and apples. Pour on top of pie crust. Top apples with butter slices.
3. Cover apples with the other pie crust. Pierce with a knife the tops of the pie.
4. Spread whisked egg on top of crust and sprinkle sugar.
5. Cover with foil.
6. For 25 minutes, cook on 390oF.
7. Remove foil cook for 10 minutes at 330oF until tops are browned.
8. Serve and enjoy.

Nutrition: Calories 372 | Carbs: 44.7g | Protein: 4.2g | Fat: 19.6g

905. Apple-Toffee Upside-Down Cake

⏱ Prep Time 10 m | ⏱ Cooking Time 30 m | 9 Servings

Ingredients:

- ¼ cup almond butter
- ¼ cup sunflower oil
- ½ cup walnuts, chopped
- ¾ cup + 3 tablespoon coconut sugar
- ¾ cup water
- 1 ½ teaspoon mixed spice

- 1 cup plain flour
- 1 lemon, zest
- 1 teaspoon baking soda
- 1 teaspoon vinegar
- baking apples, cored and sliced

Directions:

1. Preheat the air fryer to 3900F.
2. In a skillet, melt the almond butter and 3 tablespoons sugar. Pour the mixture over a baking dish that will fit in the air fryer. Arrange the slices of apples on top. Set aside.
3. In a mixing bowl, combine flour, ¾ cup sugar, and baking soda. Add the mixed spice.
4. In a different bowl, mix the water, oil, vinegar, and lemon zest. Stir in the chopped walnuts.
5. Combine the wet ingredients to the dry ingredients until well combined.
6. Pour over the tin with apple slices.
7. Bake for 30 minutes or until a toothpick inserted comes out clean.

Nutrition:

Calories: 335| Carbohydrates: 39.6g | Protein: 3.8g| Fat: 17.9g

906. Banana-Choco Brownies

⏱ Prep Time 15 m | ⏱ Cooking Time 30 m | 12 Servings

Ingredients:

- cups almond flour
- teaspoons baking powder
- ½ teaspoon baking powder
- ½ teaspoon baking soda
- ½ teaspoon salt
- 1 over-ripe banana

- large eggs
- ½ teaspoon stevia powder
- ¼ cup coconut oil
- 1 tablespoon vinegar
- 1/3 cup almond flour
- 1/3 cup cocoa powder

Directions:

1. Preheat the air fryer for 5 minutes.
2. Add together all ingredients in a food processor and pulse until well combined.
3. Pour into a skillet that will fit in the deep fryer.
4. Place in the fryer basket and cook for 30 minutes at 3500F or if a toothpick inserted in the middle comes out clean.

Nutrition:

Calories: 75 |Carbohydrates: 2.1g| Protein: 1.7g |Fat: 6.6g

907. Blueberry & Lemon Cake

⏱ Prep Time 10 m | ⏱ Cooking Time 17 m | 4 Servings

Ingredients:

- eggs
- 1 cup blueberries
- Zest from 1 lemon
- Juice from 1 lemon
- 1 tsp. vanilla

- Brown sugar for topping (a little sprinkling on top of each muffin-less than a teaspoon)
- 1/2 cups self-rising flour
- 1/2 cup Monk Fruit (or use your preferred sugar)
- 1/2 cup cream
- 1/4 cup avocado oil (any light cooking oil)

Directions:

1. In mixing bowl, beat well-wet Ingredients. Stir in dry ingredients and mix thoroughly.
2. Lightly grease baking pan of the air fryer with cooking spray. Pour in batter.
3. For 12 minutes, cook on 330oF.
4. Let it stand in the air fryer for 5 minutes.
5. Serve and enjoy.

Nutrition:

Calories: 589| Carbs: 76.7g |Protein: 13.5g |Fat: 25.3g

908. Chocolate Chip in a Mug

⏱ Prep Time 10 m | ⏱ Cooking Time 20 m | 6 Servings

Ingredients:

- ¼ cup walnuts, shelled and chopped
- ½ cup butter, unsalted
- ½ cup dark chocolate chips
- ½ cup erythritol
- ½ teaspoon baking soda

- ½ teaspoon salt
- 1 tablespoon vanilla extract
- ½ cups almond flour
- large eggs, beaten

Directions:

1. Preheat the air fryer for 5 minutes.
2. Combine all ingredients in a mixing bowl.
3. Place in greased mugs.
4. Bake in the air fryer oven for 20 minutes at 3750F.

Nutrition: Calories: 234| Carbohydrates: 4.9g |Fat: 22.8g

909. Bread Pudding with Cranberry
⏱ Prep Time 20 m | ⏱ Cooking Time 45 m | 4 Servings

Ingredients:
- 1-1/2 cups milk
- 2-1/2 eggs
- 1/2 cup cranberries 1 teaspoon butter
- 1/4 cup golden raisins
- 1/8 teaspoon ground cinnamon
- 3/4 cup heavy whipping cream

- 3/4 teaspoon lemon zest
- 3/4 teaspoon kosher salt
- tbsp. and 1/4 cup white sugar
- 3/4 French baguettes, cut into 2-inch slices
- 3/8 vanilla bean, split and seeds scraped away

Directions:
1. Lightly grease baking pan of the air fryer with cooking spray. Spread baguette slices, cranberries, and raisins.
2. In a blender, blend well vanilla bean, cinnamon, salt, lemon zest, eggs, sugar, and cream. Pour over baguette slices. Let it soak for an hour.
3. Cover pan with foil.
4. For 35 minutes, cook on 330oF.
5. Let it rest for 10 minutes.
6. Serve and enjoy.

Nutrition:
Calories: 581 | Carbs: 76.1g | Protein: 15.8g | Fat: 23.7g

910. Cherries 'n Almond Flour Bars
⏱ Prep Time 15 m | ⏱ Cooking Time 35 m | 12 Servings

Ingredients:
- ¼ cup of water
- ½ cup butter softened
- ½ teaspoon salt
- ½ teaspoon vanilla
- 1 ½ cups almond flour

- 1 cup erythritol
- 1 cup fresh cherries, pitted
- 1 tablespoon xanthan gum
- eggs

Directions:
1. In a medium bowl, make a mixture of the first 6 ingredients to form a dough.
2. Press the batter onto a baking sheet that will fit in the air fryer.
3. Place in the fryer and bake for 10 minutes at 3750F.
4. Meanwhile, mix the cherries, water, and xanthan gum in a bowl.
5. Scoop out the dough and pour over the cherry.
6. Return to the fryer and cook for another 25 minutes at 3750F.

Nutrition:
Calories: 99 | Carbohydrates: 2.1g | Protein: 1.8g | Fat: 9.3g

911. Cherry-Choco Bars
⏱ Prep Time 5 m | ⏱ Cooking Time 15 m | 8 Servings

Ingredients:
- ¼ teaspoon salt
- ½ cup almonds, sliced
- ½ cup chia seeds
- ½ cup dark chocolate, chopped
- ½ cup dried cherries, chopped
- ½ cup prunes, pureed

- ½ cup quinoa, cooked
- ¾ cup almond butter
- 1/3 cup honey
- cups old-fashioned oats
- tablespoon coconut oil

Directions:
1. Preheat the air fryer to 3750F.
2. In a bowl, combine the oats, quinoa, chia seeds, almond, cherries, and chocolate.
3. In a saucepan, heat the almond butter, honey, and coconut oil.
4. Pour the butter mixture over the dry mixture. Add salt and prunes.
5. Mix until well combined.
6. Pour over a baking dish that can fit inside the air fryer.
7. Cook for 15 minutes.
8. Allow settling for an hour before slicing into bars.

Nutrition:
Calories: 321 | Carbohydrates: 35g | Protein: 7g | Fat: 17g

912. Choco-Peanut Mug Cake
☉ Prep Time 10 m | ☉ Cooking Time 20 m | 6 Servings

Ingredients:

- ¼ teaspoon baking powder
- ½ teaspoon vanilla extract
- 1 egg
- 1 tablespoon heavy cream

- 1 tablespoon peanut butter
- 1 teaspoon butter, softened
- tablespoon erythritol
- tablespoons cocoa powder, unsweetened

Directions:

1. Preheat the air fryer for 5 minutes.
2. Combine all ingredients in a mixing bowl.
3. Pour into a greased mug.

4. Place in the air fryer oven basket and cook for 20 minutes at 4000F or if a toothpick inserted in the middle comes out clean.

Nutrition:

Calories: 293 | Carbohydrates: 8.5g | Protein: 12.4g | Fat: 23.3g

913. Coco-Lime Bars
☉ Prep Time 10 m | ☉ Cooking Time 20 m | 3 Servings

Ingredients:

- ¼ cup almond flour
- ¼ cup coconut oil
- ¼ cup dried coconut flakes
- ¼ teaspoon salt
- ½ cup lime juice

- ¾ cup coconut flour
- 1 ¼ cup erythritol powder
- 1 tablespoon lime zest
- eggs

Directions:

1. Preheat the air fryer for 5 minutes.
2. Combine all ingredients in a mixing bowl.

3. Place in the greased mug.
4. Bake in the air fryer oven for 20 minutes at 3750F.

Nutrition:

Calories: 506 | Carbohydrates: 21.9g| Protein: 19.3g | Fat: 37.9g

914. Coconut 'n Almond Fat Bombs
☉ Prep Time 5 m | ☉ Cooking Time 15 m | 12 Servings

Ingredients:

- ¼ cup almond flour
- ½ cup shredded coconut
- 1 tablespoon coconut oil

- 1 tablespoon vanilla extract
- tablespoons liquid stevia
- egg whites

Directions:

1. Preheat the air fryer for 5 minutes.
2. Combine all ingredients in a mixing bowl.
3. Form small balls using your hands.

4. Place in the air fryer oven basket and cook for 15 minutes at 4000F.

Nutrition:

Calories: 23 | Carbohydrates: 0.7g | Protein: 1.1g | Fat: 1.8g

915. Coconutty Lemon Bars
☉ Prep Time 10 m | ☉ Cooking Time 25 m | 12 Servings

Ingredients:

- ¼ cup cashew
- ¼ cup fresh lemon juice, freshly squeezed
- ¾ cup coconut milk
- ¾ cup erythritol
- 1 cup desiccated coconut

- 1 teaspoon baking powder
- eggs, beaten
- tablespoons coconut oil
- A dash of salt

Directions:

1. Preheat the air fryer for 5 minutes.
2. In a mixing bowl, combine all ingredients.
3. Use a hand mixer to mix everything.

4. Pour into a baking bowl that will fit in the air fryer.
5. Bake for 25 minutes at 3500F or until a toothpick inserted in the middle comes out clean.

Nutrition:

Calories: 118 | Carbohydrates: 3.9g | Protein: 2.6g| Fat: 10.2g

916. Coffee 'n Blueberry Cake

⏱ Prep Time 15 m | ⏱ Cooking Time 35 m | 6 Servings

Ingredients:

- 1 cup white sugar
- 1 egg
- 1/2 cup butter, softened
- 1/2 cup fresh or frozen blueberries
- 1/2 cup sour cream
- 1/2 teaspoon baking powder
- 1/2 teaspoon ground cinnamon
- 1/2 teaspoon vanilla extract
- 1/4 cup brown sugar
- 1/4 cup chopped pecans
- 1/8 teaspoon salt
- 1-1/2 teaspoons confectioners' sugar for dusting
- 3/4 cup and 1 tablespoon all-purpose flour

Directions:

1 In a small bowl, whisk well pecans, cinnamon, and brown sugar.
2 In a blender, blend well all wet Ingredients. Add dry ingredients except for confectioner's sugar and blueberries. Blend well until smooth and creamy.
3 Lightly grease baking pan of the air fryer with cooking spray.
4 Pour half of the batter in pan. Sprinkle small of the pecan mixture on top. Pour the remaining batter. And then topped with the remaining pecan mixture.
5 Cover pan with foil.
6 For 35 minutes, cook on 330oF.
7 Serve and enjoy with a dusting of confectioner's sugar.

Nutrition:

Calories: 471 | Carbs: 59.5g | Protein: 4.1g | Fat: 24.0g

917. Coffee Flavored Cookie Dough

⏱ Prep Time 10 m | ⏱ Cooking Time 20 m | 12 Servings

Ingredients:

- ¼ cup butter
- ¼ teaspoon xanthan gum
- ½ teaspoon coffee espresso powder
- ½ teaspoon stevia powder
- ¾ cup almond flour
- 1 egg
- 1 teaspoon vanilla
- 1/3 cup sesame seeds
- tablespoons cocoa powder
- tablespoons cream cheese, softened

Directions:

1. Preheat the air fryer for 5 minutes.
2. Combine all ingredients in a mixing bowl.
3. Press into a baking dish that will fit in the air fryer.
4. Place in the air fryer oven basket and cook for 20 minutes at 4000F or if a toothpick inserted in the middle comes out clean.

Nutrition:

Calories: 88 | Carbohydrates: 1.3g | Protein: 1.9g | Fat: 8.3g

918. Sweet Potato Tater Tots

⏱ Prep Time 10 m | ⏱ Cooking Time 23 m | 4 Servings

Ingredients:

- 1sweet potatoes, peeled
- 1/2 tsp. Cajun seasoning
- Olive oil cooking spray
- Sea salt to taste

Directions:

1 Boil sweet potatoes in water for 15 minutes over medium-high heat.
2 Drain the sweet potatoes then allow them to cool
3 Peel the boiled sweet potatoes and return them to the bowl.
4 Mash the potatoes and stir in salt and Cajun seasoning. Mix well and make small tater tots out of it.
5 Place the tater tots in the Air Fryer basket and spray them with cooking oil.
6 Place the Air Fryer basket inside the Air Fryer toaster and close the lid.
7 Select Air Frying mode at a temperature of 400 ° F for 8 minutes.
8 Turn the trays over and continue cooking for another 8 minutes.
9 Serve fresh.

Nutrition: Calories: 184 Cal | Protein: 9 g | Carbs: 43 g | Fat: 17 g

919. Fried Ravioli

⏱ Prep Time 10 m | ⏱ Cooking Time 15 m | 4 Servings

Ingredients:

- 1 package ravioli, frozen
- 1 cup breadcrumbs
- 1/2 cup parmesan cheese
- 1 tbs. Italian seasoning
- 1 tbs. garlic powder
- Eggs, beaten
- Cooking spray

Directions:

1 Mix breadcrumbs with garlic powder, cheese, and Italian seasoning in a bowl.
2 Whisk eggs in another bowl. Dip each ravioli in eggs first then coat them with crumbs mixture.
3 Place the ravioli in the Air Fryer basket. Place the air Fryer basket inside the oven and close the lid.
4 Select the Air Fry mode at 360°F temperature for 15 minutes.
5 Flip the ravioli after 8 minutes and resume cooking. Serve warm.

Nutrition: Calories: 124 Cal | Protein: 4.5 g | Carbs: 27.5 g | Fat: 3.5 g

920. Eggplant Fries
⏱ Prep Time 10 m | ⏱ Cooking Time 20 m | 4 Servings

Ingredients:
- 1/2 cup panko breadcrumbs
- 1/2 tsp. salt
- 1 eggplant, peeled and sliced
- 1 cup egg, whisked

Directions:
1. Toss the breadcrumbs with salt in a tray.
2. Dip the eggplant in the whisked egg and coat with the crumb's mixture.
3. Place the eggplant slices in the Air Fryer basket. Put the basket inside the Air Fryer toaster oven and close the lid.
4. Select the Air Fry mode at 400°F temperature for 20 minutes.
5. Flip the slices after 10 minutes then resume cooking. Serve warm.

Nutrition:
Calories: 110 Cal| Protein: 5 g |Carbs: 12.8 g | Fat: 11.9 g

921. Stuffed Eggplants
⏱ Prep Time 10 m | ⏱ Cooking Time 38 m | 4 Servings

Ingredients:
- Eggplants, cut in half lengthwise
- 1/2 cup shredded cheddar cheese
- 1/2 can (7.5 oz.) chili without beans
- 1 Tsp. kosher salt

FOR SERVING
- Tbsp. cooked bacon bits
- tbsp. sour cream
- Fresh scallions, thinly sliced

Directions:
1. Place the eggplants halves in the Air Fryer toaster oven and close the lid.
2. Select the Air Fry mode at 390°F temperature for 35 minutes.
3. Top each eggplant half with chili, cheese, and salt.
4. Place the halves in a baking pan and return to the oven. Select the Broil mode at 375°F temperature for 3 minutes.
5. Garnish with bacon bits, sour cream, and scallions. Serve.

Nutrition:
Calories: 113 Cal |Protein: 9.2 g| Carbs: 13 g| Fat: 21 g

922. Bacon Poppers
⏱ Prep Time 10 m | ⏱ Cooking Time 15 m | 4 Servings

Ingredients:
- 1 strips bacon, crispy cooked
- Dough:
- 2/3 cup water
- 1 tbsp. butter
- 1 tbsp. bacon fat
- 1 tsp. kosher salt
- 2/3 cup all-purpose flour
- Eggs
- oz. Cheddar cheese, shredded
- ½ cup jalapeno peppers
- A pinch pepper
- A pinch black pepper

Directions:
1. Whisk butter with water and salt in a skillet over medium heat. Stir in flour, then stir cook for about 3 minutes.
2. Transfer this flour to a bowl, then whisk in eggs and rest of the ingredients.
3. Fold in bacon and mix well. Wrap this dough in a plastic sheet and refrigerate for 30 minutes. Make small balls out of this dough.
4. Place these bacon balls the Air Fryer toaster oven and close the lid.
5. Select the Air Fry mode at 390°F temperature for 15 minutes. Flip the balls after 7 minutes then resume cooking. Serve warm.

Nutrition:
Calories: 240 Kcal| Protein: 14.9 g |Carbs: 7.1 g |Fat: 22.5 g

923. Stuffed Jalapeno
⏱ Prep Time 10 m | ⏱ Cooking Time 10 m | 4 Servings

Ingredients:
- 1 lb. ground pork sausage
- 1 (8 oz.) package cream cheese, softened
- 1 cup shredded Parmesan cheese
- 1 lb. large fresh jalapeno peppers halved lengthwise and seeded
- 1 (8 oz.) bottle Ranch dressing

Directions:
1. Mix pork sausage ground with ranch dressing and cream cheese in a bowl.
2. But the jalapeno in half and remove their seeds.
3. Divide the cream cheese mixture into the jalapeno halves. Place the jalapeno pepper in a baking tray.
4. Set the Baking tray inside the Air Fryer toaster oven and close the lid.
5. Select the Bake mode at 350°F temperature for 10 minutes. Serve warm.

Nutrition:
Calories: 168 Kcal |Protein: 9.4 g | Carbs: 12.1 g |Fat: 21.2 g

924. Creamy Mushrooms

⏱ Prep Time 10 m | ⏱ Cooking Time 15 m | 24 Servings

Ingredients:

- 20 mushrooms
- 1 orange bell pepper, dice d
- 1 onion, diced
- Slices bacon, diced
- 1 cup shredded Cheddar cheese
- 1 cup sour cream

Directions:

1 First sauté the mushroom stems, with onion, bacon, and bell pepper in a pan.
2 After 5 minutes of cooking, add 1 cup cheese and sour cream. Cook for 2 minutes.
3 Place the mushroom caps on the Air Fryer basket crisper plate.
4 Stuff each mushroom with the cheese-vegetable mixture and top them with cheddar cheese.
5 Insert the basket back insider and select Air Fry mode for 8 minutes at 350°F.
6 Serve warm.

Nutrition:

Calories: 101 Kcal | Protein: 8.8 g | Carbs: 25 g | Fat: 12.2 g

925. Italian Corn Fritters

⏱ Prep Time 10 m | ⏱ Cooking Time 3 m | 4 Servings

Ingredients:

- Cups frozen corn kernels
- 1/3 cup finely ground cornmeal
- 1/3 cup flour
- ½ tsp. salt
- ¼ tsp. pepper
- ½ tsp. baking powder
- Onion powder, to taste
- Garlic powder, to taste
- ¼ tsp. paprika
- Tbsp. green chilies with juices
- Tbsp. almond milk
- ¼ cup chopped Italian parsley

Directions:

1 Beat cornmeal with flour, baking powder, parsley, seasonings in a bowl. Blend 3 tbsp. almond milk with 1 cup corn, black pepper, and salt in a food processor until smooth.
2 Stir in the flour mixture then mix until smooth. Spread this corn mixture in a baking tray, lined with wax paper.
3 Set the baking tray inside the Air Fryer toaster oven and close the lid.
4 Select the bake mode at 350°F temperature for 2 minutes. Slice and serve.

Nutrition:

Calories: 146 Kcal | Protein: 6.3 g| Carbs: 18.8 g| Fat: 4.5 g

926. Artichoke Fries

⏱ Prep Time 8 m | ⏱ Cooking Time 13 m | 6 Servings

Ingredients:

- 1 oz. can artichoke hearts
- 1 cup flour
- 1 cup almond milk
- ½ tsp. garlic powder
- ¾ tsp. salt
- ¼ tsp. black pepper, or to taste
- For Dry Mix:
- 1 ½ cup panko breadcrumbs
- ½ tsp. paprika
- ¼ tsp. salt

Directions:

1 Whisk the wet ingredients in a bowl until smooth and mix the dry ingredients in a separate bowl.
2 First, dip the artichokes quarters in the wet mixture then coat with the dry panko mixture.
3 Place the artichokes hearts in the Air Fryer basket. Insert the basket inside the Air Fryer toaster oven and close the lid.
4 Select the Air Fry mode at 340°F temperature for 13 minutes. Serve warm.

Nutrition:

Calories: 199 Cal | Protein: 9.4 g | Carbs: 15.9 g | Fat: 4 g

927. Crumbly Beef Meatballs

⏱ Prep Time 8 m | ⏱ Cooking Time 20 m | 6 Servings

Ingredients:

- Lbs. of ground beef
- Large eggs
- 1-1/4 cup panko breadcrumbs
- 1/4 cup chopped fresh parsley
- 1 tsp. dried oregano
- 1/4 cup grated Parmigianino Regina
- 1 small clove garlic chopped
- Salt and pepper to taste
- 1 tsp. vegetable oil

Directions:

1 Thoroughly mix beef with eggs, crumbs, parsley, and rest of the ingredients.
2 Make small meatballs out of this mixture and place them in the basket.
3 Place the basket inside the Air Fryer toaster oven and close the lid.
4 Select the Air Fry mode at 350°F temperature for 13 minutes.
5 Toss the meatballs after 5 minutes and resume cooking.
6 Serve fresh.

Nutrition: Calories: 221 Cal | Protein: 25.1 g | Carbs: 11.2 g | Fat: 16.5 g

928. Pork Stuffed Dumplings

⏱ Prep Time 15 m | ⏱ Cooking Time 12 m | 3 Servings

Ingredients:

- 1 tsp. canola oil
- Cups chopped book Choy
- 1 tbsp. chopped fresh ginger
- 1 tbsp. chopped garlic
- Oz. ground pork
- 1/4 tsp. crushed red pepper
- 18 dumpling wrappers
- Cooking spray
- 1 Tbsp. rice vinegar
- 1 tsp. lower-sodium soy sauce
- 1 tsp. toasted sesame oil
- 1/2 tsp. packed light Sugar
- 1 tbsp. finely chopped scallions

Directions:

1. In a greased skillet, sauté bok choy for 8 minutes, then add ginger and garlic. Cook for 1 minute.
2. Transfer the bok choy to a plate.
3. Add pork and red pepper then mix well. Place the dumpling wraps on the working surface and divide the pork fillings on the dumpling wraps.
4. Wet the edges of the wraps and pinch them together to seal the filling.
5. Place the dumpling in the Air Fryer basket.
6. Set the Air Fryer basket inside the Air Fryer toaster oven and close the lid.
7. Select the Air Fry mode at 375°F temperature for 12 minutes.
8. Flip the dumplings after 6 minutes then resume cooking.
9. Serve fresh.

Nutrition:

Calories: 172 Cal| Protein: 2.1 g |Carbs: 18.6 g |Fat: 10.7 g

929. Panko Tofu with Mayo Sauce

⏱ Prep Time 10 m | ⏱ Cooking Time 20 m | 4 Servings

Ingredients:

- 1 tofu cutlets
- For the Marinade
- 1 tbsp. toasted sesame oil
- 1/4 cup soy sauce
- 1 tsp rice vinegar
- 1/2 tsp garlic powder
- 1 tsp. ground ginger

Make the Tofu:

- 1/2 cup vegan mayo
- 1 cup panko breadcrumbs
- 1 tsp. of sea salt

Direction:

1. Whisk the marinade ingredients in a bowl and add tofu cutlets. Mix well to coat the cutlets.
2. Cover and marinate for 1 hour. Meanwhile, whisk crumbs with salt and mayo in a bowl.
3. Coat the cutlets with crumbs mixture. Place the tofu cutlets in the Air Fryer basket.
4. Select the Air Fry mode at 370°F temperature for 20 minutes. Flip the cutlets after 10 minutes then resume cooking.
5. Serve warm.

Nutrition:

Calories: 151 Cal |Protein: 1.9 g | Carbs: 6.9 g | Fat: 8.6 g

930. Garlicky Bok Choy

⏱ Prep Time 10 m | ⏱ Cooking Time 10 m | 2 Servings

Ingredients:

- bunches baby book Choy
- Spray oil
- 1 tsp. garlic powder

Directions:

1. Toss bok choy with garlic powder and spread them in the Air Fryer basket.
2. Spray them with cooking oil.
3. Place the basket inside the Air Fryer toaster oven and close the lid.
4. Select the Air Fry mode at 350°F temperature for 6 minutes. Serve fresh.

Nutrition:

Calories: 81 Cal |Protein: 0.4 g | Carbs: 4.7 g |Fat: 8.3 g

931. Walnut Brownies

⏱ Prep Time 15 m | ⏱ Cooking Time 35 m | 6 Servings

Ingredients:

- Eggs 2
- Brown sugar 1 cup
- Vanilla ½ teaspoon
- Cocoa powder 1/4 cup
- Walnuts 1/2 cup, chopped
- All-purpose flour – 1/4 cup
- Butter – 1/2 cup, melted
- Pinch of salt

Directions:

1. Sprinkle a baking dish with cooking spray and set aside. In a bowl, whisk together eggs, butter, cocoa powder, and vanilla. Add walnuts, flour, sugar, and salt and stir well. Pour batter into the baking dish. Place steam rack into the instant pot. Place baking dish on top of the steam rack. Seal pot with the air fryer lid. Select bake mode and cook at 320 F for 35 minutes. Serve.

Nutrition:

Calories 340 Carbs 30g Fat 23g Protein 5g

932. Seasoned Cauliflower Chunks

⏱ Prep Time 10 m | ⏱ Cooking Time 15 m | 4 Servings

Ingredients:

- 1 cauliflower head, diced into chunks
- ½ cup unsweetened milk
- Tbsp. mayo
- ¼ cup all-purpose flour
- ¾ cup almond meal
- ¼ cup almond meal

- 1 tsp. onion powder
- 1 tsp. garlic powder
- 1 tsp. of sea salt
- ½ tsp. paprika
- Pinch of black pepper
- Cooking oil spray

Directions:

1. Toss cauliflower with rest of the ingredients in a bowl then transfers to the Air Fryer basket.
2. Spray them with cooking oil.
3. Set the basket inside the Air Fryer toaster oven and close the lid.
4. Select the Air Fry mode at 400°F temperature for 15 minutes.
5. Toss well and serve warm.

Nutrition:

Calories: 137 Cal |Protein: 6.1 g |Carbs: 26 g |Fat: 8 g

933. Almond Butter Brownies

⏱ Prep Time 10 m | ⏱ Cooking Time 15 m | 4 Servings

Ingredients:

- 1/2 cup Almond butter
- 1/2 teaspoon Vanilla
- 1 tablespoon Almond milk
- 2 tablespoons Coconut sugar
- 2 tablespoons Applesauce
- 2 tablespoons Honey

- 1/4 teaspoon Baking powder
- 1/2 teaspoon Baking soda
- 2 tablespoons Cocoa powder
- 3 tablespoons Almond flour
- 1 tablespoon Coconut oil
- 1/4 teaspoon Sea salt

Directions:

1. Sprinkle baking pan with cooking spray and set aside. In a small bowl, mix together almond flour, baking soda, baking powder, and cocoa powder and set aside. Add coconut oil and almond butter into the microwave-safe bowl and microwave until melted. Stir. Add honey, milk, coconut sugar, vanilla, and applesauce into the melted coconut oil mixture and stir well. Add flour mixture and stir to combine. Pour batter into the baking pan. Place steam rack into the instant pot. Place baking pan on top of the steam rack. Seal pot with the air fryer lid. Select bake mode and cook at 350 F for 15 minutes. Serve.

Nutrition:

Calories 170 Carbs 22g Fat 8g Protein 2g

934. Brownie Muffins

⏱ Prep Time 10 m | ⏱ Cooking Time 15 m | 6 Servings

Ingredients:

- 1/4 cup Cocoa powder
- 1/2 cup Almond butter
- 1 cup Pumpkin puree

- 8 drops Liquid stevia
- 2 scoops Protein powder

Directions:

1. Mixed all the ingredients into the mixing bowl and beat until smooth. Pour batter into the 6 silicone muffin molds. Place the dehydrating tray into the multi-level air fryer basket and place the basket into the instant pot. Place muffin molds on a dehydrating tray. Seal pot with the air fryer lid. Select bake mode and cook at 350 F for 15 minutes. Serve.

Nutrition:

Calories 70 Carbs 6g Fat 2g Protein 8g

935. Delicious Lemon Muffins

⏱ Prep Time 10 m | ⏱ Cooking Time 15 m | 6 Servings

Ingredients:

- 1 Egg
- 3/4 teaspoon Baking powder
- 1 tsp. grated Lemon zest
- 1/2 cup Sugar
- 1/2 teaspoon Vanilla

- 1/2 cup Milk
- 2 tablespoons Canola oil
- 1/4 teaspoon Baking soda
- 1 cup Flour
- 1/2 teaspoon Salt

Directions:

1. In a mixing bowl, beat egg, vanilla, milk, oil, and sugar until creamy. Add remaining ingredients and stir to combine. Pour batter into the 6 silicone muffin molds. Place the dehydrating tray into the multi-level air fryer basket and place the basket into the instant pot. Place muffin molds on a dehydrating tray. Seal pot with the air fryer lid. Select bake mode and cook at 350 F for 15 minutes. Serve.

Nutrition:

Calories 202 Carbs 34g Fat 6g Protein 4g

936. Vanilla Strawberry Soufflé

⏱ Prep Time 10 m | ⏱ Cooking Time 15 m | 4 Servings

Ingredients:
- 3 Egg whites
- 1 1/2 cup Strawberries
- 1/2 teaspoon Vanilla
- 1 tablespoon Sugar

Directions:
1. Spray 4 ramekins with cooking spray and set aside. Add strawberries, sugar, and vanilla into the blender and blend until smooth. Add egg whites into the bowl and beat until medium peaks form. Add strawberry mixture and fold well. Pour egg mixture into the ramekins. Place the dehydrating tray into the multi-level air fryer basket and place the basket into the instant pot. Place ramekins on the dehydrating tray. Seal pot with the air fryer lid. Select bake mode and cook at 350 F for 15 minutes. Serve.

Nutrition:
Calories 50 Carbs 8g Fat 0.5g Protein 3g

937. Healthy Carrot Muffins

⏱ Prep Time 15 m | ⏱ Cooking Time 20 m | 6 Servings

Ingredients:
- 1 Egg
- 1 teaspoon Vanilla
- 1/4 cup Brown sugar
- 1/4 cup Granulated sugar
- 1/2 tablespoon Canola oil
- 1/4 cup Applesauce
- 1 cup All-purpose flour
- 1 1/2 teaspoons Baking powder
- 1/2 teaspoon Nutmeg
- 1 teaspoon Cinnamon
- 3/4 cup Grated carrots
- 1/4 teaspoon Salt

Directions:
1. Into a large bowl put all the ingredients then mix until thoroughly combined. Pour batter into 6 silicone muffin molds. Place the dehydrating tray into the multi-level air fryer basket and place the basket into the instant pot. Place muffin molds on the dehydrating tray. Seal pot with the air fryer lid. Select bake mode and cook at 350 F for 20 minutes. Serve.

Nutrition:
Calories 165 Carbs 33g Fat 2g Protein 3g

938. Cinnamon Carrot Cake

⏱ Prep Time 10 m | ⏱ Cooking Time 25 m | 4 Servings

Ingredients:
- 1 Egg
- 1/2 teaspoon Vanilla
- 1/2 teaspoon Cinnamon
- 1/2 cup Sugar
- 1/4 cup Canola oil
- 1/4, chopped Walnuts
- 1/2 teaspoon Baking powder
- 1/2 cup Flour
- 1/4 cup Grated carrot

Directions:
1. Sprinkle a baking dish with cooking spray and set aside. In a mixing bowl, beat sugar and oil for 1-2 minutes. Add vanilla, cinnamon, and egg and beat for 30 seconds. Add remaining ingredients and stir to combine. Pour batter into the prepared baking dish. Place steam rack into the instant pot. Place baking dish on top of the steam rack. Seal pot with the air fryer lid. Select bake mode and cook at 350 F for 25 minutes. Serve.

Nutrition: Calories 340 Carbs 39g Fat 19g Protein 5g

939. Blueberry Muffins

⏱ Prep Time 15 m | ⏱ Cooking Time 20 m | 6 Servings

Ingredients:
- 2 Eggs
- 1 1/2 cups Blueberries
- 1 cup Yogurt
- 1 cup Sugar
- 1 tablespoon Baking powder
- 2 cups Flour
- 2 teaspoons Fresh lemon juice
- 2 tablespoons, grated Lemon zest
- 1 teaspoon Vanilla
- 1/2 cup Oil
- 1/2 teaspoon Salt

Directions:
1. Using a small bowl, mix flour, salt, and baking powder. Set aside. In a large bowl, whisk together eggs, lemon juice, lemon zest, vanilla, oil, yogurt, and sugar. Add flour mixture and blueberries into the egg mixture and fold well. Pour batter into 9 silicone muffin molds. Place the dehydrating tray into the multi-level air fryer basket and place the basket into the instant pot. Place 6 muffin molds on the dehydrating tray. Seal pot with the air fryer lid. Select bake mode and cook at 375 F for 20 minutes. Cook remaining muffins. Serve.

Nutrition: Calories 343 Carbs 50g Fat 13g Protein 5.9g

940. Almond Raspberry Muffins

⏱ Prep Time 10 m | ⏱ Cooking Time 35 m | 6 Servings

Ingredients:
- 2 Eggs
- 1 teaspoon Baking powder
- 5 ounces Almond meal
- 2 tablespoons Coconut oil
- 2 tablespoons Honey
- 3 ounces Raspberries

Directions:
1. In a bowl, mix together almond meal and baking powder. Add honey, eggs, and oil and stir until thoroughly combined. Add raspberries and fold well. Pour batter into the 6-silicone muffin molds. Place the dehydrating tray into the multi-level air fryer basket and place the basket into the instant pot. Place 6 muffin molds on the dehydrating tray. Seal pot with the air fryer lid. Select bake mode and cook at 350 F for 35 minutes. Serve.

Nutrition: Calories 227 Carbs 13g Fat 17g Protein 7g

941. Chocolate Cupcakes

⏱ Prep Time 10 m | ⏱ Cooking Time 25 m | 6 Servings

Ingredients:

- 1 Egg
- 1/2 cup Cocoa powder
- 1 cup Chocolate chips
- 1 cup Granulated sugar
- 2 cups All-purpose flour
- 1/2 cup Canola oil
- 1 teaspoon Vanilla
- 1/2 cup Milk
- 1 cup Yogurt
- 1 teaspoon Baking soda

Directions:

1. Using a large bowl, mix together flour, baking soda, cocoa powder, chocolate chips, and sugar. In a large bowl, beat egg with oil, vanilla, milk, and yogurt until smooth. Add flour mixture into the egg mixture and stir to combine. Pour batter into the 9-silicone cake molds. Place the dehydrating tray into the multi-level air fryer basket and place the basket into the instant pot. Place 6 cake molds on a dehydrating tray. Seal pot with the air fryer lid. Select bake mode and cook at 380 F for 25 minutes. Cook remaining cupcakes. Serve.

Nutrition: Calories 436 Carbs 59g Fat 19g Protein 7g

942. Moist Chocolate Cake

⏱ Prep Time 10 m | ⏱ Cooking Time 30 m | 4 Servings

Ingredients:

- 1 Egg
- 1/3 cup Canola oil
- 1/2 teaspoon Baking soda
- 5 tablespoons Cocoa powder
- 1/2 cup All-purpose flour
- 1 tablespoon Warm coffee
- 1/2 teaspoon Vanilla
- 1/3 cup Sour cream
- 1/2 cup Granulated sugar

Directions:

1. Sprinkle a baking dish with cooking spray and set aside. Using a bowl, mix together flour, baking soda, and cocoa powder and set aside. In a small bowl, whisk together egg, vanilla, coffee, sour cream, sugar, and oil. Pour egg mixture into the flour mixture and mix until well combined. Pour batter into the baking dish. Place steam rack into the instant pot. Place baking dish on top of the steam rack. Seal pot with the air fryer lid. Select bake mode and cook at 350 F for 30 minutes.

Nutrition: Calories 385 Carbs 41g Fat 24g Protein 5g

943. Chocolate Cookie

⏱ Prep Time 10 m | ⏱ Cooking Time 25 m | 4 Servings

Ingredients:

- 1 Egg yolk
- 1/4 teaspoon Vanilla
- 1 tablespoon Granulated sugar
- 2 tablespoons Brown sugar
- 2 tablespoons, chopped Walnuts
- 1/4 cup Chocolate chips
- 1/8 teaspoon Baking soda
- 1/3 cup All-purpose flour
- 2 tablespoons, softened Butter
- 1/8 teaspoon Salt

Directions:

1. Sprinkle two ramekins with cooking spray and set aside. In a mixing bowl, mix together butter, brown sugar, and granulated sugar. Add vanilla and egg yolk and mix until combined. Add flour, salt, and baking soda and stir to combine. Add walnuts and chocolate chips and stir well. Pour cookie dough into the ramekins. Place the dehydrating tray into the multi-level air fryer basket and place the basket into the instant pot. Place ramekins on a dehydrating tray. Seal pot with the air fryer lid. Select bake mode and cook at 350 F for 25 minutes. Serve.

Nutrition: Calories 423 Carbs 44g Fat 24g Protein 7g

944. Almond Cranberry Muffins

⏱ Prep Time 10 m | ⏱ Cooking Time 30 m | 6 Servings

Ingredients:

- Eggs – 2
- Swerve – 1/4 cup
- Almond Flour – 1 1/2 cups
- Vanilla – 1 teaspoon
- Cranberries – 1/2 cup
- Cinnamon – 1/4 teaspoon
- Baking powder – 1 teaspoon
- Sour cream – 1/4 cup
- Pinch of salt

Directions:

1. In a bowl, beat sour cream, vanilla, and eggs. Add remaining ingredients except for cranberries and beat until smooth. Add cranberries and fold well. Pour batter into the 6-silicone muffin molds. Place the dehydrating tray into the multi-level air fryer basket and place the basket into the instant pot. Place 6 muffin molds on the dehydrating tray. Seal pot with the air fryer lid. Select bake mode and cook at 325 F for 25-30 minutes. Serve.

Nutrition: Calories 218 Carbs 17g Fat 16g Protein 8g

945. Chocolate Coffee Cake

⏱ Prep Time 10 m | ⏱ Cooking Time 15 m | 2 Servings

Ingredients:

- Egg – 1
- Black coffee – 1 tablespoon
- Instant coffee – 1/2 teaspoon
- Butter – 1/4 cup
- Cocoa powder – 2 teaspoons
- Flour – 1/4 cup
- Sugar – 1/4 cup

Directions:

1. Sprinkle a baking dish with cooking spray and set aside. In a bowl, beat egg, butter, and sugar. Add black coffee, instant coffee, and cocoa powder and beat well. Add flour and stir to combine. Pour batter into the baking dish. Place steam rack into the instant pot then place baking dish on top of the rack. Seal pot with the air fryer lid. Select bake mode and cook at 330 F for 15 minutes. Serve.

Nutrition: Calories 388 Carbs 37g Fat 25g Protein 4g

946. Walnut Muffins

⏱ Prep Time 10 m | ⏱ Cooking Time 15 m | 2 Servings

Ingredients:

- 1Egg yolk
- 2 tablespoons, chopped Walnuts
- 1/8 teaspoon Vanilla
- 1 tablespoon Sour cream
- 2 tablespoons, melted Butter
- 3 tablespoons Maple syrup
- 3 tablespoons Milk
- 1/8 teaspoon Ground cinnamon
- 1/2 teaspoon Baking powder
- 2 tablespoons Brown sugar
- 1/2 cup All-purpose flour
- 1/8 teaspoon Salt

Directions:

1. Sprinkle 2 ramekins with cooking spray and set aside. In a medium bowl, mix together flour, cinnamon, baking powder, brown sugar, and salt. In a separate bowl, whisk together the egg yolk, vanilla, sour cream, butter, maple syrup, and milk. Pour egg mixture into the flour mixture and stir until thoroughly combined. Add walnuts and fold well. Pour batter into the ramekins. Place the dehydrating tray into the multi-level air fryer basket and place the basket into the instant pot. Place ramekins on dehydrating tray. Seal pot with the air fryer lid. Select bake mode and cook at 380 F for 15 minutes. Serve.

Nutrition:
Calories 525 Carbs 65g Fat 26g Protein 7g

947. Lemon Poppy seed Cake

⏱ Prep Time 15 m | ⏱ Cooking Time 23 m | 8 Servings

Ingredients:

- 1 c flour
- 1 teaspoon baking powder
- 1/8 teaspoon baking soda
- 4 tablespoon butter softened
- 1/2 c sugar
- 1 egg
- 1/2 c yogurt whole milk, vanilla is best
- 1 tablespoon poppy seeds
- 1/2 teaspoon vanilla
- 1 tablespoon lemon juice
- 1/2 scoop Vital Proteins Strawberry Lemon Collagen Beauty Water optional

Directions:

1. Put flour, baking soda and baking powder in a bowl and mix.
2. In another bowl add softened butter, sugar, egg, and yogurt, vanilla and lemon juice. Use a mixer on low to mix.
3. Slowly add dry ingredients into a wet ingredient bowl and mix on low until well combined.
4. Fold in poppy seeds and 1 scoop of Vital Proteins if you're adding that.
5. Spray inside of a 6 cup Bundt pan. Spoon mixture into your Bundt pan, spread evenly (do not fill more than 3/4 full).
6. Cover with tin foil. Put a trivet or small glass cup/bowl at the bottom of Instant Pot.
7. Pour in 2 cups of water around the bowl. Fold another pc. Of aluminum foil diagonally like a bandana to make a sling for the Bundt pan, place underneath so there are handles to lift it in at the top sides.
8. Place Bundt pan on top of trivet and closet lid.
9. Set Instant Pot or pressure cooker to manual, pressure, high, for 25 minutes. Allow to naturally release.
10. Lift lid and remove foil from Bundt pan. Take out of Instant Pot and let it set until it cools a bit.
11. Carefully flip over onto a cutting board or cake plate. Warm a bit of vanilla frosting or combine a bit of water with powdered sugar to make a frosting. Drizzle on top, add lemon zest on top if desired.

Nutrition:
Calories: 180 Fat: 7g Carbohydrates: 25g Protein: 3g

948. Chocolate Pudding Cake

⏱ Prep Time 15 m | ⏱ Cooking Time 6 m | 6 Servings

Ingredients:

- 2/3 cup chopped dark chocolate
- 1/2 cup applesauce
- 2 eggs
- 1 teaspoon vanilla
- Pinch of salt
- 1/4 cup arrowroot
- 3 tablespoons cocoa powder (plus more for dusting)
- Powdered sugar for topping (optional)

Directions:

1. Place a trivet inside the Instant Pot and pour in 2 cups of water. Measure the chocolate into a heatproof ramekin, and set on the trivet. Turn the Instant Pot on to "Sauté", and melt the chocolate over the simmering water. Remove ramekin from Instant Pot once the chocolate is melted.
2. Combine the applesauce, eggs, and vanilla in a small mixing bowl. Whisk until well blended. Add the dry ingredients (salt through cocoa powder) and slowly mix in until no dry streaks remain. Stir in melted chocolate.
3. Liberally grease a 6 inches cake pan with butter or coconut oil. Dust the bottom and sides of the cake pan with cocoa powder. Pour in the cake batter, and set the pan on the trivet above the hot water in the Instant Pot.
4. Cook on high pressure for 4 minutes. Quick release pressure when the timer goes off. Remove the cake pan from Instant Pot and let cool 10 minutes before transferring to a serving plate. Dust with powdered sugar (optional).

Nutrition:
Calories: 155 Fat: 8.3g Carbohydrate: 17.5g Protein 3.6g

949. Crème Brûlée
⏱ Prep Time 15 m | ⏱ Cooking Time 35 m | 4 Servings

Ingredients:
- 1/3 cup granulated sugar, plus 4 tablespoons for topping
- 4 large egg yolks
- 1 1/2 cups heavy cream
- 1 teaspoon vanilla extract
- Pinch fine salt

Directions:
1. Place 1/3 cup of the granulated sugar and 4 large egg yolks in a medium bowl and whisk to combine. While whisking constantly, pour in 1 1/2 cups cream. Add 1 teaspoon vanilla extract and a pinch of fine salt and whisk to combine. Pour through a fine-mesh strainer into a large liquid measuring cup — this will make it easier to fill the ramekins.
2. Divide the base into 4 (4-ounce) ramekins. Cover each ramekin tightly with aluminum foil.
3. Place 1 cup water in an Instant Pot or electric pressure cooker. Set a trivet or pressure cooker baking sling inside the pot. Nestle the ramekins on the trivet.
4. Lock on the lid and make sure the pressure valve is set to seal. Use the manual function to set to cook for 7 minutes on "Low" pressure. It will take about 10 minutes to come up to pressure.

When the cook time is up, let the pressure naturally release for 15 minutes. Quick release any remaining pressure and carefully remove the lid.

5. Place the ramekins on a baking sheet. Refrigerate until thoroughly chilled, at least 4 hours or overnight.
6. About 10 minutes before serving, remove the ramekins from the refrigerator. Sprinkle each ramekin with 1 tablespoon granulated sugar and shake the ramekin to spread the sugar out into an even layer.
7. Arrange an oven rack in the highest position and preheat the broiler. Place the baking sheet with the ramekins on the rack and broil until golden brown and bubbling, rotating them frequently so that they broil evenly, 3 to 5 minutes total. Serve immediately.

Nutrition:
Calories: 275 Fat: 21.2g Carbohydrate: 18.7g Protein: 3.6g

950. Arroz con Leche
⏱ Prep Time 15 m | ⏱ Cooking Time 20 m | 12 Servings

Ingredients
Rice:
- ¾ cup long grain rice white
- 1 ¼ cups water
- 2 cups whole milk
- 1/8 Teaspoon kosher salt

After cooking:
- 1 can sweetened condensed milk 14 ounces
- 1 teaspoon vanilla extract
- Ground cinnamon for topping

Directions:
1. Rinse the rice using a mesh strainer until the water runs clean. I like the brand Mahatma.
2. Add the milk, water, rice and salt to the Instant Pot and stir.
3. Set the Instant Pot on the Porridge setting (20 minutes).
4. Allow for a 10 minute NPR (natural pressure release) and then release the remaining pressure and open the pot.
5. Add the can of condensed milk and the teaspoon of vanilla extract to the rice. Mix it all together. Serve warm and enjoy!

Nutrition:
Calories: 188 Carbohydrates: 32g Protein: 4g Fat: 4g

951. Key Lime Pie
⏱ Prep Time 15 m | ⏱ Cooking Time 15 m | 8 Servings

Ingredients
- For Crust
- 1 cup graham crackers or vanilla cookies
- 4 tablespoons unsalted butter melted
- For Key Lime Filling
- 3 egg yolks large
- 2/3 cup key lime juice (approx. 8-9 key limes)
- 1 tablespoon key lime zest (approx.) 2-3 key limes
- 1 (14 ounces) can sweetened condensed milk
- 2 tablespoons sugar (omit if you like it super tangy)
- Topping (optional)
- 1/2 cup heavy cream
- 1/4 cup sugar
- 1 teaspoon key lime zest for garnish optional

Directions:
1. Spray a 7" spring form pan with nonstick spray
2. Ground the crackers in the food processor. In a bowl, mix the graham cracker crumbs with the melted butter
3. Press this mixture into the bottom and sides of the spring form pan. Freeze while making the filling
4. Place the egg yolks and sugar in a bowl. Using a mixer on medium-high speed, mix until the yolks turn pale yellow and thicken (about 2-3 minutes)
5. Add the condensed milk and keep mixing. Add the key lime juice and zest. Mix until combined
6. Pour this mixture on top of the prepared crust. Cover the spring form pan with aluminum foil
7. Make a sling with aluminum foil: Break a long piece of foil and fold into 3. The idea is to get a long thin rectangle (helps remove the pie from the instant pot quicker)
8. Pour 1 cup of water in the instant pot. Place trivet on top. Put the sling in and place the pie on top. Cover with lid and lock in place
9. Cook on manual high pressure for 15 minutes (15 MHP). Let the pie cool for 10 minutes before releasing the pressure (10 NPR)
10. Remove the pie from the instant pot using the sling and cool and remove the aluminum foil cover. Center should be a bit jiggly. Refrigerate for 3-4 hours or until set
11. For Topping: Whip cream and slowly add the sugar until the cream becomes stiff. Pipe on top of pie and decorate with zest. Enjoy!

Nutrition:
Calories: 212 Fat: 14g Carbohydrates: 20g Protein: 2g

952. Dulce De Leche
⏰ Prep Time 5 m | ⏱ Cooking Time 35 m | 10 Servings

Ingredients
- 1 (14- ounce) can sweetened condensed milk

Directions:
1. Transfer sweetened condensed milk to a glass jar with a sealed lid. Place the trivet in the bottom of the Instant Pot Pressure Cooker and place the jar on the trivet. Fill the Instant Pot with water until it is about an inch beneath the lid of the jar (above where the condensed milk is and below the lid). Close the Instant Pot, making sure the valve is closed, and choose Manual, High Heat, 35 minutes. It will take about 30 minutes to heat up since there is a considerable amount of water in the pot.
2. When it's done cooking, quick release the steam, and open the pot. Using tongs, remove the jar from the water, or allow it to cool before removing.
3. Transfer the jar to a wire rack and cool completely before opening the lid. The dulce de leche will be bubbling inside the jar for a bit of time. Do not open the jar, as pressure has built. Wait until it cools!

Nutrition:
Calories: 172 Fat: 4.7g Carbohydrate: 29.1g Protein 4.2g

953. Blueberry Muffins
⏰ Prep Time 15 m | ⏱ Cooking Time 15 m | 6 Servings

Ingredients:
- ¼ cup blueberries
- ½ teaspoon vanilla extract
- ¼ teaspoon lemon zest
- ½ cup all-purpose flour
- ¾ teaspoon baking powder
- 3 tablespoons sour cream
- 1 teaspoon sanding sugar, for topping (optional)
- 1 egg white
- 1/8 teaspoon salt
- 3 tablespoons vegetable oil
- ¼ granulated sugar

Directions:
1. In a small bowl, whisk together the flour, baking powder and salt.
2. In a medium bowl, whisk together the sugar and oil.
3. Into the sugar and oil mixture. Whisk the egg white sour cream and vanilla. Don't over mix.
4. Add the dry mixture to the wet, and mix until just incorporated
5. Fold in the blueberries and lemon zest
6. Divide the batter evenly among 4 silicone muffin cups, filling them about two-thirds full.
7. Sprinkle each muffin with sanding sugar.
8. Bake for 12 minutes or until a toothpick inserted into the center of a muffin comes out clean and serve warm.

Nutrition:
Calories: 202 Carbs: 29g Fat: 8g Protein: 3g

954. Homemade Nutella Pie
⏰ Prep Time 10 m | ⏱ Cooking Time 10 m | 4 Servings

Ingredients:
- 8 ounces whipped topping
- 5 tablespoons melted butter
- 25 Oreo cookies
- 13 ounces Nutella
- 8 ounces cream cheese

Directions:
1. Ground Oreo cookies and put them in a bowl. Pour melted butter over cookie mixture and stir well. Pour the mixture in a pan and press with a cup and place in freezer for 20 minutes. Now pour some Nutella over the pie crust and place in freezer again. Take a bowl add cream cheese and remaining Nutella and beat until creamy, mix with whipped topping and pour into the mixture and spread evenly. Refrigerate for 2 hours before serving.

Nutrition:
Calories: 179 Carbs: 27g Fat: 7g Protein: 3g

955. Keto Chocolate Muffins
⏰ Prep Time 15 m | ⏱ Cooking Time 25 m | 6 Servings

Ingredients:
- 3 eggs
- 1 teaspoon vanilla extract
- ½ cup coco powder
- ½ cup sugar free chocolate chips
- 1 cup almond flour
- 3 ounces butter
- 2/3 cup heavy cream
- 1 ½ teaspoon baking powder
- ½ cup erythritol

Directions:
1. Take a bowl add almond flour, coco powder, erythritol and baking powder, then add vanilla extract, eggs and heavy cream and mix well. After that add butter and mix again, then add chocolate chips and stir. Grease muffin cups and prepare 12 cups filled with mixture. Bake into preheated oven 175c for 20 minutes. Allow them to cool and serve.

Nutrition:
Calories: 158 Carbs: 4g Fat: 15g Protein: 5g

956. Cream Cheese Pancakes
⏰ Prep Time 10 m | ⏱ Cooking Time 15 m | 6 Servings

Ingredients:
- Butter for grease
- Vanilla extract or cinnamon
- 4 ounces cream cheese
- 4 eggs

Directions:
1. Take an electric blender adds cream cheese and eggs into it and beat well until mixture turn smooth. Set mixture aside for few minutes. Now heat skilled and grease with butter. Take 1/8 cup of mixture and pour it into skilled. Cook for a minute and then flip and cook another side for a minute and dish out in plate. Make 12 to 14 pancakes and serve with sprinkle cinnamon or sugar dust and enjoy.

Nutrition: Calories: 344 Carbs: 3g Fat: 29g Protein: 17g

957. Sweet Cream Canes

🕐 Prep Time 5 m | 🕐 Cooking Time 15 m | 4 Servings

Ingredients:

- 500ml custard
- 1 egg
- Sugar glass (to decorate)
- 1 plate of puff pastry 250grs

Directions:

1. You cut the puff pastry into 1cm wide strips.
2. You roll the strips in the molds.
3. You paint the surface with beaten egg and place them in the fryer to brown it, without oil.
4. After filling with the cream you sprinkle them with the glass sugar and that's it!
5.

Nutrition: Calories: 50 Carbs: 12g Fat: 0g Protein: 0g

958. Fast Crème Brulee

🕐 Prep Time 10 m | 🕐 Cooking Time 15 m | 8 Servings

Ingredients:

- 6 tablespoons sugar
- 3 cups heavy whipping cream
- 7 large Egg Yolks
- 2 cups water
- 2 tablespoons Vanilla Extract

Directions:

1. In a mixing bowl, add the yolks, vanilla, whipping cream and half of the swerve sugar. Use a whisk to mix them until they are well combined.
2. Pour the mixture into the ramekins and cover them with aluminum foil.
3. Open the cooker, fit the reversible rack into the pot and pour in the water.
4. Place 3 ramekins on the rack and place the remaining ramekins to sit on the edges of the ramekins below.
5. Close the lid, secure the pressure valve and select Pressure mode on high for 8 minutes. Press Start.
6. Once the timer has stopped, do a natural pressure release for 10 minutes, then a quick pressure release to let out the remaining pressure.
7. With a napkin in hand, remove the ramekins onto a flat surface and then into a refrigerators to chill for at least 6 hours.
8. After refrigerators, remove the ramekins and remove the aluminum foil.
9. Equally, sprinkle the remaining sugar on it and return to the pot. Close the crisping lid, select Bake mode, set the timer to 4 minutes on 380 F. Serve the crème brulee chilled with whipped cream.

Nutrition: Calories: 135 Carbs: 21g Fat: 4g Protein: 4g

959. Strawberry Ricotta Cheesecake

🕐 Prep Time 10 m | 🕐 Cooking Time 25 m | 6 Servings

Ingredients:

- 1 teaspoon lemon Extract
- 3 tablespoons Sour Cream
- 1 ½ cups water
- 10 strawberries, halved to decorate
- ½ cup Ricotta Cheese
- 10 ounces Cream Cheese
- ¼ cup sugar
- One lemon, zested and juiced
- 2 eggs, cracked into a bowl

Directions:

1. In the electric mixer, add the cream cheese, quarter cup of sugar, ricotta cheese, lemon zest, lemon juice and lemon extract. Turn on the mixer and mix the ingredients until a smooth consistency is formed. Adjust the sweet taste to liking with more sugar.
2. Reduce the speed of the mixer and add the eggs. Fold it in at low speed until it is fully incorporated. Make sure not to fold the eggs in high speed to prevent a cracker crust. Grease the spring form pan with cooking spray and use a spatula to spoon the mixture into the pan. Level the top with the spatula and cover it with foil.
3. Open the cooker, fit in the reversible rack and pour in the water. Place the cake pan on the rack. Close the lid, secure the pressure valve and select pressure mode on high pressure for 15 minutes. Press Start
4. Meanwhile, mix the sour cream and one tbsp. of sugar. Set aside.
5. Once the timer has gone off, do a natural pressure release for 10 minutes, then a quick pressure release to let out any extra steam and open the lid?
6. Remove the rack with pan, place the spring form pan on a flat surface and open it. Use a spatula to spread the sour cream mixture on the warm cake. Refrigerate the cake for 8 hours. Top with strawberries, slice it into 6 pieces and serve while firming.

Nutrition: Calories: 280 Carbs: 21g Fat: 19g Protein: 4g

960. Classic New York Cheesecake

⏱ Prep Time 10 m | ⏱ Cooking Time 45 m | 6 Servings

Ingredients:

- ½ cup brown sugar
- ¼ cup sour cream
- 4 tablespoons butter, melted
- 16 ounces cream cheese, softened
- 2 tablespoons sugar
- 1 ½ cups finely crushed graham crackers
- 2 eggs
- 1 cup water
- Fresh Strawberries, cut in half lengthwise for garnish
- ½ teaspoon salt
- 1 ½ teaspoons Vanilla extract
- 1 tablespoon all-purpose flour

Directions:

1. Line a cake pan with parchment paper and grease with cooking spray the paper.
2. In a medium mixing bowl, mix the graham cracker crumbs, sugar and butter. Spoon the mixture into the pan and press firmly into with a spoon.
3. In a deep bowl and with a hand mixer, beat the beat the cream cheese and brown sugar until well-mixed. Whisk in the sour cream to be smooth and stir in the flour, vanilla and salt.
4. Crack the eggs in and beat but not to be overly smooth. Pour the mixture into the pan over the crumbs.
5. Next, pour the water into the pot. Put the pan on the reversible rack and put the rack in the pot. Seal the pressure lid, choose Pressure, set to high and set the time to 35 minutes. Choose Start.
6. Once done baking, perform a natural pressure release for 10 minutes. Carefully open the lid.
7. Remove the pan from the rack and allow the cheesecake to cool for 1 hour. Cover the cheesecake with foil and chill in the refrigerator for 4 hours to serve. Decorate with strawberry halves.

Nutrition: Calories: 350 Carbs: 30g Fat: 23g Protein: 6g

961. Mini Cheesecakes

⏱ Prep Time 15 m | ⏱ Cooking Time 10 m | 2 Servings

Ingredients:

- ¾ cup erythritol
- eggs
- teaspoon vanilla extract
- ½ teaspoon fresh lemon juice
- 16 oz. Cream cheese, softened
- tablespoon sour cream

Directions:

1. In a blender, add the erythritol, eggs, vanilla extract and lemon juice and pulse until smooth.
2. Add the cream cheese and sour cream and pulse until smooth.
3. Place the mixture into 2 (4-inch) springform pans evenly.
4. Press "power button" of air fry oven and turn the dial to select the "air fry" mode.
5. Press the time button and again turn the dial to set the cooking time to 10 minutes.
6. Now push the temp button and rotate the dial to set the temperature at 350 degrees f.
7. Press "start/pause" button to start.
8. When the unit beeps to show that it is preheated, open the lid.
9. Arrange the pans in "air fry basket" and insert in the oven.
10. Place the pans onto a wire rack to cool completely.
11. Refrigerate overnight before serving.

Nutrition:
Calories 886 Fat 86 g Saturated fat 52.8 g Cholesterol 418 mg Carbs 7.2 g Sugar 1.1 g Protein 23.1 g

962. Vanilla Cheesecake

⏱ Prep Time 15 m | ⏱ Cooking Time 14 m | 6 Servings

Ingredients:

- cup honey graham cracker crumbs
- tablespoons unsalted butter, softened
- (453.592g). Cream cheese, softened
- ½ cup sugar
- large eggs
- ½ teaspoon vanilla extract

Directions:

1. Line a round baking pan with parchment paper.
2. For crust: in a bowl, add the graham cracker crumbs, and butter.
3. Place the crust into baking dish and press to smooth.
4. Press "power button" of air fry oven and turn the dial to select the "air fry" mode.
5. Press the time button and again turn the dial to set the cooking time to 4 minutes.
6. Now push the temp button and rotate the dial to set the temperature at 350 degrees f.
7. Press "start/pause" button to start.
8. When the unit beeps to show that it is preheated, open the lid.
9. Arrange the baking pan of crust in "air fry basket" and insert in the oven.
10. Place the crust aside to cool for about 10 minutes.
11. Meanwhile, in a bowl, add the cream cheese, and sugar and whisk until smooth.
12. Now, place the eggs, one at a time and whisk until mixture becomes creamy.
13. Add the vanilla extract and mix well.
14. Place the cream cheese mixture evenly over the crust.
15. Press "power button" of air fry oven and turn the dial to select the "air fry" mode.
16. Press the time button and again turn the dial to set the cooking time to 10 minutes.
17. Now push the temp button and rotate the dial to set the temperature at 350 degrees f.
18. Press "start/pause" button to start.
19. When the unit beeps to show that it is preheated, open the lid.
20. Arrange the baking pan of crust in "air fry basket" and insert in the oven.
21. Place the pan onto a wire rack to cool completely.
22. Refrigerate overnight before serving.

Nutrition:
Calories 470 Fat 33.9 g Saturated fat 20.6 g Cholesterol 155 mg Carbs 34.9 g Sugar 22 g Protein 9.4g

963. Ricotta Cheesecake
🕐 Prep Time 15 m | 🕐 Cooking Time 25 m | 8 Servings

Ingredients:
- oz. Ricotta cheese
- eggs
- ¾ cup sugar
- tablespoons corn starch
- tablespoon fresh lemon juice
- teaspoons vanilla extract
- teaspoon fresh lemon zest, finely grated

Directions:
1. In a large bowl, place all ingredients and mix until well combined.
2. Place the mixture into a baking pan.
3. Press "power button" of air fry oven and turn the dial to select the "air fry" mode.
4. Press the time button and again turn the dial to set the cooking time to 25 minutes.
5. Now push the temp button and rotate the dial to set the temperature at 320 degrees f.
6. Press "start/pause" button to start.
7. When the unit beeps to show that it is preheated, open the lid.
8. Arrange the pan in "air fry basket" and insert in the oven.
9. Place the cake pan onto a wire rack to cool completely.
10. Refrigerate overnight before serving.

Nutrition:
Calories 197 Fat 6.6 g Saturated fat 3.6 g Cholesterol 81 mg Carbs 25.7 g Sugar 19.3 g Protein 9.2 g

964. Pecan Pie
🕐 Prep Time 15 m | 🕐 Cooking Time 35 m | 2 Servings

Ingredients:
- ¾ cup brown sugar
- ¼ cup caster sugar
- 1/3 cup butter, melted
- large eggs
- 1¾ tablespoons flour
- tablespoon milk
- 1 teaspoon vanilla extract
- 1 cup pecan halves
- 1 frozen pie crust, thawed

Directions:
1. In a large bowl, mix together the sugars, and butter.
2. Add the eggs and whisk until foamy.
3. Add the flour, milk, and vanilla extract and whisk until well combined.
4. Fold in the pecan halves.
5. Grease a pie pan.
6. Arrange the crust in the bottom of prepared pie pan.
7. Place the pecan mixture over the crust evenly.
8. Press "power button" of air fry oven and turn the dial to select the "air fry" mode.
9. Press the time button and again turn the dial to set the cooking time to 22 minutes.
10. Now push the temp button and rotate the dial to set the temperature at 300 degrees f.
11. Press "start/pause" button to start.
12. When the unit beeps to show that it is preheated, open the lid.
13. Arrange the pan in "air fry basket" and insert in the oven.
14. After 22 minutes of cooking, to set the temperature at w85 degrees f for 13 minutes.
15. Place the pie pan onto a wire rack to cool for about 10-15 minutes before serving.

Nutrition:
Calories 501 Fat 35 g Saturated fat 10.8 g Cholesterol 107 mg Carbs 44.7 g Sugar 36.7 g Protein 6.2g

965. Fruity Crumble
🕐 Prep Time 15 m | 🕐 Cooking Time 20 m | 4 Servings

Ingredients:
- ½ lb. (226.8g) Fresh apricots, pitted and cubed
- cup fresh blackberries
- 1/3 cup sugar, divided
- 1 tablespoon fresh lemon juice
- 7/8 cup flour
- Pinch of salt
- 1 tablespoon cold water
- ¼ cup chilled butter, cubed

Directions:
1. Grease a baking pan.
2. In a large bowl, mix well apricots, blackberries, 2 tablespoons of sugar, and lemon juice.
3. Spread apricot mixture into the prepared baking pan.
4. In another bowl, add the flour, remaining sugar, salt, water, and butter and mix until a crumbly mixture forms.
5. Spread the flour mixture over apricot mixture evenly.
6. Press "power button" of air fry oven and turn the dial to select the "air fry" mode.
7. Press the time button and again turn the dial to set the cooking time to 20 minutes.
8. Now push the temp button and rotate the dial to set the temperature at 390 degrees f.
9. Press "start/pause" button to start.
10. When the unit beeps to show that it is preheated, open the lid.
11. Arrange the pan in "air fry basket" and insert in the oven.
12. Place the pan onto a wire rack to cool for about 10-15 minutes before serving.

Nutrition:
Calories 307 Fat 12.4 g Saturated fat 7.4 g Cholesterol 31 mg Carbs 47.3 g Sugar 23.7 g Protein 4.2 g

966. Cherry Clafoutis

🕐 Prep Time 15 m | 🕐 Cooking Time 25 m | 4 Servings

Ingredients:

- 1½ cups fresh cherries, pitted
- tablespoons vodka
- ¼ cup flour
- tablespoons sugar
- Pinch of salt
- ½ cup sour cream
- egg
- 1 tablespoon butter
- ¼ cup powdered sugar

Directions:

1. In a bowl, mix together the cherries and vodka.
2. In another bowl, mix together the flour, sugar, and salt.
3. Add the sour cream, and egg and mix until a smooth dough forms.
4. Grease a cake pan.
5. Place flour mixture evenly into the prepared cake pan.
6. Spread cherry mixture over the dough.
7. Place butter on top in the form of dots.
8. Press "power button" of air fry oven and turn the dial to select the "air fry" mode.
9. Press the time button and again turn the dial to set the cooking time to 25 minutes.
10. Now push the temp button and rotate the dial to set the temperature at 355 degrees f.
11. Press "start/pause" button to start.
12. When the unit beeps to show that it is preheated, open the lid.
13. Arrange the pan in "air fry basket" and insert in the oven.
14. Place the pan onto a wire rack to cool for about 10-15 minutes before serving.
15. Now, invert the clafoutis onto a platter and sprinkle with powdered sugar.
16. Cut the clafoutis into desired size slices and serve warm.

Nutrition:
Calories 241 Fat 10.1 g Saturated fat 5.9 g Cholesterol 61 mg Carbs 29 g Sugar 20.6 g Protein 3.9 g

967. Apple Bread Pudding

🕐 Prep Time 15 m | 🕐 Cooking Time 44 m | 8 Servings

Ingredients:

For bread pudding:
- 10½ oz. Bread, cubed
- ½ cup apple, peeled, cored and chopped
- ½ cup raisins
- ¼ cup walnuts, chopped
- 1½ cups milk
- ¾ cup water
- tablespoons honey
- teaspoons ground cinnamon
- teaspoons cornstarch
- teaspoon vanilla extract
For topping:
- 1 1/3 cups plain flour
- 3/5 cup brown sugar
- tablespoons butter

Directions:

1. In a large bowl, mix together the bread, apple, raisins, and walnuts.
2. In another bowl, add the remaining pudding ingredients and mix until well combined.
3. Add the milk mixture into bread mixture and mix until well combined.
4. Refrigerate for about 15 minutes, tossing occasionally.
5. For topping: in a bowl, mix together the flour and sugar.
6. With a pastry cutter, cut in the butter until a crumbly mixture forms.
7. Place the mixture into 2 baking pans and spread the topping mixture on top of each.
8. Press "power button" of air fry oven and turn the dial to select the "air fry" mode.
9. Press the time button and again turn the dial to set the cooking time to 22 minutes.
10. Now push the temp button and rotate the dial to set the temperature at 355 degrees f.
11. Press "start/pause" button to start.
12. When the unit beeps to show that it is preheated, open the lid.
13. Arrange 1 pan in "air fry basket" and insert in the oven.
14. Place the pan onto a wire rack to cool slightly before serving.
15. Repeat with the remaining pan.
16. Serve warm.

Nutrition:
Calories 432 Fat 14.8 g Saturated fat 7.4 g Cholesterol 30 mg Carbs 69.1 g Sugar 32 g Protein 7.9 g

968. Raisin Bread Pudding

🕐 Prep Time 15 m | 🕐 Cooking Time 12 m | 3 Servings

Ingredients:

- cup milk
- 1 egg
- 1 tablespoon brown sugar
- ½ teaspoon ground cinnamon
- ¼ teaspoon vanilla extract
- tablespoons raisins, soaked in hot water for about 15 minutes
- bread slices, cut into small cubes
- 1 tablespoon chocolate chips
- 1 tablespoon sugar

Directions:

1. In a bowl, mix together the milk, egg, brown sugar, cinnamon, and vanilla extract.
2. Stir in the raisins.
3. In a baking pan, spread the bread cubes and top evenly with the milk mixture.
4. Refrigerate for about 15-20 minutes.
5. Press "power button" of air fry oven and turn the dial to select the "air fry" mode.
6. Press the time button and again turn the dial to set the cooking time to 12 minutes.
7. Now push the temp button and rotate the dial to set the temperature at 375 degrees f.
8. Press "start/pause" button to start.
9. When the unit beeps to show that it is preheated, open the lid.
10. Arrange the pan over the "wire rack" and insert in the oven.
11. Serve warm.

Nutrition:
Calories 143 Fat 4.4 g Saturated fat 2.2 g Cholesterol 628 mg Carbs 21.3 g Sugar 16.4 g Protein 5.5 g

969. Donuts Pudding

☺ Prep Time 15 m | ☻ Cooking Time 1 h | 6 Servings

Ingredients:
- glazed donuts, cut into small pieces
- ¾ cup frozen sweet cherries
- ½ cup raisins
- ½ cup semi-sweet chocolate baking chips
- ¼ cup sugar
- teaspoon ground cinnamon
- 1 egg yolks
- 1½ cups whipping cream

Directions:

1. In a large bowl, mix together the donut pieces, cherries, raisins, chocolate chips, sugar, and cinnamon.
2. In another bowl, add the egg yolks, and whipping cream and whisk until well combined.
3. Add the egg yolk mixture into doughnut mixture and mix well.
4. Line a baking dish with a piece of foil.
5. Place donuts mixture into the prepared baking pan.
6. Press "power button" of air fry oven and turn the dial to select the "air fry" mode.
7. Press the time button and again turn the dial to set the cooking time to 60 minutes.
8. Now push the temp button and rotate the dial to set the temperature at 360 degrees f.
9. Press "start/pause" button to start.
10. When the unit beeps to show that it is preheated, open the lid.
11. Arrange the pan in "air fry basket" and insert in the oven.
12. Place the pan onto a wire rack to cool for about 10-15 minutes before serving.
13. Serve warm.

Nutrition:
Calories 537 Fat 28.7g Saturated fat 12.2g Cholesterol 173mg Carbs 65.1g Sugar 32.8 g Protein 6.5 g

970. Apricot Crumble With Blackberries

☺ Prep Time 30 m | ☻ Cooking Time 20 m | 4 Servings

Ingredients
- ½ cups fresh apricots, de-stoned and cubed
- cup fresh blackberries
- ½ cup sugar
- 1 tbsp lemon juice
- 1 cup flour
- Salt as needed
- 1 tbsp butter

Directions

1. Add the apricot cubes to a bowl and mix with lemon juice, 2 tbsp sugar, and blackberries. Scoop the mixture into a greased dish and spread it evenly. In another bowl, mix flour and remaining sugar.
2. Add 1 tbsp of cold water and butter and keep mixing until you have a crumbly mixture. Preheat air fryer on bake function to 390 f and place the fruit mixture in the basket. Top with crumb mixture and cook for 20 minutes.

Nutrition:
Calories: 546, Protein: 7g, Fat: 5.23g, Carbs: 102.53g

971. Apple & Cinnamon Pie

☺ Prep Time 30 m | ☻ Cooking Time 10 m | 9 Servings

Ingredients
- 2 apples, diced
- 1 oz butter, melted
- 1 oz sugar
- 1 oz brown sugar
- tsp cinnamon
- 1 egg, beaten
- large puff pastry sheets
- ¼ tsp salt

Directions

1. Whisk white sugar, brown sugar, cinnamon, salt, and butter, together. Place the apples in a baking dish and coat them with the mixture. Place the baking dish in the toaster oven, and cook for 10 minutes at 350 f on bake function.
2. Meanwhile, roll out the pastry on a floured flat surface, and cut each sheet into 6 equal pieces. Divide the apple filling between the pieces. Brush the edges of the pastry squares with the egg.
3. Fold them and seal the edges with a fork. Place on a lined baking sheet and cook in the fryer at 350 f for 8 minutes. Flip over, increase the temperature to 390 f, and cook for 2 more minutes.

Nutrition:
Calories: 140, Protein: 1.28g, Fat: 6.33g, Carbs: 21.19g

972. Berry Crumble With Lemon

☺ Prep Time 30 m | ☻ Cooking Time 20 m | 6 Servings

Ingredients
- 1 oz fresh strawberries
- 1 oz fresh raspberries
- 1 oz fresh blueberries
- 1 tbsp cold butter
- 1 tbsp lemon juice
- 1 cup flour
- ½ cup sugar
- 1 tbsp water
- A pinch of salt

Directions

1. Gently mass the berries, but make sure there are chunks left. Mix with the lemon juice and 2 tbsp. Of the sugar.
2. Place the berry mixture at the bottom of a prepared round cake. Combine the flour with the salt and sugar, in a bowl. Add the water and rub the butter with your fingers until the mixture becomes crumbled.
3. Arrange the crisp batter over the berries. Cook in the fryer at 390 f for 20 minutes on bake function. Serve chilled.

Nutrition:
Calories: 250, Protein: 3.2g, Fat: 10.28g, Carbs: 38.09g

973. Vanilla-Lemon Cupcakes With Lemon Glaze
⏱ Prep Time 30 m | ⏱ Cooking Time 13-16 m | 6 Servings

Ingredients
- 1 cup flour
- ½ cup sugar
- 1 small egg
- 1 tsp lemon zest
- ¾ tsp baking powder
- ¼ tsp baking soda
- ½ tsp salt
- 1 tbsp vegetable oil
- ½ cup milk
- ½ tsp vanilla extract
Glaze:
- ½ cup powdered sugar
- 1 tsp lemon juice

Directions
1. Preheat air fryer on bake function to 350 f, and combine all dry muffin ingredients, in a bowl. In another bowl, whisk together the wet ingredients. Gently combine the two mixtures. Divide the batter between 6 greased muffin tins. Place the muffin tins in the toaster oven and cook for 13 to 16 minutes.
2. Meanwhile, whisk the powdered sugar with the lemon juice. Spread the glaze over the muffins.

Nutrition:
Calories: 204, Protein: 3.6g, Fat: 6.01g, Carbs: 34.06g

974. Handmade Donuts
⏱ Prep Time 25 m | ⏱ Cooking Time 15 m | 4 Servings

Ingredients
- 1 oz self-rising flour
- 1 tsp baking powder
- ½ cup milk
- ½ tbsp butter
- 1 egg
- 1 oz brown sugar

Directions
1. Preheat air fryer on bake function to 350 f, and beat the butter with the sugar, until smooth. Beat in eggs, and milk. In a bowl, combine the flour with the baking powder. Gently fold the flour into the butter mixture.
2. Form donut shapes and cut off the center with cookie cutters. Arrange on a lined baking sheet and cook in the fryer for 15 minutes. Serve with whipped cream or icing.

Nutrition:
Calories: 370, Protein: 8.89g, Fat: 11.16g, Carbs: 57.94g

975. Apple Treat With Raisins
⏱ Prep Time 15 m | ⏱ Cooking Time 10 m | 4 Servings

Ingredients
- 2 apples, cored
- ½ oz almonds
- ¾ oz raisins
- 1 tbsp sugar

Directions
1. Preheat air fryer on bake function to 360 f and in a bowl, mix sugar, almonds, raisins. Blend the mixture using a hand mixer. Fill cored apples with the almond mixture. Place the prepared apples in your air fryer basket and cook for 10 minutes. Serve with powdered sugar.

Nutrition:
Calories: 188, Protein: 2.88g, Fat: 5.64g, Carbs: 35.63g

976. Almond Cookies With Dark Chocolate
⏱ Prep Time 145 m | ⏱ Cooking Time 35 m | 4 Servings

Ingredients
- 1 egg whites
- ½ tsp almond extract
- ⅓ cups sugar
- ¼ tsp salt
- 1 tsp lemon juice
- 1 ½ tsp vanilla extract
- Melted dark chocolate to drizzle

Directions
2. In a mixing bowl, add egg whites, salt, and lemon juice. Beat using an electric mixer until foamy. Slowly add the sugar and continue beating until completely combined; add the almond and vanilla extracts. Beat until stiff peaks form and glossy.
3. Line a round baking sheet with parchment paper. Fill a piping bag with the meringue mixture and pipe as many mounds on the baking sheet as you can leaving 2-inch spaces between each mound.
4. Place the baking sheet in the fryer basket and bake at 250 f for 5 minutes on bake function. Reduce the temperature to 220 f and bake for 15 more minutes. Then, reduce the temperature to 190 f and cook for 15 minutes. Remove the baking sheet and let the meringues cool for 2 hours. Drizzle with dark chocolate and serve.

Nutrition:
Calories: 170, Protein: 7.24g, Fat: 0.19g, Carbs: 34.06g

977. Air Fried Banana With Sesame Seeds
⏱ Prep Time 15 m | ⏱ Cooking Time 8-10 m | 5 Servings

Ingredients
- ½ cups flour
- 2 bananas, sliced
- 1 tsp salt
- 1 tbsp sesame seeds
- 1 cup water
- 2 eggs, beaten
- 1 tsp baking powder
- ½ tbsp sugar

Directions
1. Preheat air fryer on bake function to 340 f.
2. In a bowl, mix salt, sesame seeds, flour, baking powder, eggs, sugar, and water. Coat sliced bananas with the flour mixture; place the prepared slices in the air fryer basket; cook for 8-10 minutes. Serve chilled.

Nutrition:
Calories: 327, Protein: 9.73g, Fat: 7.55g, Carbs: 57.33g

978. Vanilla Brownies With Chocolate Chips
⏱ Prep Time 25 m | ⏱ Cooking Time 20 m | 2 Servings

Ingredients
- 1 whole egg, beaten
- ¼ cup chocolate chips
- 1 tbsp white sugar
- ⅓ cup flour
- 1 tbsp safflower oil
- 1 tsp vanilla
- ¼ cup cocoa powder

Directions
1. Preheat air fryer on bake function to 320 f and in a bowl, mix the beaten egg, sugar, oil, and vanilla. In another bowl, mix cocoa powder and flour. Add the flour mixture to the vanilla mixture and stir until fully incorporated. Pour the mixture into the baking pan and sprinkle chocolate chips on top. Cook for 20 minutes. Chill and cut into squares to serve.

Nutrition: Calories: 321, Protein: 8.56g, Fat: 20.03g, Carbs: 30.78g

979. Cinnamon & Honey Apples With Hazelnuts
⏱ Prep Time 13 m | ⏱ Cooking Time 10 m | 2 Servings

Ingredients
- 4 Apples
- 1 oz butter
- 1 oz breadcrumbs
- Zest of 1 orange
- 1 tbsp chopped hazelnuts
- 1 oz mixed seeds
- 1 tsp cinnamon
- 1 tbsp honey

Directions
1. Preheat air fryer on bake function to 350 f and core the apples. Make sure also to score their skin to prevent from splitting. Combine the remaining ingredients in a bowl; stuff the apples with the mixture and cook for 10 minutes. Serve topped with chopped hazelnuts.

Nutrition: Calories: 1174, Protein: 22.74g, Fat: 82.57g, Carbs: 106.11g

980. Pan-Fried Bananas
⏱ Prep Time 15 m | ⏱ Cooking Time 8-12 m | 8 Servings

Ingredients
- 2 bananas
- 1 tbsp vegetable oil
- 1 tbsp corn flour
- 1 egg white
- ¾ cup breadcrumbs

Directions
Preheat air fryer on toast function to 350 f. Combine oil and breadcrumbs in a bowl. Coat the bananas with the corn flour, brush with egg white, and dip in the breadcrumb mixture. Arrange on a lined baking sheet and cook for 8-12 minutes.

Nutrition: Calories: 162, Protein: 1.93g, Fat: 5.6g, Carbs: 29.09g

981. Delicious Banana Pastry With Berries
⏱ Prep Time 15 m | ⏱ Cooking Time 10-12 m | 2 Servings

Ingredients
- 2 bananas, sliced
- 1 tbsp honey
- 1 puff pastry sheets, cut into thin strips
- Fresh berries to serve

Directions
1. Preheat air fryer on airfry function to 340 f and place the banana slices into the cooking basket. Cover with the pastry strips and top with honey. Cook for 10-12 minutes on bake function. Serve with fresh berries.

Nutrition: Calories: 253, Protein: 2.02g, Fat: 0.58g, Carbs: 66.38g

982. Easy Mocha Cake
⏱ Prep Time 30 m | ⏱ Cooking Time 15 m | 2 Servings

Ingredients
- ¼ cup butter
- ½ tsp instant coffee
- tbsp black coffee, brewed
- 1 egg
- ¼ cup sugar
- ¼ cup flour
- 1 tsp cocoa powder
- A pinch of salt
- Powdered sugar, for icing

Directions
1. Preheat air fryer on bake function to 330 f and grease a small ring cake pan. Beat the sugar and egg together in a bowl. Beat in cocoa, instant and black coffees; stir in salt and flour. Transfer the batter to the prepared pan. Cook for 15 minutes. Dust with powdered sugar and serve.

Nutrition: Calories: 377, Protein: 6.54g, Fat: 28.13g, Carbs: 25.65g

983. Choco Lava Cakes
⏱ Prep Time 20 m | ⏱ Cooking Time 10 m | 4 Servings

Ingredients
- ½ oz butter, melted
- ½ tbsp sugar
- ½ tbsp self-rising flour
- ½ oz dark chocolate, melted
- 2 eggs

Directions
1. Grease 4 ramekins with butter. Preheat air fryer on bake function to 375 f. Beat eggs and sugar until frothy. Stir in butter and chocolate; gently fold in the flour.
2. Divide the mixture between the ramekins and bake in the fryer for 10 minutes. Let cool for 2 minutes before turning the cakes upside down onto serving plates.

Nutrition:
Calories: 428, Protein: 6.92g, Fat: 35.54g, Carbs: 21.06g

984. Mouthwatering Chocolate Soufflé
⏲ Prep Time 25 m | ⏲ Cooking Time 14-18 m | 2 Servings

Ingredients
- 2 eggs, whites and yolks separated
- ¼ cup butter, melted
- 1 tbsp flour
- 1 tbsp sugar
- 1 oz chocolate, melted
- ½ tsp vanilla extract

Directions
1   Beat the yolks along with the sugar and vanilla extract; stir in butter, chocolate, and flour. Preheat air fryer on bake function to 330 f and whisk the whites until a stiff peak forms. Working in batches, gently combine the egg whites with the chocolate mixture. Divide the batter between two greased ramekins. Cook for 14-18 minutes.

Nutrition:
Calories: 455, Protein: 4.64g, Fat: 28.1g, Carbs: 46.38g

985. Maple Pecan Pie
⏲ Prep Time 1 h 10 m | ⏲ Cooking Time 30 m | 4 Servings

Ingredients
- ¾ cup maple syrup
- 2 eggs
- ½ tsp salt
- ¼ tsp nutmeg
- ½ tsp cinnamon
- 1 tbsp almond butter
- 1 tbsp brown sugar
- ½ cup chopped pecans
- tbsp butter, melted
- 1 8-inch pie dough
- ¾ tsp vanilla extract

Directions
1. Preheat air fryer on toast function to 350 f, and coat the pecans with the melted butter. Place the pecans in the fryer and toast them for 5 minutes. Place the pie crust into the baking pan, and scatter the pecans over.
2. Whisk together all remaining ingredients in a bowl. Pour the maple mixture over the pecans. Set air fryer to 320 f and cook the pie for 25 minutes on bake function.

Nutrition:
Calories: 2403, Protein: 19.26g, Fat: 136.07g, Carbs: 278g

986. Tangerine Cake
⏲ Prep Time 30 m | ⏲ Cooking Time 20 m | 8 Servings

Ingredients
- ¾ cup sugar
- cups flour
- ¼ cup olive oil
- ½ cup milk
- 1 tbsp. Cider vinegar
- ½ tbsp. Vanilla extract
- Juice and zest from 2 lemons
- Juice and zest from 1 tangerine
- Tangerine segments

Directions:
1. Mix in flour with sugar and turn.
2. Mix oil with vinegar, milk, vanilla extract, tangerine zest and lemon juice, then beat properly.
3. Put flour, turn properly, get mix into a cake pan, get in air fryer and cook at 360°f for 20 minutes.
4. Serve with tangerine segments over.

Nutrition:
Calories: 225, Protein: 3.75g, Fat: 7.58g, Carbs: 34.88g

987. Blueberry Pudding
⏲ Prep Time 35 m | ⏲ Cooking Time 25 m | 6 Servings

Ingredients
- 1 cups flour
- 1 cups rolled oats
- 1 cups blueberries
- stick butter
- 1 cup walnuts
- tbsp. Maple syrup
- tbsp. Rosemary

Directions:
1. Spray blueberries smeared baking pan and keep.
2. Mix rolled oats with walnuts, flour, butter, rosemary and maple syrup, beat properly, put mix over blueberries, put all in air fryer and cook at 350° for 25 minutes.
3. Allow to cool, slice.
4. Serve.

Nutrition:
Calories: 778, Protein: 14.16g, Fat: 27.75g, Carbs: 136.5g

988. Cocoa And Almond Bars
⏲ Prep Time 34 m | ⏲ Cooking Time 4 m | 6 Servings

Ingredients
- ¼ cup cocoa nibs
- 1 cup almonds
- 1 tbsp. Cocoa powder
- ¼ cup hemp seeds
- ¼ cup goji berries
- ¼ cup coconut
- 6 dates

Directions:
1   Blend almonds in food processor, put hemp seeds, cocoa powder, cocoa nibs, coconut, goji and beat properly.
2   Put dates, beat properly, spray on a lined baking sheet, get in air fryer and cook at 320°f for 4 minutes.
3   Slice into equal segment and allow in fridge for 30 minutes.
4   Serve.

Nutrition:
Calories: 76, Protein: 2.53g, Fat: 3.86g, Carbs: 11.82g

989. Chocolate And Pomegranate Bars
⏰ Prep Time 2h 10 m | ⏰ Cooking Time 10 m | 6 Servings

Ingredients
- ½ cup milk
- 1 tbsp. Vanilla extract
- 1 and ½ cups dark chocolate
- ½ cup almonds
- ½ cup pomegranate seeds

Directions:
1. Warm pan with milk over medium heat, put chocolate, turn for 5 minutes, remove heat, put half of the pomegranate seeds, vanilla extract and half of the nuts and turn.
2. Put mix into a lined baking pan, spray, spread a pinch of salt, nuts, and remaining pomegranate, get in air fryer and cook at 300° f for 4 minutes.
3. Allow in fridge for 2 hours then serve.

Nutrition:
Calories: 139, Protein: 2.37g, Fat: 8.17g, Carbs: 13.39g

990. Tomato Cake
⏰ Prep Time 40 m | ⏰ Cooking Time 30 m | 4 Servings

Ingredients
- ½ cups flour
- 1 tbsp. Cinnamon powder
- 1 tbsp. Baking powder
- 1 tbsp. Baking soda
- ¾ cup maple syrup
- 1 cup tomatoes
- ½ cup olive oil
- tbsp. Apple cider vinegar

Directions:
1. Mix in flour with baking soda, baking powder, maple syrup and cinnamon in a bowl then turn properly.
2. Mix in tomatoes with vinegar and olive oil in another bowl and turn properly.
3. Blend the 2 mixtures, turn properly, put into round pan, get into the fryer and cook at 360°f for 30 minutes.
4. Allow to cool, divide.
5. Serve.

Nutrition:
Calories: 519, Protein: 3.66g, Fat: 27.44g, Carbs: 66.54g

991. Berries Mix
⏰ Prep Time 11 m | ⏰ Cooking Time 6 m | 4 Servings

Ingredients
- tbsp. Lemon juice
- ½ tbsp. Maple syrup
- 1 and ½ tbsp. Champagne vinegar
- 1 tbsp. Olive oil
- 1 lb. (453.592g) Strawberries
- 1 and ½ cups blueberries
- ¼ cup basil leaves

Directions:
1. Mix in lemon juice with vinegar and maple syrup in a pan, boil over medium heat, put oil, strawberries and blueberries, turn, get in air fryer and cook at 310°f for 6 minutes.
2. Dust basil over then serve.

Nutrition:
Calories: 138, Protein: 1.21g, Fat: 3.95g, Carbs: 26.74g

992. Passion Fruit Pudding
⏰ Prep Time 50 m | ⏰ Cooking Time 40 m | 6 Servings

Ingredients
- cup paleo passion fruit curd
- passion fruits
- ½ oz. Maple syrup
- eggs
- oz. Ghee
- and ½ oz. Almond milk
- ½ cup almond flour
- ½ tbsp. Baking powder

Directions:
1. Mix in the half of the fruit curd with passion fruit seeds and pulp in a bowl, turn and slice into 6 heat proof ramekins.
2. Beat eggs with ghee, the rest of the curd, maple syrup, baking powder, flour and milk then turn properly.
3. Share mix into the ramekins also, get in the fryer and cook at 200° f for 40 minutes.
4. Allow pudding to cool.
5. Serve.

Nutrition:
Calories: 214, Protein: 6.33g, Fat: 9.92g, Carbs: 26.95g

993. Air Fried Apples
⏰ Prep Time 27 m | ⏰ Cooking Time 17 m | 4 Servings

Ingredients
- 4 big apples
- A handful raisins
- 1 tbsp. Cinnamon
- Raw honey

Directions:
1. Infuse each apple with raisins, spray cinnamon, sprinkle honey, get into air fryer and cook at 367°f for 17 minutes.
2. Allow to cool
3. Serve.

Nutrition:
Calories: 100, Protein: 0.55g, Fat: 0.33g, Carbs: 26.8g

994. Pumpkin Cookies
⏰ Prep Time 25 m | ⏱ Cooking Time 15 m | 4 Servings

Ingredients
- 2 and ½ cups flour
- ½ tbsp. Baking soda
- 1 tbsp. Flax seed
- 3 tbsp. Water
- ½ cup pumpkin flesh

- ¼ cup honey
- 2 tbsp. Butter
- 1 tbsp. Vanilla extract
- ½ cup dark chocolate chips

Directions:
1. Mix flax seed with water in a bowl, turn and allow for a while.
2. Mix flour with baking soda and salt in another bowl.
3. Mix in honey with pumpkin puree, vanilla extract, flaxseed and butter in third bowl.
4. Blend flour with chocolate chips and honey mix and turn.
5. Measure 1 tablespoon of cookie dough on a lined baking sheet. Do same with remaining dough, get into air fryer and cook at 350° f for 15 minutes.
6. Allow to cool.
7. Serve.

Nutrition:
Calories: 72, Protein: 1.94g, Fat: 2.14g, Carbs: 11.36g

995. Figs And Coconut Butter Mix
⏰ Prep Time 10 m | ⏱ Cooking Time 4 m | 3 Servings

Ingredient
- 2 tbsp. Coconut butter
- 12 figs
- ¼ cup sugar
- 1 cup almonds

Directions:
1. Melt butter in pan over medium heat.
2. Put figs, almonds and sugar. Toss, get into air fryer and cook at 300°f for 4 minutes.
3. Share into bowls then serve cold.

Nutrition:
Calories: 186, Protein: 1.27g, Fat: 8.19g, Carbs: 29.87g

996. Lemon Bars
⏰ Prep Time 35 m | ⏱ Cooking Time 25 m | 6 Servings

Ingredients
- 4 eggs
- 2 ¼ cups flour
- Lemon juice
- 1 cup butter
- 2 cups sugar

Directions:
1. Mix ½ cup sugar with butter and 2 cups flour in a bowl, turn properly, push to the bottom of a pan, get into the fryer and cook at 350°f for 10 minutes.
2. Mix in remaining flour, with the remaining sugar, lemon juice and eggs, beat properly and sprinkle over crust.
3. Put in the fryer at 350°f for 15 minutes still, allow to cool, slice bars.
4. Serve.

Nutrition:
Calories: 660, Protein: 11.17g, Fat: 37.59g, Carbs: 70.28g

997. Orange Sponge Cake
⏰ Prep Time 50 m | ⏱ Cooking Time 15 m | 6 Servings

Ingredients
- 9 oz sugar
- 9 oz self-rising flour
- 9 oz butter
- 3 eggs
- 1 tsp baking powder
- 1 tsp vanilla extract
- Zest of 1 orange

Frosting:
- 4 egg whites
- Juice of 1 orange
- 1 tsp orange food coloring
- Zest of 1 orange
- 7 oz superfine sugar

Directions
1. Preheat breville on bake function to 160 f and place all cake ingredients, in a bowl and beat with an electric mixer. Transfer half of the batter into a prepared cake pan; bake for 15 minutes. Repeat the process for the other half of the batter.
2. Meanwhile, prepare the frosting by beating all frosting ingredients together. Spread the frosting mixture on top of one cake. Top with the other cake.

Nutrition:
Calories: 828, Protein:11.46 g, Fat: 39.77g, Carbs: 107.89g

998. Cashew Bars

⏱ Prep Time 25 m | ⏱ Cooking Time 15 m | 6 Servings

Ingredients

- 1/3 cup honey
- ¼ cup almond meal
- 1 tbsp. Almond butter
- 1 ½ cups cashews
- 4 dates
- ¾ cup coconut
- 1 tbsp. Chia seeds

Directions:

1 Mix honey with almond butter and almond meal in a bowl and turn properly.
2 Put coconut, dates, cashew and chia seeds and turn properly still.
3 Pour mix on a lined baking sheet and compress properly.
4 Get it in fryer and cook at 300° f for 15 minutes.
5 Allow to cool, slice into medium bars then serve.

Nutrition:
Calories: 483, Protein: 8.18g, Fat: 35.96g, Carbs: 39.44g

999. Fried Cream

⏱ Prep Time 10-20 m | ⏱ Cooking Time 15-30 m | 8 Servings

Ingredients:

For the cream:
- 500 ml of whole milk
- 3 egg yolks
- 150 g of sugar
- 50 g flour
- 1 envelope Vanilla Sugar
  Ingredients for the pie:
- 2 eggs
- Unlimited Breadcrumbs
- 1 tsp oil

Directions:

1 First prepare the custard; once cooked, pour the cream into a dish previously covered with a transparent film and level well. Let cool at room temperature for about 2 hours.
2 Grease the basket and distribute it all over.
3 When the cream is cold, place it on a cutting board and cut it into dice; Pass each piece of cream first in the breadcrumbs, covering the 4 sides well in the beaten egg and then in the pie.
4 Place each part inside the basket. Set the temperature to 1500C.
5 Cook for 10 to 12 minutes, turning the pieces after 6 to 8 minutes.
6 The doses of this cream are enough to make 2 or even 3 kitchens in a row.

Nutrition:
Calories 355, Fat 18.37g, Carbohydrates 44.94g, Sugars 30.36g, Protein 4.81g, Cholesterol 45mg

1000. Apple, cream, and hazelnut crumble

⏱ Prep Time 10-20 m | ⏱ Cooking Time 15-30 m | 6 Servings

Ingredients:

- 4 golden apples
- 100 ml of water
- 50g cane sugar
- 50g of sugar
- ½ tbsp cinnamon
- 200 ml of fresh cream
- Chopped hazelnuts to taste

Directions:

1 In a bowl, combine the peeled apples, cut into small cubes, cane sugar, sugar, and cinnamon.
2 Pour the apples inside the basket, add the water. Set the air fryer to 1800C and simmer for 15 minutes depending on the type of apple used and the size of the pieces.
3 At the end, divide the apples in the serving glasses, cover with previously whipped cream and sprinkle with chopped hazelnuts.

Nutrition:
Calories 828.8, Fat 44.8 g, Carbohydrate 120.6 g, Sugars54.2 g, Protein4.4 g , Cholesterol 29.5 mg

1001. Fregolotta with hazelnuts

⏱ Prep Time 10-20 m | ⏱ Cooking Time 15-30 m | 8 Servings

Ingredients:

- 200g of flour
- 150g of sugar
- 100 g melted butter
- 100g hazelnuts
- 1 egg
- ½ sachet of yeast

Directions:

1. Do not finely chop the hazelnuts. In a large bowl, pour all the ingredients (the butter once melted should be cooled before using), mix lightly, without the dough becoming too liquid.
2. Place parchment paper on the bottom of the basket and pour the mixture into it. Spread it evenly.
3. Set the air fryer to 1800C and simmer for 15 minutes and then turn the cake.
4. Cook for an additional 5 minutes.
5. Let cool and sprinkle the cake with icing sugar.

Nutrition:
Calories 465, Carbohydrates 37g, Fat 25g, Sugars 3g, Protein 20g, Cholesterol 0mg

CPSIA information can be obtained
at www.ICGtesting.com
Printed in the USA
LVHW022241181220
674519LV00011B/553

9 781801 329149